COMPLEMENTARY/ALTERNATIVE MEDICINE

An Evidence-Based Approach

1

COMPLEMENTARY/ ALTERNATIVE MEDICINE

An Evidence-Based Approach

JOHN W. SPENCER, Ph.D.

Private Clinical Research Consultant
Silver Spring, Maryland
Former Senior Policy Analyst
Office of Alternative Medicine
National Institutes of Health
Bethesda, Maryland

JOSEPH J. JACOBS, M.D., M.B.A.

Medical Director
Office of Vermont Health Access
Waterbury, Vermont
Former Director
Office of Alternative Medicine
National Institutes of Health
Bethesda, Maryland

With Foreword by **Nancy Dickey, M.D.**

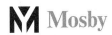 Mosby

A Harcourt Health Sciences Company

St. Louis   London   Philadelphia   Sydney   Toronto

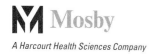

A Harcourt Health Sciences Company

Mosby, Inc.
11830 Westline Industrial Drive
St. Louis, Missouri 63146

Library of Congress Cataloging-in-Publication Data

Complementary/alternative medicine: an evidence-based approach/
[edited by] John W. Spencer, Joseph J. Jacobs.
    p.   cm.
    ISBN 0-8151-2989-0
    1. Alternative medicine.   2. Evidence-based medicine.
I. Spencer, John W. (John William)   II. Jacobs, Joseph J., M.D.
    [DNLM: 1. Alternative Medicine. 2. Evidence-Based Medicine. WB
890C7365 1999]
R733.C6526 1999
615.5—dc21
DNLM/DLC   98-36023

00 01 02 / 9 8 7 6 5 4 3

Contributors

DAVID A. BARON, D.O., F.A.C.N.
Medical Director and Chief Psychiatrist
Kirkbride Center
Philadelphia, Pennsylvania
Clinical Professor of Psychiatry
Temple University School of Medicine
Philadelphia, Pennsylvania

TACEY ANN BOUCHER, B.A.
Research Assistant, Center for Addiction
  and Alternative Medicine Research
Minneapolis Medical Research Foundation
Minneapolis, Minnesota

MILTON BULLOCK, M.D.
Medical Director, Center for Addiction and
  Alternative Medicine Research
Minneapolis Medical Research Foundation
Director, Division of Addiction and
  Alternative Medicine
Department of Medicine
Hennepin County Medical Center
Minneapolis, Minnesota

CHUNG-KWANG CHOU, Ph.D.
Director, Department of Radiation Research
City of Hope National Medical Center
Duarte, California

ANN C. COTTER, M.D.
Medical Consultant, Center for Research in
  Complementary and Alternative Medicine
Kessler Medical Rehabilitation Research and
  Education Corporation
West Orange, New Jersey

PATRICIA D. CULLITON, M.A., Dipl.Ac.
Co-Director, Center for Addiction and
  Alternative Medicine Research
Minneapolis Medical Research Foundation
Director, Alternative Medicine Clinic
Department of Medicine
Hennepin County Medical Center
Minneapolis, Minnesota

BRUCE J. DIAMOND, Ph.D.
Clinical Research Scientist, Center for
  Research in Complementary and Alterna-
  tive Medicine
Kessler Medical Rehabilitation Research and
  Education Corporation
West Orange, New Jersey

ELLEN M. DiNUCCI, M.A.
Project Coordinator, Complementary and
  Alternative Medicine Program at Stanford
Stanford Center for Research in Disease
  Prevention
Palo Alto, California

M. ERIC GERSHWIN, M.D.
The Jack and Donald Chia Professor
    of Medicine
Chief, Division of Rheumatology, Allergy
    and Clinical Immunology
Co-Director, Center for Complementary and
    Alternative Medicine Research in Asthma,
    Allergy and Immunology
Department of Internal Medicine
University of California
Davis, California

ROBERT M. HACKMAN, Ph.D.
Executive Director, Center for
    Complementary and Alternative Medicine
    Research in Asthma, Allergy and
    Immunology
Department of Nutrition
University of California
Davis, California

THOMAS L. HARDIE, Ed.D., RN., C.S., N.P.
Assistant Professor, Department of Nursing
University of Delaware
Newark, Delaware

WILLIAM L. HASKELL, Ph.D.
Professor of Medicine
Deputy Director, Stanford Center for
    Research in Disease Prevention
Principal Investigator, Complementary
    and Alternative Medicine Program
Stanford University School of Medicine
Palo Alto, California

MICAH HILL
Research Assistant, Complementary and
    Alternative Medicine Program at Stanford
Stanford Center for Research in Disease
    Prevention
Palo Alto, California

JAMES M. HORNER, M.D.
Chief, Division of Endocrinology
Associate Professor, Department
    of Pediatrics
Medical College of Ohio
Toledo, Ohio

JOSEPH J. JACOBS, M.D., M.B.A.
Medical Director, Office of Vermont Health
    Access
Waterbury, Vermont
Former Director
Office of Alternative Medicine
National Institutes of Health
Bethesda, Maryland

FREDI KRONENBERG, Ph.D.
Director, Center for Complementary and
    Alternative Medicine in Women's Health
College of Physicians and Surgeons
Columbia University
New York, New York

MAY LOO, M.D.
Clinical Assistant Professor
Department of Pediatrics
Stanford University
Palo Alto, California
Former Founder and Director
Attention Deficit Disorder Clinic
Santa Clara County Valley Medical Center
Santa Clara, California

FREDERIC M. LUSKIN, Ph.D.
Postdoctoral Research Fellow, Stanford
    Center for Research in Disease Prevention
Complementary and Alternative Medicine
    Program
Stanford University School of Medicine
Palo Alto, California

FARSHAD F. MARVASTI
Research Assistant, Stanford Center for
    Research in Disease Prevention
Complementary and Alternative Medicine
    Program
Stanford University School of Medicine
Palo Alto, California

ANGELE McGRADY, Ph.D. L.P.c.C.
Professor, Department of Psychiatry
Professor, Department of Physiology
    and Molecular Medicine
Medical College of Ohio
Toledo, Ohio

PATRICIA AIKINS MURPHY, C.N.M., Dr.Ph.
Consulting Epidemiologist, Center for
    Complementary and Alternative Medicine
    in Women's Health
College of Physicians and Surgeons
Columbia University
New York, New York

SANGEETHA NAYAK, Ph.D.
Research Scientist, Center for Research
    in Complementary and Alternative Medi-
    cine
Kessler Medical Rehabilitation Research
    and Education Corporation
West Orange, New Jersey

KATHRYN A. NEWELL, M.A.
Project Coordinator, Stanford Center
    for Research in Disease Prevention
Complementary and Alternative Medicine
    Program
Stanford University School of Medicine
Palo Alto, California

JAMES A. PEIGHTEL, M.D.
Assistant Clinical Professor, Department
    of Psychiatry
Chief, Counseling Center
Temple University
Philadelphia, Pennsylvania

ARON PRIMACK, M.D., M.A., F.A.C.P.
Medical Director, Center for Health Plans
    and Providers
Health Care Financing Administration
Baltimore, Maryland

CHERIE REEVES, M.S.
Center Manager, AIDS Research Center for
    Alternative and Complementary Medicine
Bastyr University
Bothell, Washington

RU-LONG REN, M.D.
Visiting Investigator, Department
    of Radiation Research
City of Hope Medical Center
Duarte, California

NANCY E. SCHOENBERGER, Ph.D.
Assistant Program Director
Center for Research in Complementary and
    Alternative Medicine
Kessler Medical Rehabilitation Research and
    Education Corporation
West Orange, New Jersey

SAMUEL C. SHIFLETT, Ph.D.
Principal Investigator and Director
Center for Research in Complementary and
    Alternative Medicine
Kessler Medical Rehabilitation Research and
    Education Corporation
West Orange, New Jersey

JOHN W. SPENCER, Ph.D.
Private Clinical Research Consultant
Silver Spring, Maryland
Former Senior Policy Analyst
Office of Alternative Medicine
National Institutes of Health
Bethesda, Maryland

LEANNA J. STANDISH, N.D, Ph.D.
Principal Investigator, AIDS Research
    Center for Alternative and Complemen-
    tary Medicine
Bastyr University
Bothell, Washington

JUDITH S. STERN, Sc.D.
Professor of Nutrition and Internal Medicine
Co-Director, Center for Complementary and
    Alternative Medicine Research in Asthma,
    Allergy and Immunology
Department of Nutrition
University of California
Davis, California

ANN GILL TAYLOR, R.N., Ed.D., F.A.A.N.
Professor of Nursing, School of Nursing
Center for the Study of Complementary
    and Alternative Therapies
Charlottesville, Virginia

CHRISTINE WADE
Research Manager, Center for
   Complementary and Alternative Medicine
   in Women's Health
Columbia University
College of Physicians and Surgeons
New York, New York

ROBERTA C.M. WINES
Lead Medical Interviewer, AIDS Research
   Center for Alternative and Complemen-
   tary Medicine
Bastyr University
Bothell, Washington

DIANE ZEITLIN, B.A., L.M.T.
Research Associate, Center for Research in
   Complementary and Alternative Medicine
Kessler Medical Rehabilitation Research and
   Education Corporation
West Orange, New Jersey

Foreword

As the delivery of health care in the United States becomes ever more complex, an interesting paradox is occurring—individuals are seeking an increasing amount of care from alternative or complementary sources. These sources of care often are based on cultural or historical foundations but frequently have no scientific or research undergirding. Patients learn of these alternative methods from physicians, news media, family, and friends. Although many patients do not inform their physicians that they are also using complementary or alternative interventions, some do seek the advice of their physicians. Hence there is a need for a source of information about what is known, what the identified hazards are, and where a strong anecdotal basis exists that requires further research for confirmation.

This book compiles a substantial array of information, including sources for additional reading and original research confirmation. From the introductory chapter that defines terms and sets parameters to the glossary and appendixes that provide a litany of CAM therapies from acupuncture to therapeutic touch and a listing of CAM organizations and resources, this book is substantially complete.

The organization of information is easy to follow, with chapters that deal with particular symptom or disease complexes and the corresponding forms of complementary medicine. More important than simply listing or discussing the possible forms of complementary medicine used in a particular disease complex, the authors have attempted to evaluate the scientific validity of the information currently available. When conclusions in the literature are based on anecdotes, this is noted. Where research has been done, the findings are reported and the methodological strengths and weaknesses of the studies are explained as well. For example, in the chapter on spinal cord injuries, there is a report of the use of Qi Gong to treat paralysis and other neurological disorders. Researchers in China have reported superb study results. However, a well-known Qi Gong master from China was unable to improve functioning in post-stroke hemiplegia patients in the United States. Through communication of this type of information, Drs. Spencer and Jacobs provide the tools necessary for physicians to judge the effectiveness of alternative treatments that their patients are using or considering.

In the coming months and years, much work is likely to be done in terms of gathering information, evaluating existing data, and identifying target areas for needed research in complementary medicine. However, physicians and other health care providers are in need of solid information to help them provide their patients with effective guidance even as newer and more complete information is being compiled. The ongoing work of the NIH's Office of Alternative Medicine will help ensure evaluation and dissemination of new research results. Meanwhile, *Complementary/Alternative Medicine: An Evidence-Based Approach* offers a source book that can assist a physician to educate patients, evaluate treatments that might be complicating an existing treatment regimen, and perhaps find some sources of complementary medicine that will fit with his or her practice.

According to the Council on Scientific Affairs of the American Medical Association, 1997, physicians should evaluate the scientific perspectives of unconventional theories for treatment and practice, looking particularly at potential utility, safety, and efficacy of these modalities. This book should help physicians to do just that.

Nancy W. Dickey, M.D.

Preface

In 1993 we, along with others, helped put in place the administrative components to form what would eventually be the Office of Alternative Medicine (OAM) at the National Institutes of Health (NIH). As clinicians working for the Indian Health Service in New Mexico, we had previously been exposed to and were aware of many "alternative, spiritual-indigenous" therapies of the American Indians. Joe Jacobs, being a Mohawk, grew up using many of these native healing practices. The congressional mandate of 1991 to form the OAM was the first major attempt to recognize and evaluate complementary/alternative medicine (CAM) at a national level. It sparked much rhetoric and debate among the medical and scientific communities; at the center of this debate was whether CAM could or should be evaluated because of past perceptions of mysticism and outright frauds. At times during this sojourn we felt as though we were on board as the crew of the Starship *Enterprise!*

One of the most important and immediate concerns was the status of research data about CAM. Would it "pass muster" by being valid, reliable, and methodologically sound so that it would be acceptable to both physicians and scientists? Books on healthful lifestyles and diverse healing therapies had been available to the public for many years. What we soon discovered, however, was that there was little or no information regarding (1) whether alternative therapies were useful by any standard of quality research; (2) whether alternative therapies measured up to their promoted claims; and (3) most important, whether alternative therapies were safe to use.

Thus it became clear that there is a need for an objective and fair but focused evaluation of CAM therapies. We were interested in therapies that might be useful for treating certain illnesses, as well as where gaps of knowledge might still exist. We understood the difficulty of gathering, accurately portraying, and writing a book disseminating this information because of polarities between proponents and critics of CAM. In writing this book, we have attempted to organize it around major medical themes or conditions (see the following section, "Organization of the Book"). We chose contributors who had access to CAM scientific databases and were equally committed to presenting the research evidence on CAM objectively and accurately. To that end, we wrote this book for a wide readership. It is intended for individuals who are interested in learning more about the field of CAM and those who want to intelligently discuss the merits of various CAM therapies with their physicians. In addition, this book is directed toward physicians and health care providers who want to be equally enlightened and knowledgeable about any scientific information on CAM in this changing health care environment.

We have several goals in writing *Complementary/Alternative Medicine: An Evidence-Based Approach.*

- We want it both to be informative and to serve as a reference for physicians and scientists regarding which CAM treatment studies or processes need closer and more focused scrutiny. However, we recognize that this is a huge and not very well-defined, nascent field of health care; therefore, we did not intend to include all of its components in a book of this size.
- We want this book to emphasize that basic, preclinical research is an important preliminary step toward incorporating different types and levels of information through recording the specific processes CAM may produce and their treatment effect(s), either positive or negative.
- Finally, we wish to "raise the bar" of debate about CAM by allowing the public to evaluate its relevance and verifiability. New and innovative ways to record data about patients' treatment experiences that may go beyond current conventional science should not be ignored. Neither should the individual patient and his or her beliefs about healing.

We hope this book will provide a structure for readers to evaluate, build upon, and improve their knowledge and research of CAM. The Starship *Enterprise* sought out and investigated uncharted territories and therefore expanded our curiosities about the universe. Likewise, the evaluation of CAM has the potential for studying areas of health care never adequately or fully explored, with the hope of developing new and useful knowledge about the healing process. Critics may claim that our journey is a waste of time and money, and a mistake; but we argue that to not understand and to not explore fully CAM's potential in the healing process is an even greater mistake.

ORGANIZATION OF THE BOOK

Complementary/Alternative Medicine: An Evidence-Based Approach is organized around three major themes. The first section, **Basic Foundations** (Chapters 1 and 2), is devoted to the major issues in CAM. **Chapter 1** focuses on important themes necessary to the development of CAM as a valid treatment process. In **Chapter 2** the necessary steps from basic to clinical research are traced so that both a perspective and a rationale can be developed for understanding how investigations at a preclinical level can eventually mesh with clinical trials on humans.

The second and largest section, **Clinical Research** (Chapters 3 through 14), presents information regarding clinical treatment outcomes in CAM. **Chapters 3 through 5** focus on how the common chronic conditions of asthma/allergies, cardiovascular disease, and diabetes are viewed regarding CAM treatments. Two important relevant components are discussed—prevention and quality of life. While no pure substitutes exist for insulin therapy, CAM may be useful for both improving on the effect of injected insulin and lowering blood glucose levels. **Chapter 6** provides information on both prevention efficacy and treatment strategies for cancer. Diets and the use of herbal remedies should help to develop new ways of thinking about this multifaceted, complex disease. Of interest in **Chapter 7** is the rather large database of stroke or spinal cord injury impairments, mood, affect, cognition, and motor control issues that may be responsive to certain CAM therapies. **Chapter 8** details the very few studies that evaluate mental health issues and CAM. The recent collection of studies on the use of herbs for the treatment of depression, and the many behavioral therapies used for the treatment of anxiety, stress, and depression, are promising developments. **Chapter 9** reviews the use of acupuncture for the treatment of substance abuse. This particular therapeutic approach shows some mixed results. The large number of studies utilizing other CAM approaches for the treatment of addictions is compelling and needs further development and study for its potential integration into conventional clinical practice. Using a nursing care model and each patient's unique perspective, **Chapter 10** reveals that CAM plays a large and influential role in the treatment of many kinds of pain. **Chapters 11 through 14** focus on populations that constitute a significant number of health consumers. For **women** who have HIV/AIDS, the similarities and differences between conventional and naturopathic treatments are highlighted, and the issue(s) of individualization of each patient is a central focus. The broad class of CAM therapies used by women for treating AIDS is compelling. Preliminary work evaluating the use of herbs with certain gynecologic problems appears to be encouraging, but more studies are needed. For **children,** one important issue is their vulnerability to risk and the more complicated interactions that exist between development and healing, either physical or mental. For the **elderly,** recent surveys indicate that CAM has its own specific set of issues and problems but, more important, remains quite popular even in the absence of treatment efficacy.

The final section, **Looking Ahead,** reviews emerging areas of CAM, which will need to be considered by U.S. health care practice into the twenty-first century. Integration, as Jacobs points out, between conventional medicine and CAM will occur only when CAM advocates understand, use, and participate with the managed care industry and assist with the development of credible treatment efficacy studies. The outgrowth of this emphasis will result in more broadly meeting the health needs of the consumer.

ACKNOWLEDGMENTS

Many people have provided varying degrees of assistance in the writing of this book. We are deeply appreciative of the efforts of the following: Amy Ai, Ph.D., University of Michigan; William Stuart, Ph.D., University of Maryland; Dale C. Smith, Ph.D., Uniformed Services University of the Health Sciences; Juan Lin, Ph.D.; Alan Salamy, Ph.D., University of California at San Francisco; Eric Lang, Ph.D., Sociometrics Corporation. Mr. Elliott Green, Mr. Robert Michael, and Ms. Beth Clay provided ideas and or material contained throughout this book. Rita Calderon, C.S.W.; Ann Fonfa, B.P.S.; and Ellen Silverstone of SHARE helped with ideas for the last chapter. We are especially grateful to Jean Neiner and Christine Ambrose at Mosby for their initial foresight and encouragement for this project, and to Pui Szeto also at Mosby for her useful editorial comments. Finally, we thank the real "complementary" people in our lives, Pat, MJ, Michael, Alex, and Catherine.

John W. Spencer
Joe J. Jacobs

Contents

7   Complementary/Alternative Therapies in the Treatment of Neurologic Disorders, 170

Bruce J. Diamond, Samuel C. Shiflett, Nancy E. Schoenberger, Sangeetha Nayak, Ann C. Cotter, and Diane Zeitlin

PART I   Basic Foundations

CHAPTER 1

Essential Issues in Complementary/Alternative Medicine

John W. Spencer

The debate between proponents and critics of *complementary/alternative medicine* (CAM) has renewed both old and new arguments and biases. This controversy is at an important juncture in medical health care in the United States because it involves the potential acceptance or rejection of certain "healing" therapies by medical science or consumers, or both. Opinions of many patients and researchers are divided on whether these unproved treatments can or ever will be demonstrated to be cost-effective, accessible, and, most important, medically useful and safe. Over the past 6 years the *zeitgeist* for a more holistic approach to health has reemerged. One of the major reasons for this renewed interest is that there continues to be an undercurrent of dissatisfaction among consumers about the effectiveness of conventional medicine in treating certain types of chronic diseases (i.e., cancer), along with managing the side effects of various medications. But is CAM the answer? What will be expected or demanded of these various CAM practices before they can be realistically integrated into "mainstream" medicine? Will many of these approaches eventually fade away, either because they are not helpful or because they are fraudulent? Who will ultimately decide which treatments are helpful and safe? How can the integration of CAM with conventional medicine occur? Answers to these questions will be provided throughout this textbook by using results from clinical and preclinical scientific studies for bases of opinion.

One of the ways that CAM will be accepted and integrated into conventional medicine is through the use of an *evidence-based analysis*,[53] which is featured throughout this book. While this process can provide a much-needed focus on certain ways to manage the care of patients, it also assumes (1) that an adequate scientific methodology is in place; (2) that any treatment effects (potentially even small ones) be measured and clinically meaningful, and most important; (3) that some application be made to the clinical practice itself. Of what use are large amounts of scientifically focused clinical research trials if they never have any impact on or relevance to the practice of medicine (health) by influencing questions such as who gets referred, under what conditions, and whether there is any clinical benefit? Most physicians are more influenced by reports from patients, family, or friends of a medical treatment's potential outcome: the main

3

aim of physicians is to cure patients. An evidence-based approach must be implemented in a clinical practice, however, to determine whether it has any utility for assisting both providers and patients.

It is equally important to recognize that writing about the CAM process itself, especially using terminology not familiar to mainstream medical readers, can be fraught with difficulties and complexities. New sensitivities in medical language need to continue to evolve along with the process of study and the acceptance or rejection of CAM therapies in conjunction with conventional medicine.

This introductory chapter identifies six areas to help medical providers and consumers understand this multifaceted, polarized health care debate: definition, historical considerations, clinical issues, methodology, regulation, and training and education. The issues discussed are not mutually exclusive but interact with and have varying degrees of influence on one another.

DEFINITION
What Is CAM?

CAM is the use and practice of therapies or diagnostic techniques that may not be part of any current Western health care system, culture, or society. The emphasis is on prevention or treatment, or both, using "mind and body" (in certain but not all cases) as a total entity in healing, rather than focusing on illness or disease, by means of either natural substances or other procedures or techniques, many of which still await scientific proof of benefit or safety, or both. Reimbursement through health insurance plans for use of many of these approaches is slowly evolving and changing, but their formal integration *as a standard practice in health care or patient care*—and thus their being taught as such within medical and nursing schools—has not yet occurred.

The above definition of CAM is made up of many different components. Each individual therapy can be included in any definition, and the patient is an important focal point of health. Another important descriptor that can help shape CAM into a clinical practice mode is the extent to which it is both safe and useful.

The terms "alternative" and "complementary" are not adequate descriptors because they limit a broad class of therapies and their use can depend on the clinical setting relative to conventional treatments. Most people in the United States—perhaps 70%—have never used any of these therapies. "Alternative" (or other terms such as "untested," "unproved," "unconventional," or "unorthodox") includes therapies that generally replace or substitute for an orthodox treatment, whereas "complementary" means the therapy is used in tandem with conventional treatments (e.g., treatment of hypertension or diabetes using medication plus biofeedback or relaxation procedures). Biofeedback assists or complements the medication so that it can be used in lower doses, minimizing drug side effects while maximizing treatment effects.

The use of chiropractic manipulation illustrates the difficulty in attempting to form an all-encompassing definition for CAM. Manipulation is used for the treatment of low back pain. There is good scientific evidence based on several clinical trials and studies, including a report of results from a consensus conference, that chiropractic procedures can significantly reduce associated pain.[4,9] A measurable physical response can be defined and directly linked with muscle-nerve interactions with known mechanisms of action that can be used to describe how manipulation produces its effect. The question might be asked, "Just how alternative is this practice?" General medicine, however, still may consider it an "alternative" to surgery.

When chiropractic manipulation is used to treat medical conditions for which there is little scientific data to support usage and for which no rationale exists that would explain its physiologic action, the definition and usage of CAM become more controversial. For example, is there a proven reason for the use of chiropractic manipulation to treat psychiatric depression or otitis media? A second part of the definition must include how CAM usage is framed or applied for a specific treatment.

Societal consideration, including educational and management characteristics about CAM, form a further part to the definition. CAM is proposed to be part of a social process and might be considered and defined as those practices that do not form a part of any major system for managing health and disease. This may be too self-limiting, however, because what may be considered CAM in one setting may not be in another.

Some have suggested that CAM therapies should be considered an ongoing, evolving process in which each therapy moves through and into classifications or categories based on usage and subsequent integration.[92] CAM could be referred to as ancillary, limited, marginal, "quasi-," or preliminary. As consumer demands change and more information becomes available about treatment efficacy and safety, the particular therapy or practice could move from one and through other classifications.

Recently the Office of Alternative Medicine (OAM) at the National Institutes of Health (NIH) convened a panel to provide a definition and description of CAM activities.[61] CAM was described as "seeking, promoting and treating health," but it was noted that the boundaries between CAM and other more dominant or conventional systems were not always clearly defined. The suggestion was made that CAM's definition remain flexible.

The definition(s) of CAM as described either in this textbook or in clinical or research settings is incomplete. Changes to any definition will continue to occur as more information about the entire CAM process is studied, better understood, and subsequently integrated within conventional and CAM clinical practices.

HISTORICAL CONSIDERATIONS
Ancient Times to the Twentieth Century

In ancient China a system of medical care developed as part of philosophical teaching. Principles were recorded in and subsequently translated from *The Yellow Emperor's Classic of Internal Medicine*[87] as follows:

> It is said that in former times the ancient sages discoursed on the human body and that they enumerated separately each of the viscera and each of the bowels. They talked about the origin

of blood vessels and about the vascular system, and said that where the blood vessels and the arteries (veins) met there are six junctions. Following the course of each of the arteries there are the 365 vital points for acupuncture. Those who are experts in using the needle for acupuncture follow Yin, the female principle, in order to draw out Yang. And they follow Yang, the male principle, in order to draw out Yin. They used the right hand in order to treat the illness of the left side, and they used the left hand in order to treat the illness of the right side.

Normal activities of the human body resulted as balance between yin and yang. A breakdown of yin and yang balance was thought to be the general pathogenesis of all diseases. A patient with depression would be in a state of excessive yin, whereas a patient with mania would have excessive yang. Restoration of yin and yang balance led to recovery from illness.

Diagnosis involved close observation, listening, questioning, and recording various physiologic activities (Fig. 1-1). Much of traditional Chinese medicine (TCM) as practiced today contains many of these same assumptions, including the respect for and unique aspect of the individual patient.

Chinese materia medica, an important part of TCM, is composed of materials derived from plants, animals, and minerals. The best-known, classic Chinese textbook on

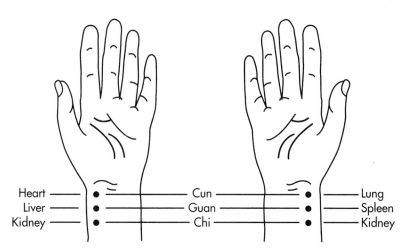

Fig. 1-1   Location of pulses on the radial artery.   Point guan is on the radial artery opposite the styloid process of the radius. The middle finger locates this, and the index and ring fingers palpate points cun and chi, respectively. The kidney pulse on the right is the kidney yang or vital gate. At least 28 qualities of the pulse, such as "superficial," "deep," and "short," relate to certain medical diseases or syndromes (internal, cold, excess). The seasons influenced the pulse, as did age, sex, and constitution. (From Hillier SM, Jewell JA: *Health care and traditional medicine in China: 1800-1982,* London, 1983, Routledge & Kegan Paul.)

materia medica is *Bencao Gangmu*, written by Li Shi-Zhen during the Ming Dynasty (1552-1578). It listed 1892 medical substances and contained more than 1000 illustrations and 10,000 detailed descriptions. Through trial and error, worthless and less effective agents were eliminated from further consideration. The Chinese have accumulated a vast experience on disease prevention and treatment by using the Chinese materia. The 1990 edition of *The Pharmacopoeia of the People's Republic of China* collected 506 single drugs and 275 kinds of complex preparations. At present there are about 100 preparations or drugs being studied in pharmacology, chemical analysis, and clinical evaluation.[55] Ethnobotany as currently practiced owes much to the early accumulation of this information.

A similar but distinct system, Ayurveda, developed on the Indian subcontinent more than 5000 years ago. An integrated approach to both prevention and treatment of illness was emphasized. Again, "imbalance" was a major part of the explanation of disease. A focus of awareness or level of consciousness was proposed to exist within each individual. This "inner" force was a major part of the practice of good health. Mental stress was thought to be involved in producing poor health, and techniques such as meditation were developed to aid in healing. Other components included lifestyle interventions of diet, herbs, exercise, and yoga.

In the second century A.D. the Greek physician Galen's ideas shaped what would eventually become modern scientific medicine. In his influential guide, *Anatomical Procedures*, Galen noted the following reasons to study the human body[74]:

> Anatomic study has one use for the man of science who loves knowledge for its own sake, another for him who values it only to demonstrate that nature does naught in vain, a third for one who provides himself from anatomy with data for investigating a function physical or mental and yet another for the practitioner who has to remove splinters and missiles efficiently, to exercise parts properly, or to treat ulcers, fistulae and abscesses.

Galen's ideas eventually became the groundwork for evaluating and treating patients by focusing on the use of visual and physical objectivity. This was subsequently emphasized in medical education during the twelfth century A.D. Greek philosophy and medicine were eventually incorporated into parts of Arabic and Latin cultures in the western Mediterranean.

During the Newtonian era of the eighteenth century there was an emphasis on an objective approach to observations of any phenomenon. The replacement of the "rational philosophy" of the ancient tradition with the implementation of a stronger experimental documentation was continuing. Anomalous events that could not be explained by a theory were questioned or ignored.[36]

Three examples reflect this paradigm shift and also illustrate foundational arguments that still exist today between proponents and critics of CAM. First, Anton Mesmer, a French scientist, observed that after electrical stimulation of nerves and muscles, "forces" such as twitching could be recorded. He concluded that there was a magnetic fluid that flowed throughout the body; disease was the result of too much or too little fluid in one part of the body. Mesmer was discredited by his peers for being unable to reproduce any result that would verify his suggestions. His clinical results were thought to result from "mental suggestion." Second, John Wesley, a Methodist minister, collected many "written ideas" for maintaining health and/or healing based on what people told him was useful or produced healing. No theory or observation could support any of his claims. Third, Samuel Hahnemann tested many common herbal and medicinal substances to establish what medical symptoms they might produce in humans. He experimented by diluting a solution and then subjecting it to vigorous shaking, called succussion. The dilution limit (i.e., that point when volume of solvent did not contain a single molecule of the solute) was often exceeded. He treated sick patients by prescribing the medicine that most closely matched the symptoms of their illness, but in doses so small that it was questioned whether they were therapeutic. Most of his results were not reproducible, and the subjectivity of his "therapies" was questioned.

By the mid-1800s, medicine in the United States was a mix of many different contributions and philosophies from various countries. A great change occurred in the way medicine was practiced with the advent and use of vaccines and antibiotics.[39] A second, equally important change occurred at the beginning of the twentieth century. Abraham Flexner, a U.S. educator, was charged with evaluating medical education. His report, *Medical Education in the United States and Canada,* was in part responsible for the diminution of the practice of CAM in this country.[46] Although the study was intended to upgrade medical education in general, medical schools with a biomedical focus were favored and positioned to receive most of the money from large philanthropic organizations and foundations. Four years after the release of his report there was a decrease of approximately 40% in the number of medical schools. Remaining institutions generally favored a biomedical approach. Other important changes included the enactment of state licensing laws (through the efforts of the American Medical Association [AMA]) and the passage of the Pure Food and Drug Act of 1906.[82]

An important trend in medicine, which influenced CAM, occurred at the beginning of the twentieth century. Manual manipulation evolved as a major ancillary health therapy to general medicine.[36] This intervention was initially promoted by Andrew Still and David Palmer. Still was an osteopath who advocated bone setting and manipulation of painful joints. Disease was thought to result as misplaced bones within the spinal cord. Palmer helped start a system called chiropractic, in which all diseases were thought to be due to impingement of nerves passing through the spine. Most osteopaths were trained with some emphasis on basic science and surgery. Osteopaths used findings from biomedical research and were able to use much of what biomedical science was discovering, including microscopic analysis of bacteria, antibiotics, analgesics, and antiinflammatory drugs. Chiropractors were slower to expand into scientific inquiry, although more recently this has changed through scientific evaluation of their procedures.[4]

Ethnologic Contributions

The cross-cultural, as distinct from the historical, record of systems of healing is voluminous. Anthropologists have studied a wide variety of "folk medical systems" (e.g., shamanism and magic). The variety of specific, native cultural theories of illness—and thus of curing—is wide. However, it is possible to identify features common to other, nonmodern medical systems, especially those recorded in cultures of the developing world. These theories are typically embedded in overarching native religious systems.[20] Among the causes of disease that are frequently described are the following:

- Loss of one's soul(s) in whole or part
- Spirit possession
- Intrusion of human-filled object, where mana is an impersonal, supernatural force
- Intrusion of illness-causing spirit
- Violation of taboos, especially those having to do with correct relations to deities, including one's ancestors
- Spirit attack, including by capricious "jokester" spirits
- Homeopathic and/or contagious magic
- Disturbances or violation of social rules and relationships

Today the alternative medical practitioner in many cultures is likely to be as much guru, shaman, and charismatic figure as physician in the mainstream Western secular sense.

Illness and healing can take on a cultural meaning that is relative to specific treatments[48] or diagnostic issues,[81] or both. For example, the healer/clinician in any society offers treatment to patients who bring stories of their own illnesses and special concerns made up of mental, emotional, and ethical components. The structure of the illness is really the manner in which it is meaningful to patient, family, and healer. Illness is a form of suffering that involves both body and self-awareness of pain or discomfort bound by various cultural or religious beliefs, or both, and involves a host of properties, many of them psychologic. Symptoms of illness or enduring illness in one society may not be as relevant in another.

Throughout this book the reader should notice that a continual dichotomy, difference, or differing emphasis exists between conventional medicine and its treatment of the individual patient using modern scientific technology and the more culture-bound approach, often emphasized in many CAM therapies, in which, more often, illness and sickness are tied to personal beliefs and complaints and patient judgments of illness effects at many levels of life.

Involvement of the National Institutes of Health

In 1991, Congress appropriated funds to start an Office of Alternative Medicine at the NIH. The establishment of the OAM was seen as demonstrating the depth of interest by Congress and the general public in expanding the range of available health treatment modalities, especially for conditions that sometimes were treated unsuccessfully by conventional medicine, such as cancer. Others viewed it as a waste of taxpayers' money, especially because of the negative stigma associated with alternative medicine and quackery. However, within this same time frame, the Office of Technology Assessment (OTA) published a lengthy report[86] expressing the need for more clinical research evaluating alternative treatments for cancer.

As a first step, to "investigate and validate" alternative treatments as mandated by Congress, in 1993 the OAM released its first Request for Applications (RFA) for a one-time, 1-year, exploratory grant that could not exceed $30,000. The purpose of these grants was to develop a foundation of scientific data that could lead to more extensive studies, possibly through funding by specific institutes at the NIH.[79] More than 450 applications were received and reviewed. Subsequently, 42 pilot projects were funded. Table 1-1 illustrates the broad range of therapies and health conditions that were evaluated.

Most of the studies have now been completed, and approximately 25% are published in peer-reviewed journals. One lesson learned from this first program was the difficulty of completing any research project with the limited financial resources made available through individual grants. This was most obvious in the costly areas of subject recruitment and data analysis.

In addition, the OAM has now funded 11 centers to study and conduct research on various types of health problems including pain, arthritis and allergies, human immunodeficiency virus (HIV) and acquired immunodeficiency virus (AIDS), cancer, women's health, drug abuse and alcoholism, stroke and neurologic conditions, aging, more general medical conditions, as well as a more specialized center to evaluate chiropractic procedures. Also, the World Health Organization (WHO) has designated the OAM itself as a collaborating center in traditional medicine. This involvement with WHO will provide for the study of more traditional healing practices and make relevant findings available to both the public and scientists in the United States.

The involvement of the NIH has renewed interests, debates, and controversies about CAM. Private foundations have increased their efforts to fund research projects and sponsor a greater number of scientific meetings. New journals relevant to CAM include *Alternative Therapies, Alternative Therapies in Clinical Practice, Alternative Therapies in Health and Medicine, Journal of Alternative and Complementary Therapies,* and *Mind-Body Medicine.* Many self-help books devoted to health and healing and emphasizing CAM are increasingly available in bookstores. The Internet contains hundreds of Web sites concerning CAM. The quality of this information is mixed, and little scientific evidence is presented for claims made.

TABLE 1-1	CAM Therapy Evaluations
CAM Therapy Used	**Medical Condition Treated**
Acumoxa	Breech birth
Acupuncture	Unipolar depression
Acupuncture	Osteoarthritis
Acupuncture	Dental pain
Acupuncture	Attention deficit
Acupuncture/herbs	HIV (sinusitis)
Acupuncture/herbs	HIV (survey)
Antioxidant vitamins	Cancer cell function
Ayurvedic herbals	Brain chemistry
Ayurvedic medicine	Health status survey
Biofeedback	Diabetes mellitus, type II
Biofeedback	Pain survey
Dance therapy	Cystic fibrosis
Electrochemical DC	Cancer (preclinical)
EEG normalization	Mild health trauma
Energetic therapy	Basal cell carcinoma
Ethnomedicine	Survey (hepatitis)
Herbal	Hot flashes
Herbal	Skin warts
Herbal	Premenstrual syndrome
Homeopathy	Health status survey
Homeopathy	Mild brain injury
Hypnosis	Bone fracture healing
Hypnosis	Low back pain
Macrobiotic diet	Cancer
Manual palpation	Device evaluation
Massage	Bone marrow transplant
Massage	Infant growth
Massage	HIV
Massage	Postsurgical pain
Music therapy	Head injury
Prayer	Substance abuse
Qi Gong	Pain
T'ai chi	Balance disorder
Therapeutic touch	Stress, immune function
Transcranial electrostimulation	Chronic pain
Visual imagery	Asthma
Visual imagery	Breast cancer (2 studies)
Visual imagery	Immune function
Visual imagery	Drug use
Yoga (hatha)	Obsessive/compulsive disorder

From Exploratory Grant Program funded by the OAM/NIH, September, 1993, Bethesda, Md.
DC, Direct current; *EEG*, electroencephalogram; *HIV*, human immunodeficiency virus.

CLINICAL ISSUES
Demographics of Usage of CAM Therapies

The description of CAM use and prevalence is generally accomplished by a direct interview or by survey. Data obtained should include numbers of patients using a particular therapy and demographic information. Additional data, not always presented, might include use and ways the particular therapy could be integrated with traditional medicine; follow-up data on long-term effects; cost issues; and an objective analysis of results using appropriate, valid measures.

A survey can be misleading if interviewer or subject bias exists. Questions that are unclear, not validated, or not clinically relevant should be avoided. Subjects with preconceived or negative views about CAM are not good candidates. Incorrect information may be collected and results skewed when variables such as age, sex, ethnicity, education, and income are not carefully indexed. Usage does not imply that the therapy is always efficacious for specific groups or sample populations. Surveys simply measure "impressions" of individuals and are limited to what information they provide. Surveys, however, can be the "first step" toward uncovering a general degree of documentation about CAM usage.

The use of complementary therapies appears to be widespread in the United States, and even moreso throughout Europe and Asia. For example, Fisher and Ward[34] reported between 20% and 50% usage of complementary therapies in Europe. Consumer surveys indicate that in the Netherlands and Belgium the usage is as high as 60%, and in Great Britain 74% were willing to pay additional insurance premiums to cover complementary therapies. One CAM therapy, homeopathy, has grown in popularity, especially in France.

Physicians and medical students have been surveyed about their knowledge and usage of CAM, especially in countries outside the United States. Reilly[66] provided one of the early surveys. He reported that physicians had positive attitudes toward their patients' usage.

The most commonly used therapies included hypnosis, manipulation, homeopathy, and acupuncture. Interestingly, the personal use of CAM therapies by physicians was linked to greater interest in training. In Germany it has been reported[42] that 95% of physicians themselves used herbal therapy or homeopathy. Of 89 physicians surveyed in Israel, 54% reported that certain complementary therapies might be clinically useful, and 42% had referred patients for specific treatments.[70] German medical students indicated a significant interest in learning about acupuncture (42%) and homeopathy (55%) and thought that these therapies had a potential for being effective.[7] Further, in Canada, a cross section of 200 general practitioners revealed that 73% thought they should have some knowledge about certain alternative treatments.[88] Chiropractic procedures were popular and efficacious treatments for musculoskeletal and chronic pain.

Ernst and colleagues[30] combined and evaluated 12 separate surveys of perceived effectiveness of complementary therapies among physicians. The individual surveys were conducted throughout Europe and the Middle East and included the United Kingdom, New Zealand, Germany, the Netherlands, Sweden, and Israel. On a scale of 1 (low) to 100 (high) the average score was 46, indicating that the therapies were considered to be moderately effective. Younger physicians viewed complementary medicine as promising. The most popular therapies were manipulation, acupuncture, and homeopathy. Respondents' views regarding whether the use of complementary therapies would be more effective than a placebo were not evaluated.

An extensive description of either the practice or research of CAM in Europe and other countries such as China and India is beyond the scope of this chapter and textbook, although this does not lessen its importance. In many ways CAM has fared much better in terms of its acceptance and integration with conventional medicine in Europe, partially because of different, less restrictive regulations. Recently recommendations have been made for the reexamination of health care and service delivery in the United Kingdom, since it has been reported[83] that 750,000 consultations may occur annually and 40% of medical practices may provide access to CAM. The interested reader might consult Vincent and Furnham[90] for additional information on CAM practice outside the United States.

The trend of CAM usage in the United States is *hypothesized* to be on the increase, especially since the 1980s, although certain CAM practice areas may have reached a numeric plateau. Cassileth[18,19] was among the first to report on the use of certain "unorthodox" therapies for the treatment of cancer (see Chapter 4). In a recent survey Eisenberg and colleagues[28] focused on the use of "unconventional" treatments for general medical conditions. They interviewed 1539 adults and recorded that 34% had used at least one alternative therapy in the previous year. The greatest usage was by middle-aged individuals (25 to 49 years of age). The major complaints most often cited included back problems, anxiety, depression, and headaches. Therapies most often used included chiropractic, relaxation, imagery, and self-help groups. Seventy-two percent of the respondents did not inform their physician that they were using unconventional approaches; it was estimated that expenditures associated with the use of these therapies was close to $14 billion, of which $10 billion was paid by the patient.

Survey and clinical usage of CAM therapies in the United States has been reported for such divergent conditions as chronic polyarthritis treated by acupuncture,[58] epilepsy treated by prayer,[24] and voice disorders treated by laryngeal massage.[25]

A focused regional survey of U.S. family physicians' knowledge and usage of, training in, and—a particularly important variable—evidence expected of complementary medicine for acceptance as a legitimate practice, revealed interesting trends.[14] A range of attitudes was reported. Diet and exercise, biofeedback, and counseling or psychotherapy were most often utilized in the medical practice (Table 1-2).

TABLE 1-2	Percentage of Responding Physicians (n=176) Using Alternative Medicine and Classifying Various Alternative Medicines as Legitimate or Alternative		
Types of Alternative Medicine	Legitimate Medical Practice	Have Used in Practice	Alternative Medicine
Counseling or psychotherapy	97.2	30.8	12.4
Biofeedback	92.5	53.8	18.4
Diet and exercise	92.1	96.6	12.1
Behavioral medicine	91.5	58.9	16.8
Hypnotherapy	73.7	30.8	30.6
Massage therapy	57.5	35.1	42.0
Acupuncture	55.9	13.5	48.9
Chiropractic	48.9	27.2	45.7
Vegetarianism	45.9	22.2	53.3
Art therapy	39.1	12.9	42.4
Acupressure	38.4	12.9	52.6
Prayer	32.8	30.8	53.4
Homeopathic medicine	26.9	5.3	62.2
Herbal medicine	22.6	6.9	67.7
Megavitamin	21.1	13.5	60.8
Traditional Oriental medicine	18.3	1.8	56.1
Electromagnetic applications	17.5	7.1	52.0
Native American medicine	16.9	3.5	60.1

From Berman BM et al: Physicians' attitudes toward complementary or alternative medicine: a regional survey, *J Am Board Fam Pract* 8:361, 1995.
NOTE: Therapies are listed in order of acceptance as a legitimate medical practice.

Most physicians sampled thought that standards of acceptance for conventional medicine using scientific rules of evidence should be equally applied to complementary medicine

Why Patients Use CAM

Reasons patients choose and use CAM are multifaceted, complex, personal, and biased. CAM patients may have strong negative opinions about conventional medicine.[49] Some mistrust institutions and new technologies. Conventional medicine is viewed as an impersonal and a profit-motivated system. When conventional treatments are not helpful, the physician is often blamed. When there is a problem in communication with their health care provider, patients may start "doctor shopping" and request additional tests to reassure themselves that earlier opinions were in error. CAM therapies may at this point be more likely to be tried.

There are important predictive parameters of useful communication between doctor and patient.[69] They include (1) the kind of disease being treated, (2) the difficulty or complexity of the treatment; (3) the interpretation placed on the treatment by the patient (i.e., attitude), and (4) the involvement by the patient in the decision-making process of the treatment. In a study evaluating the influence of attitudes,[35] two separate and matched groups of patients seen by either a general (GP) or an alternative practitioner (AP) were evaluated to determine influence of attitudes. It was reported that the AP group was more skeptical about whether conventional medicine worked, and they believed that alternative medicine would improve their health.

Both physician and patient need to work toward better communication with each other. Education is useful because there can be a high degree of referrals for alternative therapies. In community settings in Washington, New Mexico, and southern Israel, 60% of all physicians made referrals at least once in the preceding year and 38% in the previous month. Patients requested these referrals because of a closer alliance with their cultural beliefs, the lack of success of conventional treatments, and the belief of the physician that patients had a "nonorganic" or "psychologic" symptomology. It is important to note that there was no correlation between the rate of referral and the physicians' level of knowledge, beliefs about effectiveness, or understanding of alternative therapies.[17]

Safety Issues in the Clinical Use of CAM

Montbriand[60] suggested stringent safety and procedural controls for CAM similar to those for conventional medicine. For example, in herbal medicine little information exists regarding standardization of preparation, correct dosage, antidotes or risk warnings, and most important, clinical and research evidence that it is useful for any specific health condition. Risk information is important because it aids the patient in making informed, intelligent choices. These controls must be more equitably considered for many CAM therapies. For example, the Food and Drug Administration (FDA) has published final rules on labeling requirements for vitamins, minerals, herbs, or amino acids that supplement diets and requires the label to include a "supplement fact" statement.[32]

Several investigators have reviewed both direct and indirect adverse effects of certain CAM therapies.[29,45] Areas included were (1) cervical manipulations for which the most common complications were vascular accidents; (2) acupuncture with the associated risk of infections such as hepatitis C, osteomyelitis, and endocarditis by nonsterilized needles in skin or blood vessels; tissue trauma; pneumothorax; and hemothorax; (3) herbal medicine, which included varied reactions from dermatitis to anaphylactic shock, renal fibrosis, and renal failure; and (4) homeopathy, in which adverse reactions were rare, perhaps less than 3%, but toxic concentrations of arsenic and cadmium could be found in certain preparations.

A systematic evaluation of reported adverse effects of CAM in which the research methodology was strong (e.g., randomized, controlled trials with blinding procedures) revealed that herbal treatments were most often cited.[45] Also, the use of a botanic dietary supplement with antioxidant properties (Chaparral) has important associated risks.[73] Varying degrees of hepatotoxicity were noted in 13 of 18 patient cases examined. Symptoms included jaundice and an increase in serum liver chemistry values. Symptom resolution occurred 1 to 17 weeks after Chaparral was discontinued. Since many herbal products contain heavy-metal contaminants, long-term adverse effects must be more thoroughly described. The effect herbal preparations may have, when given with orthodox medications, on minimizing or preventing treatment effects needs further study and clarification.

Ultimately, the choice by patients to use a CAM therapy will result from the evaluation of different sources of information. This should include clear product information. It is important that health care professionals provide nonjudgmental, simple, updated, and accurate data about complementary therapies. Any clinical research evaluation(s) made and described should include the use of appropriate ethical guidelines (i.e., informed consent).[78] The WHO[97] has developed guidelines that should be followed for safe acupuncture treatments and include information about standards for needle structure, size, materials, packaging, and sterilization procedures.

Clinical practice guidelines and provider practice acts, which are described in the next section, ensure that the practice of CAM contain both professional and ethical components.

Clinical Practice Guidelines for CAM

Clinical practice guidelines are official statements from professional societies, government agencies, hospitals, or health plans. They either describe how to care for patients with specific health problems, or illustrate usage of specific procedures.[95] They are intended to improve patient care by focusing where potential suboptimal medical care might exist.[33] The guidelines are generally developed after scientifically based methods reveal effectiveness. Examples of practice guidelines already formulated and issued with relevance to CAM include spinal manipulation for the treatment of low back pain and hypnosis, relaxation, biofeedback, and massage therapy for treating acute postoperative or procedure-related pain.[4]

Recently a nine-member panel recommended that guidelines developed for CAM be based on creditable scientific evidence and that the field of CAM should encourage well-designed clinical studies for this purpose.[96] Clinical trials should evaluate each specific CAM therapy for its effectiveness and safety, including the role of the placebo (nonspecific effects). Further, the design of the studies should focus on target conditions, sample populations appropriate in size and gender, and validated outcome measurements. The OAM at the NIH was encouraged to act as a conduit between agencies and institutes, disseminating new information about research, bibliographies of studies purporting treatment effectiveness, and other research databases in CAM. Information should be released to consumers regarding treatment options for various health conditions. Also, standards should be developed for both evaluating and credentialing clinical competency. Each discipline (e.g., homeopathy, massage, or acupuncture) should undertake this mandate. The report recommends postponing any clinical guidelines until more clinical research in CAM is undertaken and results made available.

Legislation and Provider Practice Acts

A review of legislation in CAM is available.[68] There has been an important "convergence" between consumer usage of certain CAM therapies and practitioners attempting to gain practice rights. An important consideration is that statutory requirements for the practice of CAM broadly differ between states; regardless of the state in which the CAM therapy is practiced, however, that state must recognize and establish which credentials are required; a business license or national credential is not sufficient for practice.[27]

Provider Practice Acts

Acupuncture. Currently in the United States acupuncture is regulated by law or practice acts in 35 states and the District of Columbia.[59] Licensure is granted in 27 states. Some states require that any nonphysician practicing acupuncture be supervised by a licensed physician. The scope of practice varies greatly across states.

Homeopathy. Homeopathy practice acts exist in Arizona, Connecticut, and Nevada. The scope of practice varies but includes the usage of substances of animal, vegetable, or mineral origin given in microdosages and prepared according to the homeopathic pharmacology. All three states use licensure as a means to authorize practice. Arizona and Nevada have independent examining boards. In Delaware and New Hampshire, the practice of homeopathy is regulated by the state although under no board.

Massage. Provider practice acts for massage exist in 22 states. The scope of practice and use of methods are diverse. However, most statues include directives of treatment of tissue (soft or superficial) or muscle, or both. Techniques may include, but are not limited to, friction, kneading, or vibration. Types of health conditions treated, depending on the practice act, include maintaining good health, improving muscle tone, and reducing stress. Licensure, now required in 25 states and the District of Columbia, is the most common form of practice rights.

Naturopathy. Practice acts for naturopathy exist in 12 states. The legislative definition of naturopathy includes the focus on the use of "natural" forms of health care treatment(s). Each state defines scope of practice differently, utilizing several adjunctive therapies including acupuncture, biofeedback, and nonprescriptive medications. Except for the District of Columbia, licensure is the authorization for practice.

CAM therapists, like other health care providers, need to work within their scope of practice as defined by their state statutes. In the area of herbal or nutritional medicine, suggesting specific remedies for a specific medical condition may constitute a legal violation.[27] If there is no state-authorized scope of practice, the practitioner should "educate" and "inform" clients about the use of certain CAM therapies rather than diagnose or treat specific medical conditions.

Recently the Health Coverage Availability and Affordability Act of 1996 (H.R. 3103) was introduced and debated in Congress. This legislation may have important ramifications for the practice of CAM. The bill essentially extends freedom of choice and allows greater opportunity of access by consumers to food, drugs, devices, and procedures not yet approved by FDA. The bill allows for an individual to receive treatment from specific health care providers including alternative practitioners. The patient must be reassured that the practitioner agrees to provide treatment and is practicing within his or her scope of practice. If the treatment involves a drug or device not approved by FDA, the patient is to be informed of potential side effects and told that no claim exists for treatment efficacy, and an informed-consent form must be signed. The bill is also designed to prevent dishonest billing practices or outright scams.

A large part of the debate and controversy regarding the use of CAM therapies in the United States will be shaped through the enactment of statues at the state and federal levels. For an excellent review of the many legal issues raised by the practice of CAM, see Cohen.[23]

METHODOLOGY

Although strong research methodology can lead to outcome results that are both accurate and reproducible, a debate exists between advocates of CAM and conventional scientists and physicians about which kinds of research designs are appropriate or even needed to determine efficacy.[54]

One reason for the disparity between CAM and conventional medical research is their completely opposite theoretical models. The biomedical approach focuses on a disease orientation, which suggests that a specific agent leads to a specific illness or disorder. Hypothesis testing and linear reasoning with logic and causation are the main components. CAM therapies are based more in a philosophy that uses a comprehensive approach concerned with multidimensional factors which cannot always be studied independently. Causation and mechanisms of therapeutic action or how something "works" is not always seen as important. One central goal of CAM is to improve on the "wellness" of the patient. Rather than just removing a disease-producing agent, quality of life is emphasized by treating functional or somatic problems with ancillary and important psychological, social, emotional, and spiritual aspects.

Many CAM research studies (a) appear to be not focused, (b) do not use hypothesis testing or large number of subjects, and (c) tend to rely more on verbal reports from the patients.[44] The quality of most CAM studies, as judged by Western-trained scientists, is not considered very good.[64] In particular, research evaluating acupuncture and homeopathy has previously been described as weak.[47,89]

Strengths and weaknesses of clinical research in a particular area can be studied using a scientific consensus development approach. The OAM and the NIH recently sponsored such a conference evaluating the quality of research on acupuncture.[1] An independent, nonfederal panel reviewed the scientific evidence. It was concluded that there were few well-performed research studies assessing efficacy of acupuncture with either placebo or sham controls. Future research was encouraged to evaluate and include (1) enrollment procedures, (2) eligibility criteria, (3) clinical characteristics of the subjects, (4) methods for diagnosis, and (5) accurate description of protocols, including types and number of treatments, outcomes used, and statistical analysis. Needle acupuncture was reported to be most efficacious for postoperative and chemotherapy-associated nausea and vomiting and for nausea associated with pregnancy. It was somewhat efficacious for postoperative dental pain, but for the remaining health areas the panel found that most of the scientific literature was "mixed" regarding positive treatment outcomes; in many cases determination could not be made because of poor study design. The panel also reported that the incidence of adverse effects with the use of acupuncture was lower than with many drugs. Future proposed areas to study included (1) the demographics of use of acupuncture; (2) efficacy, including evaluating if different theories of acupuncture produce different treatment outcomes; and (3) ways to integrate research and acupuncture findings into the health care system.

These conference findings highlight the important factors to be considered when evaluating differences between conventional and CAM approaches.[8] For example, a patient receiving acupuncture may, because of varied treatment reactions, have the contact points changed throughout the procedure, making it more difficult to describe any specificity of effect of procedures, points used, or therapist-patient interactions, or a combination of these. However, since CAM therapists are an integral part of the therapy, their communication with patients is crucial. In this instance, the overall description of changes produced by acupuncture may be more important initially than isolating the many factors involved.

Table 1-3 presents types of evidence required for the validation of research. Each of the items listed—when appropriate, possible, and realistic—should be part of any practice or research protocol, regardless of clinical orientation, CAM or conventional. The use of this type of evidence is important to the consumers who use CAM therapies and to the federal and state agencies that attempt to regulate practices and need to integrate research findings, which should be collected under valid and objective conditions.

Subject Selection

Some methodologists insist that adequate numbers of subjects by gender, age, education, and similarity of medical condition be minimal conditions for inclusion. Each sub-

TABLE 1-3	Types of Evidence Useful in the Evaluation of CAM Therapies
Types of Evidence	**Validation Questions**
Experimental evidence	Is the practice efficacious when examined experimentally?
Clinical (practice) evidence	Is the practice effective when applied clinically?
Safety evidence	Is the practice safe?
Comparative evidence	Is it the best practice for the problem?
Summary evidence	Is the practice known and evaluated?
Rational evidence	Is the practice rational, progressing, and contributing to medical and scientific understanding?
Demand evidence	Do consumers and practitioners want the practice?
Satisfaction evidence	Is it meeting the expectations of patients and practitioners?
Cost evidence	Is the practice inexpensive to operate and cost-effective? Is it provided by payers?
Meaning evidence	Is the practice the right one for the individual?

ject should have an equal chance of either receiving or not receiving treatment (randomization). This ensures that the study will have more equated samples with which to evaluate, and, overall, less variance in the analyzed outcome; that a no-treatment-or-placebo control group be used; that patient and examiner be unaware of group placement (blinding), and that the medical condition to be treated is clearly diagnosed with specified criteria for each subject/group. Certain medical journals now require that parameters explicitly related to randomization be described.[37]

Ethically, conceptually, and practically, randomized trials may present problems in research design, especially for CAM.[38,90] For example, if a therapy is new and safe, a good chance exists that it may also work. Patients may not want to participate in or may "resent" being in a study in which they potentially may be "randomized" into a "control group." Their "belief" that they might be in a nontreatment group may impact attitude and possibly outcome. Quite often the clinical trial may seem artificial and pose no relevance to clinical practice itself. Randomized controlled trials are not designed to evaluate individual differences. Some patients may respond to a treatment, and others may not. This is a serious concern of many CAM practitioners who argue that randomization actually "biases out" any positive finding.

The following approaches may be taken to help obviate some of these concerns:
1. To ensure homogeneity of groups,[94] patients can be evaluated, first, using a standard, conventional physician interview with conventional diagnostic techniques and, *second*, by a CAM practitioner, with eventual subcategorizing of each patient based on findings important to the *specific therapy* under evaluation. For example, if acupuncture were being evaluated, pulse and tongue characteristics would be doc-

umented; if homeopathy were being evaluated, a collection of symptoms with specific remedies would be documented. The treatment protocol is balanced because *both* conventional and individual symptom pattern diagnoses are incorporated. One obvious difficulty is the large number of patients required, along with associated expense and time required to complete the protocol.

2. In a simpler design each patient serves as his or her own control. Variables such as gender, genetic factors, social strata, and personality are matched, and each subject is evaluated over time, generally before, during, and after treatment. In certain designs a "crossover" to the treatment can be studied. The important variable of "washout" of effects allowing adequate time for "residual" treatment effects to dissipate should be an integral part of the design.

3. In an "n-of-1" design,[40] each patient is studied individually by one physician, and results are instantaneously recorded. Individual clinical trial packages can be developed, including standardized questionnaires and measurement devices. When necessary, if similarities in patient profiles and other variables occur, data may be "pooled together," although care should be taken when equating. Using this design, the authors reported that 81% of the trials were completed, and the results caused physicians to be more confident in their practice management. The n-of-1 design could be used to begin early studies of certain CAM therapies by, first, individually profiling patients' responsiveness in clinical practice settings and then entering results into a registered database. Subsequently, larger-scale clinical trials could be developed.

A relevant issue in the selection of subjects for research is the actual number used in either treatment or nontreatment groups. Most studies evaluating treatment efficacy in CAM use too few subjects per group. The mythical number of 50 per group is either inappropriate or not always feasible. The best way to ensure that the results are accurate and reproducible is to use a power analysis to determine actual sample size needed, pre or post hoc.[21,22]

Subject Expectation and the Role of the Placebo

When patients are treated for any illness or health condition, there are the following explanations for improvement[85]:

1. The treatment itself may be responsible for change.
2. Most illnesses including pain simply remit on their own over time and heal (natural history), or extreme symptoms simply return to a closer approximation of the original health state (regression to the mean).
3. Patients improve on their own simply because they "think" someone is doing something for them (Hawthorne effect), or they mistakenly think the symptoms and complaints are related to a disease or illness but in actuality these symptoms are related more to psychosocial stress.

4. The patients were originally misdiagnosed by physician or caregiver and in fact did not have a particular illness.
5. Some unexplained, nonspecific effect operates, such as either a positive or negative attitude toward ancillary caregivers, or the patient develops or has a positive attitude or belief that the treatment will be either beneficial (placebo) or negative, that is, not beneficial (nocebo). This latter effect has possible relevance to CAM because under certain conditions it may be the major basis for responsiveness to CAM treatments.

The term "placebo" refers to a sham treatment that physicians may use to "please" (its Latin meaning) either anxious patients or those who are difficult to treat. It contains no inert, active pharmaceutical substance(s). In clinical trials research it is considered a "nontreatment" and given with the assumption that because of its inactivity, patients will not respond as they would to active treatments.

Beecher[10] postulated that placebos can actually change patient functioning structurally and physiologically. Also, Levine and colleagues[52] have demonstrated that the "placebo" response might be partially endorphin mediated, since naloxone, which blocks endorphin release, could in some cases reverse "placebo treatment effects" for reducing postoperative dental pain. A specific transmitter-mediated "placebo central nervous system (CNS) pathway," while an intriguing possibility, has not been established. Placebos do have their own pharmacokinetics, including dose response,[65] side effects,[15] and residual long-term effects.[56]

One of the more interesting aspects of placebo responses is understanding the varied conditions under which they might work.[93] In any clinical study a certain number of patients will respond positively to placebos. Generally the number varies across studies, but it may range from 30% to 70%. Oh[63] has suggested that placebos appear to work in patients with pain and disorders of autonomic sensation such as nausea, psychoneuroses, phobias, and depression and in disorders of neurohumoral control, including blood pressure and bronchial airflow. Attempts to clearly define and predict which subjects might potentially be "placebo responders" based on gender, personality, attitudes about drugs, doctors, nurses, or hospitals has not yielded consistent results. A positive expectation of treatment outcome, a favorable response to a specific practitioner, and a high degree of compliance may be aspects deserving closer attention.[85] It has been suggested that placebos may operate by decreasing patient anxiety.[31] Others have shown that highly anxious patients maximize their responsiveness to placebos.[72] Placebos may simply work through classical conditioning.[90] However, none of these explanations has been consistently verified, and it is likely that, while they play a part in placebo responding, they also remain incomplete and speculative.

Benson[11] has offered an alternative to the term placebo responding—"remembered wellness." After either an active or a passive therapeutic intervention, he suggests, there is an occurrence of a memory of past events which helps to trigger a physical response. The patient remembers a time when things such as peace, strength, and confidence were an active part of consciousness and good health. This process involves the individual's own "belief" system. It includes prior learning, previous experiences (environment), and genetic interactions (biologic factors).

According to Benson, a good way to access "remembered wellness" is through relaxation. The quieting of both the mind and the body assists in healing. Relaxation has been demonstrated in clinical research studies to reduce physiologic responses such as sweat, those of muscle and nerve (electroencephalographic), temperature, and heart rate and thus subsequently treat anxiety,[77] high blood pressure, pain, headaches, and a variety of other illnesses.[12,41,84]

Benson has described the continually evolving definition of the interaction(s) between mind/brain and body. Clinical and preclinical basic studies conducted in this area now reveal provocative relationships with the CNS and the immune system. The seminal work of Ader and Cohen[2] reporting ways in which the immune system was modifiable through conditioning of the immune suppression response helped to shape the field of psychoneuroimmunology. Other work[3] has emphasized the important role of stress management and its positive effects on cardiovascular and stroke-related illnesses and in disease prevention.

"Belief in some type of a treatment outcome," either positive or negative, becomes an integral part of a multiinteractive process that has specific relationships with CAM. Spiritual belief and its impact on healing in mental health areas have recently been reviewed and found to be of importance.[50] Patients who are committed to a more religious orientation report a better overall satisfaction with life and lower levels of depression and stress. Also, clinical psychologists report that many of their patients use reli-

ZIPPY BILL GRIFFITH

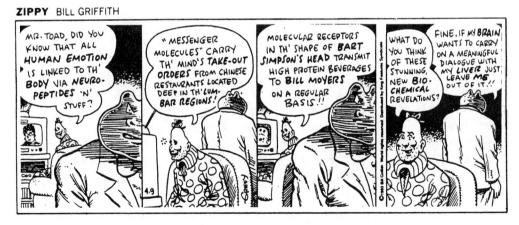

Fig. 1-2 Zippy cartoon: "My Kidney, My Self." (Courtesy of Bill Griffith. Reprinted with special permission of King Features Syndicate.)

gious language such as prayer when discussing the many emotional issues around treatment of mental health problems.[71] The potential of spiritual healing using a patient's belief system may have huge, untapped ramifications in other health-related areas outside psychiatry and psychology.

Subject Assessment

One of the major weaknesses in research evaluating CAM therapies has been the use of incomplete, biased, or, often, invalidated treatment outcome measurements. This is important because statements about degree of efficacy are severely limited and the ability to form clinical generalizations is reduced.

One outcome measurement used in CAM studies is the self-report. With certain guidelines it can produce helpful information.[76] Generally, direct questions with yes-or-no answers are asked, boxes are checked, or a ranking scale is used. A concern with this type of analysis can be the truthfulness of the respondent. Factors that can influence accuracy include motivation, deception, willingness to please, medical condition, and psychometric properties such as reliability and validity of the particular items used.

Rather than using a single outcome measure, most CAM therapies could use multi-dimensional assessments to maximize external validity. Meaningful clinical effects can be described by monitoring the instances when a treatment is both beneficial and safe and by determining longevity. In addition to evaluating major medical parameters such as basic laboratory studies or physiologic functioning, ancillary functions including quality of life, hospital visits, abilities to work (e.g., functional capacities), are all useful.

Measurements should reflect each patient's individual concerns about *his or her* illness. A more appropriate term, "subjective health status," may be more useful than "quality of life" because the latter measure is difficult to define, understand, and accurately measure.[51]

The use of multivariant analysis in certain instances may be helpful. For example, the predictive value of CAM therapeutic approaches in patients who had previously undergone coronary artery bypass graft (CABG) surgery has been evaluated.[5] A structural equation model was used to test the hypothesis that patients' health care practices improved psychological adjustment following CABG. Eight-five percent of all patients practiced CAM. Patients who used prayer, exercise, or diet modification in their lifestyle had less depression and general psychologic distress (Fig. 1-3). This is an important finding because it demonstrates how multiple variables can be appropriately evaluated in CAM research and produce meaningful outcome statements. It is also clinically significant for individual patients who want to improve their health after surgery and demonstrates the importance of belief as a cofactor in health recovery.

An approach to patient measurement and evaluation in CAM that may be less costly than conducting large-scale, controlled randomized trials is the use of systematic clinical auditing. Documentation is made of certain characteristics about patients,

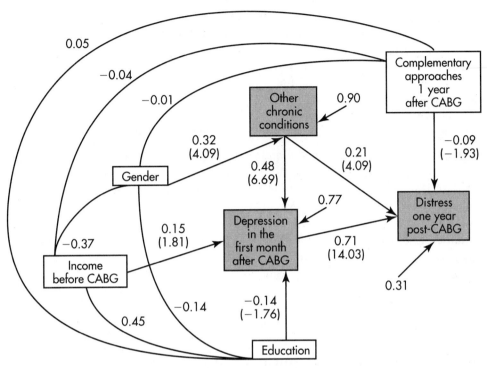

Fig. 1-3 A model of complementary approaches predicting current distress in cardiac patients after surgery. Straight lines with arrows between boxes represent a direct effect, with appropriate correlation coefficients and student *t* values in parentheses. A curved line between boxes shows bivariate associations with correlations. Arrow directed at a darker box (endogenous variable) is random error. *CABG*, Coronary artery bypass graft (surgery). (From Amy Ai, personal communication, April 1997.)

including diagnosis, type of therapy used, and outcome results using categories in large samples of individuals. This observational information describes the clinical practice by questionnaires usually sent out during set periods after hospital admission. Patients (N=1597) have been evaluated over a 1-year period at a hospital for TCM in Germany.[57] Each patient was initially seen by both a German and a Chinese physician, and general data and documentation collected. Approximately 66% of the patients had chronic pain, with the most common diagnoses including diseases of the nervous system and musculoskeletal complaints. Most patients were treated with either acupuncture or Chinese herbal remedies. At discharge, 38% improved more than 50%, 32% had improved less than 50%, 24% had no change in their condition, and 6% reported an increase in symptoms. Interestingly, according to the authors, 97.1% of the patients gave valid health information.

When using the clinical audit, researchers should be aware that data collected may be subject to bias through the use of self-reports, thus limiting accuracy of information. Criteria for inclusion and exclusion of all patients must be explicitly stated, and any coding of diagnoses to be entered also should reflect precise, accurate parameters. Through development and testing, this approach in the future may be one way of collecting in large samples useful information about CAM.

Reporting Meaningful and Informative Results for the Clinician

Databases. One of the difficulties in evaluating CAM research has been finding adequate, published research. Often it is either simply nonexistent or poorly performed and reported, or it remains untranslated in foreign journals and databases. Medline, which is located at the National Library of Medicine (NLM) of the NIH, is the major source of medical science research in the United States. There are currently less than 30 *standardized Medical Subject Heading (MeSH) codes* or terms which can access or index research articles in CAM. Most articles tracked and reported in the journals indexed have undergone peer review, although this does not guarantee that the results are without error! Also, many of the more provocative issues in CAM appear to be published in and by alternative or complementary medical journals, many of which may never be read by most physicians or scientists. It is imperative that when better methodologies are developed and used in the evaluation of CAM, they be published in mainline, conventional medical journals (e.g., see Ai and Spencer's report[6] explaining the use of structural equations in the evaluation of CAM in back and musculoskeletal rehabilitation).

One internationally focused database, the Cochrane Collaboration, is currently forming a comprehensive registry of randomized control trials and systematic reviews.[67] The goal of the Cochrane Collaboration is to make easier decisions about potential treatments and their efficacy and safety using an evidence-based approach. Within this database there is a complementary therapy research evaluation section. Other relevant, ancillary databases for CAM include PSYCHLIT or CISCOM, which is the database for the Research Council for Complementary Medicine in England and uses, in part, the British Library. CISCOM covers papers since the mid-1960s. Other data sources include the OAM's bibliographic databases of information on CAM literature and clinical trials and the Combined Health Information database. Also, data-archived bases, distinct from bibliographic (text-based) resources, are important because they can be used for standard case-level statistical analysis, subgrouping investigations, and modifying data from original analyses. Additional information about other CAM databases may be found elsewhere[13] (see Appendix C).

Meta-analysis. Databases are useful for accessing individual research articles. Meta-analysis provides general reviews of numerous research papers. Research data from several clinical trials are analyzed and interpreted together. The two main objectives are to quantify any potential effect a treatment may have and to evaluate the consistency of treatment effects across more than just one sample of patients. To be included in a meta-analysis, specified criteria include (1) subject size, (2) statistic used, (3) hypothesis present, and (4) types of outcome measures used.[61] The relevance of meta-analysis to CAM is that it becomes an acceptable format for including and determining which specific research studies accurately focus on specific parameters (e.g., the evaluation of treatment efficacy).

When evaluating groups of research articles, it is important to determine who selects the studies and on which criteria the selection is based. How far back should the evaluation be made? What and who will determine how treatment efficacy will be described and set? How can and should publication bias be handled? That is, does a bias exist against the publication of negative findings? If so—and this is most relevant in the field of CAM—is it likely that in the absence of any negative findings, the collated positive findings are reporting an effect that is falsely truncated? Sixteen studies reporting the significant effects of an herbal preparation or type of massage for the treatment of migraine headache may not be meaningful if 75 studies found no effect. This type of error poses a significant threat to the internal validity of the research design itself.

Meta-analysis can lead to better generalizations about treatment outcome. It is not the complete answer, and care must be taken to avoid placing too much emphasis on any one type of methodologic analysis.

Clinical Significance. Statistically based research is important for determining certain relationships, but it may have little to do with clinical significance. For example, how does treatment affect things beyond changing the course of a disease? Is quality of life affected? A patient with a serious chronic disease such as cancer may have side effects from the chemotherapy, such as hiccups or diarrhea from medication for the treatment of AIDS. While CAM may not resolve the disease process, its potential for reducing or removing medication side effects or providing for a less adverse effect of chemotherapy or radiation therapy might be more fully evaluated.

The requisite clinical issue is, to what extent does a CAM therapy move patients outside the range of a dysfunctional health population to or within the range of more functional populations?[43] Clinical significance results as a change associated with the return to parameters of a "normative group" and, equally important, impacts individual well-being. In addition, all clinicians have their own opinions about whether a therapy is helpful. This should and can be factored into studies in which statistical distributions of *both* observed data and clinicians' prior beliefs about the therapy and outcome can be parts of the evaluation quotient.[17]

Transfer of Clinical Information. As a first step, high-quality research should provide physicians with information about which CAM therapies are useful. Reliable clinical research information supports good clinical decision making. Textbooks and journals are not always adequate because they do not bear on the relevance of daily practice. Using a database of 406 references in which physicians were questioned regarding their needs, the majority requested information about effects of certain treatments, guidance on usage, personal psychological support, affirmation, commiseration, and feedback.[75]

With more patients asking questions about CAM, deficiencies in current information are apparent. Whatever the tool selected, it should be electronic, portable, and fast and easy to use. A summary of clinical studies in specific health categories treated by a complementary therapy with outcomes and specified rankings would be useful. Further, databases can be set up so that when an individual patient is seen, information can be recorded in a protocol along with subjective comments and then electronically collated. The goal should be better management of clinical information. This would enhance both time of treatment and quality of interaction and improve relationships among health care providers, patients, and the general public.

REGULATION

FDA's function is to oversee the safety of foods, drugs, and medical devices sold in the United States. It does this primarily by convening review panels of scientists to evaluate submitted protocols by companies, individuals, or federal grants in which there might be an issue of safety. FDA does not regulate the practice of medicine, but it does regulate the products used in the practice of medicine. The regulatory approach taken by the agency is determined by the type of product (food, drug, device) and its intended use as described in the labeling. FDA also sponsors workshops and conferences for the purpose of disseminating information concerning the risks and benefits of CAM.

In 1994 the Dietary Supplements Health and Education Act was passed. This legislation had profound effects on the regulation and marketing of herbal products in the United States. Herbs or other botanicals could be sold as dietary supplements and were not subject to the rigorous regulation that applied to drugs. A disclosure was included: "This product is not intended to diagnose, treat, cure, or prevent any disease."

However, a botanic product currently marketed as food could be regulated as a drug if the manufacturer sought a claim that the product was used to treat or prevent a human disease. In this case it would be required that the botanic product be tested in well-defined clinical trials for both safety and efficacy.

Generally botanic products are not evaluated by the strict preclinical toxicology and pharmacology guidelines that are in place for conventional drugs. Instead, the focus of the clinical trials is on the efficacy of the products. A number of herbal formulations are presently undergoing clinical trials. It is important for the clinician or physician to understand that to date efficacy has not been established and that any herbal product should be used with caution. FDA has established a hotline for information about herbal products (1-800-FDA-4010) and one for reporting any adverse effect(s) after taking any herbal product (1-800-FDA-1088).

In response to petitions submitted by the acupuncture community and a recent workshop, FDA has reclassified acupuncture needles for general use from Class III, a category in which clinical studies are required to establish safety and effectiveness, to Class II, a category that involves less stringent control by FDA but does require good manufacturing and proper labeling. Manufactures are required to label FDA needles for single use only. Acupuncture needles for clinical practice would be restricted to qualified practitioners as determined by state practice laws.

The five areas with best documentation for acupuncture efficacy according to past workshops convened by FDA include pain, substance abuse, emesis, paralysis due to stroke and other CNS damage, and pulmonary disease. As mentioned previously, the NIH, also evaluating acupuncture research, found treatment efficacy but mostly in the area of pain control and nausea and vomiting.

FDA is currently attempting to establish guidelines for the regulation of homeopathic products. FDA takes the position that homeopathic remedies which are used in the treatment of disease are by definition "drugs" and should be regulated. In recent years, FDA has exempted homeopathic products from the regular drug reviewing process if such products have been reviewed and approved by the Homeopathic Pharmacopoeia of the United States. In rare cases in which the homeopathic remedies were promoted to treat serious illness such as AIDS or cancer, FDA would require the investigator to submit a detailed description or protocol that would undergo some form of review and clinical research.

TRAINING AND EDUCATION

A growing "movement" to provide some instruction of CAM within the medical school curriculum has gained momentum in the past few years. Currently there are 63 medical schools that offer elective course(s) in CAM, including one that offers postgraduate training (see the box on p. 30).

All courses are supported entirely by extramural resources or donated faculty time, or both. Dock[26] noted more than 90 years ago:

> There is a large number of reformers going about the country longing to give medical students more work. Some think that what a young doctor needs is a course of lectures on ethics, others, lectures on medical history, and so on.

There has never been adequate time in the curriculum for all the things a medical student needs to know. One of the most common complaints made by external curriculum review committees is that the curriculum is too dense—that there are too many hours of lecture devoted to too much detail. The goal of curriculum reform in actuality is to free time for more self-directed activities rather than adding more courses.

U.S. Medical Schools Currently Offering Courses in CAM

Albert Einstein College of Medicine
Boston University School of Medicine
Case Western Reserve University School
    of Medicine
Chicago Medical School
City University of New York
Columbia University College
    of Physicians and Surgeons
Cornell Medical College
Duke University School of Medicine
East Tennessee State University James H.
    Quillen College of Medicine
Eastern Virginia Medical School
Emory University School of Medicine
Georgetown University School
    of Medicine
Harvard Medical School
Howard University College of Medicine
Indiana University School of Medicine
Jefferson Medical College of Thomas Jef-
    ferson University
Johns Hopkins School of Medicine
Marshall University School of Medicine
Mayo Medical School
Medical College of Pennsylvania-
    Hahnemann
Michigan State University
Morehouse School of Medicine
Mount Sinai School of Medicine
New York Medical College
Northeastern Ohio Universities College of
    Medicine
Northwestern University
Ohio State University College of Medicine
Pennsylvania State University College of
    Medicine
Rush Medical College
Southern Illinois University School of
    Medicine
St. Louis University School of Medicine
Stanford University School of Medicine
State University of New York at Buffalo
    School of Medicine
State University of New York
    at Syracuse School of Medicine

Temple University School of Medicine
Tufts University School of Medicine
Uniformed Services University
    of the Health Sciences
Universidad Central del Caribe School of
    Medicine, Puerto Rico
University of Arizona School
    of Medicine*
University of California, Los Angeles
    School of Medicine
University of California, San Francisco
    School of Medicine
University of Cincinnati School
    of Medicine
University of Colorado Health Sciences
    Center
University of Connecticut School
    of Medicine
University of Illinois at Chicago
University of Iowa College of Medicine
University of Louisville School of Medicine
University of Maryland School of Medicine
University of Medicine and Dentistry
    of New Jersey Medical School
University of Miami School of Medicine
University of Michigan School of Medicine
University of Minnesota, Minneapolis
University of New Mexico
University of North Carolina, Chapel Hill
    School of Medicine
University of Pennsylvania School
    of Medicine
University of Texas, Dallas, Southwestern
University of Vermont College of Medicine
University of Virginia School of Medicine
University of Washington School
    of Medicine
University of Wisconsin Medical School
Virginia Commonwealth University
    School of Medicine
Wayne State University School
    of Medicine
Wright State University School
    of Medicine
Yale University School of Medicine

Information from *http://cpmcnet.columbia.edu/dept/rosenthal*. A disclaimer notes in part "the information and resources listing on this site are not intended to be fully systematic or complete." Additional course information can also be found at this site.
*Also offers postgraduate training in "integrative" medicine.

Course offerings in CAM within medical schools will meet resistance. One part of the difficulty is scheduled instruction time, but another is the lack of clear clinical and scientific evidence that the therapies are useful. However, a good justification for courses which introduce CAM to medical students is that patients will self-refer to CAM practitioners while undergoing treatment by physicians. If the physician understands something about the CAM practitioner's therapeutic interventions, the activities can be potentially complementary, integrative, and more useful. At the very least, harmful interactions can be avoided.

Required courses in CAM will not in the near future be part of the first 2 years of the medical student's training. However, opportunities do exist during clinical rotations, where it is appropriate to have students learn about the application of various CAM techniques and their potential integration with conventional treatment strategies. As CAM gains acceptance and questions are included on the national licensing examinations, CAM emphasis may be included in the predoctoral curriculum.

In June 1996, the OAM sponsored a conference on CAM in medical and nursing education. Participants shared their experiences of teaching CAM in a wide variety of formats. The different models for teaching CAM included the following:

- Presenting a series of visiting lectures for weekly discussions.
- Offering seminars including interfacing particular health maintenance approaches such as T'ai chi in which students could learn through participation.
- Offering Continuing Education credit and formal lectures describing CAM and specific methodology skills necessary to evaluate CAM so that physicians can more completely discuss its value with their patients.

Although there seemed to be widespread agreement on the general value of CAM instruction in medical schools, there was less agreement on the practical problems of time and funding. CAM will be conceded as important but will most likely remain as an elective and limited in most curricula. Areas within the medical schools where it may become potentially integrated are behavioral and family medicine because these areas have patients who are most likely to try certain CAM therapies.

SUMMARY

This chapter has detailed six issues that impact the practice of CAM. They have evolved from many other areas and, in part, interact with each other and have many commonalties. Historical antecedents reveal that CAM is partially rooted in ancient cultures and beliefs, as well as more modern, eclectic groups of practices. Many have been integrated with conventional medicine, including the use of certain plant products (foxglove in digitalis and *Rauwolfia* plants for antihypertensive drugs); diet, exercise, and vitamins for prevention and treatment of heart disease; joint manipulation for pain.[36] Definitions of CAM must be broad and flexible for change. Most of medical science, including physicians, has been slow to accept CAM, primarily because little information exists to demonstrate that these therapies are helpful and safe. There is a need for the physician to become more knowledgeable about CAM therapies as more consumers are increasingly using CAM. Practice guidelines will help make the profession more credible. To date, the quality of CAM research has generally been poor. What will be required is a science-based evaluation that looks toward more focused and creative ways to evaluate targeted areas in CAM.[80] A potential area might be practice-based data. Outcome types of research seem important and relevant. Standardizing what is known about herbal medicine from a broad range of activities, including active substances used throughout the world, and listing which ones are most successful for treatment would be useful. Closer evaluation, replication, extension, and further development of other research strategies, some of which are described in later chapters, will be needed. This is true both for the evaluation of treatments and for better evaluating *diagnostic* methods and techniques. Of particular importance in CAM is the notion of *integration*. That is, when appropriate, it is suggested that a blending of conventional and CAM occur so that medical treatment interventions and results can be optimized. The acceptance of CAM will depend in part on how well it is able to demonstrate that it is both useful and safe for usage by consumers.

REFERENCES

1. Acupuncture. National Institutes of Health Consensus Development Conference Statement, Nov 3–5, 1997, Bethesda, Md.
2. Ader R, Cohen N: Behaviorally conditioned immunosuppression, *Psychosom Med* 37:333, 1975.
3. Adler N, Matthews K: Health psychology: why do some people get sick and some stay well? *Annu Rev Psychol* 45:229, 1994.
4. Agency for Health Care Policy and Research: Acute pain management: operative or medical procedures and trauma, Pub No AHCPR 92-0032, Rockville, Md, 1992.
5. Ai A, Peterson C, Bolling SF: Psychological recovery following coronary artery bypass graft surgery: the use of complementary therapies, *J Alternat Complement Med: Res Paradigm Pract Policy* 3(4):343, 1997.
6. Ai A, Spencer J: The use of structural equation models for analyzing the multi factors associated with neuromuscular rehabilitation, *J Back Musculoskel Rehabil* April 10(2):97, 1998.
7. Andritzky W: Medical students and alternative medicine: a survey, *Gesundneitswescn* 6:345, 1995.
8. Anthony HM: Some methodological problems in the assessment of complementary therapy. In Lewith GT, Aldridge D, editors: *Clinical Research Methodology for Complementary Therapies*, London, 1993, Hodder and Stoughton.
9. Assendelft WJ et al: The relationship between methodological quality and conclusions in reviews of spinal manipulation. *JAMA* 274(24):1942, 1995.
10. Beecher HK: The powerful placebo, *JAMA* 159:1602, 1955.
11. Benson, H: *Timeless healing: the power of biology and belief,* New York, 1996, Scribner.
12. Benson H, Crassweller SE: Relaxation response: bridge between psychiatry and medicine, *Med Clin North Am* 61:929, 1977.
13. Berman BM, Larsen D, editors: Alternative medicine: expanding medical horizons—a report to the National Institutes of Health on alternative medical systems and practices in the United States, Pub No 94-066, Bethesda, Md, 1994.

14. Berman BM et al: Physicians' attitudes toward complementary or alternative medicine: a regional survey, *J Am Board Fam Pract* 8:36l, 1995.
15. Blackwell B, Bloomfield SS, Buncher CR: Demonstration to medical students of placebo responses and non-drug factors, *Lancet* 1:1279, 1972.
16. Borkan J et al: Referrals for alternative therapies, *J Fam Pract* 39(6):545, 1994.
17. Brophy JM, Lawrence J: Placing trials in context using Bayesian analysis, *JAMA* 273(11):871, 1995.
18. Cassileth BR: Contemporary unorthodox treatments in cancer medicine: a study of patients. *Ann Intern Med* 101:105, 1984.
19. Cassileth BR et al: Survival and quality of life among patients receiving unproven as compared with conventional cancer therapy. *N Engl J Med* 324:1180, 1991.
20. Child A: *Illness and healing.* In *Religion and magic in the life of traditional peoples*, Englewood Cliffs, NJ, 1993 Prentice Hall.
21. Cohen J: The differences between proportions. In *Statistical power analysis for the behavioral sciences*, New York, 1977, Academic.
22. Cohen J: A power primer, *Psychol Bull* 112(1):155, 1992.
23. Cohen MJ: *Complementary and alternative medicine: legal boundaries and regulatory perspectives*, Baltimore, 1998, Johns Hopkins University.
24. Danesi MA, Adetunji JB: Use of alternative medicine by patients with epilepsy: a survey of 265 epileptic patients in a developing country, *Epilepsia* 35(2):344, 1994.
25. D'Antoni ML, Harvey PL, Fried MP: Alternative medicine: does it play a role in the management of voice disorders? *J Voice* 9:(3):308, 1995.
26. Dock G: Medical ethics and etiquette, *Physician Surgeon* 28:481, 1906.
27. Dumoff A: Protecting your practice, *Alternat Complement Ther* May/June, p 186, 1996.
28. Eisenberg DM et al: Unconventional medicine in the United States: prevalence, costs and patterns of use. *N Engl J Med* 328:246, 1993.
29. Ernst E: Direct risks associated with complementary therapies. In Ernst E, editor: *Complementary medicine: an objective appraisal*, Oxford, 1996, Butterworth-Heinemann.
30. Ernst E, Resch KL, White AR: Complementary medicine: what physicians think of it—a meta-analysis, *Arch Intern Med* 155:2405, 1995.
31. Evans FJ: The placebo response in pain reduction, *Adv Neurol* 4:289, 1974.
32. Federal Register, No 49859, September 23, 1997.
33. Field MJ, Lohr KN, editors: *Guidelines for clinical practice: from development to use*, Washington, DC, 1992, National Academy.
34. Fisher P, Ward A: Complementary medicine in Europe, *Br Med J* 309(6947):107, 1994.
35. Furnham A, Forey J: The attitudes, behaviors and beliefs of conventional vs complementary, alternative medicine. *J Clin Psychol* 50(3):458, 1994.
36. Gevitz N: Unorthodox medical theories. In Bynum WF, Porter R, editors: *Companion encyclopedia of the history of medicine*, London, 1993, Routledge.
37. Glass RM, Flanagin A: New requirements for authors submitting manuscripts to *JAMA*, *JAMA* 277:74, 1997.
38. Gordon G: Is there a need to devise clinical trials that do not depend on randomized controlled testing? *Adv J Mind Health* 9(2), 1993.
39. Gordon JS: The paradigm of holistic medicine. In *Health for the whole person*, Boulder, Co, 1980, Westview.
40. Guyatt GH et al: The n-of-l randomized controlled trial: clinical usefulness, *Ann Intern Med* 112:293,1990.
41. Hatch JP, Fisher JG, Rugh JD: *Biofeedback studies in clinical efficacy*, New York, 1987, Plenum.
42. Himmel W, Schulte M, Kochen MM: Complementary medicine: are patients' expectations being met by their general practitioners? *Br J Gen Pract* 43(371):232, 1993.
43. Jacobson NS, Truax P: Clinical significance: a statistical approach to defining meaningful change in psychotherapy research, *J Consult Clin Psychol* 59(1):12, 1991.
44. Jonas W: Evaluating unconventional medical practices, *J NIH Res* 5:64, 1993.
45. Jonas W: Safety in complementary medicine. In Ernst E, editor: *Complementary medicine: an objective appraisal*, Oxford, 1996, Butterworth-Heinemann.

46. King LS: The Flexner Report of 1910, *JAMA* 251(8):1079, 1984.
47. Kleijnen J, Knipschild P, Rietter G: Clinical trials of homeopathy, *Br Med J* 302(316):23, 1991.
48. Kleinman A: *The illness narrative: suffering, healing and the human condition,* New York, 1988, Basic Books.
49. Konner M: *Medicine at the crossroads,* New York, 1994, Vintage Books.
50. Larson D, Milano M: Religion and mental health: should they work together? *Alternat Complement Ther* March/April, p 91, 1996.
51. Leplege A, Hunt S: The problem of quality of life in medicine, *JAMA* 278(1):47, 1997.
52. Levine JD, Gordon NC, Fields HL: The mechanism of placebo analgesia, *Lancet* 2:654, 1978.
53. Lewith GT: The use and abuse of evidence-based medicine: an example from general medicine. In Ernst E, editor: *Complementary medicine: an objective appraisal,* Oxford, 1996, Butterworth-Heinemann.
54. Lewith GT, Aldridge D, editors: *Clinical research methodology for complementary therapies,* London, 1993, Hodder and Stoughton.
55. Liu CA, Xiao PG: *An introduction to Chinese materia medicine,* Beijing, 1993, Peking Union Medical College, Beijing Medical University.
56. Max MB et al: Amitriptyline relieves diabetic neuropathy pain in patients with normal or depressed mood, *Neurology* 37:89, 1987.
57. Melchart D et al: Systematic clinical auditing in complementary medicine: rationale, concept and pilot study, *Alternat Ther Health Med* 3(1):33, 1997.
58. Michle W: Chronic polyarthritis treatment with alternative medicine: how frequent is self therapy with alternative methods? *Fortschr Med* 113(7):81, 1995.
59. Mitchell BB: *Acupuncture and oriental medicine laws,* Washington, DC, 1997, National Acupuncture Foundation.
60. Montbriand MJ: Freedom of choice: an issue concerning alternative therapies chosen by patients with cancer, *Oncol Nurs Forum* 20(8):1195, 1993.
61. Nony P et al: Critical reading of the meta-analysis of clinical trials, *Therapie* 50:339, 1995.
62. O'Connor B et al: Defining and describing complementary and alternative medicine, *Alternat Ther Health Med,* 3(2):49, 1997.
63. Oh VM: The placebo effect: how can we use it better? *Br Med J* 309:69, 1994.
64. Patel M: Problems in the evaluation of alternative medicine, *Soc Sci Med* 25(6):669, 1987.
65. Pogge RC: The toxic placebo. I. Side and toxic effects reported during the administration of placebo medicine, *Med Times* 91:1, 1963.
66. Reilly DT: Young doctors' views on alternative medicine, *Br Med J* 287:337, 1983.
67. Robinson A: Research practice and the Cochrane Collaboration, *Can Med Assoc J* 152(6):883, 1995.
68. Sale DM: Overview of legislative developments concerning alternative health care in the United States. Research project under a grant from the John Fetzer Institute, Kalamazoo, Mich, 1994, The Institute.
69. Schr A, Messerli-Rohrback V, Schubarth P: Conventional or complementary medicine: what criteria for choosing do patients use? *Schweiz Med Wochenschr Suppl* 62:18, 1994.
70. Schachter L, Weingartern MA, Kahan EE: Attitudes of family physicians to nonconventional therapies: a challenge to science as the basis of therapeutics, *Arch Fam Med* 2(12):1268, 1993.
71. Shafranske EP, Malony HN: Clinical psychologists' religious and spiritual orientations and their practice of psychotherapy. *Psychotherapy* 27(1):72, 1990.
72. Shapiro AK, Shapiro E: Patient-provider relationships and the placebo effect. In Matarazzo JD et al, editors: *Behavioral health: a handbook of health enhancement and disease prevention,* New York, 1984, Wiley-Interscience.
73. Sheikh N, Philen RM, Love LA: Chaparral associated hepatotoxicity, *Arch Intern Med* 157:913, 1997.
74. Singer C: *Galen on Anatomical Procedures,* New York, 1956, Oxford University.
75. Smith R: What clinical information do doctors need? *Br Med J* 313:1062, 1996.
76. Sobell LC, Sobell MD, Nirneberg TD: Assessment and treatment planning with substance abusers, *Clin Psychol Rev* 8:19, 1988.
77. Spencer J: Maximization of biofeedback following cognitive stress preselection in generalized anxiety, *Percept Mot Skills* 63:239, 1986.

78. Spencer J: The use of human subjects in clinical research. In Primack A, Spencer J, editors: The collection and evaluation of clinical data relevant to alternative medicine and cancer. Conference report, 20–23, Bethesda, Md, June, 1996, National Institutes of Health.

79. Spencer J, Beckner W, Jacobs J: *Demographics of the first exploratory grant program in alternative medicine at the NIH*. Paper presented at 29th Proceedings of the United States Public Health Commissioned Officers Meetings, Baltimore, April, 1994.

80. Spencer J, Jonas W: And now...alternative medicine, *Arch Fam Med* March/April 6:155, 1997.

81. Spencer J, Thomas J: Psychiatric diagnostic profiles in hospitalized adolescent and adult Navajo Indians, *Soc Psychiatry Psychiatr Epidemiol* 27:226, 1992.

82. Starr P: *The social transformation of American medicine*, New York, 1982, Basic Books.

83. Steering Committee for Prince of Wales Initiative, Integrated Health Care: A way forward, *J Alternat Complement Med* 4(2):209, 1998.

84. Surwit D: Diabetes: mind over metabolism. In *Mind body medicine: how to use your mind for better health*, Yonkers, NY, 1993, Consumer Reports Books.

85. Turner J et al: The importance of placebo effects in pain treatment and research, *JAMA* 271(20):1609, 1994.

86. U.S. Congress, Office of Technology Assessment: Unconventional cancer treatments, Pub No OTA-H-405, Washington, DC, 1990, US Government Printing Office.

87. Veith I: *The Yellow Emperor's classic of internal medicine*, ed 2, Birmingham, Ala, 1988, Gryphon.

88. Verhoef MJ, Sutherland LR: General practitioners' assessment of and interest in alternative medicine in Canada, *Soc Sci Med* 41(4):511, 1995.

89. Vincent CA: Acupuncture as a treatment for chronic pain. In Lewith GT, Aldridge D, editors: *Clinical research methodology for complementary therapies*, London, 1993, Hodder and Stoughton.

90. Vincent C, Furnham A: *Complementary medicine: a research perspective*, Chichester, NY, 1997, John Wiley & Sons.

91. Voudouris NJ, Peck CL, Coleman G: The role of conditioning and verbal expectancy in the placebo response, *Pain* 43:121, 1990.

92. Wardwell WI: Alternative medicine in the United States, *Soc Sci Med* 38(8):1061, 1994.

93. White L, Tursky B, Schwarz GE: *Placebo theory research and mechanism*, New York, 1985, Guilford.

94. Wiegant FAC, Kramers CW, van Wijk R: The importance of patient selection. In Lewith GT, Aldridge D, editors: *Clinical research methodology for complementary therapies*, London, 1993, Hodder and Stoughton.

95. Woolf SH: Practice guidelines: a new reality in medicine. I. Recent developments, *Arch Intern Med* 150:1811, 1990.

96. Woolf SH et al: Clinical practice guidelines in complementary and alternative medicine: an analysis of opportunities and obstacles, *Arch Fam Med* 6:149-154, 1997.

97. World Health Organization: World Health Organization guidelines for sage acupuncture treatment. Geneva, 1995, World Health Organization.

SUGGESTED READINGS

Benson H: *The relaxation response,* New York, 1975, William Morrow.

Benson H: *Beyond the relaxation response,* New York, 1984, Berkley Books.

Berman B, Larson DB, editors: *Alternative medicine: expanding medical horizons,* Washington, DC, 1995, US Government Printing Office.

Castleman M: *The healing herbs,* Emmaus, Pa, 1991, Rodale.

Frawley D: *Ayurvedic healing,* Salt Lake City, 1990, Morson.

Fritz S: *Mosby's fundamentals of therapeutic massage,* St Louis, 1995, Mosby Lifeline.

Fromm E, Nash MR, editors: *Contemporary hypnosis research,* New York, 1992, Guilford.

Goldberg B: *Alternative medicine,* Puyallup, Wash, 1994, Future Medicine.

Hogarth M, Hutchinson D: *An Internet guide for the health professional,* Sacramento, Calif, 1996, New Wind.

Jonas W, Jacobs J: *Healing with homeopathy* New York 1996, Warner Books.

Mann F: *Textbook of acupuncture,* London, 1987, Heineman Medical.

Micozzi M: *Fundamentals of complementary and alternative medicine,* New York, 1996, Churchill Livingstone.

Moyers B: *Healing and the mind,* New York, 1993, Doubleday.

Murray M, Pizzorno J: *Textbook of natural medicine,* vols 1 and 2, Seattle, 1989, John Bastyr College.

Selye H: *Stress without distress,* New York, 1975, Signet.

Shapiro A, Shapiro E: *The powerful placebo: from ancient priest to modern physician,* Baltimore, 1997, Johns Hopkins University.

Upledger JE, Vredevoogd JD: *Craniosacral therapy,* Seattle, 1994, Eastland.

Ying ZZ, DeHui J: *Clinical manual of Chinese medicine and acupuncture,* New York, 1997, Churchill Livingstone.

CHAPTER 2

Preclinical Studies in Complementary/Alternative Medicine

Chung-Kwang Chou and Ru-Long Ren

Preclinical studies are important for complementary/alternative medicine (CAM) and may act as a bridge to the understanding of findings subsequently developed from clinical studies. First, CAM includes lifestyle practices, clinical tests, or therapeutic modalities that are generally promoted for the prevention, diagnosis, or treatment of diseases.[5,18] Therefore determination of their safety and effectiveness should be considered a priority. When their efficacy and safety are proven through detailed preclinical studies, including in vitro, in vivo, and clinical trials, CAM therapies can become a part of mainstream medicine, and as long as the efficacy and safety of such treatments remain unproved, those methods and agents should be abandoned to save money and avoid unnecessary harm to the public. For example, Laetrile (amygdalin) was thought to have anticancer effects. It achieved great popularity in the 1970s and was eventually legalized for use in 27 states. Public interest resulted in a National Cancer Institute–supported study that showed no effect for Laetrile against cancer.[37]

Second, some CAM treatments have already been used in clinics as effective methods, but due to lack of systemic preclinical studies, their optimal method may not be established and their maximum effects may not be achieved. For example, electrochemical treatment (ECT) for cancer has been used in China and Europe in thousands of patients. It has been shown that ECT is an effective, safe alternative therapy for some cancers.[31,41,59,60] However, ECT is not a well-established method. We believe that if an optimal method is established and the mechanisms of ECT cell death are understood through a number of preclinical studies, ECT will provide a more effective and understandable alternative therapy for some localized cancers.

This work was supported in part by the National Cancer Institute grant CA 33572 and the Army Breast Cancer Research Grant DAMD 17-96-1-6184.

The major objective of this chapter is to describe the development of certain preclinical studies in CAM. We define preclinical studies as basic research and clinical trials (Phases I to III). First, we give an overview of preclinical evaluations in conventional medicine; then we describe ECT and hyperthermia to illustrate the progression from basic research to clinical trials.

STEPS OF PRECLINICAL EVALUATIONS IN CONVENTIONAL MEDICINE

In most countries tests of drugs and medical devices are regulated by legislation and closely monitored by government agencies. In the United States federal consumer protection laws require that drugs and devices used for the prevention, diagnosis, or treatment of disease be demonstrated as both safe and effective before being marketed.[35] To meet these requirements, preclinical and clinical evaluations of a new treatment must undergo a number of steps in the evaluation of its potential effectiveness and safety. The regulatory agencies also require full disclosure of how products are manufactured and devices are designed, and how they function. In this section we describe the process of the discovery, development, and regulation of a new drug.*

The process of discovering and developing a drug involves substantial time, effort, and resources. Berkowitz and Katzung[3] and Grever and Chabner[20] have described the procedures. The first step in the development of a new drug is to discover or synthesize a potential new drug molecule. Most new drug candidates are identified through empiric, random screening of biologic activity of a large number of natural products as a result of rational chemical modification of a known molecule, or by designing a molecule based on an understanding of biologic mechanisms and chemical structure. A variety of biologic in vitro and in vivo assays (at the molecular, cell, organ, and whole animal levels) are used to define the activity and selectivity of the drug. Subsequently, through these studies more potent, less toxic derivatives often can be developed.

The second step in the development of a new drug is to conduct pharmacologic studies that include safety and toxicity tests. Candidate drugs that survive the initial screening and profiling procedures must be carefully evaluated for potential risks before beginning clinical testing. Preclinical toxicology is frequently the third step in the progression of a new drug from discovery to initial Phase I clinical trials in humans. The major kinds of preclinical toxicologic studies include (1) acute toxicity; (2) subacute and chronic toxicity; (3) effects on reproductive functions, including teratogenicity; (4) carcinogenicity; and (5) mutagenicity.[3,20,21,54] The major objectives of the preclinical toxicologic studies include the definition of the qualitative and quantitative organ toxicities, the reversibility of these effects, and the initial safe starting dose proposed for humans. Several quantitative estimates are desirable. These include the "no-effect" dose, which is the smallest dose that is observed to kill any

---

*References 1, 3, 9, 20, 32, 62.

animal, and the median lethal dose, which is the dose that kills approximately 50% of the animals.

It is important to recognize the limitations of preclinical testing. There is no guarantee that the human subject will accommodate a new drug in the same way as an animal species. Extrapolation of toxicity data from animals to humans is not completely reliable. For any given compound, the total toxicity data from all species have a very high predictive value for its toxicity in humans; however, there are limitations on the amount of information that is practical to obtain. In addition, since large numbers of animals are needed to obtain preclinical data, toxicity testing is time-consuming and expensive; for statistical reasons, rare adverse effects are unlikely to be detected, just as in clinical trials.

The fourth step in the development of a new drug is human evaluation—testing in humans begins after sufficient acute and subacute animal toxicity studies have been completed. Chronic safety testing in animals is usually conducted concurrent with clinical trials. Evaluation in humans includes three formal phases of clinical trials. Only after showing positive Phase III results on efficacy and safety can the new drug be permitted to be marketed for further postmarketing surveillance.[1,3,52]

The objective of *Phase I trials* is to determine a dose that is appropriate for use in Phase II trials. There are several different types of Phase I trials.[52] These trials are non-blind, or "open." A small number of healthy volunteers or patients with advanced disease resistant to standard therapy are included in such trials. However, it is important that the patients have normal organ functions because important pharmacokinetic parameters, such as absorption of drugs, the half-life of maximum tolerated dose, and metabolism, are often determined in this phase of trials. Many predictable toxicities are detected. The effects of the drug as a function of dosage are established in Phase I trials. It should be pointed out that because of the small sample size of Phase I trials, the pharmacokinetics parameters are generally determined imprecisely.

In *Phase II trials* the treatment is normally disease-type specific, and the aim is to identify the disease types suitable for treatment. The drug is studied for the first time in patients with the target disease to determine the efficacy of the drug. A broader range of toxicities may be detected in this phase. A small number of patients are studied in great detail. A single-blind design is often used.

Phase III is the controlled clinical trial in which the new treatment will be compared with a conventional therapy. Based on the information gathered in Phases I and II, this trial will further establish drug safety and efficacy in a much larger number of patients. Certain toxic effects, especially those caused by sensitization, may become apparent for the first time during this phase. Double-blind and crossover techniques are frequently employed. Phase III studies can be difficult to design and execute and are usually expensive, because of the large numbers of patients involved and the massive amount of data that must be collected and analyzed.

ELECTROCHEMICAL TREATMENT

Electrochemical treatment of cancer involves inserting platinum electrodes into tumors of conscious patients. A constant voltage of less than 10 V is applied to produce a 40- to 80-mA current between the anodes and cathodes for 30 minutes to several hours, delivering 100 coulombs (C) per cubic centimeter. As a result of electrolysis, electrophoresis, and electroosmosis, cells near the electrodes are killed by the microenvironmental changes. During the last 4 years we have been studying this method at the City of Hope National Medical Center in Duarte, California.

Nordenström[40-42] was the first in recent years to use direct current (DC) for the treatment of human tumors. He treated 26 lung metastases in 20 patients. Twelve of the 26 metastases regressed totally. Two patients with 5 of the 26 tumors were still alive 10 years later. In Japan, Nakayama[38] and Matsushima and colleagues[30] have treated human cancer with ECT combined with chemotherapy and radiation. Matsushima and co-workers[31] summarized 26 cases treated with ECT, including two cases of breast cancer (the majority of the 26 cases were inoperable because of poor general condition of the patient or an advanced cancer stage). There was improvement of symptoms (pain relief) in almost 50% of the patients. A decrease in tumor size to some degree was observed in 21 measurable lesions, two tumors disappeared completely, and no tumor cells remained in one case in which a histopathologic examination was performed. These results showed the usefulness of ECT alone to treat tumors, since the two tumors that completely disappeared had not responded to other, previous treatments. The main complication was pain during treatment; however, this complication spontaneously disappeared and did not require specific treatments.

In 1987, Nordenström introduced ECT to China. Because of the large patient load, authority of physicians, and minimal legal considerations in China, physicians were able to use ECT on thousands of patients with various kinds of cancers.[59] Xin[60] summarized the results of 2516 cases on 23 types of tumors. The primary cases were cancer of the lung (593 cases), the liver (388), the skin (366), and the breast (228). The 5-year survival rates were 31.7%, 17%, 67%, and 62.7%, respectively. In addition, ECT produces minimum trauma as compared with surgery. Also, unlike radiation therapy or chemotherapy, there are no serious side effects, and treatment can be repeated. Chinese physicians concluded that ECT is a simple, effective local therapy. The local control rates were considered satisfactory compared with those of conventional therapy. This method has been approved by the Chinese Ministry of Public Health and is used in approximately 1000 hospitals.[59]

Preclinical Issues

Although ECT is already prevalent in clinical practice in China and a number of clinical studies have shown that ECT has an antitumor effect, ECT has not been widely accepted in world clinics. The reason is that ECT is not a well-established method. The data lack essential preclinical studies, and reliable control of the clinical trials is missing. Review of literature pertaining to this topic shows that precise guidelines regarding electrode insertion and electrical parameters (i.e., voltage, current, treatment duration) are not available. Therefore ECT can be a feasible treatment for some cancer patients, but we are not certain that the method presently used has achieved its optimal effectiveness. More basic research to address preclinical issues is necessary before ECT can be used for patients in the United States. Compared with the steps of preclinical evaluation of conventional medicine, the following research priorities must be given to ECT preclinical evaluation.

Methodology Studies

To make ECT a reliable, effective method for treating cancers, a standardized treatment must be determined. At this time, published clinical studies have shown various electrode insertion methods and distributions; different electrode placements have been used in Europe and China. Optimal electrode distribution has not been determined.

Electrode Insertion. Nordenström[41] of Sweden introduced the biologically closed electric-circuit (BCEC) concept. He named it the third circuit in the human body, after cardiovascular and lymphatic circuits. The BCEC circulates through the vascular interstitial closed circuit (VICC). In Nordenström's view[43] ECT is an artificial activation of the BCEC through the VICC. The flow of ionic current triggers interactions between the induced electromagnetic fields and the cancer tissue. Therefore Nordenström has been treating his lung cancer patients with the anode inserted in the tumor center and cathode in normal tissue several centimeters away from the tumor boundary. European researchers and physicians have followed this method. In China Xin and colleagues[61] modified the technique, putting both anode and cathode into the tumor, with the anode in the center and cathodes in the periphery. Chinese physicians have found that placing both the anodes and cathodes in tumors not only protected the normal tissue but also had a greater effect on the tumor.

To resolve the discrepancies of whether both the anode and cathode should be inserted within the tumor or whether the cathode should be in normal tissue, a detailed animal study should be conducted to test whether induced cell damage occurs around the anode and cathode during ECT. We believe that the morphologic responses of the ECT-treated cells near the anode and cathode should be studied to understand their pathologic mechanism. By comparing the cellular changes in tumors with those of normal muscles after ECT, this preclinical study would determine whether the placement of the cathode in normal tissue can cause problems.

Electrode Configuration. Another important preclinical issue in the study of ECT is electrode configuration. The studies described earlier would answer the question of where the electrodes should be inserted and how many electrodes should be used. After several thousand patient treatments, Chinese physicians found that, for superficial tumors, if the electrodes were vertically inserted into the tumor, there were many cases of recurrence at the base of the tumor because the electric field generated at the tip is too small to destroy cells at the base of the tumor. However, by horizontally inserting an adequate number of electrodes at the tumor base, much better results were produced. We also observed this phenomenon in our animal studies.[14] Our preliminary mouse study,[14] using either two or five vertical electrodes or two horizontal electrodes going through the central part of the tumor, did not produce a high cure rate (Figs. 2-1 and 2-2). Later, in our rat study we adapted the tumor base method by inserting either six or seven electrodes at the tumor base perpendicular to the long axis of the tumor. Eighteen of 24 rats were cured for more than 6 months (Figs. 2-3 and 2-4). From the Chinese clinical experience and our animal results, we believe that inserting electrodes at the base of the tumor is the best method of ECT treatment of superficial tumors.

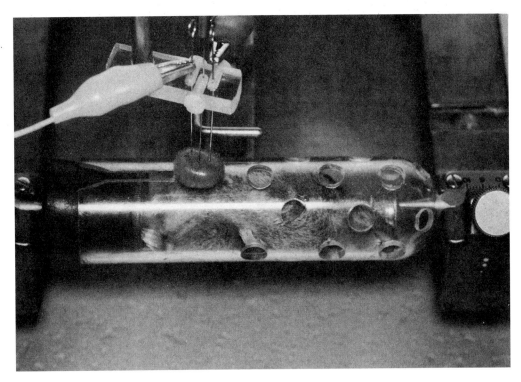

Fig. 2-1   Two platinum electrodes were vertically inserted into C3H/HeJ mice RIF-1 tumor at a spacing between 4 and 10 mm, depending on tumor size. A thermocouple for temperature measurement was in the central position.

Spacing. How many electrodes should be used? This depends on the tumor size and nature. Since the effective volume of the treatment is limited to the vicinity of the electrodes, it was thought that to cover the tumor region with an adequate number of electrodes is essential. In China it was reported that the effective volume around each electrode is about 3 cm in diameter; therefore spacing between electrodes is usually kept at less than 2 cm. However, it is not known for what type of tumor this range is effective. Japanese practitioners have used 3- to 4-cm spacing, while in Slovenia, the cathode (not the anode) was inserted in the skin tumor and a plate electrode was pasted on the skin at 3 to 4 cm from the edge of the melanoma skin lesion.[47] Since each cancer tumor has its own tissue conductivity, the effective volume differs for each different tumor; therefore the tissue conductivity must be determined. Rat tumor morphologic changes after ECT can be used to study the effect of spacing.

Preclinical Safety and Toxicity Test

Although ECT is already clinically prevalent in China and Chinese physicians have concluded that ECT is a simple, effective local therapy, the dosage guidelines have not been determined. To conduct preclinical safety and toxicity tests, priority studies should focus on dosage guidelines. Excessive dosage will cause pain, burns, and slow

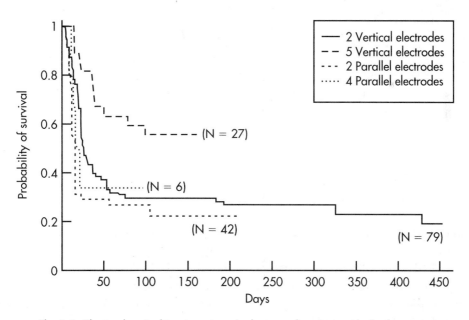

Fig. 2-2 Electrochemical treatment survival curves showing results for four groups of C3H/HeJ mice. The best results were with four electrodes inserted parallel to the body. (Modified from Chou CK et al: *Bioelectromagnetics* 18:14, 1997.)

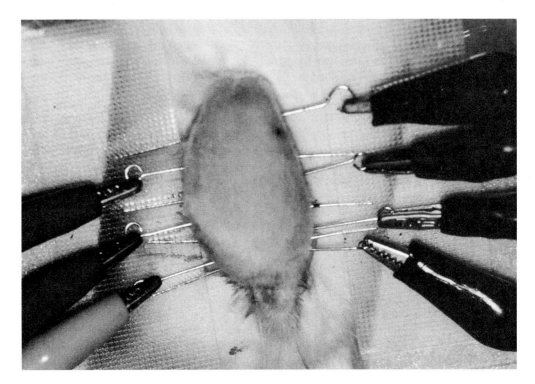

Fig. 2-3   Electrodes were inserted at the base of the Fisher 344 rat fibrosarcoma. Insertion was perpendicular to the long axis of the tumor, and an arrangement of alternating cathodes and anodes was used.

healing. Inadequate dosage will result in ineffective treatment, which is life threatening for cancer patients. Therefore proper dosage is essential for ECT. Electrical dosage in tumors varies with many factors, such as tissue conductivity and electrode configuration. Each of these factors should be examined in detail.

Dosage. Nordenström[41] stated that "because few indications existed to guide an optimal choice of voltage and amount of electric energy to be given, an arbitrary amount of current of 100 coulombs per centimeter of tumor diameter (at 10 V potential) was chosen to be the preliminary dose." Xin[60] treated his patients with 40 to 80 mA current, 8 to 10 V, at 100 C/cm^3. The 100 C/cm^3 value is more appropriate than the per-centimeter-diameter value, since the dose should be related to the volume, not the diameter, of the tumor. Although 100 C has been used widely, the dosage guidelines used by Nordenström and Xin are arbitrary and there is no scientific basis for these values.

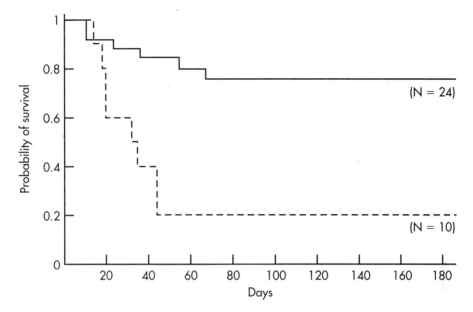

Fig. 2-4 Survival probability curves of the two groups of Fisher 344 rats that received electrochemical treatment. Ten rats were treated with two arrays of electrodes, and 24 rats were treated with multiple electrodes at the tumor base. The difference in survival was significant (log-rank test; $p = 0.001$). (Modified from Chou CK et al: *Bioelectromagnetics* 18:14, 1997.)

Electrical dose (coulombs) is a product of current (A) and time (sec). Higher current reduces treatment time but also causes pain. Lower current prolongs the treatment. Therefore a compromise with acceptable current density over a reasonable time is desirable. However, notable is the arbitrary definition of dose in coulombs per cubic centimeter. From the data published in China, apparently the charge is obtained by multiplying the DC passed between two electrodes by the time the current is applied, and dividing by the volume of the tumor. Clearly, the charge density is not uniform throughout the treated tumors. The charge density (i.e., dose distribution) is not appreciated. Many factors may affect the dose distribution. The charge density could be the source of the varying results when needles are implanted parallel or perpendicular to the body surface, or when changes in the numbers of needles and needle spacing are made. It would be advantageous to design dose experiments where one would be dealing with uniform charge density distribution rather than the highly nonuniform distributions obtained with needle electrodes. The lack of dosage guidelines has become a bottleneck in ECT development.

Safety and Toxicity. Electrochemical treatment must be carefully evaluated for potential risks before clinical use. Unlike chemical agents, ECT is a local therapy and no foreign agent is injected into the body. We can ignore some toxicity tests, such as effects on reproductive functions, including teratogenicity, carcinogenicity, and mutagenesis.

Based on published clinical data, ECT is used mainly in the treatment of patients who are not candidates for conventional therapy because of age or overall medical condition, or both. Compared with surgery, ECT is less traumatic; therefore recovery is quicker. There are no serious side effects from ECT as compared with radiation therapy or chemotherapy. However, since ECT destroys both normal and tumor tissue, there is a potential risk, depending on patient sensitivity, for certain parameters (e.g., voltage, current) to influence either quality or quantity of treatment. To bridge the gap between the animal studies and clinical evaluation, Phase I clinical trial is necessary. The following risks should be documented in preclinical tests:

- Local pain is the main acute complication during electrode insertion and ECT procedure.
- Tumor necrosis and ulceration are usually observed when superficial lesions are treated with ECT. The absorption of necrosis tissues may cause fever and leukocytosis after ECT.
- If the skin is not well insulated, it can be burned by the chemical reaction. The healing time depends on the size and location of the lesion. Platinum electrode bases should be insulated to prevent skin injury at the entrance site.
- During electrode insertion, blood vessels and nerves may be punctured. Therefore bleeding and pain may be observed during electrode insertion.

Mechanism Studies

Besides methodology and dosage studies, more basic research, such as study of mechanisms, is necessary before ECT can be accepted for the treatment of patients in the United States. Mechanisms of ECT antitumor effects remain uncertain. Very probable and often mentioned mechanisms are biochemical reactions in the vicinity of the electrodes and direct electric-current effects on tumor cells. Among the biochemical reactions are changes in the pH and ion compositions of the extracellular matrix, both of which exert an influence on cell growth and survival.[33,34,57]

It has been known that ECT involves electrolysis, electrophoresis, and electroosmosis. Electrolysis results in the decomposition of electrolytes and pH alteration. During electroosmosis, water moves from the anode to the cathode, a process that dehydrates cells near the anode and hydrates cells near the cathode. Water volume change within the cell disturbs the cell structure and its function. In addition to the changes in pH and water volume, Cl_2, which is formed at the anode as a result of Cl^- electron loss, may play a role in cell growth inhibition by its oxidizing effect. In addition, the platinum ions, possibly formed by electrolysis of the platinum electrodes, may play a role in ECT killing effects. Although ECT-induced cell death may involve complicated processes, the pH alteration and ion movement are the most obvious and important factors in ECT.[28] Therefore in basic research we should first focus on pH and ion alteration in tumor cell killing.

In ECT preclinical mechanism studies, morphologic studies help to better understand the mechanisms. Both light and electron microscopy were used to study the morphologic changes in human KB cells treated with DC. Figs. 2-5 and 2-6 show scanning electron microscopic pictures of control and treated (0.05 C/ml) human KB cancer cells. Control cells are in a polygonal shape. Microvilli are abundant on cell surfaces. After ECT cells shrink, the number of microvilli decrease, and there are holes on cell surfaces. Transmission electron microscopy shows a normal tumor cell with rich mitochondria and polysomes in cytoplasm. After 0.2 C/ml ECT, there are decreased microvilli, mild mitochondria swelling, polysome disaggregation, lysosome distention, and nuclear chromatism aggregated focally in cells. At a higher level (0.4 C/ml), plasma membrane bursts and the distended organelles escape. Microscopic studies reveal morphologic changes at ECT levels corresponding to inhibition of cell proliferation.

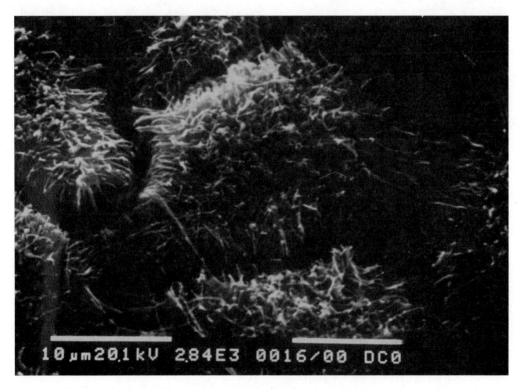

Fig. 2-5 Scanning electron micrograph showing normal human oropharyngeal carcinoma (KB) cells. Microvilli are abundant on cell surfaces.

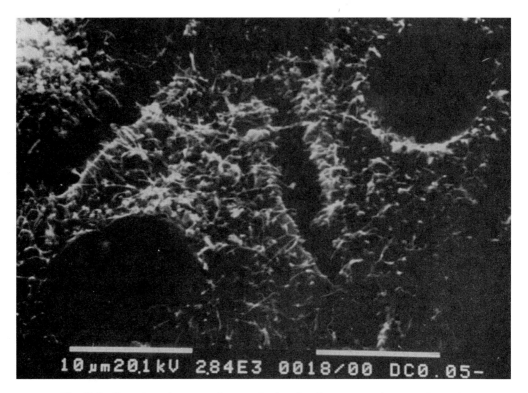

Fig. 2-6 Scanning electron micrograph showing human oropharyngeal carcinoma (KB) cells treated with 0.05 coulombs/ml electromechanical treatment (ECT). After ECT, cells shrink, microvilli collapse, and there are holes on cell membrane.

Clinical Trials

Although ECT has been used in some countries as an alternative method for cancer treatment, it is necessary to conduct clinical trials in the United States to verify its value. According to a U.S. Food and Drug Administration (FDA) investigational device exemption regulation, ECT was considered a significant-risk device. Therefore we submitted a clinical protocol to both the Institutional Review Board at the City of Hope and the FDA for Phase I clinical trial approval. A quality assurance of the equipment must be submitted to ensure the safety of its operation. The Phase I study asked for 25 recurrent, superficial, measurable malignant tumors for treatment. The purpose of these clinical trials is to evaluate the tumor response of ECT and record the acute and late toxicities of ECT in the treatment of superficial tumors.

We have treated five patients at the City of Hope as of March 1998. The first patient had a diagnosis of $T_4N_0M_0$ carcinoma of the larynx. His treatment was laryngectomy and a full course of radiation therapy. ECT was used for multiple painful, subcutaneous metastases. He developed complete response in treated sites and tolerated ECT well. The second patient had lung cancer with subcutaneous multiple scalp and distant metastases. ECT was given to a scalp nodule to relieve pain. The patient had complete response with excellent pain relief that lasted for 3 months; then there was tumor regrowth at the tumor margin. The third patient had a diagnosis of large, metastasized osteosarcoma of the left forearm. ECT achieved less than 50% response attributable to incomplete treatment. There was no complication from ECT. The fourth patient had a large, ulcerated T_4 breast cancer. Despite multiple-course chemotherapy, the patient developed multiple, extensive, painful, ulcerated local recurrences on the left-side chest wall. ECT was used to treat one of the nodules (6 cm) on the left upper arm. She developed an ulcer at the site of the tumor where the tumor was destroyed as a result of ECT. The fifth patient developed a painful left axial node metastasis (6 × 7 cm). She was given two courses of ECT. She had partial response and had excellent pain relief. From these five preliminary patient results it appears that ECT is effective, safe, and well tolerated. After the Phase I study is completed, we will conduct Phase II and III clinical trials.

HYPERTHERMIA

Numerous reports have shown a synergistic effect of heat and radiotherapy or of heat and chemotherapy.[11] The effective temperature range of hyperthermia treatments is very small: 41° C to 45° C. At lower temperatures the effect is minimal. At temperatures higher than 45° C, normal cells are damaged. During hyperthermic treatment, temperatures in tumors are usually higher than those in normal surrounding tissue because of the difference in blood flow. In addition, it is generally believed that tumors are more sensitive to heat. This is explained by the hypoxic, acidic, and poor nutritional state of tumor cells.[27] The synergism of radiation and hyperthermia is accomplished by thermal killing of hypoxic and S-phase (DNA syntheses) cells that are resistive to radiation. Hyperthermia has been used in combination with chemotherapy because heating increases membrane permeability and the potency of some drugs.

Historical Perspectives

The interest in the use of heat in cancer treatment can probably be attributed to a clinical observation in 1866 made by M. Busch, a German physician. He described a patient with a neck sarcoma, which disappeared after the patient had a high fever associated with erysipelas. Similar reports were made by others some 20 years later. These findings led to studies using bacterial toxins extracted from the bacteria-causing erysipelas. In 1893, W. C. Coley, a surgeon in New York, administered to cancer patients bacterial toxins extracted from *Streptococcus* and *Serratia marcescens*. In 1898, F. Westermark, a Swedish gynecologist, used a coil containing hot water as a controlled, localized source of heat in the treatment of uterine tumors. Such early studies and observations were followed by many reports of tumors responding to both whole-body and localized hyperthermic treatments that were induced by a variety of techniques.

Among the heating methods, electromagnetic (EM) heating earned an important role. After the German physicist Heinrich Hertz demonstrated the physical nature of EM waves and described their characteristic features, EM heating became a very popular but controversial treatment method for various diseases. As technology developed, higher-frequency EM fields were used. Shortwave diathermy became the standard approach with frequencies of up to 100 MHz by 1920 and from 100 up to 3000 MHz by 1930. Meanwhile, many of the early reports describing the use of various forms of diathermy claimed frequency-specific effects for the EM energy involved; it was Mittleman and colleagues[36] who, recognizing the need for careful dosimetry, measured the temperatures and related them to absorbed energy.

Although details of many experimental studies were published during the first half of the twentieth century, the biologic evidence was insufficient and interest in the clinical use of hyperthermia declined, principally because of lack of sufficient preclinical studies. In the 1960s, Cavaliere and colleagues[6] carried out a series of biochemical studies into the effects of elevated temperature on normal and malignant rodent cells. They observed that heat caused a greater inhibition of respiration in tumor tissues than in normal tissues and concluded that neoplastic cells were more sensitive to heat than their normal counterparts. These preclinical studies did provide a stimulus to further research in the field. In the past 30 years there has been a systematic investigation of the possible anticancer effects of hyperthermia with a variety of experimental studies being reported and critical analyses of a vast collection of clinical reports. The results confirm that temperature elevations of only a few degrees have profound effects on cells and tissues and that hyperthermia undoubtedly has an antitumor effect. Numerous biologic studies, mostly involving temperatures in the range of 41° C to 46° C, have demonstrated a clear rationale for expecting hyperthermia to have a greater effect on tumors than on normal tissue. In addition, there has been significant progress in the application of heating systems and noninvasive thermometry techniques for clinical hyperthermia. The development and potential usefulness of hyperthermia as a technique to treat cancer has been demonstrated.[17,45,50,55] In the United States the FDA has approved five hyperthermia systems (BSD 1000, Cheung Laboratory HT 100A, Cook VH 8500, Clini-Therm Mark I and IV, and Labthermic Sonotherm 1000), which meet the FDA premarket evaluation standard for clinical use.

Preclinical Issues

In vitro, in vivo, and clinical studies have shown that hyperthermia, in conjunction with radiation therapy and chemotherapy, is effective for treating cancer.[53] A summary of 25 nonrandomized studies from 1980 to 1988, including one study involving 1556 superficial tumors treated with radiotherapy and those treated with radiation therapy plus hyperthermia, shows that the average complete response rates for tumors were 34% and 64%, respectively. Clearly, hyperthermia is beneficial. However, a multiinstitution randomized Phase III study[46] conducted in the United States did not clearly show that hyperthermia in combination with radiation therapy can improve tumor response when compared with radiation therapy alone. Inadequate heat delivery is considered to be the reason for failure. Some reports have shown that the effective temperature range of hyperthermia treatment is very small: 41° C to 45° C; at lower temperatures the effect is minimal. At temperatures higher than 45° C, normal cells are damaged.[15,48] The clinical use of hyperthermia has been hampered by a lack of adequate equipment to effectively deliver heat to deep-seated and even large superficial lesions and by a lack of thermometry techniques that provide reliable information on heat distribution in the target tissues. Therefore, besides the biologic considerations, the hyperthermia preclinical studies should mainly solve the problems of how to generate heat and how to control elevated temperatures in tumors. In this section the main methods of hyperthermia treatment are reviewed and the steps necessary to evaluate the amount of heat delivered for each method are briefly discussed. In addition, we use our intracavitary applicator development as an example to discuss how much preclinical work should be performed before an applicator can be used in a clinic.

Methods

The first step in preclinical studies is to develop an effective heating method. In the past two decades several techniques have been developed for heat induction. Heating methods include whole-body heating by hot wax, hot air, a hot-water suit, or infrared irradiation, and partial-body heating by either radio-frequency (RF) EM fields (including microwaves), ultrasound, heated blood, or fluid perfusion.[11]

Whole-Body Heating. For disseminated disease, whole-body hyperthermia (WBH) in conjunction with chemotherapy and radiation therapy has been studied by many groups.[2,4,51] Methods of WBH include hot wax, hot water, water blanket, water suit, extracorporeal heated blood, and radiant heat. The high morbidity and labor-intensive methods associated with WBH have caused concerns. Except for the extracorporeal blood-heating technique, which requires extensive surgical procedures, all other methods depend on conduction of heat from the body surface to the core. The preclinical studies have indicated that the core temperature should be kept below 41.8° C; above that temperature the brain and liver can be damaged.[19]

Local Heating. Local hyperthermia is produced by coupling energy to tissue through three commonly accepted modalities: RF coupling at frequencies ranging from 100 kHz to 100 MHz, microwave coupling at higher frequencies (300 to 2450 MHz), and mechanical coupling by means of ultrasound (1 to 3 MHz).

External techniques. Two RF methods have been used to provide subcutaneous heating. In the first method the tissues were placed between two capacitor plates and heated by displacement currents. This method is simple, but overheating of the fat, which is caused by the perpendicular electrical field, remains a major problem for obese patients. A water bolus is necessary to minimize fat heating.

The second RF method is inductive heating by magnetic fields that are generated by solenoidal loops or "pancake" magnetic coils to induce eddy currents in tissue. Because the induced electrical fields are parallel to the tissue interface, heating is maximized in muscle rather than in fat. However, the heating pattern is generally toroidal with a null at the center of the coil.

In the microwave frequency range energy is coupled into tissues by waveguides, dipoles, microstrips, or other radiating devices. The shorter wavelengths of microwaves, as compared with longer wavelengths of RF, provide the capability to direct and focus energy into tissues by direct radiation from a small applicator. Engineering developments have focused on the design of new microwave applicators. A number of applicators of various sizes operate over a frequency range of 300 to 1000 MHz.[23,26,39] Most of them are dielectrically loaded and have a water bolus for surface cooling.

Intracavitary techniques. Certain tumor sites in hollow cavities may be treated by intracavitary techniques. The advantages of intracavitary hyperthermia include (1) better energy deposition because of the proximity of an applicator to a tumor and (2) the reduction of normal tissue exposure as compared with externally induced hyperthermia. There have been clinical and research studies on hyperthermia in combination with either radiation therapy or chemotherapy in cancers of the esophagus, rectum, cervix, prostate, and bladder.

Microwaves and lower-frequency RF energy (13.65 to 2450 MHz) have been used for intracavitary hyperthermia. The main problem is that tumor temperature values are unknown. Most temperatures were measured on the surface of the applicators, which can be very different from those in the tumor. Furthermore, thermocouples or thermistors have been used to measure temperatures by many investigators who did not know the perturbation problem caused by the metallic sensors.[7] One solution to this problem is to measure tissue temperature in animals and then extrapolate the results to humans.[13]

Interstitial techniques

RESISTIVE HEATING. Tissues can be heated by alternating RF currents conducted through needle electrodes. The operating frequency should be higher than 100 kHz to prevent excitation of nerve action potentials. Interstitial techniques for radiation implants, as primary or boost treatments, have been practiced successfully by radiation oncologists for many years. Other advantages of this technique include better control of temperature distributions within the tumor as compared with those of externally induced hyperthermia, and sparing of normal tissue, especially the overlying skin.[58]

MICROWAVE TECHNIQUE. Small microwave antennas inserted into hollow plastic tubing can produce satisfactory heating patterns at frequencies between 300 and 2450 MHz.[22] A frequency commonly used in the United States is 915 MHz. A small coaxial antenna can irradiate a volume of approximately 60 cm^3. With a multinode coaxial antenna the extent of the heating pattern can be extended to approximately 10 cm in a three-node antenna.[25] For large tumors a single microwave antenna cannot heat the entire tumor to a therapeutic temperature. It is necessary to use an array of microwave antennas. Because the antennas couple to each other, the spacing, phasing, and insertion depth affect the heating patterns of array applicators.[8,63]

FERROMAGNETIC SEED IMPLANTS. The technique of ferromagnetic seed implants is applicable for delivering thermal energy to deep-seated tumors. When exposed to RF magnetic fields (~100 kHz), the implants absorb energy and become heated. At the Curie point the implants become nonferromagnetic and no longer produce heat. The surrounding tissue is then heated by thermal conduction. The influence of blood flow and tissue inhomogeneities of the tumor, which may affect the temperature distribution, can be compensated for by the self-regulation of the implants; thus it is possible to maintain a temperature close to that of the Curie point.[29] Another method that exposes magnetic fluid in a tumor to an RF magnetic field (0.3 to 80 MHz) has shown to be feasible for inducing selective heating.[24]

Applicator Development

The temperature elevation in tumors and tissues is determined by the energy deposited and the physiologic responses of the patient, as well as by blood flow and thermal conduction in the tissues. When EM methods are used, many factors affect the energy deposition, such as frequency, intensity, and polarization of the applied fields, as well as the geometry and size of the applicator.[10] Along with these factors, which affect heat delivering and coupling, the importance of designing an ideal applicator cannot be overemphasized. However, it is impossible to develop effective heat delivering and coupling applicators without sufficient preclinical tests. The following example describes the steps we employed before the applicator was used in patients.

Design of the Esophageal Applicator. The closed-end applicator, which was 76 cm long, consisted of a 6-mm-diameter polyurethane tube with a 2.67-mm, Teflon-lined center channel for an antenna and six 1.23-mm-diameter, Teflon-lined peripheral channels for nonperturbing temperature sensors or intraluminal radiation seeds. The microwave antenna was a 90-cm monopole made from flexible QMI-6000 cable (2.1-mm outer diameter [OD]) with a length of 10 cm from the tip to the center of a 1-mm gap. The center conductor was connected to the outer conductor at the tip, not at the gap, to give better heating results. The antenna can accommodate up to 130 W at 1 gigahertz (GHz).

Heating Pattern Evaluations. Once an applicator was designed, heating patterns in human simulated (phantom) tissues had to be determined. A 28 × 28 × 8.5 cm Plexiglas box was filled with muscle phantom material[12] and covered with polyester silk screen. The surface temperature of the phantom interface was recorded by a thermographic camera. To simulate a clinical application, the applicator was placed on a thin plastic sheet on the phantom with the tip of the antenna at a depth of 13 to 18 cm. The applicator was then covered with a large mass of phantom muscle. After 30 to 45 seconds of 50-W, 915-MHz microwave exposure, the phantom was separated and a second thermogram obtained with the applicator removed. The thermograms before and after exposure were recorded. Fig. 2-7 shows thermograms of a 10-cm monopole. The point of maximum heating rate is 5 cm anterior to the junction. The heating length (>50% heating rate) is longer than 15 cm; the voltage standing-wave ratio is 3.5.

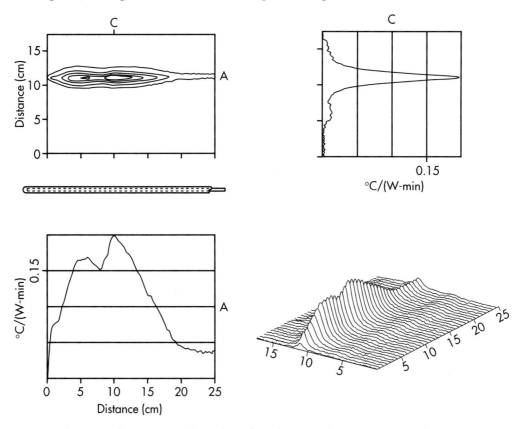

Fig. 2-7   Thermograms of esophageal applicator with antenna No. 5 showing quantitative heating patterns. (Modified from Chou CK et al. In Blank M, editor: *Electricity and magnetism in biology and medicine,* San Francisco, 1993, San Francisco Press.)

Animal Study

After the heating tests in phantoms, we conducted heating tests on animals.[13] Yucatan and domestic pigs were used. The chest region was exposed and Teflon tubes for inserting Luxtron fiberoptic probers were attached to the esophageal muscle at various locations relative to the microwave antenna junction; five sensors were near the aorta side and five were on the opposite side. A Teflon tube was attached longitudinally along the outer surface of the esophagus for temperature mapping. Temperatures inside the applicator and the helical tubing were also mapped. Forty watts of 915-MHz power was applied. When a steady state was reached, temperatures were recorded. The esophagus was removed during autopsy to determine any obvious tissue effects. Histologic study was performed with light and electron microscopy.

Fig. 2-8 shows the temperature of pig No. 5, which received treatment with 40 W of forward power (11 W reflect). Curve 1 shows temperatures in the esophageal wall near the aorta; curve 6 shows temperatures in the esophageal wall on the opposite side.

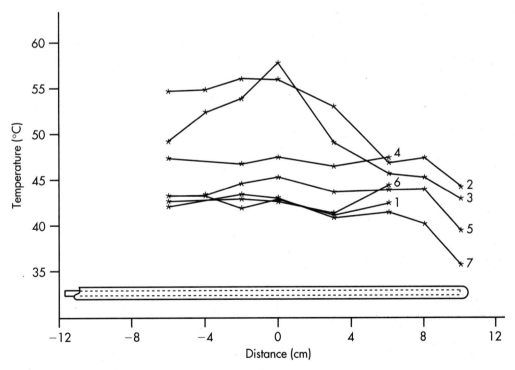

Fig. 2-8   Temperature data of pig No. 5 with esophageal applicator. Power, 40 W forward and 11 W reflected. (Modified from Chou CK et al. In Blank M, editor: *Electricity and magnetism in biology and medicine,* San Francisco, 1993, San Francisco Press.)

The aorta side was in general similar to the other side. Curves 2 and 3 show the temperatures in the peripheral lumens inside the applicator; data of curve 4 were measured in the helical tube on the surface of the applicator. Curve 5 data were measured by a bare Luxtron 2000 sensor in the esophagus outside the applicator that measured the inner surface temperatures of the esophagus. Between 5.5 cm and 8.0 cm from the applicator, these temperatures ranged from 43.3° C to 45.3° C. Curve 7 shows the temperatures outside the esophageal wall. The maximum temperature inside the esophageal muscle, which was measured 6 cm distal to the gap, was 44.4° C; this result was consistent with the thermogram. The temperatures in the peripheral lumens proximal to the gap were higher than the distal temperatures; this is because of antenna self-heating attributable to current loss and is different from the RF heating. Postmortem examination of the esophagus showed edema 5 to 6 cm distal to the antenna gap. This was consistent with the animal temperature measurement and the thermograms.

Light microscopy showed vacuolization and swollen oval cellular nuclei in the heated area. Collagen in the lamina propria from the heated area seemed to be stretched, and the collagen bundles were parallel to the epithelial surface. Nuclei of fibroblasts in the collagen fabric were elongated along its fibers in the heated region of the esophagus; organization of this collagen was less complicated than in the control. Electron microscopy of epithelial cells in the heated area showed the presence of numerous vacuoles in its cytoplasm and cell boundaries.

Clinical Trials

Through comprehensive basic studies, we found that the designed applicator could provide good heat distribution and penetration for esophageal intracavitary hyperthermia. These results provided sufficient data to design protocols from which to evaluate the efficacy and safety of a clinical trial.

To evaluate the efficacy and tolerance of intracavitary hyperthermia combined with external radiation therapy and low-dose brachytherapy in the management of esophageal cancer, 25 patients with primary esophageal cancer received treatment following a clinical trial protocol.[49] Hyperthermia was applied with the previously described applicators. Temperature measurements were obtained while moving fiberoptic temperature sensors at 1.0-cm intervals in each of the applicator's six peripheral channels (Fig. 2-9). The 1- and 2-year overall survival rates were 72% (18/25) and 32% (8/25), respectively, and the disease-free survival rates were 47% and 30%, respectively. The toxicity was mild. The acute toxic effect was pain in swallowing. The major late complication was mild esophageal fibrosis and difficulty in swallowing. No serious side effects such as fistulas or perforations were seen. These results indicate that this method is safe and feasible for treating esophageal carcinoma. It encourages us to further continue the Phases II and III studies.

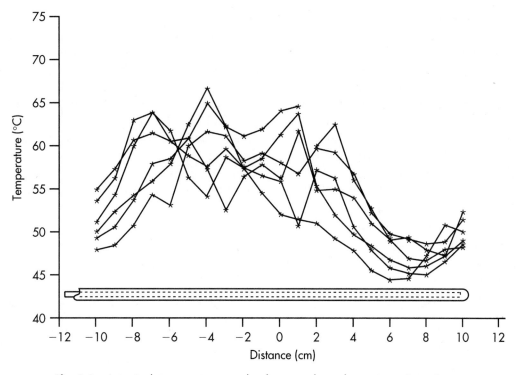

Fig. 2-9   A typical temperature graph of an esophageal cancer patient given treatment with intracavitary hyperthermia. Temperatures were obtained by moving fiberoptic temperature sensors at 1.0-mm intervals in the six peripheral channels of the applicator. Power, 42/8.5 W. (Modified from Ren RL et al: *Int J Hyperthermia* 14:245, 1998.)

Current Status and the Future

Although several thousand cancer patients have received treatment with hyperthermia, it has not become part of the routine cancer treatment modalities. In most centers the use of hyperthermia is still part of a developing project. However, through centuries of practice, it is becoming more clear that (1) hyperthermia has a significant potential as an adjuvant therapy and (2) to obtain good clinical results, we need not only better and more flexible heating systems, but also the ability to better plan and implement the individual patient treatments. The clinical use of heat has been hampered due to lack of adequate equipment to effectively deliver heat in deep-seated and even large superficial lesions and a lack of thermometry techniques that provide reliable information on heat distribution in the target tissue.

Despite the slow pace of investigation into thermal effects in U.S. clinics, several important studies are ongoing and strong interest persists in Europe and Asia. Recently, positive clinical results have emerged from well-controlled Phase III randomized trials (including melanomas, head and neck tumors, and breast tumors) in which good quality assurance has been implemented.[16,44,55] According to the literature, there is no doubt that hyperthermia would provide a significant, worthwhile improvement in cancer control if we continue our preclinical scientific studies in a more careful manner. We believe that future preclinical studies should pay more attention to the following areas of research: (1) better biologic knowledge with regard to effects of thermal cytotoxicity in normal and tumor tissue, sequencing of modalities, impact of thermotolerance, and so forth and (2) better physics and engineering support with regard to homogeneity of the power deposition, improved methods of treatment planning, and better ratio of power deposition to tumor volume, noninvasive thermometry control, and the like.

SUMMARY

As long as conventional medicine has its limitations, people will continue to seek help from CAM. Usually the origins of CAM are not scientific but are traditionally or culturally based. If a CAM therapy has initial proof that it is useful, scientists should conduct systematic preclinical studies to understand its mechanisms and variables for controlling its effectiveness. The discussion of conventional medicine, ECT, and hyperthermia treatment in this chapter provides readers with insights concerning scientific details and endeavors necessary to subsequently practicing these treatment methods in hospitals and clinics. Pyrites cannot stand the fire test, but gold can: preclinical study is the fire test of CAM.

REFERENCES

1. American Medical Association: Prescription practices and regulatory agencies. In American Medical Association, editor: *Drug evaluations annual,* Chicago, 1992, The Association.
2. Anhalt D et al: The CDRH helix: an *in vivo* evaluation, *Int J Hyperthermia* 6:241, 1990.
3. Berkowitz BA, Katzung BG: Basic and clinical evaluation of new drugs. In Katzung BG, editors: *Basic and clinical pharmacology,* Norwich, Conn, 1995, Appleton & Lange.
4. Bull JMC et al.: Chemotherapy resistant sarcoma treated with whole body hyperthermia (WBH) combined with 1-3-Bis (2-chloroethyl)-1-nitrosourea (BUCN), *Int J Hyperthermia* 8:297, 1992.
5. Cassileth BR, Chapman CC: Alternative cancer medicine: a ten-year update, *Cancer Invest* 14:396, 1996.
6. Cavaliere R et al: Selective heat sensitivity of cancer cells, *Cancer* 20:1351, 1967.
7. Cetas TC: Temperature. In Lehmann JF, editor: *Therapeutic heat and cold,* Baltimore, 1990, Williams & Wilkins.
8. Chan KW et al.: Changes in heating patterns of interstitial microwave antenna arrays at different insertion depths, *Int J Hyperthermia* 5:499, 1989.

9. Chappell WR, Mordenti J: Extrapolation of toxicological and pharmacological data from animals to humans, *Adv Drug Res* 20:1, 1991.
10. Chou CK: Evaluation of microwave hyperthermia applicators, *Bioelectromag*netics 13:581, 1992.
11. Chou CK: Electromagnetic heating for cancer treatment. In Blank M, editor: *Electromagnetic fields: biological interactions and mechanisms,* Washington, DC, 1995, American Chemical Society.
12. Chou CK, et al: Formulas for preparing phantom muscle tissue at various radio frequencies, *Bioelectromagnetics,* 5:435, 1984.
13. Chou CK et al.: Intracavitary hyperthermia and radiation of esophageal cancer. In Blank M, editor: *Electricity and magnetism in biology and medicine,* San Francisco, 1993, San Francisco Press.
14. Chou CK et al.: Electrochemical treatment of mouse and rat fibrosarcomas with direct current, *Bioelectromagnetics* 18:14, 1997.
15. Dahl O, Mella O: Hyperthermia and chemotherapeutic agents. In Field SB, Hand JW, editors: *An introduction to the practical aspects of clinical hyperthermia,* London, 1990, Taylor & Francis.
16. Datta NR et al.: Head and neck cancers: results of thermoradiotherapy versus radiotherapy, *Int J Hyperthermia* 6:479, 1990.
17. Dunlop PRC, Howard GCW: Has hyperthermia a place in cancer treatment? *Clin Radiol* 40:76, 1989.
18. Eisenberg DM et al: Unconventional medicine in the United States: prevalence, cost, and patterns of use, *N Engl J Med* 328:246, 1993.
19. Engelhardt R: Hyperthermia and drugs, *Recent Results Cancer Res* 104:136, 1987.
20. Grever MR, Chabner BA: Cancer drug discovery and development. In DeVita VT, Jr, Hellman S, Rosenberg SA, editors: *Cancer: principles and practice of oncology,* ed 5, Philadelphia, 1997, Lippincott-Raven.
21. Grever MR, Schepartz S, Chabner BA: The National Cancer Institute: cancer drug discovery and development program, *Semin Oncol* 19:622, 1992.
22. Iskander MF, Tumeh AM: Design optimization of interstitial antennas, *IEEE Trans Biomed Eng* 36:238, 1989.
23. Johnson RH, Preece AW, Green JL: Theoretical and experimental comparison of three types of electromagnetic hyperthermia applicator. *Phys Med Biol* 35:761, 1990.
24. Jordan A et al: Inductive heating of ferromagnetic particles and magnetic fluids: physical evaluation of their potential for hyperthermia, *Int J Hyperthermia* 9:51,1993.
25. Lee DJ et al: A new design of microwave interstitial applicators for hyperthermia with improved treatment volume, *Int J Radiat Oncol Biol Phys* 12:2003, 1986.
26. Lee ER et al.: Body-conformable, 915-MHz microstrip array applicators for large surface area hyperthermia, *IEEE Trans Biomed Eng* 39:470, 1992.
27. Lepock JR, Kruuv J: Mechanisms of thermal cytotoxicity. In Gerner EW, Cetas TC, editors: *Hyperthermic Oncology,* vol 2, Tucson, Ariz, 1992, Arizona Board of Regents, p. 9
28. Li KH et al: Effects of direct current on dog liver: possible mechanisms for tumor electrochemical treatment, *Bioelectromagnetics* 18:2, 1997.
29. Mack CF et al: Interstitial thermoradiotherapy with ferromagnetic implants for locally advanced and recurrent neoplasms, *Int J Radiat Oncol Biol Phys* 27:109, 1993.
30. Matsushima Y, Amemiya R, Liu JS: Direct current therapy with chemotherapy for the local control of lung cancer, *Nippon Gan Chiryo Gakki Sh* 24:2341, 1989.
31. Matsushima Y et al: Clinical and experimental studies of anti-tumoral effects of electrochemical therapy (ECT) alone or in combination with chemotherapy, *Eur J Surg Suppl* 574:59, 1994.
32. Mattison N, Trimble AG, Lasagna L: New drug development in the United States: 1963 through 1984, *Clin Pharmacol* 43:290, 1988.
33. Miklavcic D, Sersa G, Kryzanowski M: Tumor treatment by direct electric current: tumor temperature and pH, electrode material and configuration, *Bioelectrochem Bioenerg* 30:209, 1993.
34. Miklavcic D, Sersa G, Novakovic S: Tumor bioelectric potential and its possible exploitation for tumor growth retardation, *J Bioelectricity* 9:133, 1990.
35. Miller HI, Young FE: Drug approval process at the Food and Drug Administration: new biotechnology as paradigm of science-based activist approach, *Arch Intern Med* 149:655, 1989.
36. Mittleman E, Osborne SL, Coulter JS: Short-wave diathermy power absorption and deep tissue temperature, *Arch Phys Ther* 22:133, 1941.

37. Moertel CG et al: A clinical trial of amygdalin (Laetrile) in the treatment of human cancer, *N Engl J Med* 306:201, 1982.

38. Nakayama T: Anti-tumor activities of direct current therapy combined with fractional radiation or chemotherapy, *J Jpn Soc Med Radio* 48:1269, 1988.

39. Nikawa Y, Okada F: Dielectric loaded lens applicator for microwave hyperthermia, *IEEE Trans Microwave Theory Tech* 39:1173, 1991.

40. Nordenström BEW: Preliminary clinical trials of electrophoretic ionization in the treatment of malignant tumors, *IRCS Med Sc* 6:537, 1978.

41. Nordenström BEW: *Biologically closed electric circuits,* Stockholm, 1983, Nordic Medical.

42. Nordenström BEW: Electrochemical treatment of cancer. I. Variable response to anodic and cathodic fields, *Am J Clin Oncol* 12:530, 1989.

43. Nordenström BEW: The paradigm of biologically closed electric circuits (BCEC) and formation of an international association (IABC) for BCEC systems, *Eur J Surg Suppl* 574:7, 1994.

44. Overgaard J et al: Randomized trial of hyperthermia as adjuvant to radiotherapy for recurrent or metastatic malignant melanoma, *Lancet* 345:540, 1995.

45. Perez CA, Emami B: Clinical trials with local irradiation and hyperthermia: current and future perspectives, *Radiol Clin North Am* 27:525, 1989.

46. Perez CA et al.: Randomized phase III study comparing irradiation and hyperthermia with irradiation alone in superficial measurable tumors, *Am J Clin Oncol* 14:133, 1991.

47. Plesnicar A et al: Electric treatment of human melanoma skin lesions with low-level direct electric current: an assessment of clinical experience following a preliminary study in five patients, *Eur J Surg Suppl* 574:45, 1994.

48. Raaphrost GP: Fundamental aspects of hyperthermic biology. In Field, SB, Hand JW, editors: *An introduction to the practical aspects of clinical hyperthermia,* London, 1990, Taylor & Francis.

49. Ren RL et al: A pilot study of intracavitary hyperthermia combined with radiation in the treatment of esophageal carcinoma, *Int J Hyperthermia* 14:245, 1998.

50. Seegenschmiedt HM et al: Superficial chest wall recurrences of breast cancer: prognostic treatment factors for combined radiation therapy and hyperthermia, *Radiology* 173:551, 1989.

51. Shen RN et al: Whole body hyperthermia: a potent radioprotector in vivo, *Int J Radiat Oncol Biol Phys* 20:525, 1991.

52. Simon RM: Clinical trials in cancer. In DeVita VT, Jr, Hellman S, Rosenberg SA, editors: *Cancer: principles and practice of oncology,* ed 5, Philadelphia, 1997, Lippincott-Raven.

53. Sneed P, Phillips TL: Combining hyperthermia and radiation: how beneficial? *Oncology* 5(3):99, 1991.

54. Suffiness M, Newman DJ, Snader K: Discovery and development of antineoplastic agents from natural sources, *Bioorg Marine Chem* 3:131, 1989.

55. Valdagni R, Amichetti M: Report of long-term follow-up in a randomized trial comparing radiation therapy and radiation therapy plus hyperthermia to metastatic lymph nodes in stage IV head and neck patients, *Int J Radiat Oncol Biol Phys* 28:163, 1994.

56. Van der Zee J et al: Low-dose reirradiation with hyperthermia: a palliative treatment for patients with breast cancer recurring in previously irradiated areas, *Int J Radiat Oncol Biol Phys* 15:1407, 1988.

57. Vodovnik L, Miklavcic D, Sersa G: Modified cell proliferation due to electrical currents, *Med Biol Eng Comput* 30:21, 1992.

58. Vora N et al: Primary radiation combined with hyperthermia for advanced (stage III-IV) and inflammatory carcinoma of breast, *Endocuriether Hyperthermia Oncol* 2:101, 1986.

59. Xin YL: Organization and spread of electrochemical therapy (ECT) in China, *Eur J Surg Suppl* 574:25, 1994.

60. Xin YL: Advances in the treatment of malignant tumors by electrochemical therapy (ECT), *Eur J Surg Suppl* 574:31, 1994.

61. Xin YL et al: Electrochemical treatment of lung cancer, *Bioelectromagnetics* 18:8, 1997.

62. Young FE, Nightingale SL: FDA's newly designated treatment: INDs, *JAMA* 260:224, 1988.

63. Zhang Y, Joines WT, Oleson JR: Prediction of heating patterns of a microwave interstitial antenna array at various insertion depths, *Int J Hyperthermia* 7:197, 1991.

SUGGESTED READINGS

Bioelectromagnetics vol 18, issue 1, 1997. This special issue includes the following reports: Li KH et al: Effects of direct current on dog liver: possible mechanisms for tumor electrochemical treatment; Chou CK et al: Electrochemical treatment of mouse and rat fibrosarcomas with direct current; and Xin YL et al: Electrochemical treatment of lung cancer.

Chou CK: Radiofrequency hyperthermia for cancer therapy. In Bronzino JD, editor: *CRC Biomedical Engineering Handbook,* Boca Raton, Fla, 1995, CRC.

Nordenström B et al, editors: *Proceedings of the IABC International Association for Biologically Closed Electric Circuits (BCEC) in Medicine and Biology, Eur J Surg* p 160 (suppl 574):7, 1994.

Seegenschmiedt HM, Fessenden P, Vernon CC: *Thermo-radiotherapy and thermo-chemotherapy,* London, 1995, Springer.

PART II   Clinical Research

CHAPTER 3

Complementary/Alternative Therapies in General Medicine: Asthma and Allergies

Robert M. Hackman, Judith S. Stern, and M. Eric Gershwin

An estimated 14 million Americans suffer from asthma, and the incidence is rising at an alarming rate. Asthma is especially prevalent in children but affects people of all ages. Mortality from asthma is increasing as the number of hospital admissions for the treatment of asthma has increased; the number of deaths attributed to asthma has nearly doubled since 1976. Moreover, despite the thoughts of William Osler that "an asthmatic does not die of asthma, but rather pants one's way into old age," the number of older Americans with reactive airway disease is also increasing, even in the absence of direct tobacco exposure.[4,21,30,128]

Asthma is a common lung disease characterized by reversible airway obstruction and airway inflammation.[21,30] It is characterized by paroxysmal bronchospasm, inflammation, hypersecretion of mucus, airway wall edema, and bronchial hyperreactivity. The reasons for the unsettling increase in incidence and mortality are complex, and successful therapeutic approaches are elusive. However, throughout the world hundreds of unproved, yet potentially applicable treatment programs are used which rely on complementary/alternative medicine (CAM) for the management of asthma and sinusitis. These programs rely on a variety of protocols including nutrition, botanic medicine, homeopathy, and acupuncture. While conventional therapy is typically directed toward reducing airway inflammation and attenuating bronchial hyperreactivity, investigation of CAM approaches toward treatment and prevention of asthma may help yield new medical modalities to address an important personal and public health problem.[39,41,128]

EPIDEMIOLOGY

Asthma is a chronic condition of varying severity, affecting approximately 3% to 5% of the population.[27,50] Over 15 million asthma-related visits are made to physicians,[77] and asthmatics experience well over 100 million patient days of restricted activity annually. Medical care costs related to asthma treatment exceed $4.6 billion a year.[77] Although the public primarily associates asthma with children, 40% of people with asthma first develop the disease after the age of 40 years.[28] In 1989, more than 479,000 hospitalizations were recorded in which asthma was the first listed diagnosis.[77]

Black children are 2.5 times more likely to have asthma than white children, and blacks of both sexes are about twice as likely as whites to die of asthma.[73,105] It is not clear why prevalence of asthma and its complications are more common among black cohorts compared with whites. Certain health-damaging behaviors, such as smoking or inhaling second-hand smoke, are more common in blacks than in whites. Blacks also have less access to health care. In addition, an underlying genetic predisposition to asthma may influence the higher incidence in blacks.[34]

According to the U.S. National Health Interview Survey on Child Health,[37] asthma is the leading cause of school absence in the United States. The data strongly suggest that childhood asthma is reaching epidemic proportions. Childhood asthma is a major reason for health care usage, totaling over 3.4 million patient visits from 1980 to 1981[84] and 149,000 hospitalizations in 1987.[78] With such an alarming rise in the incidence of childhood asthma, some investigators are calling for new perspectives on asthma care, including the use of complementary therapies to augment conventional care.[50,106]

The incidence of asthma in seniors (those 65 years of age and older) is 5.2%, and, as stated earlier, 40% of people with asthma first develop the disease after the age of 40 years. Greater disability among seniors has been linked to a history of asthma. A number of factors appear to influence the relatively high incidence of asthma among seniors. In 10% of asthmatics an acute inflammatory response to aspirin and related nonsteroidal antiinflammatory agents precipitates an attack.[110] Seniors are the most common users of aspirin and related nonsteroidal antiinflammatory agents, thus increasing their risk of aspirin-induced asthma. A second factor that may precipitate asthma, particularly among seniors, is sinusitis. Sinusitis is proposed to be a leading—and commonly undiagnosed—cause of asthma.[103]

RISK FACTORS AND PATHOGENESIS

Like most chronic diseases, asthma appears to have both genetic and environmental factors that precipitate the disease. We have shown that when appropriate quantitative genetic models are applied to data from large-scale twin studies, support exists for the notion that genetic factors are important in the etiology of asthma.[116] We have also reviewed the primary environmental factors that trigger genetically predisposed individuals to develop asthma.[116] The most significant environmental variables include allergen exposure, air pollution, cigarette exposure, respiratory viral infections, and oxygen radical damage. Perhaps increased exposure of susceptible individuals to such triggers helps explain the increase in asthma incidence and mortality.

Substantial data suggest that in asthmatics' airways T lymphocytes are activated and encourage interaction with eosinophils, contributing to ongoing airway inflammation and bronchial hyperreactivity.[26,48] The major mechanism by which lymphocytes interact with other immune/inflammatory cells is through cytokine production. Cytokines act via specific receptors and form a network by which interleukins, interferons, lymphokines, monokines, and a variety of factors are related.[15]

Exposure to certain environmental hazards such as cigarette smoke and chemical fragrances can play a significant role in potentiating asthma because they act as triggers.[105] Common triggers include viral infections, cold air, sinusitis, dust, pollens, animal dander, and foods. Many of these aggressions may result in the release of reactive oxygen species (ROS)[109] by inflammatory cells. Oxygen free radicals generated by neutrophils,[72] eosinophils,[17] and other cells[20] are implicated in asthma by a variety of mechanisms, including bronchoconstriction, induction of mucus secretion, and microvascular leakage.[6,29] Reactive oxygen species can also cause an autonomic imbalance between muscarinic-receptor–mediated contraction and beta-adrenergic–mediated relaxation of pulmonary smooth muscle.[29,79] Neutrophils from asthmatics produce increased amounts of superoxide anion compared with those from normal subjects after stimulation by either N-formyl-methionyl leucyl-phenylalanine or phorbol-myristate acetate. Selenium levels in sera from asthmatics have been found to be lower than normal, although the extent to which the antioxidant capability of the circulating blood cells is compromised is not clear.[108]

For many years the upper and lower airways of humans have been regarded as anatomically and fundamentally separate with little or no relationship. Diseases of the upper and lower airways may coexist. For example, 80% of patients with asthma have rhinitis symptoms, and 5% to 15% of patients with perennial rhinitis have asthma. A number of relationships between the upper and lower airways can be identified. The nose serves as an important filter of inspired air. Relatively large particles are captured by the hairs within the nostrils, and other noxious substances are trapped in mucus. Therefore nasal obstruction or a failure in the filter function increases the allergen/irritant burden to the lower airway, thus potentiating lower airway hyperresponsiveness.

Heating and humidification of inspired air are important functions of the nose. Such functions are largely provided by a highly vascularized mucosa of the turbinates and septum. If inspired air bypasses warming and humidification provided by the nose, cooler, drier air is delivered to the lungs, which can potentiate a phenomenon referred to as exercise-induced asthma (EIA). Exercise is an important trigger for bronchial asthma and is thought to be initiated by loss of water and heat from the lower airway. Reduction in severity of EIA can be achieved by breathing through the nose rather than the mouth during exercise.[102]

In both children and adults with asthma, certain viral upper respiratory tract infections (URIs) provoke wheezing. Respiratory syncytial virus is most common in young children, with rhinovirus and influenza virus being more prevalent in older children and adults.[12] Obstructive changes in small airway function of the lung associated with viral illness may persist for up to 5 weeks, even after clinical illness has resolved. Viral URIs also cause airway hyperreactivity.

An estimated 75% of patients admitted with status asthmaticus had abnormal sinus x-rays.[38] Although more objective evidence that sinusitis triggers or exacerbates asthma would be helpful in further clarifying this issue, the data suggest that patients who come to medical attention with difficult-to-control asthma will improve when coexistent sinusitis is cleared by medical and/or surgical treatment. This can be considered as strong suggestive evidence for an etiologic role of sinusitis in lower airway disease.[104]

CAM THERAPIES IN THE TREATMENT OF ASTHMA

Complementary and alternative medicine therapies for asthma and allergies appear to be widely used by a number of health care professionals in the United States. In a recent survey approach among health professionals subscribing to a leading CAM research journal, we found that dietary therapies were the most commonly used method of intervention for asthma[26a] (Table 3-1). This was closely followed by environmental medicine, which also includes dietary manipulation. Nutritional supplements ranked third in use prevalence. Taken together, these data suggest that nutritional therapies are the most commonly used therapies used by CAM professionals in treating asthma. Other interventions commonly cited for asthma included homeopathy, botanicals, and prayer/meditation.

History

Most current conventional asthma treatments were first alternative therapies. That is to say, most of the pharmacologic treatments used by physicians to manage asthma were initially discovered based on the traditional use history of plants and animal glands for the treatment of asthma. Many CAM remedies currently employed in the United States and Europe stem from folk remedies previously used in Europe. Most European practices originated in the Middle East and were derived over centuries from work of physicians in ancient Akkadia, Sumeria, Mesopotamia, and Egypt.[124,126] Originally rooted in the concept of magical energy in plants, systematic investigations by physicians in ancient Greece and Rome eventually developed a fairly rational pharmacopoeia by the first century A.D.

Nonbotanic Greco-Roman approaches were also used throughout Europe, including cupping, leeching, scarification, and venesection, supplemented by massage, exercises, baths, inhalations, fomentations, poultices, emetics, cathartics, and clusters.[124] Dietary prescriptions were routinely employed in the management of all diseases, and for asthma various herbs, spices, animal extracts, and food eliminations or additions were widely advocated by health experts of the time.

TABLE 3-1	Top 12 Rankings* of Complementary/Alternative Medicine (CAM) Treatments Used for Asthma Among Health Care Professionals Subscribing to a Leading CAM Research Journal			
	Utility/Usefulness		Usage (%)	
Therapy	Survey Ranking by MD	Survey Ranking by Non-MD	MD	Non-MD
Dietary	1	1	74	75
Environmental medicine	2	7	69	62
Nutritional supplements	3	2	57[†]	65
Homeopathy	4	3	39[†]	47
Botanicals	5	12	40[†]	57
Meditation/prayer	6	8	45[†]	58
Mind-body therapy	7	5	37[†]	47
Acupuncture	8	4	19[†]	33
Detoxification	9	9	32[†]	47
Massage	10	6	27[†]	48
Chiropractic	11	10	7[†]	23
Osteopathy	12	13	11	15

From Davis PA, Gold EB, Hackman RM, Stern JS, Gershwin ME: The use of complementary/alternative medicine for the treatment of asthma in the United States, *Invest Allergol Clin Immunol* 8:73, 1998.
*Ranking of 1 (most useful) to 20 (least useful) and usage (percentage of total respondents using a particular form of therapy).
MD, Doctor of Medicine.
[†]Different from non-MD, $p < 0.05$, chi-squared analysis.

Moses Maimonides, the noted thirteenth-century physician, prescribed an integrated lifestyle for the asthmatic patient. His chief dietary remedy was a spicy, herbal mixture of chicken broth that contained herbs such as fennel, parsley, oregano, mint, and onion.[24,31] It is now well known that hydration of the upper respiratory tract is helpful in alleviating some asthmatic symptoms, and robust consumption of broth is one way to accomplish such hydration. The role of vegetable and herbal extracts in soup broth remains to be examined, although onions and garlic have some protective effect against allergic reactions.

In eighteenth-century Europe, strong coffee was widely used for treatment of asthma.[127] The subsequent discovery that caffeine functions as an effective bronchodilator helped verify this practice. Although drinking tea was not particularly favored as an asthma treatment, tea leaves were the original source of theophylline, whose name means tea leaf. Another nineteenth-century European drug used to treat asthma was saltpeter, or potassium nitrate. Saltpeter was inhaled for the muscle-relaxing nitrate vapor. Potassium nitrate was also used in combination with *Datura stramonium* and other herbs in tobacco preparations.

Currently most conventional physicians are treating "alternative medicine" with caution when it comes to the treatment of asthma.[14,16,56] But out of the morass of alternative therapies, rigorous scientific exploration may reveal new, exciting approaches that may be viewed as "complementary." That is to say, therapies such as nutritional supplementation, botanic extracts, mind-body practices, and manipulation strategies may one day offer the physician and the asthma sufferer more options in their quest for a comprehensive approach to asthma[62] (Fig. 3-1).

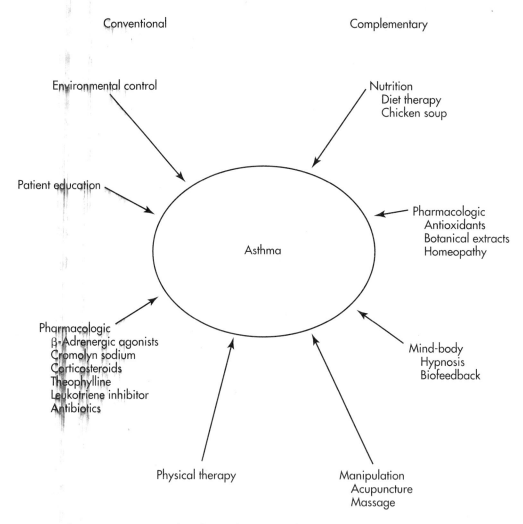

Fig. 3-1   Conventional and complementary/alternative medicine (CAM) therapies currently in use for treatment of asthma.

Nutrition

Dietary adjustments have been made throughout the ages to control asthma.[24] Unusual additions and rigorous elimination of articles of diet have had their advocates. Elimination and rotation diets are popular with some patients, who avoid items such as seafood (especially shellfish), chocolate, eggs, nuts, milk, cheeses, and certain liquors. In some cases a true food allergy can be avoided, but many patients subscribe to a limited diet without any clear evidence that the avoided foods are harmful. Undoubtedly, certain foods or additives can make asthma worse, but it is a challenge to construct a realistic elimination diet unless an obvious relationship between specific foods and an individual's asthma exists. For example, avoidance of restaurant salads or various packaged foods could be of importance in patients with sulfite sensitivity. Reports also exist of asthma-causing allergic reactions to vegetables[82] and fruits,[83] but such occurrences are rare. The concept of hypersensitivity to certain foods, most commonly, staple foods in a person's diet (e.g., in the United States, milk, eggs, soy, wheat, corn, and rice) is embraced by physicians practicing "environmental medicine" (EM). A recent report from India found that 83% of parents whose children have asthma believe that certain foods precipitate acute attacks.[55] This is in stark contrast to the estimated 8.5% of the population having true allergic reactions to food.[76] Reconciling the claim of widespread food hypersensitivity with the conventional physician's view of food allergies is impossible at the present time, since EM has not been documented in any systematic scientific manner.

The lung is particularly exposed to high levels of oxygen; thus oxygen-induced free radical damage is of concern. Antioxidants scavenge free radicals, and the role of antioxidants in pulmonary function and pathologies such as asthma has been investigated. Most of the research has focused on ascorbic acid (AA), since AA is the predominant antioxidant in the lung.

Low dietary AA intake has been associated with asthma, bronchitis, and wheezing in the National Health and Nutrition Examination Survey (NHANES II).[93] Recently, dietary analysis of patients suffering from seasonal allergic-type symptoms and asthma found that low AA intake was associated with more than a fivefold increased risk of bronchial reactivity.[104] Other epidemiologic studies have not found an association between AA intake and asthma.[114] Meta-analysis of existing human studies on dietary AA intake and asthma reports a majority of studies finding a positive association, while other studies find no relationship.[9]

In humans, acute AA supplementation (2 g) was found to improve forced expiratory volume in 1 second (FEV_1) pulmonary measures significantly better than a placebo.[11] AA supplementation has also been found to dramatically improve airway hyperresponsiveness in humans when exposed to nitrogen dioxide.[74] This double-blind, placebo-controlled study found that 500 mg of AA taken four times per day for 3 days, followed by exposure to nitrogen dioxide, resulted in complete prevention of airway reactivity when assessed by a methacholine challenge test. Recently the effect of

2 g of AA on exercise-induced asthma (EIA) was assessed in those with EIA. Nine of the 10 individuals who received AA supplements 1 hour before exercise demonstrated significant improvement in pulmonary function as assessed by FEV_1. These benefits persisted for 2 weeks following the initial treatment, while the subjects consumed 0.5 g AA per day.[22] In other human studies, AA supplementation 1 hour before testing was able to reduce the duration and intensity of acute airway constriction induced by exercise,[91] histamine,[129] or methacholine.[75] Indomethacin was found to negate the beneficial effects of AA supplementation,[75,80] suggesting a mechanism involving prostaglandin and leukotriene metabolism. In contrast, other clinical studies have not found a role of AA in airway hyperreactivity.[52,112] The different findings in the various research studies on AA and asthma may be partly due to the wide range of vitamin C supplements used in the protocols, as well as the heterogeneous population that probably combines AA-sufficient and AA-deficient individuals. Most protocols to date use acute interventions, and the effect of longer-term treatment with dietary and supplemental AA remains an intriguing research area.

We have suggested other possible links between diet and asthma.[18] Potentially important dietary variables in regard to asthma are the amount and composition of polyunsaturated fatty acid (PUFA) intake. Much attention has been focused on the omega-3 class of fatty acids, such as eicosapentaenoic acid (EPA). EPA competitively inhibits formation of prostaglandins and leukotrienes derived from omega-6 PUFA, arachidonic acid, including LTC_4, LTD_4, and LTE_4, which activate ion transport,[61] mucus secretion,[67] smooth muscle contraction, and LTB_4, which stimulates neutrophil chemotaxis.[8] In addition to being a competitive inhibitor of arachidonate, EPA is itself a substrate for the biosynthesis of leukotrienes as well as prostaglandins.[60,87]

Fish oils have been reported to aid in the relief of asthma symptoms among persons with mild asthma.[5] In a subsample of 2526 participants in the first National Health and Nutrition Examination Survey (NHANES I), a significant positive association between dietary fish oil intake and pulmonary function was reported.[94] Recently a placebo-controlled study found that addition of omega-3 polyunsaturated fatty acids in 27 patients with bronchial asthma resulted in less severe and less frequent attacks of asphyxia, and drug doses were reduced.[69] Provocation tests with allergen after 2 weeks of supplementation showed a significant decline in allergic response. In contrast, children with asthma given fish oil supplements for 12 weeks showed no significant differences in FEV_1 compared with those receiving a placebo.[64]

Fish oils are rich in EPA and docosahexaenoic acid (DHA). These fish oils limit leukotriene synthesis and biologic activities by substituting substrate fatty acids as alternatives to arachidonic acid. Both EPA and DHA inhibit the conversion of arachidonic acid by the cyclooxygenase pathway to prostanoid metabolites and reduce the production of platelet-activating factor (PAF), which may be a possible mechanism of action to explain the apparent benefits of fish oil intake in those with asthma. However, obtaining sufficient fish oil from dietary sources may be problematic for many individuals,[105] since two to four servings weekly of cold-water fish such as salmon or mackerel are recommended. Supplements may be the best way to ensure adequate intake of essential fatty acids.

Zinc is a key nutrient with respect to modulation of immune function and has been implicated in asthma. Recently plasma zinc levels were found to be significantly lower among 22 asthma patients compared with 33 healthy controls (0.80 ± 0.01 mg/L among asthmatics vs. 0.89 ± 0.02 mg/L among controls (mean ± SE).[46] Plasma copper levels and the plasma zinc/copper ratio were also elevated in asthmatics compared with controls (1.28 ± 0.03 mg/L and 1.61 ± 0.04 vs. 1.06 ± 0.02 mg/L and 1.21 ± 0.02, respectively (mean ± SE). Both zinc and copper are involved in Zn/Cu–superoxide dismutase (SOD), a key antioxidant enzyme involved in free radical scavenging as well as in cytokine expression. Manganese-SOD has also been implicated in asthma. In a rat model of allergic asthma, Mn-SOD, but not Zn/Cu-SOD, showed significant induction when an asthmatic episode was evoked.[70] Pretreatment with recombinant human SOD resulted in a dramatic suppression of the asthmatic episode, with elimination of Mn-SOD induction.

Low dietary zinc intakes have been positively associated with bronchial hyperreactivity among persons with seasonal allergic symptoms and asthma.[105] Marginal dietary zinc intake may occur in many Americans,[115] and inadequate intake may modulate the severity of asthma, as we have proposed.[49] More specifically, we have suggested that physicians check zinc status of their patients as part of a comprehensive medical examination into the causes of asthma. Further, we suggest that dietary therapies and nutritional supplementation might be employed to replenish marginal or deficient zinc status. Excessive zinc intake due to occupational exposure has been reported to cause asthma[66]; although this level of exposure is unlikely in a normal population, it does illustrate the potential hazard of overconsumption of zinc if used to help treat asthma or other clinical conditions.

A potential link between nutrition and asthma involves magnesium.[117] An epidemiologic study of 2415 randomly selected persons in the United Kingdom found that airway hyperreactivity as measured by methacholine challenge was significantly lower among those consuming high-magnesium diets.[10] After adjusting for age, sex, and the effects of atopy and smoking, a 100-mg/day-higher intake of magnesium was related to a 28-ml-higher FEV_1, and an 18% reduction in relative odds of airway hyperreactivity. Low dietary intake of magnesium has been further associated with increased airway hyperreactivity among patients with asthma.[105] Intravenous magnesium is well known for its bronchodilating effect,[81,90] but evidence of the potential of dietary magnesium to impact asthma symptoms is still evolving. The bronchodilating effect of magnesium may be due to interference with calcium handling by bronchial smooth muscle cells.[33] An intriguing question for CAM research is whether dietary magnesium supplementation can attenuate severity of asthma symptoms.

Probiotics may also be a useful area of investigation in regard to nutritional influences on asthma. Consumption of microorganisms in yogurt and other beneficial bacteria is associated with a reduction in susceptibility to a variety of diseases. In recent studies we have found that daily consumption of 450 g of yogurt with live cultures (Dannon) is associated with a fivefold increase in gamma interferon by stimulated lymphocytes.[42] Since gamma interferon inhibits immunoglobulin E (IgE) synthesis, and since hyperproduction of IgE is implicated in asthma, probiotic supplementation may attenuate this sequence of events and reduce the severity of asthmatic symptoms. Further research is needed to confirm this hypothesis.

Asian Herbs

Chinese knowledge of botanic medicine dates back to the discovery of the herbal therapeutic *Ma huang* around 3000 B.C. It was initially used as a stimulant but was also used for respiratory afflictions and other diseases.[125] The active ingredient in Ma huang was subsequently found to be ephedrine, an effective bronchodilator. Ma huang has been central to asthma treatment in traditional forms of Chinese medicine. Numerous composite preparations that are used in treatment of asthma rely on this botanical. For example, Ma huang is combined with gecko lizard tails in Ge Jie Anti-Asthma Pill; other traditional mixtures are prescribed under such names as Minor Blue Dragon Combination.[124,125] Some preparations contain a compound with disodium cromoglycate–like activity, but many other favorite traditional Chinese remedies without Ma huang have yet to show proven value. Traditional antiasthma agents such as *Bupleurum* and *Pinellia*, and *Magnolia* have not been found to be effective.[125]

Extracts of *Gingko biloba* have been shown to inhibit PAF, thus offering a scientific explanation for the use of this herb for treatment of asthmatic coughs.[7] Other traditional agents are known to antagonize PAF, including various fungal derivatives such as gliotoxin from a wood fungus and kadsurenone from *haifentenga*, a Chinese medication found in *Piper futokadsura*, and an extract of *Tussilago farfara*. This latter herb is known in the West as coltsfoot, and has long been used in both the West and in China as a mild antitussive. A comprehensive review of Chinese herbal medicines used to treat asthma has been published,[13] and the reader is directed to this exhaustive review for details beyond those provided in this chapter.

Traditional Chinese medicine may have introduced steroid therapy in a crude fashion through use of fetal and placental extracts and urine of pubescent children, practices sometimes used in the treatment of asthma. Although none of the Chinese herbal medications used to treat asthma have been found to have corticosteroid activity, it is quite possible that many components have antiinflammatory activity. For example, licorice has been extensively studied and does have such activity. *Ledebouriella seseloides*, *Rehmannia glutinosa*, and *Paeonia lactflora* also have antiinflammatory activity.[124]

In Japan a form of traditional practice, Kampo, has its origins in traditional Chinese medicine. Saiboku-To, a mixture of herbs that has been used for more than 200 years for treatment of asthma, is one such Kampo formula. Recent analytic studies suggested possible mechanisms for its effectiveness in treating asthma.[44,65] Another modern use of Saiboku-To in asthma aims at reducing the dose of steroids in steroid-dependent severe asthma.[113]

In Hawaii traditional use of *Sophora chrysophylla* has been reported for the treatment of asthma.[68] Locally termed "mamane," review of the historical use of this plant and the existing pharmacologic knowledge of other *Sophora* species suggests promising opportunities for future research.

Ayurvedic Herbs

Ayurveda is a traditional form of medicine practiced throughout the Indian subcontinent. The practice is based on more than 7000 years of traditional use history. A multiple-intervention strategy is typically used in Ayurvedic medicine, involving dietary adjustments, meditation and yogic practices, environmental alterations, and the use of herbal extracts.

Most Ayurvedic medications used for asthma are still relatively unknown to Western scientists, but one plant, *Tylophora indica asthmatica*, has been a standard remedy in the treatment of respiratory disorders in which mucus accumulation is a symptom.[126] Chewing the leaves of *T. indica* was found to be an effective therapy in relieving asthmatic symptoms in an early double-blind, placebo-controlled crossover study.[100] Subsequent investigation found that an alcoholic extract of *T. indica* produced complete to moderate relief of asthma symptoms in 58% of patients after 1 week, compared with 31% of those taking a placebo.[101] The difference between the treatment and placebo groups became more marked during the following 12 weeks. In contrast, others have reported no effect of *T. indica* in FEV_1 measurements or symptom relief scores.[40]

The traditional drug vasaka, derived from *Adhatoda vasica* or the malabar nut tree, is smoked in cigarettes for asthma and tuberculosis. *A. vasica* is the source of bromhexine and ambroxol, two mucoregulating drugs used in Europe. Leaves of *Datura stramonium*, called "d'hatura" in India, contain a bronchodilator. Traditional use of this plant as a tobacco remedy for asthma originated in India, and *D. stramonium* cigarettes eventually became popular for treating asthma and bronchitis in Europe and North America.[128]

African Herbs

Desmodium adscendens is a traditional botanic medicine used in Ghana as a treatment for asthma and other diseases associated with excessive smooth muscle contraction. Plant extracts inhibit contraction of guinea pig ileum caused by electrical field stimulation[1] and contractions of sensitized guinea pig airway smooth muscle induced by arachidonic acid or leukotriene D_4.[2,3] This botanical contains several different elements that aid in relaxation of smooth muscle, acting to inhibit or reduce nicotinamide adenine dinucleotide phosphate (NADPH)–dependent monooxygenase pathway of arachidonic acid metabolism.[3] Recently *D. adscendens* has been shown to contain triterpenoid glycosides, which function as high-affinity activators of calcium-dependent potassium channels.[71] As such, this ethnomedicine contains the most potent known potassium channel opener yet discovered.

American Herbs

North American plant derivatives were used in European respiratory therapeutics beginning in the sixteenth century. Important botanicals included guaiac wood, ipecacuanha, tobacco, and chili peppers. As discussed previously, cigarettes containing *D. stramonium* were used and, often, also included horehound, mullein, coltsfoot, lobelia, cubebs, seaweed, and marijuana. Glyceryl guaiacolate (guaifenesin), which has mucus-loosening, expectorant properties, was eventually derived from guaiac wood. The mechanism of action of guaiac is the same as that produced by subemetic doses of ipecacuanha, which causes activation of the gastropulmonary mucokinetic reflex, thereby resulting in secretion of low-viscosity mucus.[123] Capsaicin, an active ingredient in cayenne and chili peppers, stimulates the mucokinetic reflex and releases and then depletes substance P stored in nonadrenergic noncholinergic nerves. The subsequent release of mucus, and possible bronchospasm, may help to decrease mucus production and prolong dilation of bronchial muscles.

In recent years isocyanates found in pungent vegetables such as onion have been shown to be protective against allergic reactions in the guinea pig.[31] Mandrake and related solaneous plants, a source of atropinic agents, offer benefits similar to those of *D. stramonium*. The related *Atropa belladonna* was long recognized in Europe to be a potent pharmacologic agent and appears to have been favored by observant lay healers as an antiasthma remedy hundreds of years before it became popular in the nineteenth-century medical community.

Homeopathy

Homeopathy has a devoted group of users in western Europe and the United States. The treatment originated in Germany and was initially expanded to Europe and America. The homeopathic physician believes that a constellation of physical, psychologic, and emotional domains must be considered to devise an individualized therapeutic program which uses very diluted extracts of botanicals and other compounds. Each person is treated individually based on their "constitution," which creates a challenge in researching the effectiveness of specific homeopathic remedies that work in large, heterogeneous populations. Nonetheless, a number of studies in credentialed, peer-reviewed journals report the apparent effectiveness of homeopathy for certain asthmatic and allergic conditions.

Reilly and colleagues tested 28 patients with allergic asthma in a randomized, double-blind, placebo-controlled trial.[88] Before the intervention patients were tested for allergic responses using skin pricks. The largest skin test wheal was used to determine the primary allergen. Also at this time, patients were tested for FEV_1, forced vital capacity (FVC), and pulmonary reactivity to inhaled histamine. A diary was begun to log drug use for asthma, and a visual analog, scaled questionnaire was administered to assess patients' symptom intensity. Four weeks later, patients were assigned to one of the two groups; those in the homeopathy group received extremely dilute preparations of their primary allergen, while those in the placebo group received inert material. Doses were taken orally, once daily for 4 weeks, at which time follow-up measurements were taken. Patients in the homeopathy group reported significant improvements in their symptom intensity within 1 week of starting the intervention compared with those receiving the placebo, and this difference persisted for the duration of the study. Measures of FEV_1 and FVC were significantly improved in the homeopathy group, and a median 53% reduction in bronchial reactivity to histamine was found in the homeopathy group, compared with a 7% increase in histamine reactivity in the placebo group. This study, published in *Lancet* in 1994, has sparked vigorous discussion about the potential merits of homeopathy as a complementary treatment for asthma. Further research is needed to help focus such discussions.

Upon stepping back from the details of individual studies and assessing the broad field of CAM for asthma, one thing becomes clear. Despite mountains of traditional use history and current day testimonials, very little objective scientific research exists using the basic tenets of research design (Table 3-2). More research emphasis is urgently required for a number of reasons. First, a very real potential exists to make significant discoveries that help people who have asthma. Modern drugs have been successful at managing asthma symptoms but have limitations. Pharmaceuticals produce side effects, and many authorities believe that the drugs may not address the root causes of asthma. New approaches to help treat asthma at both the symptom and underlying disease levels are needed, and the areas of dietary therapies, nutritional supplements, and botanic extracts appear to offer the most promise for discoveries. A second reason for more research in CAM and asthma is that the consumer marketplace demands it. The sale of herbal remedies in the United States has been increasing at the rate of almost 20% per year since 1993. The sale of herbs is unregulated, and many false, misleading products exist. Research studies can help define which plants and plant fractions may be most useful as complementary therapies available to physicians and asthma sufferers. Quality standards in botanic extracts are desperately needed by industry, government, and biomedical groups, and research laboratories are the place to start getting such standards established.

TABLE 3-2	Research Overview of Some CAM Therapies Used for Asthma

Category	Practice	Research Strength	Key Citation (Reference No[s].)	Issues
Nutrition	Dietary: Avoid foods causing allergies	Excellent	76	Widely accepted by allopathic and CAM physicians
	AA (vitamin C) supplementation	Strong suggestive evidence	11, 22, 74	What is appropriate dosage? Do AA-depleted individuals respond differently than AA-replete persons?
	Essential fatty acids (fish oil) supplementation	Epidemiolgic association; two small studies show promise in adults; one study in children showed no effect	5, 69, 94	Should doses be standardized to specific amounts of omega-3 and omega-6 fatty acids? What are appropriate dosage and duration? Do age differences exist?
	Zinc supplementation	Low zinc intake associated with seasonal asthma and allergies	104	No human clinical studies exist
	Magnesium supplementation	Strong epidemiologic evidence relating high magnesium intake to improved pulmonary function	10	No human clinical studies on magnesium supplementation exist
Botanicals	Ma huang (ephedra)	Excellent scientific studies	125	Side effects: Nervousness, cardiac arrhythmias, hypertension
	Other Chinese and Japanese single herbs and mixtures	Strong traditional use, but weak or mixed scientific results	13, 124	Studies fail to find benefits of some mixtures; traditionally used herb mixtures have not been studied using basic principles of research design
	Tylophora indica (from India)	One small study found benefit; one small study did not	40, 101	Repeat study using animal model; is this the very best herb from India to study?

TABLE 3-2	Research Overview of Some CAM Therapies Used for Asthma—cont'd			
Category	Practice	Research Strength	Key Citation (Reference No[s].)	Issues
	Other Indian herbs	Traditional use (Ayurvedic) history but no scientific studies	126, 128	Systemic study of popular herbs required
	Native American plants	Traditional use history but no scientific studies	123	Systemic study required
Homeopathy	Ingestion of extremely diluted materials, typically botanic in origin	One significant, positive study	88	Repeat study with non-homeopaths conducting intervention; what are the active ingredients?

AA, ascorbic acid.

CAM IN THE TREATMENT OF ALLERGIES

A variety of CAM treatments exist for allergies, eczema, summer hay fever, and rhinitis. These include therapies such as Chinese herbs, clinical ecology, acupuncture, hypnosis, applied kinesiology, nutritional and botanic supplementation, and homeopathy. Very little scientific evaluation of these therapies exists. Conventional physicians point to the lack of controlled studies and suggest that any benefit ascribed to the CAM treatment is most likely the result of suggestion or a placebo response. Some studies, however, suggest that further research into the area of CAM and allergies is warranted.

Chinese Herbs

The best scientific evidence in the area of CAM and allergies comes from the study of a traditional Chinese herbal formulation used to treat atopic eczema. The formulation contained a blend of 10 herbs and had proved beneficial in open studies. Although traditional Chinese medicine considers every person as unique and botanic formulations are typically individualized for each patient, the same standard formula was used in six studies that have been published since 1992.

Initially, 40 adults with atopic eczema that was nonresponsive to conventional medical treatment were randomized into two groups for a double-blind, placebo-controlled, crossover study.[97] Herbal decoctions or placebos were consumed daily for 2 months, followed by a 1-month washout period, after which time the groups were crossed. Severity and extent of erythema and surface damage were significantly improved when subjects received the Chinese herbal formula compared with the placebo. No side effects were reported. A similarly designed study was also conducted with children who had nonexudative atopic eczema.[95] When the children received the herbal decoction, their eczema improved, compared with when they consumed the placebo. Ten of the 47 children who initially enrolled in the study withdrew, primarily because they found no relief. While such recidivism may have biased the study results, the similarity of results between the study with children and that with adults suggested that further research was warranted.

At the conclusion of the study with the children the opportunity to continue treatment was offered. All 37 children and parents chose to continue with the herbal treatments, and each child's progress was monitored for the following 12 months.[96] At the end of the year-long follow-up, 18 children showed at least 90% improvement in eczema symptoms, 5 showed moderate improvement, and 14 withdrew from the study (10 because of lack of response, 4 because of unpalatability of the decoction). Among those who completed the follow-up, 7 were able to discontinue treatment with the herbal formula and did not experience any relapse. The other 16 children were able to control their eczema with the herbs, with 12 of them able to reduce the frequency of intake from daily to once every 2 to 5 days. At recruitment into the initial blinded study, use of topical emollients averaged 60 g per day. At the end of the follow-up those who completed the study were using an average of 15 g per day. Only 4 children used 1% hydrocortisone ointment, and none applied it daily. Antihistamine use followed a similar pattern, with 17 of the 23 patients taking nightly antihistamines at the beginning of the controlled study and only 3 sporadically taking these drugs at the conclusion of the follow-up. Twenty-one of the 23 children who completed the study showed elevated IgE levels on admission to the blinded trial. By the end of the follow-up, 10 showed a decrease of greater than 10% in IgE and 3 showed more than a 10% increase. All showed a drop in peripheral blood eosinophil levels into the normal range during the 1-year follow-up. Serum aspartate aminotransferase (AST) levels exceeded 1.5 times the upper limit of normal in 2 children who enrolled in the follow-up. They were dropped from the study, and their AST levels returned to normal. The authors suggested that these 2 patients had idiosyncratic hepatotoxicity.

To investigate possible mechanisms of action of the traditional Chinese herbal formula cited above, the effect of an extract of these herbs or a placebo was tested on peripheral blood monocytes from nonatopic subjects.[57] Expression of CD23, a low-affinity IgE receptor thought to be involved in the pathology of atopic eczema, was assessed. The influence of interleukin 4 (IL-4), known to stimulate expression of CD23, was also monitored. The herbal formula was found to inhibit CD23 expression by as much as 60%, while the placebo had no effect on this parameter. Inhibition was dose dependent and was effective at a concentration as low as 250 µg/ml. When IL-4 was first added to the in vitro system, followed by the Chinese herbal extract or placebo, inhibition of CD23 was noted for the herbal extract for up to 12 hours, while no inhibition resulted from the placebo. The possibility of inhibition of CD23 expression by IL-4 due to cell death was assessed, but no effects were found for either the herbal or placebo preparation.

A more detailed study of immunologic changes among patients with atopic eczema who consumed the traditional Chinese herbal decoction has recently been published.[57] Eighteen patients consumed the formula for 8 weeks and showed an approximately 50% improvement in skin surface damage and erythema. Blood was collected from each patient at the beginning and end of the study period and measured for serum IgE complexes and total serum IgE. Peripheral blood mononuclear cells were derived and used to assess CD23 expression, IL-4 induction of CD23, and soluble interleukin 2 (IL-2) receptor. The treatment decreased serum IgE complexes but did not affect serum IgE or expression of CD23. A significant reduction in the ability of IL-4 to induce CD23 expression was found in monocytes isolated after the completion of the study, relative to pretest expression. At the start of the study soluble IL-2 levels were elevated in the serum of the patients compared with normal values. At the completion of the study soluble IL-2 values decreased significantly. Thus the benefits from the herbal remedy appear to correspond to a variety of changes in immunologic parameters. Antioxidant activity in aqueous decoctions of this Chinese herbal formula also have been reported recently.[51] Which herb(s) and which active compound(s) exert the immunologic effect await further identification, as does the role, if any, of antioxidants in modulating the immune response in this disease.

Other Asian herbs have been studied for their possible allergy treatment potential. The best study is of the dried rhizomes of *Alisma orientale*.[53] Methanol extracts were shown to significantly inhibit antibody-mediated allergic reactions in animal models of types I, II, III, and IV allergies. Four triterpenes and two sesquiterpenes isolated from the methanol fraction exhibited allergy-inhibiting effects, particularly for type III allergies.

The evidence on Chinese herbal medicine for skin disease is not entirely positive. Two cases of hepatitis have been reported in individuals consuming Chinese herbal formulas for skin conditions.[86] Both patients got better on discontinuing the use of the herbs, and recurrence of liver disease was noted on reintroduction of the formulas. Nine other cases of liver damage following the use of Chinese herbal medicines were also reported in that report, although the authors did not provide case histories on these nine. Since the herbal formulas varied in composition and concentration of the different herbs, no clear indication of which ingredient(s) might be causing the liver toxicity was found. The effects did not appear to be dose dependent, and the authors suggested that the pathologic conditions were probably idiosyncratic. Two other cases of hepatitis[47] and one case of severe cardiomyopathy[35] induced by traditional Chinese herbs taken for skin conditions have been reported. The need for consumer caution and for physician inquiry into the use of herbal remedies in their patients is clearly warranted.

Acupuncture

The role of acupuncture in the treatment of allergic rhinitis has been reported, although these reports are case studies and clinical observations. An early study[59] described 22 patients with allergic rhinitis who received a series of six acupuncture treatments. Fifty percent of subjects were "virtually symptom-free" at the end of the regimen; an additional 36% had a moderate reduction in symptoms and 14% reported no relief. Measurement of serum IgE by radioimmunoassay, percentage of nasal eosinophils, and absolute blood eosinophil count were obtained before treatment, immediately following the final treatment, and 2 months later. Immunoglobulin E levels decreased in 64% of subjects at the end of the treatment regimen and in 76% of subjects at the 2-month follow-up. Those who reported subjective relief of symptoms also showed a drop in blood and nasal eosinophils.

The effect of acupuncture compared with antihistamine treatment was evaluated in 45 patients with allergic rhinitis.[19] Half of the subjects received 7 weeks of acupuncture treatment, and half consumed oral antihistamines. Data were collected before and immediately after the final treatment and at a 3-month follow-up. Symptom severity assessed by the patients and laboratory measures of serum and nasal secretion immunoglobulin (IgA) levels, blood eosinophil levels, and nasal clearance time were collected. X-rays of the paranasal sinus were also taken. Both groups recorded improvements in symptom relief, with the acupuncture group reporting significantly greater improvement than the antihistamine group. Symptom relief persisted at the 3-month follow-up. Similarly, both groups showed improved nasal clearance times, with the effect more lasting in the acupuncture group. Both groups showed significant declines in serum and nasal IgA levels, which still existed at the 3-month follow-up. No differences were found in blood eosinophil levels or in nasal sinus x-rays.

Desensitization treatment for allergic rhinitis was tested with 102 patients using positive allergens and acupuncture points on the head and face.[122] After two treatments allergen extracts were prepared and injected intradermally. The diameter of redness and degree of swelling were significantly less than when tested before acupuncture treatment. Cases were followed for up to 2 years, and the authors reported that 72% of cases had "significant curative effect" with another 24% showing improvement.

A recent study from China[111] reported the effects from a botanic extract (10% Cantharides), which was plastered and blistered on a key acupuncture point (Dazhui, Neiguan point) among 50 people with allergic rhinitis. The treatment was deemed "effective" for 88% of cases, with pretest to posttest measures of serum IgE and nasal eosinophil and basophil secretion levels, and an allergic mucosal provocation test showing statistically significant differences. No control group was used in this study.

Although numerous other acupuncture studies* also report positive effects, these are clinical observations and lack any control groups, making the reports difficult to

*References 23, 25, 32, 36, 43, 45, 54, 92, 98, 99, 118, 119, 120, 121.

evaluate scientifically. Research studies using the principles of contemporary science are clearly warranted in this area to help clinicians and patients make informed decisions regarding the potential of acupuncture as a complementary therapy for allergic rhinitis.

Homeopathy

One of the first systematic studies on homeopathy assessed its effect on individuals with hay fever.[89] This double-blind, placebo-controlled study randomly assigned 144 patients with symptoms of grass pollenosis (hay fever) to either a treatment or placebo group for 2 weeks, followed by 2 weeks of observation. The homeopathic remedy tested was an extremely diluted solution of a mixture of 12 grass pollens in the subject's geographic locale that were commonly associated with hay fever. Both patients and doctors kept logs of hay fever-related symptom intensity. Participants also recorded their use of antihistamine medication. The homeopathy treatment group showed a significant reduction in patient- and doctor-scored symptom intensity compared with the placebo group. When the data were adjusted for pollen count, the symptom score differences were even greater. Those in the treatment group also showed a reduction of approximately 50% in their use of antihistamines. The authors took great care to emphasize the statistical rigor of their study and concluded that the effects seen in the homeopathy group were beyond the effects of a placebo alone.

A survey of 102 patients treated in a homeopathic clinic of a large medical center in Israel reported that treatment of allergy-related conditions was the main reason for using this form of health care.[85] Most of the survey respondents were children and young adults (mean age, 22.7 years) in whom conventional Western medicine had been ineffective. Asthma, skin problems, and recurrent URIs were the three most frequently noted categories for which participants sought homeopathic care. More than 80% of participants were greatly satisfied with the homeopathic approach, and half of the respondents reported that their symptoms had improved. The survey bias of a self-selected population is obvious, and it is impossible to determine whether the benefits and satisfaction of patients are due to a placebo effect or a result of the treatment. Since different patients received different homeopathic remedies, it is also impossible to assess which, if any, remedy was effective using scientifically accepted criteria. Nonetheless, such reports suggest a consumer demand for complementary therapies for allergy treatment, and rigorous study of homeopathy in the treatment of common allergic diseases is necessary to help patients and physicians more clearly identify treatments that may be beneficial.

A recent meta-analysis of 185 homeopathic trials[63] is the latest report pointing to the need for more rigorous research in this area. After applying the principles of scientific research design to the trials, 89 were found to have appropriate data for meta-analysis. The combined odds ratio was 2.45 in support of homeopathy. Four studies on the effect of a particular remedy used to treat seasonal allergies had a pooled odds ratio

TABLE 3-3	Research Overview of Some CAM Therapies Used for Treatment of Allergies			
Category	Practice	Research Strength	Key Citation (Reference No[s].)	Issues
Botanical	Specific Chinese herbal formula	Excellent results in children and adults	95, 96, 97	What are the active ingredients?
Acupuncture	Methods vary; needles only, herbal point stimulation; may or may not include herbal teas	Limited uncontrolled studies suggest some benefit	19, 59, 122	Standardize treatment; use basic principles of research design
Homeopathy	Ingestion of extremely diluted material, typically grass pollen, animal dander or other botanical	One study suggests benefits	89	Repeat study; what are the active ingredients?

of 2.03 for relief of ocular symptoms after 4 weeks of treatment. The authors concluded that their results "are not compatible with the hypothesis that the clinical effects of homeopathy are completely due to placebo." Yet, they also note a lack of sufficient scientific study of homeopathy for any single medical condition and make a strong case for systematic scientific research in this area.

A broad view of the research on CAM therapies for allergies suggests that some benefits may exist (Table 3-3). However, as with the case for CAM and asthma, more research and new research initiatives are required, to make sense of an exciting yet confusing area of emerging biomedical importance.

REFERENCES

1. Addy ME: Some secondary plant metabolites in *Desmodium adscendens* and their effects on arachidonic and metabolism, *Prostagland Leukot Essent Fatty Acids* 47:85, 1992.
2. Addy ME, Burka JF: Effect of *Desmodium adscendens* fractions on antigen- and arachidonic acid–induced contractions of guinea pig airways, *Can J Physiol Pharmacol* 66:820, 1988.
3. Addy ME, Burka JF: Effect of *Desmodium adscendens* fraction 3 on contractions of respiratory smooth muscle, *J Ethnopharmacol* 29:325, 1990.
4. Alexander HL: A historical account of death from asthma, *J Allergy* 34:305, 1963.
5. Arm JP et al: Effect of dietary supplementation with fish oil lipids on mild asthma, *Thorax* 43:84, 1988.
6. Barnes PJ: Reactive oxygen species and airway inflammation, *Free Radic Biol Med* 9:235, 1990.
7. Barnes PJ, Chung KF, Page CP: Platelet-activating factor as a mediator of allergic disease, *J Allergy Clin Immunol* 82:751, 1988.

8. Barnes N, Piper PJ, Costello J: The effect of an oral leukotriene antagonist L-649, 923 on histamine and leukotriene D_4-induced bronchoconstriction in the normal man, *J Allergy Clin Immunol* 79:816, 1987.

9. Bielory L, Gandhi R: Asthma and vitamin C, *Ann Allergy* 73:89, 1994.

10. Britton J et al: Dietary magnesium, lung function, wheezing, and airway hyperreactivity in a random adult population sample, *Lancet* 344:357,1994.

11. Bucca C et al: Effect of vitamin C on histamine bronchial responsiveness of patients with allergic rhinitis, *Ann Allergy* 65:311, 1990.

12. Busse WE: The precipitation of asthma by upper respiratory infections, *Chest* 87(suppl):44, 1985.

13. But P, Chang C: Chinese herbal medicine in the treatment of asthma and allergies, *Clin Rev Allergy Immunol* 14:253, 1996.

14. Carlson CM, Sachs MI: Is alternative medicine an alternative for the treatment of asthma? *J Asthma* 31:149, 1994.

15. Casale TB, Smart SJ: Pathogenesis of asthma: mediators and mechanisms. In Gershwin ME, Halpern GM, editors: *Bronchial asthma: principles of diagnosis and treatment*, ed 3, Totowa, NJ, 1994, Humana.

16. Chanez P et al: Controversial forms of treatment for asthma, *Clin Rev Allergy Immunol* 14:247, 1996.

17. Chanez P et al: Generation of oxygen free radicals from blood eosinophils from asthma patients after stimulation with PAF or phorbol ester, *Eur Respir J* 3:1002, 1990.

18. Chang CC et al: Asthma mortality: another opinion—is it a matter of life and . . . bread? *J Asthma* 30:93, 1993.

19. Chari P et al: Acupuncture therapy in allergic rhinitis, *Am J Acupunct* 16:143, 1988.

20. Cluzel M et al: Enhanced alveolar cell luminol-dependent chemiluminescence in asthma, *J Allergy Clin Immunol* 80:195, 1987.

21. Cockcroft DW et al: Allergen-induced increase in non-allergic bronchial reactivity, *Clin Allergy* 7:503, 1977.

22. Cohen HA, Neuman I, Nahum H: Blocking effect of vitamin C in exercise-induced asthma, *Arch Pediatr Adolesc Med* 151:367, 1997.

23. Cortes JL: The practice of allergy in the People's Republic of China, *Ann Allergy* 46:92, 1981.

24. Cosman MP: A feast for Aesculapius: historical diets for asthma and sexual pleasure, *Ann Rev Nutr* 3:1, 1983.

25. Czubalski K et al: Acupuncture and phonostimulation in pollenosis and vasomotor rhinitis in the light of psychosomatic investigations, *Acta Otolaryngol (Stockh)* 84:446, 1977.

26. De Monchy JGR et al: Bronchoalveolar eosinophilia during allergen-induced late asthmatic reactions, *Am Rev Respir Dis* 131:373, 1985.

26a. Davis PA, Gold EB, Hackman RM, Stern JS, Gershwin ME: The use of complementary / alternative medicine for the treatment of asthma in the United States, *Invest Allergol Clin Immunol* 8:73, 1998.

27. Dodge R, Burrows B: The prevalence and incidence of asthma and asthma-like symptoms in a general population sample, *Am Rev Respir Dis* 122:567, 1980.

28. Dodge R, Cline MG, Burrows B: Comparisons of asthma, emphysema, and chronic bronchitis in a general population sample, *Am Rev Respir Dis* 133:981, 1986.

29. Doelman CJ, Bast A: Oxygen radicals in lung pathology, *Free Radic Biol Med* 9:381, 1990.

30. Dolovich J et al: Late-phase airway reaction and inflammation, *J Allergy Clin Immunol* 83:521, 1989.

31. Dorsch W et al: Antiasthmatic effects of onion extracts—detection of benzyl and other isothiocyanates (mustard oils) as antiasthmatic compounds of plant origin, *Eur J Pharm* 107:17, 1985.

32. Drasnar T, Palecek D: Classical acupuncture in the treatment of rhinitis vasomotorica and rhinitis pollinosa, *Cesk Otolaryngol* 30:104, 1981.

33. Durlach J: Commentary on recent clinical advances: magnesium depletion, magnesium deficiency and asthma, *Magnes Res* 8:403, 1995.

34. Evans R et al: National trends in the morbidity and mortality of asthma in the United States: prevalance, hospitalization and death from asthma over two decades–1965-1984, *Chest* 91(suppl):65S, 1987.

35. Ferguson JE, Chalmers RJ, Rowlands DJ: Reversible dilated cardiomyopathy following treatment of atopic eczema with Chinese herbal medicine, *Br J Dermatol* 136:592, 1997.

36. Fischer MV, Behr A, von Reumont J: Acupuncture: a therapeutic concept in the treatment of painful conditions and functional disorders—report on 971 cases, *Acupunct Electrother Res* 9:11, 1984.

37. Fowler MG, Davenport MG, Garg R: School functioning of U.S. children with asthma, *Pediatrics* 90:939, 1992.

38. Fuller C et al: Sinusitis in status asthmaticus, *J Allergy Clin Immunol* 85:222, 1990 (abstract).

39. Gershwin ME, Terr A: Alternative and complementary therapy for asthma, *Clin Rev Allergy Immunol* 14:241, 1996.

40. Gupta S et al: *Tylophora indica* in bronchial asthma: a double blind study, *Indian J Med Res* 69:981, 1979.

41. Hackman RM, Stern JS, Gershwin ME: Complementary and alternative medicine and asthma, *Clin Rev Allergy Immunol* 14:321, 1996.

42. Halpern GM et al: Influence of long-term yogurt consumption in young adults, *Int J Immunother* 7:205, 1991.

43. He S, Wang S, Peng Y: Treatment of allergic rhinitis with helium neon laser on acupoints, *J Tradit Chin Med* 10:116, 1990.

44. Homma M et al: A strategy for discovering biologically active compounds with high probability in traditional Chinese herbal remedies: an application of Saiboku-To in bronchial asthma, *Anal Biochem* 202:179, 1992.

45. Jia D: Current applications of acupuncture by otorhinolaryngologists, *J Tradit Chin Med* 13:59, 1993.

46. Kadrabova J et al: Plasma zinc, copper and copper/zinc ratio in intrinsic asthma, *J Trace Elem Med Biol* 10:50, 1996.

47. Kane JA, Kane SP, Jain S: Hepatitis induced by traditional Chinese herbs: possible toxic components, *Gut* 36:146, 1995.

48. Kay AB: Asthma and inflammation, *J Allergy Clin Immunol* 87:893, 1991.

49. Keen CL, Gershwin ME: Zinc deficiency and immune function, *Annu Rev Nutr* 10:413, 1990.

50. Kemper KJ: Chronic asthma: an update, *Pediatr Rev* 17:111, 1996.

51. Kirby AJ, Schmidt RJ: The antioxidant activity of Chinese herbs for eczema and of placebo herbs. I, *J Ethnopharmacol* 56:103, 1997.

52. Kreisman H, Mitchell C, Bouhuys A: Inhibition of histamin-induced airway constriction negative results with oxtriphylline and ascorbic acid, *Lung* 154:223, 1977.

53. Kubo M et al: Studies on Alismatis rhizoma. I. Anti-allergic effects of methanol extract and six terpene components from Alismatis rhizoma (dried rhizome of *Alisma orientale*), *Biol Pharm Bull* 20:511, 1997.

54. Lai X: Observation on the curative effect of acupuncture on type I allergic diseases, *J Tradit Chin Med* 13:243, 1993.

55. Lal A, Kumar L, Malhotra S: Knowledge of asthma among parents of asthmatic children, *Indian Pediatr* 32:649, 1995.

56. Lane DJ: What can alternative medicine offer for the treatment of asthma? *J Asthma* 31:153, 1994.

57. Latchman Y et al: Association of immunological changes with clinical efficacy in atopic eczema patients treated with traditional Chinese herbal therapy (Zemaphyte), *Int Arch Allergy Immunol* 109:243, 1996.

58. Latchman Y et al: Efficacy of traditional Chinese herbal therapy in vitro: a model system for atopic eczema–inhibition of CD23 expression on blood monocytes, *Br J Dermatol* 132:592, 1995.

59. Lau BH, Wong DS, Slater JM: Effect of acupuncture on allergic rhinitis: clinical and laboratory evaluations, *Am J Chin Med* 3:263, 1975.

60. Lee TH et al: Effect of dietary enrichment with eicosapentaenoic and dicosahexanoic acids on in vitro neutrophil and monocyte leukotriene generation and neutrophil function, *N Engl J Med* 312:1217, 1985.

61. Leikauf GD et al: Alteration of chloride secretion across canine tracheal epthelium by lipoxygenase products of arachidonic acid, *Am J Physiol* 250:F47, 1986.

62. Lewith GT, Watkins AD: Unconventional therapies in asthma: an overview, *Allergy* 51:761, 1996.

63. Linde K et al: Are the clinical effects of homeopathy placebo effects? A meta-analysis of placebo-controlled trials, *Lancet* 350:834, 1997.

64. Machura E et al: The effect of dietary fish oil supplementation on the clinical course of asthma in children, *Pediatr Pol* 71:97, 1996.

65. Makino S: Preventive therapy in Japan. In Morley J, editor: *Preventive therapy in asthma,* London, 1991, Academic.

66. Malo JL, Cartier A, Dolovich J: Occupational asthma due to zinc, *Eur Respir J* 6:447, 1993.
67. Marom Z et al: Slow reacting substance, leukotriene C_4 and D_4, increase the release of mucus from human airways in vitro, *Am Rev Respir Dis* 126:449, 1982.
68. Massey DG, Chien YK, Fournier-Massey G: Mamane: scientific therapy for asthma? *Hawaii Med J* 53:350, 1994.
69. Masuev KA: The effect of polyunsaturated fatty acids on the biochemical indices of bronchial asthma patients, *Ter Arkh* 69:33, 1997.
70. Matsuyama T et al: Superoxide dismutase suppressed asthmatic response with inhibition of manganese superoxide induction in rat lung, *Nippon Kyobu Shikkan Gakkai Zasshi* 31(suppl):139, 1993.
71. McManus OB et al: An activator of calcium-dependent potassium channels isolated from a medicinal herb, *Biochemistry* 32:6128, 1993.
72. Meltzer SM et al: Superoxide generation and its modulation by adenosine in the neutrophils of subjects with asthma, *J Allergy Clin Immunol* 83:960, 1989.
73. Mitchell EA: Racial inequalities in childhood asthma, *Soc Sci Med* 32:831, 1991.
74. Mohsenin V: Effect of vitamin C on NO_2-induced airway hyperresponsiveness in normal subjects: a randomized double-blind experiment, *Am Rev Respir Dis* 136:1408, 1987.
75. Mohsenin V, Dubois AB, Douglas JS: Effect of ascorbic acid on response to methacholine challenge in asthmatic subjects, *Am Rev Respir Dis* 127:143, 1983.
76. Moneret-Vautrin DA, Kanny G, Thevenin F: Asthma caused by food allergy, *Rev Med Interne* 17:551, 1996.
77. National Heart, Lung and Blood Institute: Asthman statistics: data fact sheet, Bethesda, Md, May 1992, National Institutes of Health.
78. National Hospital Discharge Survey: Annual summary: 1987. Vital and Health Statistics, Pub PHS 89-1760, Series 13, No 99, National Center for Health Statistics, Hyattsville, Md, 1989, US Department of Health and Human Services.
79. Nijkamp FP, Henricks PA: Receptors in airway disease: beta-adrenoceptors in lung inflammation, *Am Rev Respir Dis* 141:S145, 1990.
80. Ogilvy CS, DuBois AB, Douglas JS: Effects of ascorbic acid and indomethacin on the airways of healthy male subjects with and without induced bronchoconstriction, *J Allergy Clin Immunol* 67:363, 1981.
81. Okayama H et al: Bronchodilating effects of intravenous magnesium sulphate in bronchial asthma, *JAMA* 257:1076, 1987.
82. Parra FM et al: Bronchial asthma caused by two unrelated vegetables, *Ann Allergy* 70:324, 1993.
83. Pastorello EA et al: Allergenic cross-reactivity among peach, apricot, plum, and cherry in patients with oral allergy syndrome: an in vivo and in vitro study, *J Allergy Clin Immunol* 94:699, 1994.
84. Patterns of ambulatory care in pediatrics: the National Ambulatory Medical Care Survey, United States, January 1980–December 1981 (data from the National Health Survey), Vital and Health Statistics, Pub PHS 84-1736, Series 13, No 75, National Center for Health Statistics, Hyattsville, Md, 1983, US Department of Health and Human Services.
85. Peer O, Bar Dayan Y, Shoenfeld Y: Satisfaction among patients of a homeopathic clinic, *Harefuah* 130:86, 1996.
86. Perharic L et al: Possible association of liver damage with the use of Chinese herbal medicine for skin disease, *Vet Hum Toxicol* 37:562, 1995.
87. Phinney SD et al: Reduced adipose 18:3w3 with weight loss by very low calorie dieting, *Lipids* 25:798, 1990.
88. Reilly DT et al: Is evidence for homeopathy reproducible? *Lancet* 344:1601, 1994.
89. Reilly DT et al: Is homoeopathy a placebo response? Controlled trial of homeopathic potency, with pollen in hay fever as model, *Lancet* 2:881, 1986.
90. Rolla G et al: Acute effects of intravenous magnesium sulfate for airway obstruction of asthmatic patients, *Ann Allergy* 61:388, 1988.
91. Schachter EN, Schlesinger A: The attenuation of exercise-induced bronchospasm by ascorbic acid, *Ann Allergy* 49:146, 1982.
92. Scheidhauer D, Gestewitz B: Acupuncture: a method in the treatment of vasomotor rhinitis, *Z Arztl Fortbild (Jena)* 83:37, 1989.

93. Schwartz J, Weiss ST: Dietary factors and their relation to respiratory symptoms: the Second National Health and Nutrition Examination Survey, *Am J Epidemiol* 132:67, 1990.

94. Schwartz J, Weiss ST: The relationship of dietary fish intake to level of pulmonary function in the first National Health and Nutrition Survey (NHANES I), *Eur Respir J* 7:1821, 1994.

95. Sheehan MP, Atherton DJ: A controlled trial of traditional Chinese medicinal plants in widespread non-exudative atopic eczema, *Br J Dermatol* 126:179, 1992.

96. Sheehan MP, Atherton DJ: One-year follow-up of children treated with Chinese medicinal herbs for atopic eczema, *Br J Dermatol* 130:488, 1994.

97. Sheehan MP et al: Efficacy of traditional Chinese herbal therapy in adult atopic dermatitis, *Lancet* 340:13, 1992.

98. Shevrygin BV, Karpova EP: Characteristics of acupuncture reflexotherapy in vasomotor and allergic rhinitis in children, *Vestn Otorinolaringol* 21, 1988.

99. Shevrygin BV et al: Status of the autonomic nervous system and reflexotherapy in children with vasomotor rhinitis, *Pediatriia* 46, 1989.

100. Shivpuri DN, Menon MPS, Parkash S: Cross-over double-blind study on *Tylophora indica* in the treatment of asthma and allergic rhinitis, *J Allergy* 43:145, 1969.

101. Shivpuri DN, Singhal SC, Parkash D: Treatment of asthma with an alcoholic extract of *Tylophora indica*: a cross-over, double-blind study, *Ann Allergy* 30:407, 1972.

102. Shturman-Ellstein R et al: The beneficial effect of nasal breathing on exercise induced bronchoconstriction, *Am Rev Respir Dis* 118:72, 1978.

103. Slavin RG: Chronic sinus disease and asthma. In: Gershwin ME, Halpern GM, editors: *Bronchial asthma: principles of diagnosis and treatment,* ed 3, Totowa, NJ, 1994, Humana.

104. Soutar A, Seaton A, Brown K: Bronchial reactivity and dietary antioxidants, *Thorax* 52:166, 1997.

105. Spector SL: Common triggers of asthma, *Postgrad Med* 90:50, 1991.

106. Spigelblatt LS: Alternative medicine: should it be used by children? *Curr Probl Pediatr* 25:180, 1995.

107. Stephen AM, Wald NJ: Trends in individual consumption of dietary fat in the United States: 1920-1984, *Am J Clin Nutr* 52:457, 1990

108. Stone J et al: Reduced selenium status of patients with asthma, *Clin Sci* 77:495, 1989.

109. Szczeklik A, Gryglewski RJ, Czerniawska-Mysik G: Clinical patterns of hypersensitivity to nonsteroidal anti-inflammatory drugs and their pathogenesis, *J Allergy Clin Immunol* 60:276, 1977.

110. Szczeklik A, Sladek K: Aspirin, related nonsteroidal anti-inflammatory agents, sulfites, and other food additives as precipitating factors in asthma. In Gershwin ME, Halpern GM, editors: *Bronchial asthma: principles of diagnosis and treatment,* ed 3, Totowa, NJ, 1994, Humana.

111. Tang ZM, Chen JX, Tan JS: Therapy of cantharides extract for perennial allergic rhinitis and its effect on total IgE in serum, *Chung Kuo Chung Hsi I Chieh Ho Tsa Chih* 15:334, 1995.

112. Ting S, Mansfield LE, Yarbrough J: Effects of ascorbic acid on pulmonary functions in mild asthma, *J Asthma* 20:39, 1983.

113. Toda S et al: Effects of the Chinese herbal medicine "Saiboku-To" on histamine release from and the degranulation of mouse peritoneal mast cells induced by compound 48/80, *J Ethnopharmacol* 24:303, 1988.

114. Troisi RJ et al: A prospective study of diet and adult-onset asthma, *Am J Respir Crit Care Med* 151:1401, 1995.

115. U.S. Department of Agriculture: 1986 Nationwide Food Consumption Survey: Continuing Survey of Food Intakes of Individuals–women 19 to 50 years and their children 1 to 5 years, 4 days, Report No 86-3, Hyattsville, Md, 1986, Nutrition Monitoring Division, Human Nutrition Information Service.

116. Waller NG, Teuber S, Gershwin ME: The genetics and epidemiology of asthma. In Gershwin ME, Halpern GM, editors: *Bronchial asthma: principles of diagnosis and treatment,* ed 3, Totowa, NJ, 1994, Humana.

117. Whang R: Magnesium deficiency: pathogenesis, prevalence, and clinical implications, *Am J Med* 82:24, 1987.

118. Xu J: Influence of acupuncture on human nasal mucociliary transport, *Chung Hua Erh Pi Yen Hou Ko Tsa Chih* 24:90, 1989.

119. Yang YQ: Progress on anti-allergy treatment with acupuncture, *Chung Kuo Chung Hsi I Chieh Ho Tsa Chih* 13:190, 1993.
120. Yu S, Cao J, Yu Z: Acupuncture treatment of chronic rhinitis in 75 cases, *J Tradit Chin Med* 13:103, 1993.
121. Zhao C, Yue F, Yao S: Treatment of allergic rhinitis by medicinal injection at fengmen acupoint, *J Tradit Chin Med* 10:264, 1990.
122. Zhou RL, Zhang JC: Desensitive treatment with positive allergens in acupoints of the head for allergic rhinitis and its mechanism, *Chung Hsi I Chieh Ho Tsa Chih* 11:721, 708, 1991.
123. Ziment I: *Respiratory pharmacology and therapeutics,* Philadelphia, 1978, WB Saunders.
124. Ziment I: Five thousand years of attacking asthma: an overview, *Respir Care* 31:117, 1986.
125. Ziment I: The management of common respiratory diseases by traditional Chinese drugs, *Oriental Healing Art Int Bull* 13(2):133, 1988.
126. Ziment I: Historic overview of mucoactive drugs. In Braga PC, Allegra L, editors: *Drugs in bronchial mucology,* New York, 1989, Raven.
127. Ziment I: Unconventional therapy in asthma. In Gershwin ME, Halpern GM, editors: *Bronchial asthma: principles of diagnosis and treatment,* ed 3, Totowa, NJ, 1994, Humana.
128. Ziment I: Unconventional therapy in asthma. *Clin Rev Allergy Immunol* 14:289, 1996.
129. Zuskin E, Lewis AJ, Bouhuys A: Inhibition of histamine-induced airway constriction by ascorbic acid, *J Allergy Clin Immunol* 51:218, 1973.

SUGGESTED READINGS

Gershwin ME, Halpern GM, editors: *Bronchial asthma: principles of diagnosis and treatment,* ed 3, Totowa, NJ, 1994, Humana.
Robbers JE, Speedie, MK, Tyler, VE: *Pharmacognosy and pharmacobiotechnology,* Baltimore, 1996, Williams & Wilkins.
Tyler VE: *The honest herbal: a sensible guide to the use of herbs and related remedies,* ed 3, New York, 1993, Pharmaceutical Products Press.
Tyler VF: *Herbs of choice: the therapeutic use of phytomedicinals,* New York, 1994, Pharmaceutical Products Press.

CHAPTER 4

Complementary/Alternative Therapies in General Medicine: Cardiovascular Disease

William L. Haskell, Frederic M. Luskin, and Farshad F. Marvasti, *with assistance from* Kathryn A. Newell, Ellen M. DiNucci, and Micah Hill

Atherosclerotic vascular disease (AVD) is the major cause of death and disability in most technologically advanced societies and by early in the twenty-first century will be the leading cause of death worldwide. As underdeveloped societies adopt the lifestyle typified in "advanced westernized cultures," the incidence of the disease markedly increases with substantial evidence that personal choices regarding lifestyle are more important determinants of disease risk than heredity. Two important features of the disease have become apparent in the past 30 years: (1) the disease process is multifactorial with a large number of personal characteristics and habits influencing disease initiation, progression, stabilization, or regression and (2) for many people the disease is preventable or can be delayed to very old age. Although pharmacologic and surgical procedures have dominated therapy for AVD in the United States, the prevention of the underlying disease or its clinical manifestations requires the effective management of personal health-related behaviors.

Given the multifactorial nature of the disease process, the possibility exists that a number of therapies now considered complementary or alternative can be effective in the prevention of the disease, in management of the clinical status in patients with the disease, or in assisting patients in coping with their disease. The purpose of this section is to provide a brief overview of selected complementary/alternative medicine (CAM) therapies that have been proposed as potentially beneficial in the prevention or management of AVD (coronary heart disease, peripheral vascular disease and stroke). This brief review focuses on selected CAM therapies that are currently being promoted and have received the most research or clinical attention in the United States.

ATHEROSCLEROTIC VASCULAR DISEASE
Pathophysiology

Atherosclerotic deposits or plaques develop in selected arteries when the amount of low-density lipoprotein cholesterol (LDL-C) entering the subintimal space exceeds that removed, resulting in the accumulation of LDL-C droplets in the form of cholesterol esters. The "response to injury" theory proposes that mechanical or chemical injury to the endothelium increases its permeability and exposes the subintimal and medial layers of the artery wall to the infiltration of LDL-C, monocytes, platelets, and other vasoactive factors.[68] The accumulation of LDL-C in the subintima increases the tendency for monocytes to adhere to the endothelium and migrate into the subintimal space where they take up the extra cellular lipid as they become macrophages. Modification of LDL-C by oxidation and other processes facilitates its uptake by macrophages. Continued accumulation of lipid by macrophages leads to their conversion to foam cells, the major constituent of fatty streaks and the early lipid-filled plaque. The "lipid filtration" hypothesis assumes that at increased concentrations of LDL-C in the blood, LDL-C filtrates through the endothelium into the subintimal space followed by monocytes and a series of events similar to that proposed by the "response to injury" theory.[19] Conversion of the plaque from being mainly lipid-filled to a complex structure involving smooth muscle cells, platelets, inert lipid crystals, calcification, and formation of a fibrous cap is the result of a series of events currently under intense investigation.[60] Platelets, macrophages, and modified (oxidized) LDL-C all release a variety of chemoattractants and growth factors resulting in the migration and proliferation of smooth muscle cells that contribute to the formation of raised lesions.

It now appears that many clinical cardiac events, including myocardial infarction, cardiac arrest, and unstable angina pectoris, occur when a plaque ruptures, releasing platelet aggregation factors into the artery lumen and stimulating the formation of a blood clot that can rapidly occlude the artery.[26] These so-called "culprit lesions" that rupture tend to be the early lipid-filled plaques rather than the more advanced complex lesions. Thus prevention of clinical cardiac events may be achieved by the reduction of new lesion formation, stabilization of existing lesions, reduction in the rate of existing lesion growth or progression, decrease in lesion size or regression, and the reduction of platelet aggregation or an increase in fibrinolysis.

Given the complex, multifactorial nature of the pathobiology of the events that contribute to the development, progression, regression, and stabilization of atherosclerotic lesions and thrombosis, there are a variety of mechanisms by which therapies could cause a reduction in AVD morbidity and mortality. Also, it is possible that selected therapies might reduce the occurrence or severity of clinical cardiac events by their effects on the myocardium instead of the coronary arteries, including reduction of myocardial work at rest and during exercise, an increase in myocardial electrical stability, or an enhancement of intrinsic myocardial contractility.

Epidemiology

Atherosclerotic vascular disease, clinically evident as coronary heart disease, peripheral vascular disease, or stroke, occurs most frequently in technologically advanced societies that consume a diet high in calories, animal products, and salt and low in plant-based foods and have reduced levels of energy expenditure due to a relatively low level of habitual physical activity.[83] As people from primitive, low-mechanized cultures where a plant-based diet predominates acculturate to a more "westernized" way of life, the occurrence of AVD rapidly increases and becomes the dominant cause of death within several generations.[90] Approximately as many women as men die from AVD; however, women tend to develop AVD 10 to 15 years later than men, with their early protection believed to be due primarily to the effects of endogenous estrogens.

Selected genetic predisposition for developing AVD has been identified, but environmental factors explain more of the intergroup and interindividual differences in AVD morbidity and mortality than heredity. Major factors found to be causally linked to AVD include abnormal lipoprotein profiles (elevated levels of low-density cholesterol and low levels of high-density cholesterol), elevated blood pressure, cigarette smoking, obesity, and a sedentary lifestyle. Strongly associated with the increased risk of AVD are diabetes; a diet low in fruits, vegetables, and grains and high in animal fats; elevated levels of homocystine in the blood; and chronic high levels of psychologic stress, depression, and hostility. Thus there are substantial opportunities to favorably influence the basic disease process or clinical manifestations of AVD using various complementary or alternative therapies.

CAM THERAPIES FOR ATHEROSCLEROTIC VASCULAR DISEASE

CAM therapies that have been promoted as beneficial for the prevention and treatment of AVD are numerous and varied. They include vegetarian diets, dietary supplements, herbal remedies, stress reduction/relaxation, both Western and Eastern approaches to exercise, and chelation therapy. Also, it has been proposed that entire traditional medical systems such as traditional Chinese medicine (TCM) and Ayurevda are effective in both the prevention and treatment of AVD. While many claims have been made and numerous clinical observations or case studies have been reported, few therapies have been rigorously tested by appropriately conducted randomized trials with a reduction in clinical AVD events as the primary outcome.

Claims regarding the beneficial effects of CAM therapies on AVD have been based on how the therapy influences (1) one or more AVD risk factors (e.g., elevated cholesterol, hypertension, or a high level of stress); (2) the basic disease processes of atherosclerosis/thrombosis; (3) clinical events including angina pectoris, myocardial infarction, and sudden cardiac death; and (4) psychologic status, especially depression, anxiety, and hostility.

Chelation Therapy

Introduced as a treatment for AVD in 1955, chelation therapy is the repeated administration of the amino acid, ethylenediamine tetraacetic acid (EDTA).[28] Typically, 3 g Na_2 EDTA or 50 mg/kg body weight of EDTA is infused through a vein over 4 hours several times per week up to a total of 20 infusions over 10 to 12 weeks. Due to its poor absorption by the gastrointestinal tract, EDTA is administered intravenously and it is often given with multivitamin and mineral supplementation because it tends to remove a variety of micronutrients from the body. The original clinical rationale provided by those in support of chelation therapy is that EDTA has a high affinity for divalent ions, in particular, calcium, which it binds and which then is eliminated by the kidneys in an unmetabolized form. It is theorized that calcium deposits which are found in many advanced atherosclerotic plaques will be removed, thus reducing their size and helping to increase blood flow through the artery. No study has been reported using techniques that can detect calcium deposits in atherosclerotic plaques, such as electron beam computed tomography or intravascular ultrasound. More recently, claims have been made that chelation therapy will reduce oxidation of lipoproteins, possibly by the removal of copper from the blood, and increase the dilating capacity of arteries.

A large number of clinical observations or anecdotal reports have been cited—but many of them have not been published—supporting the effectiveness of chelation therapy to reduce atherosclerosis progression in coronary and peripheral arteries, enhance disease regression, or improve clinical cardiovascular status.[28] These reports lack the scientific rigor required to attribute a causal benefit to chelation therapy. This type of reporting by proponents of chelation therapy leads to a selection bias favoring a beneficial effect. An even greater problem in the proper interpretation of these data are studies that do not have a randomized control group, since frequently, other AVD risk reduction therapies are initiated along with chelation therapy. Many patients initiating chelation therapy are advised to make changes in their diet and exercise, take dietary supplements, and participate in a program of stress reduction. Thus in studies without randomized control groups there is no way to assign improvement in patient status just to the chelation therapy.

Only a few randomized, placebo-controlled trials testing chelation therapy have been published. The first two randomized trials reported a beneficial effect of chelation therapy, but conclusions from these studies are limited because of poor study design. In a double-blind study, Kitchell and colleagues[37] administered EDTA to four patients and placebo to five patients with angina pectoris. Two of the patients receiving EDTA "improved" compared with none who received placebo. In another small trial Olszewer and colleagues[53] attempted a randomized placebo-controlled trial in 10 subjects with peripheral vascular disease but aborted the trial because of refusal of patients to be randomized; the authors reported a "profound improvement" in patients receiving EDTA.

Two well-designed, placebo-controlled, randomized trials involving patients with peripheral arterial disease failed to demonstrate any net benefit of chelation therapy. Guldager and colleagues[29] randomized 153 patients with stable intermittent claudication to either EDTA or saline (20 infusions over 5 to 7 weeks). Vitamins, minerals, and trace elements were added to the EDTA. Pain-free treadmill walking distance, maximal walking distance, ankle/brachial blood pressure index, and patient symptoms were assessed before and 3 and 6 months after the infusions. Angiography of the lower limbs was performed in a subset of patients.[76] No treatment differences were observed at either 3 or 6 months. Also, van Rij and colleagues[86] did not find any benefit of EDTA infusions on walking distance, ankle/brachial index, cardiac function, hematology, blood glucose and lipids, and symptoms in patients with intermittent claudication up to 3 months after 20 infusions of either EDTA (N = 15) or normal saline (N = 17).

Under experienced medical supervision, including the use of generally accepted exclusion criteria, administration of EDTA appears relatively safe but does not provide any biologic, chemical, or symptomatic benefit to patients with AVD.[23] Given the lack of benefit, the low but real risk for some patients, and the significant cost, chelation therapy should be discarded in favor of therapies that have been proven to have major beneficial effects on AVD.

Behavioral and Mind-Body Therapies

Behavioral and mind-body therapies have been a component of non-Western medical systems for centuries. Techniques such as yoga, meditation, Eastern exercise, and social support function to promote health and longevity by making use of the connection between mind and body. However, research into the effectiveness of these therapies is often sketchy, and further work using randomized controlled trials is necessary. Nonetheless, a body of research does exist that offers some indications as to the effectiveness of the mind-body approaches to the prevention and management of AVD.

One of the primary links creating the need for mind-body therapies is the insidious effect of stress on cardiovascular function and health. Stress and anxiety have been shown to increase blood pressure, contribute to the development of atherosclerosis, and predispose to arrhythmias that can lead to sudden death.[61] Mind-body therapies are designed to work with both the cognitive and physiologic aspects of the creation and amelioration of the stress response.[57]

Meditation. Meditation practice may be the most basic of the mind-body approaches. It is a cognitive tool whose purpose is the development of focused attention through concentration on a specified thought or object. Research has shown that meditation brings about a healthy relaxation state by dampening sympathetic response and decreasing respiration rate, heart rate, plasma cortisol, and blood pressure.[69] In a well-designed, randomized, single blind trial the blood pressure–lowering effects of transcendental meditation were compared with a program of progressive muscle relaxation and a health education control over a period of 3 months in 111 older African American men and women with moderate hypertension.[64] After controlling for age and baseline blood pressure, the meditation program produced significantly greater reduction in blood pressure than either the health education control or the program of progressive muscle relaxation (Fig. 4-1). The blood pressure–lowering effects were similar in men and women and subjects assigned to high or low risk for developing cardiovascular disease.[5]

The practice of meditation has been shown to have a salutary effect on risk factors of AVD such as hypertension,[81,88] elevated cholesterol levels, cigarette smoking,[18] oxidative stress,[64] and chronic stress.[84] The practice of meditation also creates what has been termed the "relaxation response," which is hypothesized to be the contrasting bodily mechanism to the "fight-or-flight response."[11] Several studies have shown that meditation can also have a beneficial effect on patients already suffering from cardiovascular disease.[10,41] In an interesting study, 21 patients with coronary artery disease who were taught to meditate displayed a significant improvement in exercise tolerance as well as a reduction in ischemia after 8 months of practice when compared with a "wait-list" control group.[92] In another study, a 3-year follow-up showed the effects of meditation practice to significantly reduce measured levels of anxiety and depression as well as reducing medical utilization.[46]

Guided Imagery. Imagery is the use of imagination to invoke one or more of the senses. Imagery is hypothesized as a means of communication between emotion, perception, and bodily change.[1] Laboratory experiments and controlled trials have shown imagery

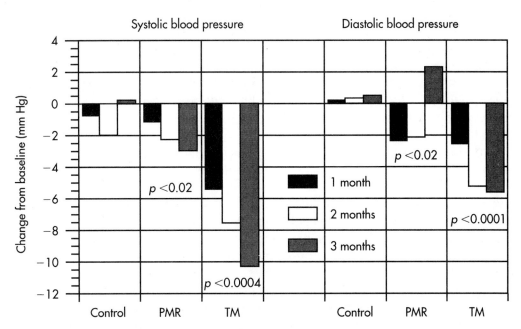

Fig. 4-1   Change in mean blood pressure over 3 months in patients with moderate hypertension assigned to control (education class), progressive muscle relaxation (PMR), or transcendental meditation (TM) groups. *P* values are for the differences in the changes in blood pressure in each treatment group versus the control group using repeated analysis of variance (ANOVA).

to be effective in reducing stress, heart rate reactivity, blood pressure, and resting heart rate.[17,22,47,55] It is speculated that one's ability to image can become evident in an altered state of consciousness, as in hypnosis, and thus lead to physiologic changes such as a reduction in sympathetic activity.[1]

In the "Ornish" multidisciplinary approach to AVD management, the practice of imagery was an important component.[54] Other studies have shown imagery to be effective in managing aspects of AVD. In one study male autonomic defibrillator recipients were given audiotapes of guided imagery exercises for use at home.[79] The treatment group demonstrated lower state and trait anxiety after 1 month of practice. In another experiment healthy subjects were trained in biofeedback-assisted imagery while experiencing a standard stressor.[71] This laboratory experiment showed significantly lower heart rate reactivity for the treatment group in comparison to controls that was maintained at 28-week follow-up.

Music Therapy. Music therapy may include the active playing of instruments, singing, chanting, or drumming and/or the passive listening to live or prerecorded music.[4] Research has shown music therapy to positively affect risk factors for AVD such as blood pressure, heart rate, and anxiety.[45,48,66] A randomized, controlled trial showed both music therapy and relaxation to be effective in reducing physiologic indicators of stress such as apical or peak heart rate and peripheral temperature in patients with AVD.[30] However, some studies have shown little or no effect for similar interventions.[7] Patients with coronary artery disease exhibited no difference in recovery rate when assigned to one of three groups listening to either taped therapeutic suggestions, taped music, or a blank tape.[13]

Eastern Exercise. Yoga and two forms of the martial arts, T'ai chi and Qi Gong, are culturally rooted in Eastern philosophic and medical systems. Each form of exercise is considered a mind-body therapy because of its multifaceted approach that often includes imagery, meditation, and physical exercise. As with meditation, the cognitive goal of practice is to develop concentrated attention that creates certain physiologic correlates. Research has shown acute physiologic changes from practice, such as decreases in sympathetic activity, oxygen consumption, blood pressure, heart rate, and respiratory rates.[6,44,62,63,81]

Yoga. Yoga, a Sanskrit term meaning union, has strong ties with spiritual and mystical traditions originating in India. The two primary forms practiced in the West are hatha yoga (physical postures and breathing) and raja yoga (the yoga of mental and spiritual mastery).[16] Yoga practice has been shown to reduce blood pressure and heart rate.[15,56,62] It is important that studies have shown yoga to be valuable in promoting cardiovascular fitness in healthy subjects. A study involving 40 male high school students revealed higher cardiovascular endurance and anaerobic power in the yoga group when compared with control-group participants after 1 year of practice.[12]

Another study[81] involved male physical education teachers who had an average of 8.9 years of physical activity before treatment. Following a 3-month yoga intervention, the subjects showed a significant reduction in systolic and diastolic blood pressure, heart rate, and respiratory rate and a decrease in autonomic arousal. Studies of yoga practice conducted with healthy women have also shown a decrease in blood pressure and heart rate in comparison to controls.[66]

T'ai chi. T'ai chi, also known as "shadow boxing,"[40] originated in China hundreds of years ago[91] and is a component of TCM. Most studies on T'ai chi have limited generalizability because they did not use randomized trials with a control group. However, positive cardiovascular change has been demonstrated when comparing a participant's own pretest and posttest performance. Reductions in heart rate, blood pressure, and urinary catecholamine levels have been shown.[36] T'ai chi may also help in promoting cardiorespiratory functioning in elderly subjects,[35,36,40] as well as in enhancing positive mood effects[35,36] and aerobic capacity.[94]

Social Support. In a study on cardiovascular reactivity, social support has been defined as the expression of positive affect, agreement, acknowledgment, and feelings through social encouragement.[27] Considered an independent risk factor for AVD, minimal social support has been associated with cardiovascular health in classic studies such as the Alameda County Study.[54] Other studies have shown a correlation between minimal social support and increased sympathetic response,[24] as well as showing that patients who lacked social resources were more at risk for mortality independent of other accepted risk factors.[89] Uchino and Garvey[85] suggested that cardiovascular reactivity to acute psychologic stress may by reduced through the availability of social support. The specific social support mechanism of religious attendance was found to create improvement in 22 of 27 studies including such AVD indices as ischemic heart disease and hypertension.[42]

Cognitive Behavioral Therapy. By attempting to modify a patient's thinking, cognitive behavioral therapy seeks to reduce AVD risk factors that are amenable to lifestyle change. These include smoking cessation, enhanced social relationships, reduced hostility, reducing "type A" behavior, increased treatment adherence, and improved nutrition.[69] Although group settings make it difficult for researchers to isolate the specific component of cognitive behavioral therapy, many studies have documented its positive effect in reducing AVD risk factors. For example, hypertensive participants experienced a significant reduction in the need for drugs.[21]

Using the statistical technique of meta-analysis, Eisenberg and colleagues[20] evaluated the effects of various cognitive behavioral therapies (such as relaxation, meditation, and biofeedback) on blood pressure levels in patients with hypertension.[20] They identified 26 randomized control trials involving 1264 patients that met their criteria of an acceptable research design. The primary results of these analyses are presented in Fig. 4-2, *A,* for systolic blood pressure and Fig. 4-2, *B,* for diastolic blood pressure. When

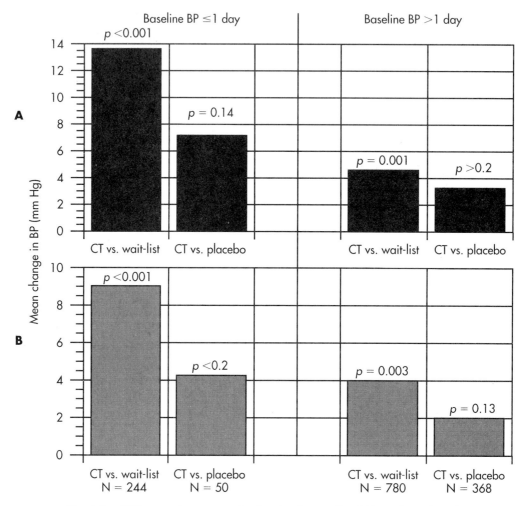

Fig. 4-2 Difference in mean reduction in, **A,** systolic (SBP) and, **B,** diastolic (DBP) blood pressure between cognitive behavioral therapy and either wait-list (no treatment) control or placebo. Data are presented for meta-analysis that grouped studies by length of baseline measurement period (>1 day vs. 1 day). *P* values are for differences in the change in blood pressure between the treatment and control or placebo group. *CT,* Cognitive therapy.

cognitive therapies are compared with no treatment or a wait-list control, a significant effect of the therapy is observed (whether the baseline blood pressure value is for 1 day or less or longer than 1 day). However, if the "placebo effect" is taken into account and cognitive therapies are compared with a placebo treatment, the net blood pressure–lowering effect is smaller and not statistically significant.

Mind-Body Therapies: Reduction in Clinical Cardiovascular Events

There is some evidence that patients with AVD assigned to a mind-body therapy will have a greater reduction in recurrent clinical events than patients assigned to usual medical care. Freidman and colleagues[25] found that counseling to alter type A behavior over a period of 4.5 years in patients following myocardial infarction significantly reduced the rate of nonfatal infarctions and cardiac death as compared with patients assigned to a noncounseling control group. This was a large, well-designed, multicenter study that included 1013 patients, and the differences were clinically significant (12.9% cardiac event rate for patients receiving counseling vs. 21.8% and 28.2% in the control group). In a smaller study of stress reduction in patients with AVD, Blumenthal and colleagues[14] reported a significant benefit of stress reduction as compared with exercise rehabilitation on myocardial ischemia and cardiac events. The stress reduction and exercise programs were conducted over 4 months, and patients were followed for an average of 38 months. As compared with a nonrandomized control group, patients in the stress reduction program had significantly fewer cardiac events during follow-up, as well as fewer episodes of ischemia. These studies, along with the large amount of data on the benefits of mind-body therapies on cardiovascular function and regulation, support their use in comprehensive programs of AVD prevention and management.

Diet, Dietary Supplements, and Herbal Therapy

Substantial data exist from epidemiologic and experimental studies in animals and humans demonstrating that what a person consumes as foods or as dietary supplements can have a major effect on AVD risk factors, disease progression, and clinical events.[72] In fact, over the past decade, such therapies for AVD as plant-based diets, dietary fiber supplementation, and antioxidant supplementation, which previously were considered alternative therapies, are now considered either complementary or a part of standard medical practice for AVD risk reduction or treatment, along with low-saturated-fat diets, aerobic exercise, and stress reduction.

Plant-Based Diets. Populations that consume diets low in animal products and high in a variety of vegetables, fruits, and grains have a lower mortality from AVD than populations that have a diet higher in animal products and processed foods.[62] Plant-based diets not only decrease low-density cholesterol, but have been shown to reduce the rate of oxidation of low-density cholesterol,[19] blood pressure,[51] and platelet aggregation.[39]

A decrease in the rate of progression of coronary artery atherosclerosis and increased disease regression was reported by Ornish and colleagues[54] in patients with AVD during a 1-year trial of a multifactor risk reduction program featuring a plant-based diet very low in fat (< 10% calories from fat, 15% to 20% from protein, and 70% to 75% from predominantly complex carbohydrates). The other treatments included moderate-intensity aerobic exercise and stress reduction/relaxation. The rate of athero-sclerosis was assessed by computer- based quantitative coronary arteriography at base-line and after 1 year. The patients in the usual-care group (N = 19) demonstrated dis-ease progression (from 42.7% to 46.1% closure of artery segments), while the treatment group (N = 22) showed regression of their disease (from 40.0% to 37.8% closure of artery segments). In another angiographically based study, Schuler and colleagues[67] reported a decrease in coronary atherosclerotic progression during 1 year in patients with AVD who participated in a low-fat diet and exercise program compared with patients assigned to the usual care of their physicians.

Several studies have assigned patients with AVD to either a plant-based diet or a usual diet or another type of control diet and determined the development of nonfatal and fatal clinical events attributable to AVD. Singh and colleagues[74] randomly assigned 406 patients with myocardial infarction or unstable angina pectoris to either a low-fat diet or a low-fat diet with increased emphasis on the intake of fruits, vegetables, nuts, and grains. After 1 year, patients assigned to the low-fat and plant-based diet had fewer cardiac events (50 vs. 82 patients; $p > 0.001$) and a lower total mortality (21 vs. 38 died; $p < 0.01$). In another study of patients soon after myocardial infarction, a "Mediter-ranean Diet" was compared with the usual postinfarction prudent diet in 606 patients.[45] Patients were randomly assigned to one of the two diets and followed for a period of up to 5 years with the primary outcome being nonfatal myocardial infarction or cardiac death. At a mean follow-up period of 27 months the patients assigned to the Mediter-ranean Diet had had 8 events, and patients consuming the prudent diet had had 33 events (risk ratio = 0.27; 95% CI = 0.12 to 0.82; $p = 0.02$). Although no randomized trial of their lifestyle risk reduction program that features a plant-based diet has been con-ducted, patients treated at the Pritikin Longevity Center have been reported to do bet-ter clinically for up to 5 years.[8] The combined diet and exercise program significantly reduces adiposity, LDL-C, and blood pressure and the need for various cardiovascular medications during the 4-week inpatient program.[8]

Dietary Supplements. Numerous attempts have been made to achieve the risk-reduc-tion benefits for AVD seen with plant-based diets by providing specific substances from plants in the form of a supplement. Given the large number of different substances found in plants, there is almost no end to the substances to be tested. Examples of promising substances delivered as a supplement include water-soluble dietary fiber, antioxidants, folic acid, and plant estrogens.

Dietary fiber. Some of the cholesterol that returns to the liver ends up in the intes-tine as part of bile acid secreted by the gallbladder. Water-soluble dietary fibers found in a number of plants reduce blood cholesterol concentrations by binding this choles-terol and excreting it from the body before it has a chance to be reabsorbed. Part of the cholesterol lowering achieved by a plant-based diet is this effect of water-soluble fiber.

A number of randomized, controlled trials have shown that supplementation with water-soluble fiber (oats, guar gum, pectin, mixed fibers) in the range of 10 to 40 g per day results in a lowering of plasma cholesterol in the range of 10% (range, 0% to 17%).[34]

Antioxidants. Antioxidants appear to influence a number of processes in the body that may help reduce the rate of development of AVD. Of particular interest has been their potential role in reducing the oxidation of LDL-C that has found its way through the endothelium and into the artery wall. Oxidation of these particles is necessary before they can be taken up by macrophages and become part of the atherosclerotic plaque. The antioxidant vitamins A, C, and E and beta carotene all appear to help protect the LDL particles against oxidation by free radicals.[19] Also, antioxidant vitamins have a favorable effect on the endothelial-mediated vasodilation, helping to restore a reduction in dilation caused by hypercholesterolemia and cigarette smoking.[32,43]

In population studies people who report a greater antioxidant supplementation use have less AVD.[19] Results of trials attempting to document a causal relation between supplementation use and reduced clinical cardiovascular events have been mixed. In two prospective cohort studies[59,77] there was a 35% to 40% reduction in the incidence of major coronary events in individuals in the highest quintile of vitamin E intake versus those in the lowest quintile. The greatest benefit was in persons taking 100 to 250 IU per day. However, only one of three recently published randomized studies of antioxidant supplementation and AVD clinical events has demonstrated benefit.[33,78,82] In a study of heavy smokers who were treated with beta carotene, vitamin E, both, or neither for 5 to 8 years, there was no benefit from supplementation.[82] There was no reduction in deaths from AVD among physicians receiving supplemental beta carotene over a 12-year period.[33] In contrast to these studies, patients with AVD treated with vitamin E (400 to 800 IU per day of alpha-tocopherol) had a 77% reduction in clinical cardiac events compared with those patients not receiving vitamin E over a median period of 510 days.[78]

In addition to the antioxidant vitamins, other substances with antioxidant properties being promoted to help protect against AVD include various bioflavonoids, the trace mineral selenium, and coenzyme Q10 (Co-Q10). Bioflavonoids are found in fruits (large amounts in berries and grapes), vegetables, tea, and wine. They appear to reduce LDL-C oxidation and improve endothelial function and may be one factor in the low AVD rate in southern France (the so-called French Paradox). Selenium is needed for the production of antioxidant enzymes and thus deficiency can cause increased oxidation of LDL-C. While some studies have shown that low selenium blood levels are associated with increased risk of AVD, no studies have shown that selenium supplementation reduces clinical AVD. Coenzyme Q10 can be produced by the body and is available in U.S. diets (especially in meat and seafood) or as a supplement. It has been shown to help protect LDL-C against oxidation,[93] and several clinical trials have shown improved clinical status in patients with congestive heart failure.[49]

Folic acid. Elevated blood levels of the amino acid homocysteine are strongly related to an increased risk of AVD, and this relationship is largely independent of other major risk factors.[50] How elevated homocysteine increases AVD has not been fully established, but it appears to influence endothelial toxicity, coagulation, and smooth muscle cell proliferation. Elevated homocysteine levels can be reduced by even moderate amounts (400 to 650 μg/day) of folic acid supplementation.[52] To date, no randomized trial has been conducted to test whether persons with elevated levels of homocysteine who take a folic acid supplement will have a reduction in the number of clinical events attributable to AVD.

Plant estrogens. Many populations that consume a plant-based diet and have lower rates of AVD tend to have a much higher intake of various plant (or phyto) estrogens than populations who consume more animal products.[2] Various plant estrogens have been identified, and they are found in numerous food products, including many grains, beans, vegetables, and fruits. Highest concentrations are found in flax seed (linseed) and soybeans, while products with lower concentrations include sunflower seeds, cranberries, and Japanese green tea.[3] Plant estrogens appear to have an effect on a large number of biochemical mechanisms that impact AVD processes, including the lowering of LDL-C, inhibition of LDL-C oxidation, and the reduction of platelet adhesion and endothelial cell proliferation.[3] No randomized studies have been reported in which the effects of plant estrogen supplementation on clinical events attributable to AVD have been evaluated.

Herbal Products. A major component of many native or traditional medical systems is the use of a wide variety of herbal products independently or in combination. In prevention/treatment systems such as TCM or Ayurveda, herbal therapies are important elements for AVD. For example, curcumin (a major component of the spice turmeric) possesses antiplatelet activities,[75] and MA-631, a complex herbal mixture, reduces LDL-C oxidation.[31] Both are herbal products used in Ayurveda. Another example is the use of green tea in TCM. One form of green tea has been shown to lower plasma cholesterol concentrations[38] and is claimed to reduce blood pressure.

Another herb considered among those that protect against some aspect of AVD is garlic. A number of trials have demonstrated that garlic supplementation reduces plasma cholesterol concentrations by 8% to 10%[87] and decreases lipoprotein oxidation susceptibility,[58] but has only a minor blood pressure–lowering effect.[73]

Difficulties in the evaluation of herbal therapies used in traditional medical systems include (1) a number of potentially active ingredients in a single herb, (2) lack of standardization or quality control of the individual herbs, and (3) the use of a combination of herbs in a single preparation. However, as various herbs are evaluated, it is very likely that a number of them will be shown to have active ingredients that are useful in AVD prevention or treatment.

SUMMARY

Atherosclerotic vascular disease is a complex biologic process that can be favorably modified by a number of therapeutic approaches. Recent advances in preventive actions (stopping smoking, a shift to a diet lower in animal fat), the pharmacologic management of various risk factors (reductions in cholesterol, blood pressure, and platelet aggregation), surgical treatment (coronary artery bypass surgery, balloon angioplasty), and more aggressive patient management (treatment by paramedics and coronary care units) have contributed to a significant reduction in age-adjusted mortality attributable to AVD in many countries. However, AVD is still the major cause of mortality in most technologically advanced countries and a major economic burden. A number of therapies still considered alternative or complementary have the potential to significantly reduce AVD when effectively integrated into a comprehensive prevention/management program. Of particular promise are the increased consumption of a plant-based diet, selective dietary or herbal supplementation, and mind-body therapies that can be learned easily and carried out without supervision. All of these therapies can be implemented as preventive for the general population or for patients with existing disease.

REFERENCES

1. Achterberg J: *Imagery in healing: shamanism in modern medicine,* Boston, 1985, Shambhala.
2. Adlercreutz H: Western diet and Western diseases: some hormonal and biochemical mechanisms and associations, *Scand J Clin Lab Invest* 50(suppl 201):3, 1990.
3. Adlercreutz H, Mazur W: Phyto-oestrogens and western diseases, *Ann Med* 29:95, 1997.
4. Aldridge D: The music of the body: music therapy in medical settings, *Advances* 9(1):17, 1993.
5. Alexander C et al: Trial of stress reduction for hypertension in older African Americans. II. Sex and risk subgroup analysis, *Hypertension* 28(2):228, 1996.
6. Ankun K, Chongxing W: Research on "anti-aging" effect of qigong, *J Tradit Chin Med* 11(2):153, 1991.
7. Bamason S, Zimmerman L, Nieveen J: The effects of music interventions on anxiety in the patient after coronary artery bypass grafting, *Heart Lung* 24(2):124, 1995.
8. Barnard RJ et al: Effects of an intensive, short-term exercise and nutrition program on patients with coronary heart disease, *J Cardiac Rehabil* 2:995, 1981.
9. Barnard RJ et al: Effects of an intensive exercise and nutrition program on patients with coronary artery disease, *J Cardiac Rehabil* 3:1830, 1983.
10. Benson H, Alexander S, Feldman C: Decreased premature ventricular contractions through use of the relaxation response in patients with stable ischemic heart disease, *Lancet* 2:380, 1975.
11. Benson H, Kotch J, Crasswelter K: The relaxation response. a bridge between psychiatry and medicine, *Med Clin North Am* 6l(4):929, 1977.
12. Bera T, Rajapurkar M: Body composition, cardiovascular endurance and anaerobic power of yogic practitioner, *Indian J Physiol Pharmacol* 37(3):225, 1993.
13. Blankfield R, Zyzanski S, Flocke S: Taped therapeutic suggestions and taped music as adjuncts in the care of coronary-artery-bypass patients, *Am J Clin Hypnosis* 37(3):32, 1995.
14. Blumenthal JA et al: Stress management and exercise training in cardiac patients with myocardial ischemia, *Arch Intern Med* 157:2213, 1997.
15. Brownstein A: Treatment of essential hypertension with yoga relaxation therapy in a USAF aviator: a case report, *Aviat Space Environ Med* 60:684, 1989.
16. Christensen A: *The American yoga association wellness book,* ed 1, New York, 1996, Kensington.

17. Collins JA, Rice VH: Effects of relaxation intervention in phase II cardiac rehabilitation: replication and extension, *Heart Lung* 26(l):31, 1997.

18. Cooper M, Aygen M: Effect of meditation on blood cholesterol and blood pressure, *J Isr Med Assoc* 95:1, 1978.

19. Diaz MN et al: Antioxidants and atherosclerotic heart disease, *N Engl J Med* 337:408, 1997.

20. Eisenberg D et al: Cognitive behavioral techniques for hypertension: are they effective? *Ann Intern Med* 118:964, 1993.

21. Emmelkamp P, Van Oppen P: Cognitive interventions in behavioral medicine, *Psychother Psychosom* 59:116, 1993.

22. Eppley K, Abrams A, Shear J: Differential effects of relaxation techniques on trait anxiety: a meta-analysis, *J Clin Psychol* 45(6):957, 1989.

23. Ernst E: Chelation therapy for peripheral artery occlusive disease: a systematic review, *Circulation* 96:1031, 1997.

24. Fontana A et al: Support, stress and recovery from coronary heart disease: a longitudinal causal model, *Health Psychol* 8:175, 1989.

25. Friedman M et al: Alteration in type A behavior and its effect on cardiac recurrences in post-myocardial infarction patients: Summary results of the recurrent coronary prevention project, *Am Heart J* 12:653, 1986.

26. Fuster V et al: The pathogenesis of coronary artery disease and the acute coronary syndromes, *N Engl J Med* 326:241, 1992.

27. Germ W et al: Social support in social interaction: a moderator of cardiovascular reactivity, *Psychosom Med* 54(3):324, 1992.

28. Grier MT, Meyers DG: So much writing, so little science: a review of 37 years of literature on edetate sodium chelation therapy, *Ann Pharmacother* 27:1504, 1993.

29. Guldager B et al: EDTA treatment of intermittent claudication: a double blind placebo-controlled study, *J Intern Med* 231:261, 1992.

30. Guzzetta C: Effects of relaxation and music therapy on patients in a coronary care unit with the presumptive diagnosis of acute myocardial infarction, *Heart Lung* 18:609, 1989.

31. Hanna AN et al: In vitro and in vivo inhibition of microsomal lipid peroxidation by MA-631, *Pharmacol Biochem Behav* 48:505, 1994.

32. Heitzer T, Just H, Munzel T: Antioxidant vitamin C improves endothelial dysfunction in chronic smokers, *Circulation* 94:6, 1996.

33. Hernnekens CH et al: Lack of effect of long-term supplementation with beta carotene on the incidence of malignant neoplasm and cardiovascular disease, *N Engl J Med* 334:1145, 1996.

34. Jensen C, Haskell WL, Whittum JH: Long-term effects of water-souble dietary fiber in the management of hypercholesterolemia in healthy men and women, *Am J Cardiol* 79:34, 1997.

35. Jin P: Changes in heart rate, noradrenaline, cortisol and mood during tai chi, *J Psychosomatic Res* 33:197, 1989.

36. Jin P: Efficacy of tai chi, brisk walking, meditation, and reading in reducing mental and emotional stress, *J Psychosom Res* 36(4):361, 1992.

37. Kitchell JR et al: The treatment of coronary artery disease with disodium EDTA, *Am J Cardiol* 11:501, 1963.

38. Kono S et al: Green tea consumption and serum lipid profiles: a cross-sectional study in northern Kyushu, Japan, *Prev Med* 31:526, 1992.

39. Kwon JS et al: Effects of diets high in saturated fatty acids, canola oil, or safflower oil on platelet function, thromboxane B2 function and fatty acid composition of plasma phospholipids, *Am J Clin Nutr* 54:351, 1991.

40. Lai J-S, Lan C: Two-year trends in cardiorespiratory function among older tai chi chuan practitioners and sedentary subjects, *J Am Geriatr Soc* 43:1222, 1995.

41. Lesennan J et al: The efficacy of the relaxation response in preparing for cardiac surgery, *Behav Med* 15:111, 1989.

42. Levin J: Religion and health: is there an association, is it valid, is it causal? *Soc Sci Med* 38(11):1475, 1994.

43. Levine GN et al: Ascorbic acid reverses endothelial vasomotor dysfunction in patients with coronary artery disease, *Circulation* 93:1107, 1996.

44. Lim Y, Boone T: Effects of qigong on cardiorespiratory changes: a preliminary study, *Am J Chin Med* 21(1):106, 1993.
45. Logeril M-D et al: Mediterrean alpha-linolenic acid-rich diet, in secondary prevention of coronary heart disease, *Lancet* 343:1454, 1994.
46. Miller J, Fletcher K, Kabat-Zinn J: Three-year follow-up and clinical implications of a mindfulness meditation-based stress reduction intervention in the treatment of anxiety disorders, *Gen Hosp Psychiatr* 17:192, 1995.
47. Miller K, Perry P: Relaxation technique and postoperative pain in patients undergoing cardiac surgery, *Heart Lung* 19(2):136, 1990.
48. Mockel M, Rocker L, Stork T: Immediate physiological responses of healthy volunteers to different types of music: cardiovascular, hormonal, and mental changes, *Eur J Appl Physiol Occup Physiol* 68(6):451, 1994.
49. Morisco C, Trimarco B, Condorelli M: Effect of coenzyme Q10 therapy in patients with congestive heart failure: a long-term multicenter randomized study, *Clin Invest* 71(suppl):S134, 1993.
50. Morrison HI et al: Serum folate and risk of fatal coronary heart disease, *JAMA* 275:1893, 1996.
51. National High Blood Pressure Education Program Working Group report on primary prevention of hypertension, *Arch Intern Med* 153:186, 1993.
52. O'Keefe CA et al: Controlled dietary folate affects folate levels in nonpregnant women, *J Nutr* 125:2717, 1995.
53. Olszewer E, Sabbag FC, Carter JP: A pilot double blind study of sodium-magnesium EDTA in peripheral vascular disease, *J Natl Med Assoc* 82:173, 1989.
54. Ornish D et al: Can lifestyle changes reverse coronary artery disease? *Lancet* 336:129, 1990.
55. Osborne R, Brajkovich C: Brief imagery training: effects of psychological, physiological and neuroendocrinological measures of stress and pain, *Dissertat Abstr Int* 53(9):4938-B, 1993.
56. Patel C: Yoga and bio-feedback in the management of hypertension, *Lancet* 7837:1053, 1973.
57. Pelletier K: Friends can be good medicine. In *Sound mind, sound body*, New York, 1994, Simon & Schuster.
58. Phelps S, Harris WS: Garlic supplementation and lipoprotein oxidation susceptibility, *Lipids* 28:475, 1993.
59. Rimm EB et al: Vitamin E consumption and the risk of coronary disease in men, *N Engl J Med* 328:1450, 1993.
60. Ross R: The pathogenesis of atherosclerosis: a perspective for the 1990s, *Nature* 362:801, 1993.
61. Rozanski A, Bairey N, Krantz D: Mental stress and the induction of silent myocardial ischemia in patients with coronary artery disease, *JAMA* 318(6):1005, 1988.
62. Sachdeva U: The effect of yogic lifestyle on hypertension. CIANS-ISBM Satellite Conference Symposium: lifestyle changes in the prevention and treatment of disease–1992, Hannover, Germany, Homeostasis Health Dis 5(4-5):264, 1994.
63. Schell F, Allolio B, Schonecke 0: Physiological and psychological effects of hatha-yoga exercise in healthy women, *Int J Psychsomat* 41(1-4):46, 1994.
64. Schneider R et al: A randomized controlled trial of stress reduction for hypertension in older African Americans, *Hypertension* 26:820, 1995.
65. Schneider R et al: Lower lipid peroxide levels in practitioners of the transcendental meditation program, *Psychosom Med* 60:38, 1998.
66. Schroeder-Sheker T: Music for the dying: a personal account of the new field of music thanatology—history, theories, and clinical narratives, *Advances* 9(1):36, 1993.
67. Schuler G et al: Regular physical exercise and low-fat diet: effects on progression of coronary artery disease, *Circulation* 86:1, 1992.
68. Schwartz CJ et al: The pathogenesis of atherosclerosis: an overview, *Can Cardiol* 14:111, 1991.
69. Shapiro D: Meditation. In Strohecker J et al, editors: *Alternative medicine: the definitive guide*, Fife, Wash, 1995, Future Medicine.
70. Shapiro D et al: Reduction in drug requirements for hypertension by means of a cognitive behavioral intervention, *Am J Hypertens* 10:9, 1997.
71. Sharpley C: Maintenance and generalizability of laboratory-based heart rate reactivity control training, *J Behav Med* 17(3):309, 1994.
72. Shrapnel WS et al: Diet and coronary heart disease, *Med J Aust* 156:1, 1992.

73. Silagy CA, Neil AW: A meta-analysis of the effect of garlic on blood pressure, *J Hypertens* 12:463, 1994.

74. Singh RB et al: An Indian experiment with nutritional modulation in acute myocardial infarction, *Am J Cardiol* 69:879, 1992.

75. Sirvastava KC: Extracts from two frequently consumed spices—cumin *(Cuminumciminum)* and turmeric *(Curcuma longa)*—inhibit platelet aggregation and alter eicosanoid biosynthesis in human platelets, *Prostagland Leukot Essent Fatty Acids* 37:57, 1989.

76. Sloth-Nielson J et al: Arteriographic findings in EDTA chelation therapy on peripheral arteriosclerosis, *Am J Surg* 162:122, 1991.

77. Stampfer MJ et al: Vitamin E consumption and the risk of coronary disease in women, *N Engl J Med* 328:1444, 1993.

78. Stephens NG et al: Randomized controlled trial of vitamin E in patients with coronary disease: Cambridge Heart Antioxidant Study (CHOS), *Lancet* 347:781, 1996.

79. Stockdale L: The effects of audiotaped guided imagery relaxation exercises on anxiety levels in male automatic implantable cardioverter defibrillator recipients, *Dissertat Abstr Int* 51(9):4270-B, 1991.

80. Telles S, Nagarathna R, Nagendra H: Autonomic changes during "OM" meditation, *Indian J Physiol Pharmacol* 39(4):418, 1995.

81. Telles S et al: Physiological changes in sports teachers following 3 months of training in Yoga, *Indian J Med Sci* 47(10):235, 1993.

82. The Alpha tocophrol, Beta Carotene, Cancer Prevention Study Group: The effect of vitamin E and beta carotene on the incidence of lung cancer and other cancers in male smokers, *N Engl J Med* 330:1029, 1994.

83. Thom TJ et al: Total mortality and mortality for heart disease, cancer and stroke from 1950 to 1987 in 27 countries, NIH Pub No 92-3088, National Heart, Lung and Blood Institute, Bethesda, Md, 1992, National Institutes of Health.

84. Traver M: Efficacy of short-term meditation as therapy for symptoms of stress, *Dissertat Abstr Int* 50(12):5897-B, 1989.

85. Uchino BN, Garvey TS: The availability of social support reduces cardiovascular reactivity to acute psychological stress, *J Behav Med* 20(l):15, 1997.

86. van Rij AM et al: Chelation therapy for intermittent claudication: a double-blind randomized controlled trial, *Circulation* 90:1194, 1994.

87. Warshafsky S, Kamer RS, Sivak SL: Effect of garlic on total serum cholesterol: a meta-analyis, *Ann Intern Med* 119:599, 1995.

88. Wenneberg S et al: A controlled study of the effects of the transcendental meditation program on cardiovascular reactivity and ambulatory blood pressure, *Int J Neurosci* 89:15, 1997.

89. Williams R, Barefoot J, Califf R: Prognostic importance of social and economic resources among medically treated patients with angiographically documented coronary artery disease, *JAMA* 267:520, 1992.

90. Worth RM et al: Epidemiologic studies of coronary heart disease and stroke in Japanese men living in Japan, Hawaii and California: mortality, *Am J Epidemiol* 102:481, 1975.

91. Yan J: The health and fitness benefits of tai chi, *J Physical Educ Health Recreat* 87:61, 1995.

92. Zamarra JW et al: Usefulness of the transcendental meditation program in the treatment of patients with coronary artery disease, *Am J Cardiol* 77(10):867, 1996.

93. Zamora R et al: Comparative antioxidant effectiveness of dietary beta carotene, vitamin E, selenium and co-enzyme Q10 in rat erythocytes and plasma, *J Nutr* 121:50, 1991.

94. Zhuo D et al: Cardiorespiratory and metabolic response during tai chi chuan exercise, *Can J Sport Sci* 9:7, 1984.

SUGGESTED READINGS

Goldstrich JD: *Healthy heart: longer life,* Santa Monica, Calif, 1996, Ultimate Health.

Leonard G, Murphy M: *The life we are given,* New York, 1995, GP Putnam's Sons.

Miller M, Vogel RA: *The practice of coronary disease prevention,* Baltimore, 1996, Williams & Wilkins.

CHAPTER 5

Complementary/Alternative Therapies in General Medicine: Diabetes Mellitus

Angele McGrady and James Horner

Diabetes is a chronic disease that becomes evident as hyperglycemia and affects all aspects of metabolism. About 6 million people carry the diagnosis of diabetes in the United States. There are two types of diabetes mellitus: type I insulin dependent (IDDM) and type II non–insulin dependent (NIDDM). Type I occurs when the pancreatic beta cells are injured or destroyed by autoimmune processes or infection and become incapable of producing insulin. Symptoms develop rapidly in individuals under the age of 30 years. Type II, the most common form, is diagnosed in about 80% of diabetics. Type II develops slowly, is usually associated with obesity, begins after age 30, and is characterized by insulin resistance. The most common acute complication is hypoglycemia, low blood glucose (BG) levels, which can occur in both types of diabetes but is more frequent in IDDM. Long-term complications include microvascular deterioration and neuropathy.[39,44]

Blood glucose values are expressed in milligrams per deciliter (mg/dl) or in millimoles (mmole). Physicians monitor disease status by reviewing their patients' records of daily BG values and by a biologic assay, glycohemoglobin, which represents the average BG value for the previous 2 to 3 months. Treatment recommendations for patients with IDDM are based on provision of exogenous insulin by injection. Patients are strongly advised to monitor BG several times a day with a glucometer, exercise regularly, and maintain a well-controlled diet. For NIDDM the physician initially recommends diet, weight loss if appropriate, and exercise. The diabetic diet is based on American Diabetes Association (ADA) guidelines.[4] If this regimen does not produce euglycemia (BG level within the normal range), oral medication is prescribed and followed, sometimes, by insulin therapy. Oral hypoglycemics include first- and second-

We thank Cheryl Kern Buell for her assistance with the databases. Material was gathered from MedLine, PsycInfo, WorldCat, and Healthstar.

generation agents (sulfonylureas) metformin, and acarbose. Since many NIDDM patients are now being given treatment with insulin in addition to oral hypoglycemic agents, the future designations for IDDM and NIDDM, are likely to be type I and type II diabetes, respectively.[44] However, in this chapter the IDDM and NIDDM terminology is used, since that is the differentiation made in most articles dealing with complementary/ alternative medicine (CAM).

In both types of diabetes, self-care is the critical component of management.[17,29] At the time of diagnosis the patient is informed that self-monitoring of BG (SMBG) and regular checkups are necessary. Nutrition and exercise recommendations are sometimes conflicting and often complicated. Acute illness often challenges BG control, requiring adjustments in dosage of hypoglycemic agents. The physician caring for patients with diabetes often emphasizes the seriousness of the disease to foster adherence, while compromising empathy in the doctor-patient relationship.

Three examples emphasize the role of self-care in the treatment of the person with diabetes. First, a recent book[12] written for the diabetic patient begins with the following statement: "You're the only person who can be responsible for normalizing your diabetes." Second, the foreword to the book, written by a former president of the ADA states that "we (physicians) are finally accepting the central role of the person with diabetes in making daily decisions." Third, the results of the clinical trial comparing usual care of IDDM with intensive monitoring and insulin dosing showed conclusively that the latter decreased the incidence of long-term complications, particularly retinopathy. However, the Diabetes Control and Complications Trial (DCCT) regimen[19] was much more demanding of patients than usual care. This group of patients was highly motivated, yet one questions whether such an intensive regimen can be maintained over the long term. Thus patient behavior, psychosocial factors, and variables related to adherence should be emphasized to practitioners caring for diabetic patients.

In adolescent populations social support is important in maintenance of BG control. Supportive, cohesive families promote better metabolic control, particularly during the early years after diagnosis. Open, empathetic communication fosters good adherence. Developmental issues must be considered in adolescents who are trying to learn about their disease and take responsibility for its control.[13] A model has been developed to explain the interplay among support, perceived threat, and depression in diabetic patients. Threat is defined as the impact of diabetes on self-esteem, happiness, or life satisfaction. Lower levels of depression were associated with higher perceived support of family and friends. Patients who saw diabetes as very threatening were less satisfied with their life and had a higher incidence of depression.[15]

Locus of control is important in patients' views of the physician and their willingness to accept physicians' advice. Locus of control refers to a concept embodying whether patients believe that outcomes (like BG control) depend on their own decisions or those of powerful others, or occur largely by chance. Some patients believe they have diabetes because it is God's will.[76] In general, patients with a belief in powerful others have less knowledge of diabetes and poorer glycemic control than patients who believe that they have a major amount of control over the outcome of their diabetes.[38]

Culture and race affect the person's perception of disease and the sick role, thereby affecting self-care. Is an individual with diabetes "sick" in the sense of feeling unwell, held blameless for their condition, or permitted to decrease responsibilities?[57] In general, persons with IDDM or NIDDM are expected to incorporate their self-care into their usual responsibilities of occupation and family, and individuals react differently to those demands. In a study of two cultural groups, African Americans' self-care was the most significant predictor of dietary adherence, while social support was the most significant predictor for whites.[25] Culture may be particularly influential in acceptance of the mind-body therapies, since patients' views of mental influences on physical functions may be influenced by religion. Assessment and treatment of the patient from a biopsychosocial framework improves the doctor-patient relationship and facilitates treatment.

A British survey on the impact of beliefs on adherence found that patients with poorer glycemic control are not only at greater risk for complications but are also more likely to have psychiatric conditions such as eating disorders, depression, and anxiety. Patients who often miss their medical appointments and are poor adherers to their prescribed regimen are more likely to be living in families with high levels of conflict.[31] Negative life events are associated with onset, severity of disease, and quality of life of the person with diabetes.[72]

Because of the chronicity of diabetes, the impact of the disease on quality of life, the possibility of severe complications, and the requirements for self-care, it is very likely that diabetic patients will seek CAM therapies. This chapter discusses the role of the CAM therapies in IDDM and NIDDM, based on outcome studies obtained largely from databases. Only studies on human subjects were considered. The chapter ends with recommendations for physicians providing treatment to diabetic patients who use CAM.

What is the role of CAM in diabetes? In IDDM there are few or no functioning beta cells, and there are no proven substitutes for insulin. However, CAM therapies may be very useful adjuncts to insulin, may enhance the effect of injected insulin, and may lower BG levels. The NIDDM patient may seek CAM therapies to lower BG levels, to decrease dosage of oral hypoglycemics, and to decrease insulin resistance. For both types of patients at any stage of the disease, quality of life issues are important, particularly because the demands of the daily routine may compromise quality of life. However, SMBG and biologic assay are the only ways to test effects of adjuvant or alternative treatment similarly to standard treatments for diabetes. The goal of the CAM therapies must be to obtain preprandial BG levels between 80 and 120 mg/dl or glycosylated hemoglobin values less than 7%.[4] In addition to specific effects on BG, some CAM therapies may assist patients in managing the complications of diabetes. For example, there are ample data on the efficacy of acupuncture for pain control (see Chapter 10). For the diabetic patient with neuropathy, acupuncture may be indicated.

To be accepted by the ADA, an unproved therapy must meet specific criteria. Recommendations must be supported by data generated from well-controlled studies to meet the goals of reducing BG, lessening the incidence of complications, and maintaining euglycemia, without increasing the frequency of dangerous hypoglycemic episodes.[3] It is important to be aware that recommendations to the lay public by self-proclaimed experts in CAM do not always follow the ADA guidelines.

DIET AND NUTRITIONAL SUPPLEMENTS
Pritikin, Low-Calorie, Ornish, and Oslo Diets

The Pritikin diet, developed by Nathan Pritikin, is a largely vegetarian diet, high in complex carbohydrates and fiber, containing less than 10% fat. The diet is usually combined with aerobic exercise. Results in NIDDM showed significant improvements in BG levels and decreases in required hypoglycemic medication. Patients with newly diagnosed diabetes were the best responders; they were able to decrease or eliminate oral hypoglycemic agents. In NIDDM patients requiring insulin, results were less striking; nonetheless, decreased BG was achieved in more than one third of these patients.[9,10]

The effect of very-low-calorie diets (400 to 600 kcal/day with most of the calories in the form of high-quality protein) was tested in NIDDM. Thirty-six patients participated either in a 20-week behavioral program combined with 1200 to 1500 kcal per day or in the same behavioral program with 8 weeks on the very-low-calorie diet. Results showed that the combination of low-calorie diet and behavior modification was effective in lowering BG levels.[73]

The Ornish diet, originally designed for reversal of cardiovascular disease, is also applicable to patients with diabetes, since many patients with long-term diabetes develop hypertension and heart disease. The Ornish diet consists of a low-fat, high-fiber, basically vegetarian diet with 75% of the calories from carbohydrates. Exercise and relaxation are combined with the diet. Sixty percent of the NIDDM patients on insulin regimens adhering to the Ornish plan no longer required it.[50,51] The Oslo diet, which included increased intake of fish and reduced fat intake, was tested by a randomized trial in 219 persons with neither hypertension nor diabetes. Although it is not directly relevant to this chapter, the significant decrease in insulin resistance suggests a potential avenue toward prevention of NIDDM.[69] The "diets" described above are actually lifestyle change programs and include exercise, stress management, and sometimes group therapy. Although these programs are effective for normalizing BG, further research is needed to distinguish the specific effects of each component of these programs.

Supplements

Magnesium has been suggested to be an important nutritional supplement for persons with diabetes. Low serum magnesium level is associated with a number of diabetic complications, in particular, retinopathy and cardiovascular disease. According to an ADA panel, supplementation with magnesium is recommended for diabetics who are at risk for these complications or who are documented to have hypomagnesemia.[71]

Adding chromium picolonate to the diet of diabetic patients is a topic that has generated much controversy. The original study reporting benefits of chromium in diabetes suggested that chromium supplementation is a means of preventing NIDDM rather than a cure or a replacement for insulin or oral hypoglycemic agents.[5] Chromium functions as a cofactor for insulin action, thus regulating the activity of insulin. No recommended daily allowance exists for chromium. A group of Chinese NIDDM patients were reported to normalize glycohemoglobin on a regimen of chromium picolonate but could have been initially deficient. It is likely that only patients whose impaired glucose metabolism is related to dietary chromium will respond to supplementation, but most diabetics are not chromium deficient.[24] Side effects from taking chromium supplements are possible, in particular, severe hypoglycemia.

TRADITIONAL CHINESE MEDICINE

Traditional Chinese medicine consists of many diagnostic procedures and forms of treatment. Disease is conceptualized as resulting from a disturbance in vital energy (Qi). In a recent text on the practice of Chinese medicine, diabetes is briefly mentioned under the heading of "tiredness" or "exhaustion." Treatment recommendations are based on restoring energy to the patient; however, documentation of BG levels or other indicators of disease are sparse.[43]

More than 800 elderly Chinese diabetics were given treatment within the Chinese medicine conceptual framework, which included (1) "regular life," (2) "rational diet," (3) hypoglycemic agents including insulin, (4) working within the patients' power, and (5) physical exercise. Results showed that 12.5% of participants obtained "clinical alleviation" (fasting BG levels less than 110 mg/dl), 40% showed marked improvement (fasting BG levels less than 130 mg/dl), 44% had some improvement, and no effects were observed in 3% of the cases.[42]

Qi Gong

Qi Gong has been a component of traditional Chinese medicine for centuries. Qi Gong has been reported to produce healing in many disorders, some of which are considered to be incurable within the realm of Western medicine. One year of daily Qi Gong practice decreased fasting BG and serum insulin levels in a group of 31 NIDDM patients. These changes were statistically and clinically significant.[45]

Acupuncture

Acupuncture combined with modified diet was tested in 26 patients, 5 with IDDM and 21 with NIDDM. BG values normalized after acupuncture treatment in 80% of the NIDDM patients, but no effects were observed in the IDDM patients. Effectiveness rates between 60% and 80% from other studies are referenced in this report, but again, little benefit was obtained in IDDM patients.[14]

Herbal Medicine

Chinese medicine uses plant extracts in combination, not as single agents. Some of the herbal therapies show little consistency in preparation or combination of herbs and vary in composition among different cultural groups.[58] In many cultures herbal medicine is incorporated into comprehensive diabetic therapy, including diet, exercise, and, depending on the culture, Qi Gong, meditation, or relaxation.[68] Thus, although herbal medicine is listed as part of Chinese medicine, some of the plants described in the next section are also components of other treatment models.

The risk-benefit ratio must always be considered when testing adjunctive therapies, as it is in U.S. Food and Drug Administration–sponsored Phase I, II, or III clinical trials. Patients may be put at considerable risk by discontinuing their hypoglycemic medication to test a new substance. For example, an herbal substance was tested in 67 persons, some with IDDM and others with NIDDM. A hypoglycemic effect was claimed, but very high BG values were listed after patients were withdrawn from their medication. Final BG levels remained above 200 mg/dl.[55]

Three scientific reviews of plant medicines as hypoglycemic agents are discussed in this section.[7,8,33] Four hundred plant treatments for diabetes have been recorded; only a few have been evaluated in human studies, and fewer are reported as outcome studies on BG. Some of the herbs are useful for their effects on complications of diabetes, but there is no evidence of positive effects on BG. One example is *Gingko biloba,* for which impressive documentation exists for its ability to improve circulation. This herb may be beneficial for patients with peripheral neuropathy and retinopathy.[35]

A survey was conducted of herbalists in the Baja peninsula. Two herbs were most often mentioned by the herbalists for the treatment of diabetes: *Bidens pilosa* (Spanish needles) and *Tecoma stans* (yellow bells).[74] Despite the common usage of these two substances in Baja, no human scientific studies were identified, nor are human studies referenced in the review articles.[7,8,33]

Table 5-1 summarizes research on hypoglycemic agents conducted on individuals with diabetes in which some form of control was described. Citations indicate the primary source and the review articles in which the substance is mentioned. A case series of 15 patients is described who were treated with *Artemisia herba-alba* (wormwood) extract, common in Iraq. Results showed decreased BG and no side effects.

TABLE 5-1	Effects of Plant Substances on Blood Glucose		
Substance	**Documented Effect**	**Type of Study**	**Reference No(s).**
Artemisia herba-alba	Decreased BG	Case series	2, 33
Gymnema sylvestre	Decreased BG, decreased glycohemoglobin	Controlled	7, 33, 61
	Reduced BG, decreased glycohemoglobin	Case series	11, 33
Coccinia indica	Improved glucose tolerance	Double-blind control	6, 7, 33
Trigonella foenum graecum	Decreased BG, improved glucose tolerance, decreased glycohemoglobin	Controlled	7, 33, 62, 63
Momordica charantia	Decreased BG Improved glucose tolerance	Case series	7, 8, 33, 64, 70

BG, Blood glucose.

These results are promising, but identification of the active ingredient and controlled studies are required.[2]

The herb *Gymnema sylvestre* (gurmar) has as its active ingredient gymnemic acid, which appears to enhance the effects of endogenous and injected insulin. The herb decreased fasting BG levels and decreased insulin requirements in 27 IDDM patients and 22 NIDDM patients. In the latter, glycosylated hemoglobin and plasma proteins were significantly reduced as well. No hypoglycemia was observed in normal (nondiabetic) individuals or in diabetic persons.[11,61]

Coccinia indica improved glucose tolerance in NIDDM patients participating in a double-blind, controlled trial. Ten of 16 patients in the treated group showed marked improvement in glucose tolerance in comparison to none of the controls.[6] Glycohemoglobin values were not reported.

Trigonella foenum graecum (fenugreek seed powder), a common spice in India, was administered to 60 NIDDM patients in a prescribed diet for 24 weeks after a 7-day control period. A control group of 10 nondiabetic patients received no fenugreek but did receive the prescribed diet. Decreases in glycosylated hemoglobin, fasting BG levels, and insulin levels, in addition to improved glucose tolerance, were observed in the diabetic patients.[63] Similar results were reported for IDDM.[62]

Momordica charantia (bitter melon) is composed of compounds with antihyperglycemic effects, charantin and momordica. Significant decreases in BG and improved glucose tolerance were well documented in NIDDM patients.[70,64] Thus, although a botanic substitute for insulin seems unlikely, phytomedicine can provide therapeutic effects on BG and improve quality of life and may lead to clues for development of new oral hypoglycemic agents.

MIND-BODY THERAPIES
Emotional and Spiritual Factors

The basic tenet underlying the mind-body therapies is that cognitive, emotional, and spiritual factors affect physiology in health and disease. For the diabetic patient mind-body interventions may include supportive therapy or specific treatments targeting BG and glycohemoglobin.

Psychologic care of IDDM patients has been suggested as an integral part of the lifetime management of the disease. Different types of mental and emotional support are appropriate as follows: (1) at diagnosis, (2) to manage day-to-day challenges, and (3) when complications occur. Adjustment problems often accompany the early months after diagnosis of diabetes. When complications develop, patients need assistance in coping with the loss of some of their abilities. Family members should be considered an important part of the support system throughout the life span of the person with diabetes.[32,36]

Spiritual well-being may affect adjustment to living with a chronic illness such as diabetes. Individuals with a greater sense of spiritual well-being reported less uncertainty and psychologic distress and were better adjusted to living with diabetes.[40] In a well-designed study of therapeutic touch and intercessory prayer a majority of the participants decreased insulin usage; however, there were no significant differences between groups. Patients reported a greater sense of calm and peacefulness, both of which are positive psychologic benefits in terms of quality of life.[75]

Yoga

Yoga as practiced for thousands of years in India is considered a way of life. As such, yoga comprises diet, meditation, physical exercise, and adherence to ethical principles. The practice of yoga in the Western world is usually more limited, consisting only of breathing exercises, static postures, and relaxation.[1]

A controlled study tested the effects of 40 days of yoga and a vegetarian diet in 140 hospitalized patients with NIDDM. None of these patients was receiving hypoglycemic drugs. Outcome measures were an oral glucose tolerance test and the number of hypoglycemic medications. Results showed that the duration of disease was related to response. Patients with less than 10 years of diabetes sustained improved glucose tolerance and decreased usage of hypoglycemic agents.[37] Two other studies studied yoga in a total of 87 patients. The practice of yoga decreased fasting and postprandial BG levels, improved insulin kinetics, and also enhanced the sense of well-being in both IDDM and NIDDM patients.[20,56]

Biofeedback

The type of alternative mind-body therapy for diabetics most often reported in the Western literature is relaxation combined with biofeedback. Electromyography (EMG) and thermal biofeedback, commonly used for treatment of muscle contraction headaches and migraine headaches, respectively, are also applicable to diabetes.[60] Patients with diabetes can be treated safely with biofeedback-assisted relaxation as long as daily SMBG is maintained and medication changes are not made without physician consultation.[47]

In most of the stress-related disorders where biofeedback is recommended, relaxation therapy is used concomitantly. Two basic types of relaxation are involved: passive concentration on words or phrases designed to produce the state of relaxation or progressive or active relaxation in which muscle groups are tensed and relaxed sequentially.[18] Often, counseling or psychotherapy, particularly of the cognitive behavioral type, is also incorporated into a biofeedback-assisted relaxation protocol.

The basic premise underlying the use of relaxation therapies in diabetes is that psychologic stress has an influence on BG levels. This has been explored on a theoretical basis and through laboratory testing of diabetic individuals. A detailed analysis of this concept is beyond the scope of this chapter, but several references are provided for the interested reader.[16,28,66,67]

Biofeedback and relaxation therapies have been tested in controlled studies in IDDM and NIDDM. In these studies patients' medication regimens were maintained, and patients remained under the care of their own physicians. In an early study Surwit and Feinglos[65] compared the effects of progressive relaxation and EMG biofeedback in six NIDDM patients to usual care in another six patients. Glucose tolerance but not insulin sensitivity improved. In a study of patients with poorly controlled IDDM Feinglos et al.[23] provided EMG biofeedback and progressive relaxation to 10 patients while 10 others received no additional treatment. Treatment was provided in a hospital setting, followed by home practice of relaxation. Glycohemoglobin and total insulin dose were unchanged in either group. In another study carried out in Greece, statistically significant decreases in BG and glycosylated hemoglobin were reported in a relaxation group in comparison to an untreated control group. Both IDDM and NIDDM patients participated in this study.[52]

Thirty-eight patients with NIDDM were given treatment with intensive diabetes therapy. Half of the patients also received biofeedback-assisted relaxation. Significant improvements in glycohemoglobin levels were observed in both groups, but no additional benefit came with the biofeedback-assisted relaxation. The patients who did benefit from the relaxation treatment were those whose BG levels appeared to be stress sensitive.[41] Another study[34] of NIDDM patients also reported no advantage for the patients given treatment with EMG biofeedback and progressive relaxation.

McGrady and colleagues[48,49] tested the effects of a biofeedback and passive relaxation protocol in a total of 34 patients (17 experimental and 17 controls) with IDDM in two studies. Both EMG and thermal types of feedback were used, with passive or autogenic relaxation. Patients continued under the care of their own physicians, and no changes in insulin dosage were carried out without physician permission. Patients monitored BG daily and met with a nurse weekly to discuss BG and insulin data. Average BG value, percentage of BG values greater than 200 mg/dl, and percentage of fasting BG values greater than 120 mg/dl were all significantly reduced in the treated groups compared to controls. Figs. 5-1 and 5-2 illustrate the results documented for average BG value and percentage of fasting BG values above 120 mg/dl in the first study.[48] Furthermore, in the second study[49] glycohemoglobin values were correlated with self-reported BG values at pretest, suggesting that the self-reported values were accurate.

A third study[46] from our laboratory sought to investigate the role of the patient's mood in biofeedback-assisted relaxation in IDDM. The protocol was similar to earlier studies, except that the baseline was extended to 6 weeks to allow for additional education about diabetes and follow-up was extended to 3 months to explore changes in glycohemoglobin values. In contrast to our two earlier reports, there were no significant differences between the experimental and control groups in average BG value or any other related variable, although five of nine individuals did show decreases in BG and glycohemoglobin in comparison to one of eight controls. Analysis of the mood data was

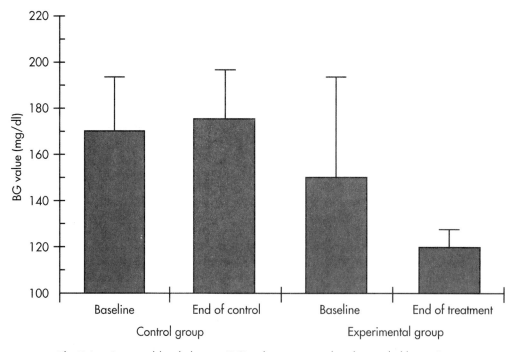

Fig. 5-1   Average blood glucose (BG) values measured and recorded by patients during 2-week pretest and 2-week posttreatment or postcontrol periods. Values are means ± SD. (Modified from McGrady A, Bailey BK, Good MP: Controlled study of biofeedback assisted relaxation in type I diabetes, *Diabetes Care* 15(5), 1991.)

of interest in that the successful patients reported lower levels of depression, anxiety, and daily hassles. The treatment failures were more depressed, more anxious, and took longer to complete the protocol. Statistically significant correlations were found between the indicators of mood, particularly depression, and BG values.

The relatively high incidence of depression in diabetic patients has been consistently documented.[26] The depressed diabetic patient is at greater risk of hyperglycemia because, enveloped in a negative mood and sense of failure, they may fail to use SMBG or to administer hypoglycemic agents appropriately. In the context of mind-body interventions, depressed patients may not practice relaxation as recommended or, when doing so, may lack sufficient concentration to realize its full benefit. Recently the serotonin reuptake inhibitors have been shown to have BG level–lowering effects in depressed diabetics.[30]

Other applications of biofeedback may be in ameliorating symptoms of complications of diabetes. For example, thermal biofeedback was shown to help 40 diabetic patients to increase the temperature of their hands and feet, thereby improving circulation.[54] A case study reported decreased symptoms of intermittent claudication in one patient given treatment with thermal biofeedback.[59]

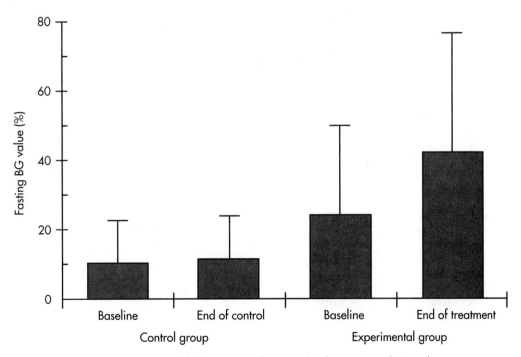

Fig. 5-2   Fasting BG values at target during 2-week pretest and 2-week post-treatment or postcontrol periods. Values are means ± SD. (Modified from McGrady A, Bailey BK, Good MP: Controlled study of biofeedback assisted relaxation in type I diabetes, *Diabetes Care* 15(5), 1991.)

The mind-body therapies hold promise for incorporation into diabetes management. Although there are negative studies, particularly in NIDDM patients, significant therapeutic effects have been reported and quality of life improves. Risk associated with these therapies is very low, as long as patients maintain SMBG and take their medication as prescribed.

Two areas require further study: predicting who will respond to mind-body therapies and the consistency of short-term benefits. Data on long-term maintenance of improved BG in patients who have undergone mind-body therapy is unavailable but extremely important to have. A key question is how much continued practice is necessary, once active treatment is complete. With regard to prediction of short-term success or failure, important factors are patient mood and adherence to treatment recommendations. In particular, depressive symptoms and mood disorder may prevent acquisition of the relaxation response[46] and may predict poorer self-care.[15,26,30]

WHAT THE PHYSICIAN NEEDS TO KNOW

"Diabetes is a nearly pure example of behavioral medicine…it is an outcome of the interplay among the underlying disease process, the environment and the behavior of the affected individual."[53] Many of the CAM therapies that have been discussed also require personal effort and commitment over the patient's lifetime.

The classic report by Eisenberg and colleagues[22] on use of unconventional medicine does not specifically mention diabetes but clearly suggests that use of CAM therapies will be higher in patients with chronic illness.[22] Information about patients' use of CAM therapies is critical to determining the potential impact of the CAM therapy on BG and the interaction between the CAM therapy and the patient's prescribed regimen. The therapeutic relationship between physician and patient is enhanced by careful questioning of patients about their self-care practices, use of CAM therapies, and review of issues of safety and efficacy.[21] There is cause for concern if proper monitoring is not performed and physicians are not informed about what the patient is doing.[27] Since a patient's decision to miss insulin shots or eliminate oral medicine will have rapid, life-threatening consequences, open communication is crucial.

Present and future physicians providing treatment for patients with diabetes must be informed about some forms of CAM. First, a source of basic information about diabetes should be recommended to newly diagnosed patients. Three excellent resources are listed at the end of this chapter. Second, the crucial role of behavior and physician-patient partnership must be emphasized to patients. Third, the diabetologist should be updated about the mind-body therapies, phytomedicine, diet programs, and some areas of traditional Chinese medicine as adjunctive therapies to control BG. Fourth, alternative methods of pain control for management of diabetic complications should be used. Fifth, the patients' culture, available social support, and quality of life must be considered in making treatment decisions.

SUMMARY

Diabetes is a chronic disorder of metabolism that is characterized by hyperglycemia and can progress to serious complications over the person's life span. The two predominate types of diabetes mellitus are type I (IDDM) and type II (NIDDM). Treatment is directed at decreasing elevated BG levels by means of oral hypoglycemic agents or by injected insulin. Outcome of therapy is determined by BG values and biologic assay. Self-care on the part of the patient is critical to day-to-day management. Social support, mood, and locus of control affect adherence to prescribed therapy, and depression seems to have a particular impact. The most common types of CAM therapies applicable to patients with diabetes are mind-body, herbal, and diet therapies. Scientific literature on many of the CAM therapies is very difficult to obtain. Nonetheless, this chapter provides support for relaxation and biofeedback, yoga, phytomedicine, and structured diet. Limited support is provided for Qi Gong and acupuncture as agents to decrease hyperglycemia. There is no substitute for insulin, but CAM therapies may reduce BG, decrease requirement for oral medicine or insulin, decrease severity of complications, and improve quality of life.

REFERENCES

1. Achterberg J et al: Mind-body intervention. In *Alternative medicine: expanding medical horizons,* Washington, DC, 1992, US Government Printing Office.
2. Ali-Waili NS: Treatment of diabetes mellitus by Artemisia herba-alba extract: preliminary study, *Clin Exp Pharmacol Physiol* 13(7):569, 1986.
3. American Diabetes Association: Unproven therapies, *Diabetes Care* 20(1):S60, 1997.
4. American Diabetes Association: Standards of medical care for patients with diabetes mellitus, *Diabetes Care* 21(1):S23, 1998.
5. Anderson RA: Chromium, glucose tolerance and diabetes, *Biol Trace Elem Res* 32:19, 1992.
6. Azad KAK, Akhtar S, Mahtab H: *Coccinia indica* in the treatment of patients with diabetes mellitus, *Bangladesh Med Res Counc Bull* 5(2):60, 1979.
7. Bailey CJ, Day C: Traditional plant medicines as treatments for diabetes, *Diabetes Care* 12(8):553, 1989.
8. Bakhiet AO, Adam SE: Therapeutic utility, constituents and toxicity of some medical plants: a review, *Vet Hum Toxicol* 37(3):255, 1995.
9. Barnard RJ et al: Response of noninsulin dependent diabetic patients to an intensive program of diet and exercise, *Diabetes Care* 5:370, 1982.
10. Barnard RJ et al: The role of diet and exercise in the management of hyperinsulinemia and associated atherosclerosis risk factors, *Am J Cardiol* 69:330, 1992.
11. Baskaran K et al: Antidiabetic effect of a leaf extract from *Gymnema sylvestre* in non–insulin-dependent diabetes mellitus patients, *J Ethnopharmacol* 30:295, 1990.
12. Bernstein RK: *Dr. Bernstein's diabetes solution,* Boston, 1997, Little, Brown.
13. Burroughs TE et al: Research on social support in adolescents with IDDM, *Diabetes Educator* 23(4):438, 1997.
14. Chen J, Wei J: Changes of plasma insulin level in diabetics treated with acupuncture, *J Tradit Chin Med* 5(2):79, 1985.
15. Connell CM et al: Impact of social support, social cognitive variables and perceived threat on depression among adults with diabetes, *Health Psychol* 13(3):263, 1994.

16. Cox DJ, Gonder-Frederick LA: The role of stress in diabetes mellitus. In McCabe PM et al, editors: *Stress, coping, and disease,* Hillsdale, NJ, 1991, Lawrence Erlbaum Association.
17. Cox DJ, Gonder-Frederick LA: Major developments in behavioral diabetes research, *J Consult Clin Psychol* 60(4):628, 1992.
18. Davis M, Eshelman ER, McKay M: *The relaxation and stress reduction workbook,* ed 4, Oakland, Calif, 1995, New Harbinger.
19. Diabetes Control and Complications Trial Research Group: The effect of intensive treatment of diabetes on the development and progression of long-term complications in insulin-dependent diabetes mellitus, *N Engl J Med* 329(14):977, 1993.
20. Divekar MV, Bhat M, Mulla A: Effect of yoga therapy in diabetes and obesity, *J Diabetes Assoc India* 28:75, 1998.
21. Eisenberg DM: Advising patients who seek alternative medical therapies, *Ann Intern Med* 127:61, 1997.
22. Eisenberg DM et al: Unconventional medicine in the United States, *N Engl J Med* 328:246, 1993.
23. Feinglos MN, Hastedt P, Surwit RS: Effects of relaxation therapy on patients with type I diabetes mellitus, *Diabetes Care* 10(1):72, 1987.
24. Finney LS, Gonzalez-Campoy JM: Dietary chromium and diabetes: is there a relationship? *Clin Diabetes* 15(1):6, 1997.
25. Fitzgerald JT et al: Differences in the impact of dietary restrictions on African Americans and Caucasians with NIDDM, *Diabetes Educator* 23(1):41, 1997.
26. Gavard JA, Lustman PJ, Clouse RE: Prevalence of depression in adults with diabetes, *Diabetes Care* 16:1167, 1993.
27. Gill GV et al: Diabetes and alternative medicine: cause for concern, *Diabet Med* 11(2):210, 1994.
28. Goetsch V: Stress and blood glucose in diabetes mellitus: a review and methodological commentary, *Ann Behav Med* 11(3):102, 1989.
29. Goodall T, Halford NK: Self-management of diabetes mellitus: a critical review, *Health Psychol* 10(1):1, 1991.
30. Goodnick PJ, Henry JH, Buki VM: Treatment of depression in patients with diabetes mellitus, *J Clin Psychiatry* 56(4):128, 1995.
31. Hawthorne K, Mello M, Tomlinson S: Cultural and religious influences in diabetes care in Great Britain, *Diabet Med* 10(1):8, 1993.
32. Holmes DM: The person and diabetes in psychosocial context, *Diabetes Care* 9(2):194, 1986.
33. Ivorra MD, Paya M, Villar A: A review of natural products and plants as potential antidiabetic drugs, *J Ethnopharmacol* 27:243, 1989.
34. Jablon SL et al: Effects of relaxation training on glucose tolerance and diabetic control in type II diabetes, *Appl Psychophysiol Biofeedback* 22(3):155, 1997.
35. Jacobs J et al: Herbal medicine. In *Alternative medicine: expanding medical horizons,* Washington, DC, 1992, US Government Printing Office.
36. Jacobson AM: The psychological care of patients with insulin-dependent diabetes mellitus, *N Engl J Med* 334(19):1249, 1996.
37. Jain SC et al: A study of response pattern of non–insulin dependent diabetics to yoga therapy, *Diabetes Res Clin Pract* 19(1):69, 1993.
38. Kohlmann CW et al: Associations between type of treatment and illness-specific locus of control in type 1 diabetes patients, *Psychol Health* 8(5):383, 1993.
39. Krall LP, Beaser RS: *Joslin diabetes manual,* ed 12, Philadelphia, 1989, Lea & Febiger.
40. Landis BJ: Uncertainty, spiritual well-being and psychosocial adjustment to chronic illness, *Issues Ment Health Nurs* 17(3):217, 1996.
41. Lane JD et al: Relaxation training for NIDDM predicting who may benefit, *Diabetes Care* 16(8):1087, 1993.
42. Lu R: Treatment of diabetes in the elderly: an analysis of 885 cases, *J Tradit Chin Med* 13(2):83, 1993.
43. Maciocia G: *The practice of Chinese medicine,* Edinburg, 1994, Churchill Livingstone.
44. Margolis S, Saudek CD: Diabetes mellitus. In *The Johns Hopkins white papers,* Baltimore, 1997, Johns Hopkins University.

45. McGee CT, Sancier K, Chow EPY: Qigong in traditional Chinese medicine. In Micozzi MS, editor: *Fundamentals of complementary and alternative medicine*, New York, 1996, Churchill Livingstone.
46. McGrady A: Role of mood in outcome of biofeedback-assisted relaxation in insulin dependent diabetes, *Appl Psychophysiol Biofeedback* 22(2):127, 1997.
47. McGrady A, Bailey B: Biofeedback-assisted relaxation and diabetes mellitus. In Schwartz MS, editor: *Biofeedback: a practitioner's guide*, ed 2, New York, 1995, Guilford.
48. McGrady A, Bailey B, Good M: A controlled study of biofeedback-assisted relaxation in type I diabetes, *Diabetes Care* 14(5):360, 1991.
49. McGrady A, Graham G, Bailey B: Biofeedback-assisted relaxation in insulin dependent diabetes: a replication and extension study. *Ann Behav Med* 18(3):185, 1996.
50. Ornish DM: *Dr. Dean Ornish's program for reversing heart disease*, New York, 1990, Random House.
51. Ornish DM et al: Can lifestyle changes reverse coronary heart disease? *Lancet* 336:129, 1990.
52. Paschali A, Karamanos B, Griggiths I: Effect of relaxation therapy on the control of diabetes mellitus. In Christodoulou GN, editor: *Psychosomatic medicine: past and future*, New York, 1987, Plenum.
53. Pohl SL, Gonder-Frederick LC, Daniel J: Diabetes mellitus: an overview, *Behav Med Update* 6(1):3, 1984.
54. Rice BI, Schindler JV: Effects of thermal biofeedback-assisted relaxation training on blood circulation in the lower extremities of a population with diabetes, *Diabetes Care* 15(7):853, 1992.
55. Sadhukhan B et al: Clinical evaluation of a herbal antidiabetic product, *J Indian Med Assoc* 92(4):115, 1994.
56. Sahay BK: Yoga and diabetes, *J Assoc Physicians India* 34(9):645, 1986.
57. Salloway JC: Medical sociology. In Sierles F, editor: *Behavioral science*, Baltimore, 1993, Williams & Wilkins.
58. Sanders D, Kennedy N, McKendrick MW: Monitoring the safety of herbal remedies: herbal remedies have a heterogeneous nature, *Br Med J* 311(7019):1569, 1995.
59. Saunders JT et al: Thermal biofeedback in the treatment of intermittent claudication in diabetes: a case study, *Biofeedback Self Regul* 19(4):337, 1994.
60. Schwartz MS: *Biofeedback: a practitioner's guide*, ed 2, New York, 1995, Guilford.
61. Shanmugasundaram ERB et al: Use of *Gymnema sylvestre* leaf extract in the control of blood glucose in insulin-dependent diabetes mellitus, *J Ethnopharmacol* 30:281, 1990.
62. Sharma RD, Raghuram TC, Sudhakar RN: Effect of fenugreek seeds on blood glucose and serum lipids in type I diabetes, *Eur J Clin Nutr* 44:301, 1990.
63. Sharma RD et al: Use of fenugreek seed powder in the management of non–insulin dependent diabetes mellitus, *Nutr Res* 16(8):1331, 1996.
64. Srivastava Y et al: Antidiabetic and adaptogenic properties of *Momordica charantia*: an experimental and clinical evaluation, *Phytother Res* 7:285, 1993.
65. Surwit RS, Feinglos MN: The effects of relaxation on glucose tolerance in noninsulin dependent diabetes, *Diabetes Care* 6(2):176, 1983.
66. Surwit RS, Schneider MS: Role of stress in the etiology and treatment of diabetes mellitus, *Psychosom Med* 55(4):380, 1993.
67. Surwit RS, Schneider MS, Feinglos MN: Stress and diabetes mellitus, *Diabetes Care* 15(10):1413, 1992.
68. The Burton Group: *Alternative medicine*, Fife, Wash, 1993, Future Medicine.
69. Torjesen PA et al: Lifestyle changes may reverse development of the insulin resistance syndrome, *Diabetes Care* 20(1):26, 1997.
70. Welihinda J et al: Effects of *Momordica charantia* on the glucose tolerance in maturity onset diabetes, *J Ethnopharmacol* 17:277, 1986.
71. White JR, Campbell RK: Magnesium and diabetes: a review, *Ann Pharmacother* 27:775, 1993.
72. Wilkerson G: The influence of psychiatric, psychological and social factors on the control of insulin-dependent diabetes mellitus, *J Psychosom Res* 31(3):277, 1987.
73. Wing RR: Very low calorie diets in the treatment of type II diabetes: psychological and physiological effects. In Wadden TA and Vanitallie TB, editors: *Treatment of the seriously obese patient*, New York, 1992, Guilford.
74. Winkelman M: Ethnobotanical treatments of diabetes in Baja California Norte, *Med Anthropol* 11(3):255, 1989.

75. Wirth DP, Mitchell BJ: Complementary healing therapy for patients with type I diabetes mellitus, *J Sci Explor* 8(3):367, 1994.
76. Zaldivar A, Smolowitz J: Perceptions of the importance placed on religion and folk medicine by non–Mexican American Hispanic adults with diabetes, *Diabetes Educator* 20(4):303, 1994.

SUGGESTED READINGS FOR PATIENTS

American Diabetes Association: *American Diabetes Association Complete Guide to Diabetes,* Alexandria, Va, 1997, The Association. An excellent, clearly written resource book for people with diabetes. Discusses team approach to care. Psychological issues relevant to diabetes are well presented.
Beaser RS: *The Joslin guide to diabetes,* New York, 1995, Simon & Schuster. Written to educate patients with diabetes about their disease. Individual chapters describe normal functioning of the pancreas, the onset of diabetes, characteristics, complications, and management. Emphasis is placed on the attainment of as normal a life as possible for the diabetic patient.
Guthrie DW, Guthrie RA: *The diabetes sourcebook,* ed 3, Los Angeles, 1997, RGA Publishing. An excellent resource book, written for people with diabetes and their families. It emphasizes self-management based on education about the disease. Appendices provide meal plans and listings of ADA state affiliates.

CHAPTER 6

Complementary/Alternative Therapies in the Prevention and Treatment of Cancer

Aron Primack

Cancer is a major disease category in today's health care for people of all ages. Even in the face of beneficial programs, such as early detection of breast cancer with improving screening techniques, the overall incidence and mortality attributable to the major cancers such as lung, breast, colon, and prostate have changed very little over the past three decades, and conventional medical treatments of today are inadequate. There has been considerable progress in genetic research explicating many of the reasons people are susceptible to cancer. Radical surgical treatment for cancer has been replaced by more focused surgical approaches in combination with other methods, including radiation therapy, brachytherapy, chemotherapy, and immunotherapy, with some improvements. Even with the burgeoning number of new chemotherapeutic agents, the general acceptance of severe toxic effects, and the many new products to ameliorate these potentially life-threatening toxicities, the medical treatment of cancer has led to little improvement in statistics over several decades. Radiation therapy often has the ability to control local areas of disease, local recurrences, and specific complications but falls short in overall cure rates and longevity.

This chapter attempts to delineate some of the treatments in complementary/alternative medicine (CAM) and their results. It is not an all-inclusive listing of treatments tried, used, or rejected. It is an attempt to inform students in the health sciences of directions that have been taken and that need to be taken for CAM to be adjudicated, understood, and incorporated into medical treatment as it becomes scientifically validated.

USAGE OF CAM THERAPIES: SURVEY RESULTS

Campion[40] pointed out that patients generally use CAM for chronic diseases such as back pain, headaches, arthritis, musculoskeletal pain, insomnia, depression, and anxiety. (However, we will learn that patients with cancer are frequent users of CAM therapy, often for the chronic symptoms that accompany this condition.) Most patients who are using CAM therapy for their diabetes, cancer, and hypertension were also seen by conventional medical practitioners. They have not circumvented the established medical system.

In a survey of 304 cancer patients in a major United States cancer center compared with 356 patients being treated with CAM, Cassileth and colleagues[42] reported the following interesting facts: 54% of the cancer center patients were also using CAM, and 40% of cancer center patients ultimately abandoned conventional therapy in favor of CAM. Sixty percent of the practitioners of CAM were physicians. Patients who used CAM were more likely to be white and well educated. The most commonly used CAM therapies were metabolic treatments, diet treatments, megavitamins, imagery, spiritual treatments, and "immune" treatments. Patients chose CAM to assume personal responsibility for their care and because there was an underlying belief that pollution and diet were the causation of the cancer and therefore avoidance of the former and modification of the latter could be put to best use in its cure. Satisfaction in the CAM treatment was reflected in the finding that 43% of patients believed their vitamin therapy helped their cancer and 58% believed it helped their overall health.

Banner and co-workers[16] found that 28% of breast and cervical cancer patients in Hawaii used traditional Hawaiian remedies within the year before the authors' survey. Fourteen percent of patients had sought help from a Hawaiian healer, and 6% said it would be their first source of medical help. Further, Lerner and Kennedy[162] performed a statistically valid sampling study using telephone interviews of 5047 patients with cancer, almost all of whom were treated at least in some way with conventional medicine, including surgery (69%), radiation therapy (33%), and chemotherapy (33%). Of these, 9% used at least one type of CAM. Women and men used CAM approximately equally (9.2% and 8.7%, respectively). CAM use rose proportionately with increased wealth, age of less than 49 years, increasing education, and increase in the size of the household. Patients generally learned of these alternative methods of treatment from physicians, but the news media or television was instrumental as well (25%), as was word of mouth from family and friends. Some types of cancer were more often associated with CAM: central nervous system cancer (21%), lymphomas (14.5%), and ovarian cancer (16%) were the most common. The longer the patient had a malignancy, the more likely it was for that patient to seek alternative therapy. If the cancer was still in evidence at 5 years, 10% were using alternative therapy; if no evidence of disease, 6%. Diet therapies were more commonly used by women, mind-body therapies by men, and drug therapies equally by both.

Lerner and Kennedy also found that 44% of the patients were using CAM after conventional therapy, presumably because there was residual disease. Twenty percent of patients were using these methods simultaneously with conventional medicine, whereas 17% were using them before conventional therapy, leading to the possibility of delayed treatment and delayed chance of cure from the conventional approach. The authors found that patients rarely discontinued their visits to their conventional therapist once they started CAM. Fifty-eight percent of these CAM users believed they were "likely to be cured" by it. Twenty-five percent of the costs for this CAM was covered through third-party health insurance.

Lerner and Kennedy concluded that

> ...it is evident that physicians must become familiar with questionable cancer therapies, must make it known to patients that they are available to discuss questionable methods, and must then, without criticism, direct patients to appropriate sources of care and additional information...

and that

> ...while some questionable therapies are harmless or inexpensive, others have toxic effects and may be costly, and none have scientifically proven efficacy. Although the percentage of usage reported is relatively low, overall large numbers of patients are involved, especially in certain groups. The physician plays a key role in encouraging or preventing the use of questionable methods, and substantial improvements in public and professional education are needed.

Specific surveys of the use of CAM in the pediatric cancer population have been made,[278,279] showing that approximately 10% of children with cancer—presumably through their parents—had previously consulted CAM practitioners, most commonly employing chiropractic, homeopathy, naturopathy, hypnotherapy with relaxation, and acupuncture. They were generally older children with better-educated mothers. Some children were given megavitamins, which could have serious negative consequences. The cancer-related medical conditions for which this therapy was sought were most commonly respiratory illness, musculoskeletal problems, dermatologic or gastrointestinal tract problems, and allergies. The use of CAM for cancer treatment is a worldwide phenomenon (Table 6-1).

Physician-Patient Issues

Why do so many people with cancer seek CAM treatment? The most common reasons include the appeal of "natural," "holistic" remedies; the possibility of improving quality and quantity of life in the face of the allopathic community saying "nothing can be done"; the need to have a sense of control over one's own life; pressure from family and friends; and mistrust of the conventional medical establishment and authority figures in general.[36] Further, allopathic medicine can be expensive. Scientific medicine demands appropriate, clear diagnosis, requiring a biopsy. Testing often includes costly radiographic imaging studies and laboratory evaluation. The therapy itself, including surgery, chemotherapy, and radiation therapy, can be very costly. CAM, with its stress

TABLE 6-1	Survey of Use of CAM for Cancer				
Author	Country	Number of Patients	Percentage who used CAM	Specific Findings	Five Most Commonly Used Types of CAM
Downer et al.[69]	Great Britain	415	16%	—	Healing relaxation, diet therapy, homeopathy, vitamin therapy
Lerner, Kennedy[162]	United States	5047	9%	—	Diet therapy, mind/body, drug therapy
Begbie et al.[23]	Australia	335	21.9%	Young adults, women, married, single, well educated, desire for "natural"	Diet therapy, psychologic, herbal remedies
Cassileth, Chapman[44]	United States	660	54%	—	Metabolic therapy, diet therapy, megavitamin therapy, imagery, spiritual, "immune" therapy
Fisher, Ward[83]	England	Not given	16% 16% 36% 24%	—	Acupuncture Homeopathy Manual therapy Phytotreatment
Hauser[115]	Europe	Survey article	Various	Well educated, recommended by relatives and friends	Diet therapy (38%), drug therapy (33%), electrotherapy (33%)
Risberg et al.[247,248]	Norway	642	20%	Younger older, geographic differences, higher educated	Healing by hands, herbal medicine, vitamin therapy, diet therapy, Iscador
Van der Zouwe et al.[312]	Holland	949	9.4%	—	
Sawyer et al.[258]	Australia	48 children	46%	66% one type, added rather than replaced conventional therapy	Positive imagery, hypnosis, relaxation, exercise, diet therapy, vitamin therapy, herbal remedies

TABLE 6-1	Survey of Use of CAM for Cancer—cont'd				
Author	Country	Number of Patients	Percentage who used CAM	Specific Findings	Five Most Commonly Used Types of CAM
Morant et al.[201]	Switzer-land	160	53%	Younger older	Herbal teas, beetroot juice plant extracts, laying on hands, homeopathy, Iscador, magnetic therapy, diet ther-apy, acupuncture, psychologic
Pawlicki et al.[229]	Poland	70	25%	Caused delay in conven-tional medi-cine use	Unknown
Munstedt et al.[205] *	Germany	206	39%	—	Mistletoe, trace minerals, megavitamins, enzymes
Helary[119]	France		52%	—	Unknown
Dady[63]	New Zealand	463	32%, advised generally along with con-ventional treat-ments	20 to 50 year olds	Diet therapy, vitamin therapy, Laetrile, magnetic resonance, faith healing

*Cancer in women.

on natural products, teas, herbs, electric stimulation, massage, and so forth, often is much less expensive per treatment. Patients often seek an "integrative" approach to treatment, using both conventional medicine and CAM simultaneously. A huge amount of money is spent on CAM, but much less per treatment. There are exceptions: megavitamin therapy, antineoplastons, and dietary therapy in specialized spas all may cost more per week than allopathic treatment. But in the main, the naturopathic treat-ment seems to be a small expense compared with allopathic medicine.[73-75]

Montbriand[198] found that 75% of her 300 informants did not tell their doctor they were using some type of alternative therapy for treatment of cancer. With such a high prevalence of alternative treatments, it is important for the conventional medical practitioners to know what their patients are doing. There is a significant chance of product interactions or of clinical effects that could confuse the patient's diagnosis. Some CAM treatments being used have potentially harmful effects, such as those listed in Table 6-2. Physicians also need to incorporate the beneficial effects of all types of treatments into their patients' treatment.[175] Lerner[161] has delineated the following guidelines for an effective physician role:

- Avoid patient abandonment, which drives patients to the alternative medical practitioner completely.
- Adopt a strategy of preemptive discussion, making it clear that this discussion is desired and valuable for the patient and the physician.
- Clearly indicate that the physician is a valuable source of information about CAM practices.
- Know the specific questionable methods that have been shown to be at best useless and at worst fraudulent.

Doctors should be clear in their goals of treatment and in the promise conventional therapy offers, but brutal honesty and fearful predictions only tend to drive the patient to other sources of potential help, often promised without statistical validity.[40] Knowing about CAM therapies, discussing these alternative therapies early in the patient's treatment, and being honest with the patient about the goals the patient has and the likelihood of help from conventional medicine and CAM can only support the physician/patient relationship. Seeking to help the whole patient, to look at patients in a humanistic way, is good medicine, whether practiced by the conventional therapist or the alternative practitioner. Approximately 5% of cancer patients abandon conventional therapy and pursue alternative methods.[186] The goals of studies of CAM treatments are often complex and blurred. Standard chemotherapy, surgery, and radiation therapy studies hinged on measurements of disease-free survival and longevity. Although there were always questions of quality of life, these were often asked secondarily. However, in CAM studies this question of the "quality of life" often becomes the key one, especially when treatments are given with only palliative intent. It will always be difficult to measure "quality of life," and it will be necessary that studies be more and more carefully designed to use measurement and survey instruments that can accurately reflect difference across groups.[272]

Clinical Research Issues

In cancer therapy there are three types of specific multipatient studies (see Chapter 2 for a detailed discussion of the phases of preclinical studies). Phase I studies are performed to determine the appropriate dose of a given material for study, not to seek anti-

TABLE 6-2 Potential Herbal Toxicities

Name of Plant or Product	Potential Active Ingredient	Toxicity	Reference in Addition to Tyler[304]
Comfrey	Pyrrolizidine alkaloids	Hepatic; primary pulmonary hypertension	Couet et al.,[59] Betz et al.,[27] D'Arcy[62]
Senecio or *Crotalaria* sp.	Pyrrolizidine akaloids	Venoocclusive disease	
Heliotropium	Unknown	Hepatic failure	
Ilex plants	Pyrrolizidine	Ascites; hepatic disease	
Psoralea corylifolia (babchi)	Psoralen	Photosensitivity	
Piper methysticum (Kavakava)	Unknown	Stimulates, then depresses central nervous system	
Catha edulis (Khat)	Unknown	Psychosis, optic atrophy, pharyngeal cancer	
Datura (thornapple, jimson weed)	Hyosciamine	Hallucinations	
Valerian and skullcap	Unknown	Liver damage	MacGregor et al.,[176] Chan et al.,[48] Willey et al.[321]
Taheebo	Unknown	Bleeding	
Aloe vera	Unknown	Laxative causing low vitamin K levels	
Arnica	Unknown	Cardiac toxicity	
Alfalfa	Canavanine (?)	Splenomegaly, pancytopenia	
Aristolochia (Virginia snakeroot)	Unknown	Nephrotoxicity; squamous cell carcinoma of stomach in rats	
Coffee enemas	Unknown	Fluid and electrolyte imbalance	
Ginseng	Sugars, steroids, saponins	Swollen, tender breasts; vaginal bleeding, hypertension	
Fungi (*Psilocybe* sp.)	Psilocybin, psilocin	Hallucinations	
Lawsonia alba (henna dyes)	Unknown	Edema of face, lips, epiglottis, pharynx, neck and bronchi; anuria, acute renal failure	
"Black powder" (p = phenylenediamine)	Unknown	Skin irritation, eczematoid dermatitis; vertigo; anemia; gastritis	
Laetrile (vitamin B_{17})	Hydrogen cyanide	Cyanide poisoning	
Glycyrrhiza glabra (licorice)	Unknown	Hypokalemia, ventricular fibrillation	
Margosa oil	Unknown	Fatty infiltration of liver; vomiting, drowsiness, metabolic acidosis	

From Tyler VE: *The new honest herbal: a sensible guide to herbs and related remedies,* Philadelphia, 1987, Stickley.

cancer effect of these therapies. Phase II studies are performed to seek potential clinical usefulness of a new drug or new drug combination. A number of patients, often with varying types of malignancies, are given a treatment at an acceptable dose level, as determined from Phase I studies. With greater than 20% potential response, these drugs can be entered into controlled Phase III studies, controlled trials, comparing the newer agent or combination with a control group using the best treatment to date. This could be another single agent, combination of treatments, or placebo.[237]

There are very few controlled scientific studies of CAM related to cancer treatment and there is a reluctance on the part of many CAM therapy practitioners to conduct such research, although some are actively engaged in careful clinical studies. Studies can be costly if they are to be controlled and well documented and if they include high-level statistical analysis. Also, it is often difficult to control these studies in a double-blind format, but that is no excuse for not keeping good records of quantifiable data including tumor size and laboratory work. CAM practitioners often rely on the subjective views of the patient rather than objective evidence such as radiographs, laboratory work, or clinical measurement. Clear survey instruments can be developed to obtain subjective information in a reproducible way from patients about their lifestyle and quality of life. This is a plea to future health care providers to obtain such data. For a discussion of requirements of research design, see Chapter 1. Presence of the following criteria should warn of questionable practices in the use of CAM, particularly for the treatment of cancer[12]:

- A lack of studies on effectiveness
- Practitioners who claim the medical community is trying to keep the cure from the public
- A treatment that primarily relies on diet and nutrition
- A claim that the "curative" treatment is harmless, painless, and without side effects
- A treatment with a "secret formula" that only a small group of practitioners can use

CAM AND PREVENTION OF CANCER

Cancer prevention is a major subspecialty of conventional oncology. The search for genetic predispositions and for carcinogens is very active, but the arena in which preventive activities can make the most headway is personal behavior modification. Because these modifications, in the form of diet and/or specific chemical use, are being made in otherwise healthy individuals, such modifications must be safe.[90]

There is a growing body of literature relating to cancer prevention and CAM. Although common lore indicates that among the major causes of cancer are civilization and pollution (i.e., the industrial world), cancer is commonly found in less polluted areas. In fact, 56% of the world's 5,000,000 cancer deaths in 1985 occurred in the developing world.[76,226,233] Three approaches for prevention of cancer are delineated by Reizenstein and co-workers[243]: control of environmental sources of carcinogens; modification of personal habits including cigarette smoking and diet; and identification of specific genotypes. Of these, only personal habit modification is under the individual's direct control. It is also thought that this one approach would lead to the greatest potential decrease in cancer incidence. A particularly novel approach to the prevention of cancer by personal habit modification relates to what I will call "cyberprevention." Shinke and colleagues[268] described using interactive, culture-sensitive computer software to reduce risks of carcinogens, mainly cigarettes and poor diets, in a small study in one Native American population.

An exciting, ongoing study to determine the potential benefit of changing behavior is the Working Well Trial being performed in work-sites across the country under the auspices of the National Cancer Institute (NCI).[1] With an assumption that 80% of cancers are attributable to lifestyle or environmental exposure, including smoking, diet, and occupational exposures, the study will attempt to influence behavior at the workplace level rather than the usual individual level. The hope is to change motivational factors and social norms in a more widespread way than that possible in the clinical setting.

DIET

A potential link between cancer and diet has been suggested for more than 50 years. As early as 1933, a supposition was voiced that overweight people had a higher cancer risk than people of normal weight. The active study of this potential relationship began in the 1960s when the World Health Organization concluded that potentially the majority of human cancers are preventable[326] in large part by dietary modification. In the 1988 Surgeon General's Report on Nutrition and Health,[310] a straight-line relationship between estimated daily dietary fat intake and breast cancer death rate was demonstrated, colon cancer was shown to be correlated with dietary fiber intake and overall body weight, several cancers were correlated with vitamin A or alcohol intake, esophageal cancer was correlated with vitamin C intake, and both stomach and esophageal cancer were associated with poor nutritional status.

Using international surveys, migration studies, cohort studies, case-control studies, and clinical trials, data are revealing this relationship between diet and cancer, especially of the colon and rectum, breast, prostate, esophagus, lung, stomach, and liver.[105,106] A high-calorie, high-fat, low-fiber diet may increase the risk of cancer.[210,327] However, the fat intake by the general population in the United States is decreasing, potentially changing the comparison between control and treatment arms of studies.[86]

Colon cancer has been positively correlated with fat intake in a number of studies. Potentially premalignant adenomatous polyps are more common in countries of high animal fat consumption.[320] In an epidemiologic study of 24 European countries using mortality data, a direct correlation was shown between the consumption of animal but not vegetable fat and colon and breast cancer, and an inverse relationship with fish oil consumption.[47] The authors surmised that fish oil is protective against these cancers and that animal fat is carcinogenic in colorectal and breast cancers.

Fish oils are potent modulators of eicosanoid production. Eicosanoids are derived from arachidonic acid[181] and include prostaglandins, thromboxanes, leukotrienes, and various hydroxy and hydroperoxy fatty acids. These have effects in inflammation, immune function, and tumor cell division. Recent epidemiologic and clinical studies point to a potential role in cancer prevention and treatment with these.[191] Some eicosanoids activate protein kinase C and appear to have potential action in animals, retarding tumor growth and inhibiting metastasis production.[185] Increased dietary fat leads to certain eicosanoids that result in increased levels of cytochrome C oxidase II (COX-II), which may play an active role in the production of breast and prostate cancer.[254]

There is ongoing controversy over the role of dietary fat, cancer production, and cancer recurrence or spread.[58,86,253] There are marked differences in prevalence rates of breast cancer and prostate cancer in various parts of the world that correlate with increasing dietary fat intake, and these rates are changing with increasing dietary fat intake over time. In Japan dietary fat intake and breast and prostate cancers have risen significantly.[328,329] Interestingly, Eskimos with their high fatty intake, predominantly omega fatty acids, still have a very low incidence of breast cancer.

The blood levels of estrogenic compounds can be altered by diet. Fiber binds estrogen in the gastrointestinal tract, resulting in lower blood levels. The hypothesis that endogenously produced estrogen is related to the development of breast cancer is at least in part substantiated by the finding that tamoxifen, an estrogen blocker, reduces recurrence rates when used as adjuvant therapy after "curative" surgery and reduces occurrence of breast cancer in the contralateral breast when used in cases of carcinoma in situ.[72]

Estradiol and estrone blood levels have been found to be related to fat intake in the diet in several studies and directly correlate with the prevalence of breast cancer.[146,267] Women who decrease the percentage of fat in their diet for 3 months lower their circulating estrogen, estrone, and estradiol levels, whereas progesterone, luteinizing hormone, and follicle-stimulating hormone levels remained unchanged.[99,237,251,252] It remains to be determined whether this would lead to lower cancer rates.[58]

Fat intake may influence breast cancer prevalence through mechanisms other than hormonal.[254] Fat-rich linoleic acid, an omega-6 fatty acid, enhances rat mammary carcinoma,[58] whereas olive oil, containing oleic acid, an omega-9 fatty acid, has no such effect. Epidemiologic studies in humans appear to be consistent with these findings in humans, and similar results are obtained with fish oil ingestion.[139,140] Eicosanoids produced by lipoxygenase activity have an enhancing role in growth, invasion, and metastases of cancers. Similar harmful effects were seen in prostate cancer cell growth.[252,253]

A low-fat diet may decrease the production of these eicosanoids and thus inhibit growth, invasion, and/or metastases of breast or prostate cancer.

The nuclear grade of carcinoma in situ of the breast and of the prostate is also found to be proportional to the fat intake, being less aggressive in Japan with its low-fat diet than in the United States.[2,216,284] Akazaki and Stemmermann[2] reported that first-generation Japanese immigrants in Hawaii have a higher tendency for latent carcinoma to become invasive and aggressive compared with Japanese in Japan.

Total fat consumption from meat is directly related to risk of advanced prostate cancer.[94,318] In a population-based, case-control nutrition intake study in Utah of 358 cases of prostate cancer surveyed and matched with 679 controls, West[318] found that dietary fat was the strongest risk factor to explain the aggressiveness of this cancer. Other factors that had no significant effect on the study population included the intake of protein, vitamin A, beta-carotene, vitamin C, zinc, cadmium, and selenium. Fat intake from dairy products or fish was free from correlation. Heinonen and colleagues[118] reported the significant reduction in prostate cancer incidence and mortality in male smokers in a large, long-term study in Finland. Further studies are needed to corroborate this finding.

Recent clinical results indicate potential applications of polyunsaturated fatty acids to cancer treatment. A double-blind study at the Harvard and Deaconess Medical Centers suggested a significant effect of postsurgical adjuvant supplementation with eicosapentaenoic acid (EPA) in limiting recurrence of colon cancer.[30] Twenty-seven patients with stage I or II colon carcinoma or potentially premalignant adenomatous polyps were randomly selected to consume 9 g daily of either fish oil with high EPA content or corn oil after excision of detectable lesions. S-phase labeling of tissue from proctoscopic mucosal biopsies, a predictor for incidence of new neoplasms, dropped from its baseline in the treated group but rose in the control group. The rate of metastases after curative breast cancer surgery also suggested a clinical benefit with the use of adjuvant supplementation with omega-3 polyunsaturated fatty acid.[32] For a potential mechanism of action, see Nanji et al.[209]

Vitamins

Observational epidemiologic studies have suggested a possible decrease in the prevalence of cancer in people who consume higher amounts of fruits and vegetables, foods high in beta-carotene, and this decrease may be through their antioxidant effect. The literature is rife with anecdotal reports of antioxidant properties of many foods or food additives. For example, the spice turmeric has been found to exhibit such properties in vitro.[261]

Animal studies suggest the value of vitamin A and retinoids in regulating epithelial cell differentiation and maintenance; animals receiving a vitamin A–deficient diet develop keratinization, squamous metaplasia, and gross tumors, with subsequent regression of this metaplasia upon reintroduction of vitamin A into the diet.[200]

Retinoids also inhibit tumor angiogenesis.[178,271] Chemoprevention of mammary carcinoma in some strains of rats and mice by vitamin A and retinoids has been shown, but hepatic toxicity may be significant, as well as dermatologic toxicity.[235] There is also a decrease in metastases if retinoids are used as adjuvant treatment after removal of the primary tumor.

Further animal studies revealed that combining retinoids with oophorectomy, with dehydroepiandosterone, or with 2-bromo-alpha-ergocryptine (an inhibitor of pituitary prolactin secretion), had an additive effect. For example, in N-methyl-N-nitrosourea–induced rat mammary carcinoma, the combination of retinoids and selenium had an additive effect in cancer prevention. However, there is still an absence of clinical studies in humans.

Matthew[184] reported that the blue-green microalgae *Spirulina*, rich in carotenoids, reversed oral leukoplakia in tobacco chewers. Complete regression of lesions was observed in 45% of the 44 evaluable patients as compared with only 7% of the placebo-treated patients, with no toxicity. However, almost half of the responders developed a recurrence within 1 year of discontinuance of its use.

An intriguing study by Torun and colleagues[298] indicated that, when compared with normal control subjects, patients with cancers from many different sites, including breast, head and neck, genitourinary tract, lung, and gastrointestinal tract, had a significantly decreased level of beta-carotene, vitamin E, and vitamin C but had a significantly increased level of malondialdehyde, a product of arachidonic acid metabolism and a potential mutagen and carcinogen whose increased level in serum may indicate increased lipid peroxidation in tissues.

In the 1995 Western Electric study[225] following 1556 employed middle-aged men from 1958, men who ate a diet rich in vitamin C and beta-carotene fared better, with less heart disease and possibly less cancer. The correlation persisted after adjustment for age, cigarette smoking, blood pressure, serum cholesterol values, alcohol consumption, and other factors.

Henneckens and co-workers[122] reported in 1996 on 22,071 male physicians 40 to 84 years of age in the United States who were evaluated in a randomized, placebo-controlled, double-blind study to determine the potential effectiveness of alternate-day beta-carotene as a cancer preventive. Eleven percent of subjects were active smokers and 39% were former smokers at the time the study began in 1982. (A second part of this study, designed to determine the effectiveness of aspirin as a cardiac disease preventive, was discontinued before the predetermined end point of the study because the aspirin had a statistically significant preventative effect.) The study was continued for more than 12 years. There were no differences in the overall incidence of early or late malignant neoplasms or in overall mortality, and no significant harmful effects were found. In addition, no decrease in specific types of cancer including lung, colon and rectum, prostate, brain, and melanoma were observed.

Omenn[223] followed 18,314 people at high risk for lung cancer because of their past or present smoking or exposure to asbestos. That study also showed no beneficial effect and, in fact, revealed an increase in lung cancer prevalence and death from lung cancer in the antioxidant-treated group. A recent randomized study of 755 former asbestos workers at high risk for cancer failed to find a decrease in sputum atypia between the beta-carotene or retinol arm and the placebo arm.[211]

In a double-blind, controlled study reported by Albanes and colleagues,[3] 29,133 eligible male cigarette smokers were randomly selected to receive beta-carotene, alpha-tocopherol, both, or placebo and were followed for more than 5 years. The beta-carotene–treated group was observed to have no decrease in cancer, but on the contrary had increases in lung, prostate, and stomach cancer. Although the alpha-tocopherol–treated patients had a decrease in prostate and colorectal cancer and no change in lung cancer, they had an increase in stomach cancer and an increase in stroke, an unexpected finding, considering vitamin E's usual effect on platelets.

Greenberg and Sporn[103] followed 1805 patients who had had a recent non-melanomatous skin cancer and were randomly selected to receive 50 mg of beta-carotene daily or placebo. With yearly evaluations to detect new skin cancers no reduction in the number of new nonmelanomatous skin cancers was detected.

In recent years cruciferous vegetables, notably broccoli, have been touted as beneficial. Although rich in antioxidants of vitamin C and beta-carotene as well as folacin, they are also a source of hundreds of phytochemicals, which may stimulate the production of anticancer enzymes and chemicals that may block the effects of estrogen, among other as yet unidentified mechanisms.[170]

The craze to add antioxidants to treatment methods must be balanced by the need for scientifically valid studies. In two complex, nonrandomized, single-arm studies using beta-interferon, retinoids, and tamoxifen as maintenance therapy in metastatic breast cancer, Recchia and colleagues[242] drew the conclusion that the combination as maintenance "is feasible and shows activity in metastatic breast cancer with an acceptable toxicity," but that further controlled studies would be needed to be able to confirm this statement.

In a randomized comparison of fluorouracil, epidoxorubicin, and methotrexate plus supportive care versus supportive care alone in patients with nonresectable gastric cancer, Pyrhonen and co-workers[241] showed that the chemotherapy-treated group had a better response rate and a prolonged survival. But subjects in *both* arms of the study received vitamins A and E; therefore no conclusions can be drawn related to the effectiveness of these antioxidants.

Chemoprevention by retinoids in upper aerodigestive tract and lung carcinogenesis has been studied by Lippman and colleagues.[165] In a Phase II study, they found a significant improvement in leukoplakia (67% in the treated group versus 10% in the control group) with the use of high-dose isotretinoin in a short-term study. Because of the significant mucocutaneous toxic effects and short remission duration of this isotretinoin treatment, their subsequent study employed prolonged low-dose treatment. After a 3-month induction phase with high-dose isotretinoin, patients were randomly selected to receive either 9-month low-dose isotretinoin or beta-carotene. With a follow-up period of up to 5 years, the authors showed highly significant results, with progression of disease in only 8% of the isotretinoin-treated group as opposed to the 55% in the beta-carotene–treated group.

Pastorino and colleagues[227] reported a Phase III controlled study of retinyl palmitate compared with placebo used as adjuvant therapy in patients who had undergone curative surgery for stage I, non–small cell lung cancer. Although there was a decrease in second primary cancers in the retinyl palmitate–treated group and an increase in the disease-free interval, there was no 5-year survival difference. The latter finding may be a result of the vigorous treatment received by those individuals in whom the second primary cancers did occur.

Trace elements may have an antioxidant effect. Copper is required to maintain antioxidant defenses in vivo. Low-copper states may produce prooxidant effects. Copper complexes have been shown to have anticancer, anticarcinogenic, and antimutagenic properties in vitro. Also, zinc has potential antioxidant effects, but its role in disease is unclear.[287] Zinc-deficient rats have an increase in single-strand DNA breaks in the liver and zinc leukocyte or plasma levels have been found to be low in cancer patients, but there is little evidence of a zinc deficiency in these patients. The finding of decreased cancer rates in people who eat greater quantities of fruit may be related to their intake of these trace elements, which are found in these foods along with vitamins and beta-carotene.

Van Zandwijk[313] reported the use of N-acetylcysteine and glomerulus-stimulating hormone as antioxidants with potential antimutagenic and anticarcinogenic properties for prevention of lung cancer as evidenced in a large European chemopreventive study. Ongoing European studies may determine the effectiveness of these agents and delineate possible toxicities.

Soybeans

Several recent review articles* suggested multiple soy products that could suppress carcinogenesis, including a protease inhibitor, the Bowman-Birk trypsin inhibitor (BBI), also found in other beans and peas; inositol hexaphosphate (phytic acid); and the sterol beta-sitosterol. Soybean isoflavones also appear to suppress carcinogenesis in animals. Other trypsin inhibitors with evidence of potential preventive effects on cancer include saponins and the phytoestrogen genistein, which may inhibit neovascularization and

---

*References 84, 116, 143, 190, and 196.

tumor cell proliferation.[19,84] BBI did not confer resistance on lung cancer cells in culture to irradiation or cisplatinum-induced cytotoxicity but did confer such protection on mouse fibroblasts treated with both of these methods.[145]

Finding reversal of the cancer prevention effects of soybean products in animal studies by feeding the animals methionine leads to the possible conclusion that methionine deficiency in these animals is the cause of the decreased cancers.[116]

Other Dietary Preventives

Recent studies indicate that high fiber and folic acid intake is protective against colon cancer. Other cancers whose prevalence is inversely related to vegetable and fruit intake include those of the oral cavity, larynx, pancreas, bladder, and cervix. Whole-grain products seem to reduce the rate of colon cancer, possibly because of their increased fiber.

Animal protein intake may increase urinary calcium loss, contributing to homocysteinemia, leading to an increase in the risk of various cancers, whereas low calcium intake has been associated with a risk of colon cancer.[320]

Folic Acid. A high dietary intake of folate appears to exert a protective action against adenomatous polyps in the colon.[94] A deficiency of folate appears to be correlated with cervical dysplasia (vide infra).

Selenium. Garlic, high in selenium, has been found to inhibit colon cancer in mice[316] potentially through its action as an antioxidant. Garlic inhibits skin tumor growth,[214] inhibiting carcinogenesis,[38] and appears to have an immunostimulatory effect.[24] An epidemiologic study revealed that the stomach cancer prevalence in the area of Georgia where there is the highest level of production of Vidalia onions, high in selenium, is significantly lower than in other parts of the state.[335] However, in one area of Japan where gastrointestinal tract carcinoma is common, high levels of selenium in the soil were not associated with a significantly high cancer mortality.[207] Gupta and co-workers[111] studied plasma selenium levels in cancer patients and found that mean plasma selenium levels fell with increasing extent of disease and that patients with recurrent cancers had lower levels than those without recurrence. Gupta and colleagues believed that the low level is a causative factor in the cancer. One NCI study reported a 16% decrease in incidence of gastric cancer, a 4% reduction in esophageal cancer, and an overall 20% reduction in other cancers in a large group of Chinese adults taking vitamin E, beta-carotene, and selenium as compared with a control group.[170] Because the study did not compare single variables, it is impossible to say what the role of each of the three additives is. Clark and co-workers[57] reported a decrease in cancer incidence in patients with a history of basal cell or squamous cell carcinoma of the skin with supplementation with selenium.

Molybdenum. Nakadaira and colleagues[207] found a correlation between molybdenum concentrations in soil sediment samples and death resulting from pancreatic cancer in women.

TREATMENT OF CANCER

The following are some methods with evidence in the literature of possible effectiveness. The listing is not meant to be all-inclusive. See Table 6-3 for information on CAM in the treatment of specific malignancies.

Acupuncture

After being employed for thousands of years in China, acupuncture is rapidly gaining popularity in the United States. Despite this long-term usage, there is no evidence of its effectiveness as treatment for cancer itself. Most claims for effectiveness are as treatment of the side effects of cancer, such as pain control, possibly through endogenous pain inhibitory systems by the production of beta-endorphins and neuropeptides which bind to opioid receptors, increase interleukin-2 (IL-2) levels, and increase natural killer cell activity.[9,28,29,39]

Measurements of CD3, CD4, and CD8 cells as well as soluble IL-2 receptor and beta-endorphin levels in the peripheral blood of patients with malignancies revealed an increase in CD3, CD4, and CD4/CD8 ratio and an increase in the beta-endorphin level after acupuncture with a concomitant decrease in soluble IL-2 receptor levels.[28,29] Theoretically these findings might lead to clinical treatments for cancer patients, but further studies are needed. A preliminary review of electroacupuncture[306] with imagery has revealed some potential usefulness.

Antineoplastons

Antineoplastons are derived from glutamine, isoglutamine, and phenylacetate salts; antineoplaston AS5 is phenylacetate itself.[37] These chemicals inhibit incorporation of glutamine[234,276] into the proteins of tumor cells, which may cause G_1 phase arrest. Antineoplaston A10 is thought to interfere with intercalation with DNA. Other antineoplastons inhibit methylation of nucleic acids.[37] Burzynski[37] believed that hypomethylation may activate tumor suppressor genes.

Antineoplaston A10 and AS2-1 have been shown to produce a deleterious effect on cell proliferation, cell morphology, cell cycle, and DNA in human hepatocellular carcinoma cell culture lines and in one patient with hepatocellular carcinoma.[300] Burzynski[37] stated that "it can be clearly observed that antineoplastons induce abnormal cells to undergo terminal differentiation and die."

Many Phase I trials have been performed in the United States and Japan. Tsuda and colleagues[300,301] reported responses in patients with ovarian cytoadenoacarcinoma, anaplastic astrocytoma, recurrent renal cell carcinoma, brain metastases from prostatic

TABLE 6-3	Specific Malignancies and CAM		
Type of Malignancy	**Treatment, if Specific**	**Results**	**Reference**
Superficial bladder cancer	Keyhole limpet hemocyanin	Increase of natural killer cell activity	Kalble, Otto,[141] Lamm et al.[156]
Cervical dysplasia and cancer		Beta-carotene and vitamins A and C levels were low	Romney et al.[249]
Cervical cancer		Deficiency of folate, beta-carotene, vitamin C, and riboflavin	Orr et al.[224]
Cervical smears abnormal		Folic acid deficiency in Bantu women; corrected with folic acid treatment	Niekerk[212]
Cervical dysplasia		Low vitamin A and selenium levels	Dawson et al.[65]
Colorectal adenomas	Use of NSAIDs or diets high in fresh fruits and vegetables	Lower incidence of adenomas	Giovannucci et al.[94]
Esophageal cancer	Animal protein supplements in a Chinese diet	Decrease in occurrence rate	Herbert[124]
Gastric cancer	Increase garlic and onion intake	Decrease in occurrence rate	You et al.[335]
Acute promyelocytic leukemia	Co-oxide in culture cells	Apoptosis and morphologic change	Chen et al.,[50] Sun et al.[289]
Melanoma	Sesame oil and safflower oil in culture	Inhibition of cell growth	Salerno, Smith[275]
Nonmelanomatous skin cancer	Beta-carotene treatment	No change in number of new lesions over 5 years	Greenberg et al.[104]
Oral leukoplakia	*Spirulina fusiformis* vs. placebo	45% regression vs. 7% with placebo	Matthew[184]
Pancreatic cancer	Mistletoe extract	No improvement in tumor size or survival	Friess et al.[87]

NSAIDs, Nonsteroidal antiinflammatory drugs.

carcinoma, brain metastases from breast cancer, lymphoma, and brainstem glioma. Their overall response rate was reported to be 32%. In a previous study in the same journal, Sugita and colleagues[288] reported treatment success in a few patients with antineoplastons. Side effects included weakness, drowsiness, febrile reactions, nausea and vomiting, skin rash, and leukopenia and thrombocytopenia. Phase I studies of phenylacetate in patients with cancer have been made,[296] and clinical Phase II studies would be needed to determine the likelihood of clinical usefulness. Although an NCI study was begun to determine the usefulness of this treatment in patients with brain tumors, after a very slow accrual of patients, disagreements over study design prohibited the study from moving forward. (See Appendix B for Web sites presenting additional clinical trial data.)

Ayurveda

Ayurveda (Sanskrit for "that which has been seen to be true about long life"[299]) treatment has been used in India for thousands of years. Smit and co-workers[273] found cytotoxicity in the flowers of *Calotropsis procera* and the nuts of *Semecarpus anacardium.* However, there are no randomized studies in humans to show the clinical effectiveness in cancer treatment.

Over the past 7 years, a form of Ayurveda medicine promoted vigorously through the Maharishi Mahesh Yogi has become quite popular[115] with animal experiments showing cytotoxicity of Maharishi-4, a mixture of low-molecular-weight substances including antioxidants such as alpha-tocopherol, ascorbate, beta-carotene, catechins, bioflavinoids, and flavoproteins in the treatment of 7, 12-dimethylbenz[a]anthracene (DMBA)–induced mammary tumors in rats[265] and in the treatment of lung metastases in Lewis lung carcinoma in mice.[228] MAK-A, one such compound, induced biochemical and morphologic differentiation in murine neuroblastoma cells in culture.[236] MAK-4 and MAK-5 may have antioxidant properaties.[71,77,215]

Toxicity has been reported with Ayurveda remedies. Hepatic venoocclusive disease was reported in patients taking *Heliostropium* species, causing rapidly progressive hepatic failure leading to death.

Chiropractic

Chiropractic is generally reserved for the treatment of pain related to nonmalignant causes. Of concern is the possibility of negative outcomes resulting from manipulative treatments of patients with undiagnosed cancer. There are few published studies of the complications of chiropractic manipulation, but in one such study misdiagnosis of the patient's condition accounted for 26 of 135 complications to this type of treatment, 16 of which were in patients with neoplasms.[154] Because of the potential of paraplegia resulting from spinal manipulation in patients with cancer, malignancy is, at least, a relative contraindication to chiropractic manipulation.[266] For example, a case of quadriplegia after chiropractic manipulation in a 4-month-old infant with congenital torticollis caused by a spinal astrocytoma has been reported.[263] At surgery for removal of the intraspinal, low-grade astrocytoma with acute necrosis was found; the necrosis was thought to be a result of the two manipulations the baby had undergone.

Diet and Nutrition

Diet has been discussed in this chapter in relation to cancer prevention, but there are several diets that are used as treatment.

So-called metabolic diets include anticancer diets with digestive enzymes, high-dose vitamin therapy including vitamins A and C, pangamic acid (so-called vitamin B_{15}), amygdalin (Laetrile), or so-called vitamin B_{17}, an alleged vitamin preparation ("Plus 198"), and vitamin E and mineral supplements, with ancillary injections of intra-tumoral enzymes. Raw food consumption is increased, protein intake is decreased, and refined foods and additives are eliminated. Coffee enemas are used. Hair and blood analyses are also performed routinely. The American Cancer Society has published its findings of serious risks to patients resulting from these "metabolic diets."[6]

Macrobiotic diets were developed by Michio Kushi[152] based on the yin-yang principle of opposites. The diet is considered part of a whole regimen and philosophy. This diet obtains 50% to 60% of its calories from whole grains, 25% to 30% from vegetables, and the rest from beans, seaweed, and vegetarian soups. These strictly vegetarian diets have been touted as successful for the prevention of cancer, as well as its treatment. Although conventional medicine has recognized the *potential* benefit of increasing vegetables in the diet for prevention, there is no compelling evidence that this diet overall has a beneficial effect for prevention or treatment of cancer. No controlled trials of these diets have been made. The diets are potentially significantly deficient in vitamins D and B_{12}, as well as protein, iron, and calories.[45,199]

Many anticancer diets have been described; they tend to be especially popular in Europe.[13,115] A partial listing of some of these follows:

- Kousmine diet: Raw vegetables and wheat that are "rich in vital energy"
- Instinctotherapy: Only raw products, including raw meat; no milk products
- Moerman diet: Lactovegetarianism plus "the eight essential substances: vitamins A, B, C, and E, iodine, sulfur, iron, and citric acid"
- Breuss cancer cure: Up to 1 L of vegetable juice daily and different teas for 42 days
- Budwig's oil-protein diet: A curd cheese and flaxseed oil mixture, fruits and fruit juices
- Anthroposophic diet: Lactovegetarianism, unrefined carbohydrates, and sour milk products
- Bristol diet: Raw and partly cooked vegetables, soybeans, peas, and beans
- Gerson therapy: Crushed fruits and vegetables, coffee enemas, and nutritional supplements

Only the Bristol diet has been studied in a prospective, controlled trial.[14] There was no benefit for breast cancer patients attending a Bristol diet center when compared with a control group. For those who were metastases free at entry into the center, the metastases-free survival rate was, in fact, significantly worse than that in the control group. Survival in relapsed cases was also inferior to controls.

Hoxsey herbal treatment includes a paste of antimony, zinc and bloodroot; arsenic; sulfur; and talc as external treatments, and a liquid mixture of licorice, red clover, burdock root, *Stillingina* root, barberry, *Cascara*, prickly ash bark, buckthorn bark, and potassium iodide for internal consumption. A mixture of procaine hydrochloride and vitamins, along with liver and cactus, is prescribed. The Office of Technology Assessment (OTA) found that "taken together, the data indicate that many of the herbs used in the Hoxsey internal tonic or the isolated components of these herbs have antitumor activity or cytotoxic effects in animal test systems."[349] The OTA indicated that a paste made from these herbs had reliable beneficial effect on the treatment of basal cell carcinoma of the skin. A report by Austin and colleagues[13] did find cures for patients placed on the Hoxsey regimen but did not find such responses for patients treated at the Gerson clinic. Review by the NCI of the "cures" from these treatments failed to reveal any evidence of effectiveness for these patients with cancer.

The Gerson diet is a no-sodium, high-potassium diet rich in carbohydrates and defatted liver capsules, and injections of liver extract are taken in association with coffee enemas. The treatment has led to serious infections from the poorly administered liver extracts, as well as electrolyte imbalance resulting from the coffee enemas. No study published in the peer-reviewed literature has indicated any beneficial effect of this diet.

The Kelley diet employs enemas, diuretics, nasal irrigation, Sitz baths, deep-breathing exercises, and external body cleansing to rid the body of toxins. In addition, an expensive, restrictive diet is followed. There have been no carefully performed studies to show the benefit. Nicholas Gonzales in New York follows a similar system (although Kelley apparently disagrees) and has produced a best-case series for the NCI but has not published his data.[238] The hair analysis is believed to be of no value.

Manner metabolic therapy, coffee enemas, laxatives, juices, "antineoplastic" enzymes, amygdalin, pangamic acid, and dozens of other products including vitamins C and E, selenium, zinc, RNA, DNA, and ground-up animal organs all have been used, and no studies have indicated effectiveness.[12,43]

Essiac ("Caisse" when spelled backwards; named after Rene Caisse, a Canadian nurse who popularized its use) is a combination of four herbs: burdock, Turkey rhubarb, sorrel, and slippery elm. Researchers at the NCI and Memorial Sloan-Kettering Cancer Center have found that it has no anticancer effect.[45]

Cancell therapy is particularly popular in Florida and the Midwest. Through these medications, the practitioners claim to return the cancerous cell to a "primitive state" from which it can be rendered inert.[45,109] U.S. Food and Drug Administration (FDA) laboratory studies revealed that these are common chemicals, including nitric acid, sodium sulfite, potassium hydroxide, sulfuric acid, and catechol. FDA found no basis for the claims of effectiveness of the Cancell treatment.[45]

Herbal Remedies

Plant products have been used for centuries as medicines. Today in most of the developing world, plant remedies are the most prevalent treatments, with recipes handed down from generation to generation. They are available and are less costly than allopathic medicine, practitioners are available, and there is generally a more culturally sensitive attitude on the part of these practitioners.

Much of our allopathic medicine is derived from plant product. An estimated 20% to 25% of U.S. prescriptions contain natural plant products.[246] Oncology drugs are no exception. Taxol and Taxetere are derived from the Western yew tree, epipodophyllo-toxins from the mandrake plant, camptothecin from the bark of a Chinese tree (bought at the rate of approximately $35,000/kg),[206] and vinca alkaloids from periwinkle plants.

Approximately 114,000 plant extracts from 35,000 species were screened for anti-cancer activity between 1960 and 1981 in a mouse leukemia model. None proved effective in clinical trials during that time; therefore interest diminished.[246] Other countries, notably Japan, France, and China, continue to screen new plant materials.

With the advent of newer models of such evaluation, including cell culture lines, a screening program at the NCI has been renewed.[164,246] The NCI maintains a repository of 22,000 samples of natural products, primarily higher plants, adding about 6000 new samples yearly.

There are significant problems with any study of herbal products. There is generally a lack of standardization of dosage and formulation. The plant contains many potentially effective compounds with their inherent synergistic and competitive possibilities making it difficult to determine which products are beneficial and which are potentially harmful. Often, naturopaths employ several such plants simultaneously, making determination of effects of any one plant impossible. The studies are frequently poorly controlled, and scientific method is seldom employed. Biopsy proof of malignancy is often absent, as is direct clear measurement of end points. Careful, well-controlled statistical studies are needed.

Currently, hundreds of herbal remedies purported to have anticancer benefits are available over the counter. Most of them have no such demonstrated benefit. Many are not reliably formulated in available products and, as noted below, some are toxic. Nevertheless, a handful have demonstrated indications of potential anticancer activity, including one, polysaccharide krestin (PSK), that has demonstrated this in Phase III studies. Some of the herbal agents that merit closer study as potentially beneficial complementary treatments for cancer are described below.

Polysaccharide Krestin

Polysaccharide krestin is a polysaccharide preparation isolated from the mushroom *Coriolus versicolor* (basidiomycetes) that consists predominantly of glucan and approximately 25% tightly bound protein.[302] It has been heavily reported in the medical literature and studied in vitro, in vivo in animal studies, and in controlled human clinical trials.[56] It is administered orally and has shown no toxicity. Murine colon cancer studies showed a suppression of growth of these cancers and augmentation of tumor-neutralizing lymph node activity of draining mesenteric nodes by PSK.[114]

PSK has shown significant effectiveness as clinical treatment, as well as adjuvant therapy. In colon cancer as adjuvant therapy, the PSK-treated patients had a 30% 8-year disease-free survival as compared with 10% for the control group. When added to radiation therapy as treatment for stage III non–small cell lung cancer, the 5-year survival was 22% compared with the control survival of 5%.[117] An 8-year disease-free survival for women with breast cancer with demonstrated vascular invasion was reported to be 75% with combination chemotherapy plus PSK compared with 58% for those with only the chemotherapy.[132,133] As adjuvant therapy added to adjuvant chemotherapy of 5-fluorouracil plus mitomycin for gastric cancer, the 5-year disease-free survival was found to be 71% compared with 59% for the adjuvant chemotherapy alone.[208] Fukushima[88] reviewed the Japanese experience with gastric carcinoma treatment and concluded that PSK and other biologic response modifiers may have a role. In patients with colorectal cancer, PSK increased disease-free survival.[297]

In a randomized study of 158 patients with esophageal cancer treated with radiation therapy, there was a statistically significant improvement in survival in those treated with PSK as well.[221] On the other hand, Suto and colleagues[291] found no survival benefit to PSK in hepatocellular carcinoma patients after treatment with various standard therapies.

PSK was found to sharply increase the motility and phagocytic activity of polymorphonuclear leukocytes, which may be significant based on other findings that the prognosis of cancer patients was positively correlated with the degree of cellular infiltration around tumor sites.[297]

Chlorella

Chlorella pyrenoidosa is a one-celled green alga rich in proteins, vitamins, nucleic acids, and chlorophyll, which is used extensively as a food supplement worldwide. It has not exhibited toxicity at any dose. The components with identified anticancer activity are water-soluble polysaccharides in the cell wall[283,307,314] and glyceroglycolipids.[202,203]

Chlorella has been shown to have antitumor activity in association with immune activation.[1,48,194,294] A study at the Medical College of Virginia of 15 patients with glioblastoma treated with chlorella with or without other therapies including radiation therapy or chemotherapy resulted in a 2-year survival of almost 40%, with four of these six patients showing no tumor progression during that time.[189]

Potential mechanisms of actions include polysaccharide ingredients binding to tumor cell membranes with subsequent effects on tumor cell growth, adhesion, invasion of normal tissues, metastasis, and vulnerability to immune attack; increase in natural killer cell activity; increase in the T-cell helper to suppressor cell ratio; and stimulation of macrophage activity.[113,213,283]

Chinese Herbs

Chinese herbal remedies form a subset of herbal medicine. Several of these have been studied in vitro for cytotoxic activity (see Table 6-4).

One specific Chinese herbal preparation deserves specific mention. PC SPES consists of reproducible extracts of seven different Chinese herbs and one American herb. This combination has been shown to have the ability to suppress tumor cell proliferation and to reduce the clonogenicity of a variety of human tumor cell lines, inducing apoptosis.[112] Specific studies in prostate cancer cell lines have revealed that exposure to PC SPES resulted in a decrease in secretion of prostate-specific antigen (PSA), as well as a less prominent decrease in intracellular PSA.[129] Preliminary study with SPES indicates a potential beneficial effect on metastatic growth and on pain resulting from cancer.[155]

Currently, clinical studies are under way to validate the anecdotal reports from patients who have had a significant drop in PSA and symptomatic improvement in patients with advanced prostate cancer. The impression is, at least, an initial response. Side effects of high doses of the herbs must be evaluated in these patients with advanced disease. There has been some evidence of an estrogenic effect. However, preliminary observations indicate some effectiveness in patients for whom diethylstilbestrol (DES) treatment failed previously. Because PC SPES contains concentrated phytoestrogenic components, precautions against thromboembolic phenomena may be appropriate.[18]

TABLE 6-4	Chinese Herbal Remedies		
Plant Source	**Type of Chemical Found**	**Cytotoxic Assay Cell Line**	**Reference**
Pteris multifida poir	Deterpens	Ehrlich ascites tumor cells	Woerdenbag et al.[323]
Pulsatilla chinensis	Triterpenoids	P-388 murine leukemia, Lewis lung cancer, human large-cell lung cancer	Ye et al.[330]
Guava leaf, mangosteen peel, pomegranate leaf	Unknown	Human cell lines	Settheetham, Ishida[262]
Antrodia cinnamomea	Zhankuic acid (steroid)	P-388 murine leukemia	Chen et al.[49]
Trichosanthes	Triterpenoid	B-16 melanoma	Takeda et al.[293]

Capsaicin. The use of hot peppers is common around the world. Often considered a food preservative or a sweating agent for people in hot climates, peppers are thought to be beneficial. Capsaicin (8-methyl-*N*-vanillyl-6-nonenamide), a major ingredient of these peppers, is used specifically for topical treatment of pain. It has also been shown to improve symptoms and reduce the size of the polyps associated with nasal hyperactivity.[78]

In mouse and human melanoma lines capsaicin has been shown to inhibit plasma membrane–reduced nicotinamide adenine dinucleotide (NADH) oxidase and cell growth, leading to apoptosis,[204] and to have potential carcinogenic activity as a result of its covalent modification of protein and nucleic acids.[290] Recent studies show that capsaicin may possess chemoprotective activity against some chemical carcinogens and mutagens.[290] On the other hand, in a case-control study in Mexico, chili pepper consumers were at a significantly higher risk of developing gastric cancer than nonconsumers.[171]

Capsaicin is among a whole host of chemical compounds, including sulfides, indoles, and vitamins, that have significant influence on the cytochrome P-450 enzymes which are responsible for the bulk of oxidation of xenobiotic chemicals.[110]

Evening Primrose Oil. In 1987, Van der Merwe and Booyens[311] reported the treatment of 21 patients with advanced malignancies with gamma-linolenic acid (GLA), based on the finding that GLA suppresses the proliferation of malignant cells in tissue culture and the observation that evening primrose oil, containing a high level of GLA, reduces the rate of growth of transplanted mammary carcinoma in rats. Subjective improvement was observed in almost all of their patients, and a survival benefit was reported in hepatocellular carcinoma patients, increasing from a mean of 40 days to 90 days, but using historical controls. Ongoing studies in Europe sponsored by Scotia Pharmaceuticals will help answer the question of clinical benefit. A single-course, 10-day infusion of lithium GLA for nonresectable pancreatic cancer is said to have significantly prolonged survival.[260] Intratumoral GLA is reported to have had significant results shrinking lesions without toxicity.[64,206]

Garlic. Garlic extract has been reported to inhibit the first stage of tumor promotion in a two-stage mouse skin carcinogenesis model in vivo,[214] to inhibit dimethylhydrazine-induced colon cancer in mice,[316] and to inhibit growth of Morris hepatomas,[61] possibly as a result of diallyl sulfide, a thioether. No clinical study in humans has been reported.

Ginseng. Yun and Choi[337] found a lower overall rate of several cancers, including lung cancer, hepatoma, and head and neck cancer, in people who took extracts or powdered ginseng but not in those who used fresh ginseng or ginseng tea. Ginseng can cause swollen, tender breasts; vaginal bleeding; and hypertension.

Mistletoe. Without empiric evidence of benefit, Steiner considered mistletoe a future cancer therapy but thought its spiritual quality would help integrate patients' "four different entities."[89] It is commonly used in Europe, especially in Germany, where yearly expenditure is more than $750,000. It has been used as a sedative and for treatment of epilepsy, headache, paralysis, hypertension, lung ailments, and debility. It is so popular that a stamp picturing the plant was issued in Guernsey, England, in 1978. Animal studies[153] in India have shown that Iscador, an extract from the semiparasitic plant *Viscum album*, was found to exhibit a dose-related inhibition of 20-methylcholanthrene-induced carcinogenesis in mice. Yoon and colleagues[334] reported the inhibitory effect of Korean mistletoe (*Viscum album coloratum*) extract on tumor angiogenesis and metastasis of hematogenous and nonhematogenous tumor cells in mice, which he believed to be a result of the induction of tumor necrosis factor–alpha.

Further studies with mistletoe (*Viscum album*) lectins[38] revealed that using these purified proteins from this plant induced apoptosis in lymphocytes in culture, as measured by the appearance of a hypodiploid DNA peak using flow cytometry. Mistletoe lectins have also been shown to have cytotoxic effects on breast cancer in cell culture.[259] In addition, it was postulated that cell killing may have been accomplished in an indirect way by damaging the cell membranes with subsequent influx of Ca^{2+} and of DNA intercalating dye propidium iodide and cell shrinkage.

Although mistletoe has been regarded as a dangerous plant, Spiller and co-workers[280] surveyed 92 people who had used this treatment, finding 11 patients symptomatic from the mistletoe treatment. The symptoms included gastrointestinal tract upset (six patients), mild drowsiness (two), eye irritation (one), ataxia (one child), and seizure (one child). Medical intervention was required in only one of these patients.

Herbal Remedy Toxicity

Plant products taken in excessive amounts may cause toxicity, just as synthesized drugs do. Even prune juice, a natural laxative, may cause diarrhea if taken in excess. Licorice may cause hypertension, as well as potassium loss. Many products can cause an allergic reaction, and many plants are carcinogenic in animals. Many herbal products are collected in their plant form, which may be contaminated with toxic insecticides, fertilizers, or infectious agents. Herbal remedies may contain lead, arsenic, mercury, tin, zinc, or arsenic, which can be toxic in their own right.[62]

Herbal remedies are often believed to be harmless because of the "natural" characteristics. Although this is generally true, potential and demonstrated toxicities occur and, especially because these herbs are often prescribed in otherwise healthy people and they are presumed to be safe, it is of particular importance to delineate some of these side effects (Table 6-2).

Two herbal products deserve specific mention: (1) Chaparral tea can cause severe liver toxicity with cholestasis and hepatocellular injury, which resolved with discontinuation and recurred with challenge[4,20] in one reported case leading to fulminant hepatic failure requiring a liver transplant.[102] There is also the possibility of renal disease resulting from chronic Chaparral tea ingestion.[274] (2) Recently the short-term use of the Chinese herb *Jin bu huan* has been found to produce life-threatening neurologic and cardiovascular effects requiring intubation in children. Long-term treatment causes liver injury of poorly defined hepatotoxic mechanism.[127,325] The chemical levo-tetrahy-dropalmatine, a potent neuroactive substance, may play a role in the toxicity because it is 34% by weight, whereas in the natural plant it is only 1.5%. This product is sold without childproof packaging. It has been banned in the United States but apparently is still available.

Other Toxicities

As has been stated before, supplementation in healthy individuals can be problematic because of the toxicities, even if they are rare, of these products. Vitamin toxicities are uncommon but well defined, including vitamin A's side effects of increased intracranial pressure and vomiting in children and its chronic use in adults potentially leading to hypercalcemia,[85] teratogenic abnormalities,[222] and rheumatologic complications.* Pennes and colleagues,[230] in a *prospective* study of patients receiving 13-*cis*-retinoic acid therapy, described the skeletal hyperostoses. The most common site of extraspinal hyperostoses is the knee.[322] These arthropathies with arthralgias and myalgias may appear, often disappearing even with continued use.

Vitamin B complex overdose can lead to cardiovascular toxicities including arrhythmias, edema, vasodilation, and allergic reactions. Megadoses of niacin can cause cardiac toxicity with arrhythmias and infarction, as well as liver toxicity and peptic ulceration. Long-term high-dose toxicities include gouty arthritis, hyperglycemia, hyperkeratosis, dry skin, and rashes.[199] Vitamin B_6 in megadose levels has caused peripheral neuropathies with resulting numbness lasting up to 3 years.

Vitamin C toxicities include the development of renal stones and a risk of rebound scurvy when high-dose treatment is discontinued. Ascorbate has been found to inhibit mitoses and to induce chromosomal aberrations in cultured Chinese hamster ovary cells. The addition of copper and manganese enhanced both actions. Iron in both the ferrous and ferric states also enhanced the chromosome-damaging capacity of ascorbate.[285,286]

Vitamin D overdose becomes evident in elevated blood calcium levels causing symptoms of anorexia, nausea and vomiting, polyuria, polydipsia, weakness, pruritus, and nervousness, potentially with irreversible calcification of soft tissue in the kidney and liver. As newer, more highly active forms of vitamin D are developed, it becomes imperative to monitor even more carefully for this potential toxicity.

---

*References 41, 85, 147, 187, 211, 230.

High-dose vitamin E therapy can interfere with blood coagulation by antagonizing vitamin K and inhibiting prothrombin production. As discussed earlier, in a recent study of vitamin E an increased number of strokes were observed in the vitamin E treatment group as compared with the control group.[3]

Immunoaugmentative Therapy

Immunoaugmentative therapy (IAT), proposed by Burton (cited by Cassileth and Hauser),[45,115] is based on balancing four protein components in the blood, relying on strengthening the patient's immune system. The use of various organ extracts from cows and pigs is claimed to selectively suppress tumors, stimulate defense cells, and revitalize several tissues. No studies have shown clinical effectiveness.[5,43,308] There is an apparent decline in the popularity of this treatment.[45]

Mind-Body Techniques

A number of laboratories have documented that psychologic techniques have affected the immune system of specific people, such as those with a high absorption ability, that is, the ability to concentrate so intently that physiologic responses occur to mental events such as fantasies or memories.[295] Screening for these inclusionary personal characteristics may be helpful before prescribing a particular adjunctive technique such as relaxation or imagery.[107]

Prayer, meditation, biofeedback, and yoga are all being used with increasing frequency in the treatment of cancer. Anecdotal cases of tumor regression in juxtaposition with prayer have been discussed, as well as the relationship of prayer in lessening anxiety.[68] Biofeedback has been beneficial in treating cancer pain as well as in regaining both urinary and fecal continence after cancer surgery.[46,150,264] *Visualization* of the cancer so that the body is able to fight it helps put the patient back into control over his or her own health care and may help with stress reduction,[269] but failure of the method to change the course of cancer puts the blame squarely on the shoulders of the patient.

The use of these treatment methods as a primary treatment has not been studied in a controlled way. Anecdotal reports of response, for example, in Bob Brody's *Athlete's Edge Against Cancer,* implies that the mind of the athlete is particularly conducive to "fighting" against cancer and that others can learn to do this as well.[44]

Distraction therapies—having pleasant thoughts or activities to distract someone from the unpleasant effects of cancer such as pain—and *cognitive behavior*—making an active effort to view the cancer in the best possible light (such as "taking 1 day at a time")—may have roles to play in the overall care of the cancer patient.

A 1989 report in *Lancet* showed a survival advantage for women who were randomly assigned to a weekly support group with self-hypnosis for pain compared with those who were not.[277] A second study failed to demonstrate such an advantage,[91] but there are other end points to be measured rather than just survival, including satisfaction with treatment or coping skills. It is important to consider these intermediate or surrogate end points when designing studies. Also, combining methods such as nutrition and relaxation or other mind-body therapies can lead to additive effects.[317] A greater self-awareness in one arena may potentiate good health practices in another.

Aromatherapy is becoming more popular in the United States. Wilkinson[319] described 51 patients in a hospice who were divided into two massage therapy arms, one using standard massage oil alone and one group with 1% essential oil, Roman chamomile, added. Although both groups showed a decrease in anxiety, the experimental aromatherapy group exhibited even lower anxiety, fewer physical symptoms, and a better quality of life.

Meditation. Transcendental meditators have been found to have higher daytime levels of the serotonin metabolite 5-hydroxyindole-3-acetic acid (5-HIAA) compared with controls, and these levels increased with meditation. Serotonin is a precursor of melatonin. Meditation and melatonin have some similar effects: analgesia, antistress effect, antiinsomnia/hypnotic effect, and decreased heart rate and blood pressure.[182]

Bioelectric Treatments

Nordenstrom[217,218,219] described electric stimulation treatment for cancer. Electroporation, a new technique to enhance antitumor effects of chemotherapeutic agents, has been expounded recently by a number of researchers.[66,95,120,121] They reported that electric current delivered to the tumor reversibly increases permeability of the cell membranes, allowing intracellular concentrations of chemotherapy to increase significantly, up to 700 times with some agents.

Chou and colleagues[55] reported beneficial treatment of fibrosarcomas in mice and rats with direct electrical current via apoptosis (see Chapter 2). A number of reports of small studies indicate the potential of electrochemotherapy in several cancer types including salivary gland and breast cancer,[67] lung cancer,[336] hepatocellular carcinoma,[130,332] and others.[151,183,338]

In a clinical study of basal cell carcinomas of two patients, using some untreated nodules as controls while applying direct electrical current to other nodules simultaneously with systemic bleomycin chemotherapy, improvement noted with the direct current was significantly greater than with bleomycin alone. Mir and co-workers[193] found that the addition of IL-2 to bleomycin/electrochemotherapy increased cure rates of subcutaneously implanted cancer in mice.

Seven patients with squamous cell carcinoma of the head and neck were treated with electroporation and very-low-dose bleomycin.[192] Of the 34 treated nodules in these seven patients, 14 showed a complete remission, and 9, partial regression. Multiple nodular disease is an odd presentation for head and neck carcinomas, and there is a question of the natural history of these patients. The results indicate a need for randomized studies with clear measurements and follow-up.

Hydrazine Sulfate

Hydrazine sulfate has been claimed to be a cure for cancer and a treatment of its devastating effects, including cachexia, for several decades. The potential mechanism of action was said to be its monoamine oxidase–like effect. Many anecdotal and some controlled studies were reported throughout the 1970s and 1980s indicating effectiveness of hydrazine as a cancer treatment,* as well as effectiveness as a treatment for the abnormal glucose tolerance found in cachectic cancer patients,[54] but other studies failed to confirm this.[160,220,281] Recently, several randomized, well-controlled studies showed no beneficial effect in lung cancer or colorectal cancer.[149,172,173] The double-blind study by Kosty and colleagues[149] included 291 newly diagnosed, untreated patients with non–small cell cancer of the lung randomly selected after optimal treatment with cisplatinum and etoposide to receive hydrazine sulfate or placebo. There was no evidence of increased response rate or survival difference as a result of the hydrazine, but there was evidence of a *poorer* quality of life in the treated group. There was no difference in the two arms of this double-blind study with regard to anorexia, weight gain, or nutritional status. In the study by Loprinzi and colleagues,[173] 127 assessable patients with advanced colorectal cancer were randomly selected to use hydrazine sulfate or placebo. There were trends for poorer survival and for poorer quality of life in the hydrazine-treated patients. There were no differences in the two arms of this randomized study relating to anorexia or weight loss. Chlebowski and colleagues[53] reported a randomized study of non–small cell lung cancer patients treated with bleomycin, vinblastine, and cisplatinum followed by either observation or hydrazine sulfate. Neither response rate nor survival was statistically different in the two arms of the study. Caloric intake and albumin maintenance levels were improved in the hydrazine arm of the study. A further double-blind, randomized study of hydrazine sulfate of patients with colorectal cancer had to be discontinued early because the mortality in the treated arm was higher than predicted. Yet, the proponents of this therapy continue to claim value and report further noncontrolled studies (e.g., Filov et al.[81]) such as the treatment of 200 patients with lung cancer and 55 patients with colorectal cancer, claiming "positive" results when 6 of 740 patients are said to have a complete remission without clear evidence of measurable, biopsy-proven disease.

Much has been said of the potential improvement of the feeling of wellness and an improvement in the cachexia suffered by cancer patients.[51,53] Chlebowski and Grosvenor[54] described the abnormal glucose tolerance and increased glucose produc-

---

*References 51, 52, 53, 79, 80, 93, 96, 97, 98, 232.

tion frequently seen in cancer patients and the improvement found with hydrazine sulfate in these measurable parameters thought to be a result of the inhibition of gluconeogenesis. However, in the first of these "randomized" studies, the control group of 30 had an addition of 40 nonrandomized treated patients, a serious flaw in the design of the study. This was not confirmed in the well-designed study by Kosty and co-workers[149] and in the other studies cited above.

Amygdalin (Laetrile)

No discussion of CAM and cancer would be complete without a mention of the drug amygdalin (Laetrile), derived from apricot and other fruit pits. Although amygdalin had been used for centuries, it was elevated to new heights under the trade name Laetrile by Ernest Krebs, Jr., in 1952, and it totally eclipsed all other unorthodox treatments. A review was undertaken that revealed six cases in which there was a possible Laetrile effect. Based on these findings, Moertel and colleagues[195] treated 178 previously untreated patients with good performance status with Laetrile; vitamins A, C, E, and B complex; and minerals, as well as with pancreatic enzymes. Only one patient, who had a gastric carcinoma with cervical lymph node metastases, had a possible short-lived, partial remission of 10 weeks. All others showed no response. There was no evidence of stabilization of disease. Blood cyanide levels were high and often in the toxic range, at levels known to kill animals and humans. In addition, the Laetrile was generally available from Mexican suppliers and was found to be contaminated with infectious agents and endotoxin. Deaths attributable to Laetrile have been reported.[27,34,123,256]

Melatonin

The pineal gland appears to have an important role in regulating the body's circadian rhythm. In animal studies, pinealectomy has been reported to cause a proliferation of cancers, and physiologic concentrations of melatonin, a hormone synthesized in the pineal gland, inhibit growth in vitro of some breast cancer cell lines.[250] Epithalamin, a low-molecular-weight, pineal-derived peptide, prolonged the life of various strains of mice and rats. It was found to decrease the incidence of spontaneous tumors, as well as radiation-induced mammary carcinoma in rats; inhibited the growth of NEU-induced transplacental carcinogenesis in rats; inhibited the growth of transplanted tumors and their metastases; and increased tumor sensitivity to cytotoxic therapies.[10] One explanation given for these actions may be the observed increase in the night peak of melatonin with epithalamin treatment.

Melatonin levels rise to a plateau between midnight and 3:00 AM in people who have a standard work-sleep lifestyle) and then fall to low levels after light appears. The pineal gland and melatonin are involved in regulation and timing of reproduction, in development, and in the aging process.[182] Some of the possible mechanisms for melatonin activity are as an anti–physical stress hormone, as an immunomodulatory agent through the release of opioid peptides and IL-2 by T-helper cells, as a scavenger of endogenous hydroxyl radicals, as an oncostatic agent inhibiting proliferation of estrogen-responsive cells (e.g., MCF-7 human breast cancer cells), and as an endogenous antiestrogen inhibiting breast cancer growth in vivo and in vitro. Studies indicate that it may act synergistically with tamoxifen.

Melatonin level has been found to have a suppressed nighttime rise in patients with breast cancer. Patients who exhibited a twofold rise in peak levels were associated with a low proliferative index, possibly indicating a more favorable outcome. A depressed or absent nocturnal peak level has also been reported in men with prostate cancer as compared to men with benign prostatic hypertrophy or to normal control subjects. Also, melatonin has produced a survival advantage and an improvement in quality of life indicators in patients with brain metastases from solid tumors.[166]

It has been suggested that melatonin is a gonadal inhibitor and that the loss of this function with the decrease of melatonin could be related to the development of hormonally sensitive cancers, such as those of the breast or the prostate. Melatonin also appears to antagonize the immunosupressor effects of corticosteroids, to increase the cytotoxic activity of natural killer cells, and to reciprocally interact with beta-endorphins. There has been evidence of in vitro cytotoxic effects on cell culture preparations of breast, ovarian, and bladder cancers. Lissoni and colleagues[167] reported on preliminary work in which melatonin appeared to enhance the effect of IL-2 in patients with solid tumors other than renal cancer and to ameliorate the IL-2 toxicity. There is also evidence that melatonin blocks macrophage activation of IL-2, producing a possible beneficial effect in the treatment of cancer-related thrombocytopenia.[168,169]

The melatonin cycle has been found to be abnormal in some cancer patients. High rather than low levels of melatonin have been reported in the morning in women with breast cancer. Abnormal levels in the cycle of melatonin have been reported in men with prostate cancer.

Based on a very small, noncontrolled trial using subjective end points related to performance status, Braczkowski and colleagues[33] wrote in the *Annals of the New York Academy of Sciences* that "melatonin has to be considered as an essential drug in the curative or palliative therapy of human neoplasms and as a drug that plays an important role in reducing the administration toxicities of some cytokines." Further studies are needed to be able to draw such a conclusion. Maestroni and Conti[177] reviewed the published literature on the effects of melatonin on tumor growth and quality of life. They concluded that "melatonin protects against IL-2 and synergizes with the IL-2 anticancer action. This combined strategy represents a well-tolerated intervention to control tumor growth. In most cases performance status and quality of life seem improved." However, these reviewed studies were noncontrolled and often anecdotal, with subjective measurements.

Lissoni and co-workers[169] reported a study of 100 people with solid tumors who were to have no further conventional chemotherapy and were randomly selected to receive either IL-2 plus melatonin or supportive care. There was no single drug arm of the study. The investigators found a 17% response rate in the immunotherapy group as compared with the expected "no response" in the supportive therapy arm of the study. In addition, the 1-year survival was significantly improved, as was the experimental arm's performance status.

An intriguing study[128] indicates that the timing of chemotherapy may play an important role. The timing of the adriamycin dose when given in combination with cis-platinum in the treatment of 31 ovarian cancer patients was a determinant in the toxicity with a morning dose being less toxic. This again points to a potential influence of the circadian rhythm system.

Shark Cartilage

The use of shark cartilage as a potential treatment of cancer has become so well known that, according to one oncologist, 80% of cancer patients in that practice had asked about this treatment in the preceding several months.[180] The scientific basis for the use of shark cartilage is based on the following: (1) a finding that sharks infrequently get cancer (but in fact they have been shown to develop melanomas and brain malignancies[174]) and that most of the bulk of the shark is cartilage and this cartilage may be protective and (2) that cartilage from calves as well as other animals contain substances that decrease angiogenesis.[35,159] Cartilage itself is resistant to invasion by most tumors.[271] The fact that cartilage is vascularized in its embryonal form and then loses this vascularization led Brem and Folkman[35] to postulate the production of a factor from cartilage that inhibits vascularization and could inhibit tumor angiogenesis. Such a cartilage-derived factor has been discovered, purified, and found to be a protein with an approximate molecular weight of 24,000 with potent anticollagenase properties and very similar to a collagenase inhibitor isolated from cultured human skin fibroblasts.

McGuire and colleagues[187] reported that shark cartilage produced a concentration-dependent decline in endothelial cell ^{3}H-thymidine incorporation using a human umbilical vein endothelial cell proliferation assay. Gomes and colleagues[100] reported that shark cartilage was instrumental in protecting cells against lesions induced by hydrogen peroxide in normal and low iron conditions, suggesting a possible scavenger role against free radicals.

No clinical controlled studies have been published using shark cartilage. A small study conducted in Cuba was reported in a segment of the television show "60 Minutes" in 1993. Fifteen evaluable patients in a study of 29 patients were said to have 3 responders. No further information was given regarding the types of cancer, the definition of response, or the reason for deeming the other patients not evaluable. The NCI chose not to sponsor further studies. A further study of 70 patients by Simone was said to be ongoing, but no reports have been generated.[131] Even if cartilage has these properties, the likelihood of the ingested material reaching the tumor at all, and in an active state, would be unlikely.[180] Further, toxicity appears to be rare. One case of presumed hepatitis attributable to shark cartilage has been reported.[11]

The complete absence of clinical studies indicating any degree of efficacy among the thousands of cancer patients treated with shark cartilage suggests that, despite early in vitro results and extensive commercial publicity, this product offers no significant benefit for cancer patients.

Bovine Tracheal Cartilage

Bovine tracheal cartilage (BTC) is an acidic glycosaminoglycan complex containing 20% chondroitin sulfate and lesser quantities of dermatan sulfate, heparan sulfate, hyaluronic acid, and other polysaccharides. Human tumor stem cell assays have shown antitumor effect in vitro.[70] In 1985, Prudden[239] reported a significant response rate of 10% to 15% in various tumor types including pancreatic, non–small cell lung, gastric, and colon cancers and glioblastoma with no follow-up series. Puccio and co-workers [240] in 1994 reported three responses among 20 patients with metastatic renal cell cancer with this same agent. No toxicity has been reported.

TREATMENT OF SIDE EFFECTS OF CANCER AND CANCER TREATMENT

Cancer and its treatment causes many types of symptoms. Pain, nausea, and weakness are all potentially disabling. People's perceptions of their discomfort are so different one from another that health care providers must treat them individually with varying methods. Physical suffering (i.e. pain) is the most commonly reported and quantifiable, albeit imprecisely and subjectively, of these side effects (see Chapter 10).

One nonrandomized, controlled trial comparing one group that heard a personal tape-recorded message from the patient's physician at the time of chemotherapy with a control group without a recording found a reduction in overall anxiety levels with the personal message, but found no difference in specific side effects of chemotherapy.[255]

Breathlessness

Breathlessness in cancer patients is a common finding and a late sign of disease. The first treatment is that of the underlying disease entity (e.g., a mass lesion such as primary lung cancer or metastases from other cancers or the finding of a pleural effusion and, if that fails, treatment of the symptom itself. Its treatment is often chest physiotherapy to remove secretions, bronchodilators, oxygen, and respiratory sedatives such as opioids, frequently with little benefit. Other symptoms are controllable; pain is generally improved but breathlessness is not.[15] An intriguing preliminary study by Filshi and colleagues[82] found significant improvement in 14 of 20 patients with various cancer types who received treatment with sternal and hand acupuncture. This beneficial result lasted over the next $1^1/_2$ to 6 hours and was independent of the patient's anxiety index. The authors acknowledged that the placebo effect could have played a significant role and that a controlled study is needed. Bailey[15] discussed breathing control techniques and nursing therapy to alleviate loss of function and to ease the psychologic burden through an integrative model. The aims of these techniques are to promote a relaxed and gentle breathing pattern; to minimize the work of breathing; to establish a sense of control; to improve ventilation at the bases of the lungs; to increase the strength, coordination, and efficiency of the respiratory muscles; to maintain mobility of the thoracic cage; and to promote a sense of well-being. They reported preliminarily that their techniques are successful in enhancing a quality of life of patients with lung cancer experiencing breathlessness.

Mucositis

A controlled clinical trial of 94 patients in the use of imagery and cognitive-behavior training designed to reduce mucositis pain during cancer treatment was performed by Syrjala and colleagues[292] The following groups of patients who had undergone bone marrow transplantation were compared: (1) treatment as usual, to act as controls, (2) therapist support, (3) relaxation and imagery training, and (4) training in a package of cognitive-behavioral coping skills that included relaxation and imagery. The authors concluded that relaxation and imagery training reduced the cancer treatment–related pain of mucositis relative to the control arm but that adding cognitive-behavioral skills did not enhance this improvement further.

Nausea and Vomiting

Keller[142] summarized several nonpharmacologic approaches to the treatment of nausea and vomiting resulting from cancer treatment in children. These included distraction, including listening to music, which was effective in decreasing the duration of the nausea but not its severity, or the use of video games, which decreased both the anticipatory and the posttreatment nausea. Hypnosis, used in children as young as 4 years old, led to a decrease in severity and duration of nausea. Progressive muscle relaxation with relaxation tapes appeared to decrease nausea. Modification of diet can be helpful. Acupuncture, acupressure, or transcutaneous electric stimulation of the P6 antiemetic acupuncture site seemed to have some effect, which was not found with treatment to a dummy acupuncture site. Nausea resulting from chemotherapy can be ameliorated by the use of hypnosis.[92] Jacknow and colleagues[134] reported the decrease in anticipatory nausea in children, a common and often treatment-limiting side effect of chemotherapy, that was sustained after only 2 months of treatment using self-hypnosis. Significantly fewer doses of as-needed antiemetics were used by the treatment group as compared with a control group in this small, randomized study of 20 patients. Hypnosis also was found to improve coping skills in cancer patients, leading to decreased symptoms.

Radiation-Induced Xerostomia

Xerostomia is a common toxic effect of radiation therapy. Acupuncture was given to 41 patients with varying degrees of xerostomia.[31] No explanation for the rationale for this treatment was given. Classic acupuncture was used as the treatment arm, and superficial, subcutaneous acupuncture 1 cm from the classic site was used as a control. There was no difference in the results between the two arms, although there was some improvement in both groups. Whether it was the normal healing that occurs or if it was a result of the acupuncture could not be determined. The authors concluded that acupuncture might be helpful in this condition and that superficial acupuncture should not be the control.

SUMMARY

CAM is widely used in the treatment of cancer by all types of people, more commonly among the educated and affluent. As insurance companies increase coverage, CAM use will rise. It is important for health care providers to be knowledgeable about these treatments and to discuss them openly with patients.

Diet has been implicated as a means of preventing cancer. Low-fat, high-fiber diets are associated with lower colon, breast, and aggressive prostate cancer risks. The use of antioxidants, for example, vitamins A, C, and E, is controversial as preventive treatment. No diets or herbal treatments have been shown to reliably achieve responses for active cancer, although the polysaccharide agent PSK has been demonstrated in Phase III studies to prolong survival when used as an adjuvant agent. Melatonin, chlorella, PC SPES, and other herbal agents have shown indications of anticancer activity in preliminary studies and merit closer investigation.

An important use of CAM in cancer patients appears to be in the treatment of side effects of the cancer and its treatment. The value of acupuncture, even in the treatment of pain, is still controversial. Hypnosis, relaxation, and imagery techniques seem to benefit patients with pain, anxiety, and nausea.

All alternative therapies, including diet, herbal products, and electric stimulation, must be studied in controlled, preferably blinded, randomized trials to prove effectiveness and to be included in the general armamentarium of treatments for patients with cancer.

REFERENCES

1. Abrams DB et al: Cancer control at the workplace: the Working Well Trial, *Prev Med* 23(1):15, 1994.
2. Akazaki K, Stemmermann GN: Comparative study of latent carcinoma of the prostate among Japanese in Japan and Hawaii, *J Natl Cancer Inst* 50:1137, 1973.
3. Albanes D et al: Effects of alpha-tocopherol and beta-carotene supplements on cancer incidence, *Am J Clin Nutr* 62(6 suppl):1427s, 1995.

4. Alderman S et al: Cholestatic hepatitis after ingestion of Chaparral leaf: confirmation by endoscopic retrograde cholangiopancreatography and liver biopsy, *J Clin Gastroenterol* 19(3):242, 1994.

5. American Cancer Society: Questionable methods of cancer management: Immuno-augmentative therapy (IAT), *CA Cancer J Clin* 41:357, 1991.

6. American Cancer Society: Questionable methods of cancer management: "nutritional therapies," *CA Cancer J Clin* 43(5):309, 1993.

7. American Cancer Society: Questionable methods of cancer management: electronic devices, *CA Cancer J Clin* 44(2):115, 1994.

8. American Cancer Society: Psychic surgery, *CA Cancer J Clin* 40(3):18, 1990.

9. Andersson S, Lundeberg T: Acupuncture: from empiricism to science—functional background to acupuncture effects in pain and disease, *Med Hypotheses* 45(3):271, 1995.

10. Anisimov VN, Khavinson Vkh, Morozov VG: Twenty years of study on effects of pineal peptide preparation: epithalamin in experimental gerontology and oncology, *Ann N Y Acad Sci* 719:483, 1994.

11. Ashar B, Vargo E: Shark cartilage-induced hepatitis, *Ann Intern Med* 125(9):780, 1996.

12. Aulas JJ, Alternative cancer treatments, *Scientific American* 275(3):162, 1996.

13. Austin S, Dale EB, DeKadt S: Long term follow-up of patients using Contreras, Hoxsey, and Gerson therapies, *J Naturopath Med* 5:74, 1995.

14. Bagneal FS et al: Survival of patients with breast cancer attending Bristol Cancer Help Centre, *Lancet* 336:606, 1990.

15. Bailey C: Nursing as therapy in the management of breathlessness in lung cancer, *Eur J Cancer Care* (Engl) 4(4):184, 1995.

16. Banner RO et al: A breast and cervical cancer project in a native Hawaiian community: Wai'anae cancer research project, *Prev Med* 24(5):447, 1995.

17. Barber DA, Harris SR: Oxygen free radicals and antioxidants: a review, *Am Pharm* NS34(9):26, 1994.

18. Barken I: Personal communication, June 1997.

19. Barnes S: Effect of genistein on in vitro and in vivo models of cancer, *J Nutr* 125(3 Suppl):777s, 1995.

20. Batchelor WB, Heathcote J, Wanless JR: Chaparral-induced hepatic injury, *Am J Gastroenterol* 90(5):831, 1995

21. Beck SL: The therapeutic use of music for cancer-related pain, *Oncol Nurs Forum* 18(8):1327, 1991.

22. Beecher HK: The powerful placebo, *JAMA* 159:1602, 1995.

23. Begbie SD, Kerestes ZL, Bell DR: Patterns of alternative medicine use by cancer patients, *Med J Aust* 18;165(10):545, 1996.

24. Beisel WR: Single nutrients and immunity, *Am J Clin Nutr* 35:416, 1982.

25. Benmeir P et al: Giant melanoma of the inner thigh: a homeopathic life-threatening negligence, *Ann Plast Surg* 27:583, 1991.

26. Berkowitz CD: Homeopathy: keeping an open mind, *Lancet* 344:701, 1994.

27. Betz JM et al: Determination of pyrrolizidine alkaloids in commercial comfrey products (*Symphytum* sp.), *J Pharm Sci* 83(5):649, 1994.

28. Bin W, Zhou RX, Zhou MS: Effect of acupuncture on interleukin-2 level and NK cell immunoactivity of peripheral blood of malignant tumor patients, *Chung Kuo Chung Hsi I Chieh Ho Tsa Chih* 14(9):537, 1994.

29. Bin W: Effect of acupuncture on the regulation of cell-mediated immunity in the patients with malignant tumors, *Chen Tzu Yen Chiu* 20(3):67, 1995.

30. Blackburn GL: Fatty acids decrease colonic epithelial cell proliferation in high-risk bowel mucosa. Second International Congress of the International Society for the Study of Fatty Acids and Lipids (ISSFAL). Congress Program and Abstracts, Symposium H, June 8, 1995.

31. Blom M et al: Acupuncture treatment of patients with radiation-induced xerostomia, *Eur J Cancer B Oral Oncol* 32B(3):182, 1996.

32. Bounoux P et al: Alpha-linolenic acid content of adipose breast tissue: a host determinant of the risk of early metastasis in breast cancer, *Br J Cancer* 70:330, 1994.

33. Braczkowski R et al: Modulation of tumor necrosis factor, *Ann N Y Acad Sci* 768:334, 1995.

34. Braico KT et al: Laetrile intoxication: report of a fatal case, *N Engl J Med* 300:238, 1979.

35. Brem H, Folkman J: Inhibition of tumor angiogenesis mediated by cartilage, *J Exp Med* 141:427, 1975.
36. Brigden ML: Unproven (questionable) cancer therapies, *West J Med* 163(5):463, 1995.
37. Burzynski SR: Potential antineoplastons in disease of old age, *Drugs Aging* 7(3):157, 1995.
38. Bussing A et al: Induction of apoptosis in human lymphocytes treated with *Viscum album L.* Is mediated by the mistletoe lectins, *Cancer Lett* 99(1):59, 1996.
39. Camp V: The place of acupuncture in medicine today, *Br J Rheumatol* 34(5):404, 1995.
40. Campion EW: Why unconventional medicine? *N Engl J Med* 328:282, 1993.
41. Carey BM et al: Skeletal toxicity with isotretinoin therapy: a clinico-radiological evaluation, *Br J Dermatol* 119:604, 1988.
42. Cassileth B et al: Contemporary unorthodox treatments in cancer medicine: a study of patients, treatments, and practitioners, *Ann Intern Med* 101:105, 1984.
43. Cassileth BR et al: Survival and quality of life among patients receiving unproven as compared with conventional cancer therapy, *N Engl J Med* 324:1180, 1991.
44. Cassileth BR, Chapman CC: Alternative cancer medicine: a ten-year update, *Cancer Invest* 14(4):396, 1996.
45. Cassileth BR, Chapman CC: Alternative and complementary cancer therapies, *Cancer* 77(6):1026, 1996.
46. Cavina E: Outcome of restorative perineal graciloplasty with simultaneous excision of the anus and rectum for cancer: a ten-year experience with 81 patients, *Dis Colon Rectum* 39(2):182, 1996.
47. Caygill CP, Charlett A, Hill MJ: Fat, fish, fish oil, and cancer, *Br J Cancer* 74(1):159, 1996.
48. Chan TY et al: Poisoning due to an over-the-counter hypnotic: Sleep-Qik (hyoscine, cyproheptadine, valerian), *Postgrad Med J* 71(834):227, 1995.
49. Chen CH, Yang SW, Shen YC: New steroid acids from *Antrodia cinnomomea*, a fungal parasite of *Cinnamomum micranthum*, *J Nat Prod* 58(11):1655, 1995.
50. Chen GO et al: In vitro studies on cellular and molecular mechanisms of arsenic trioxide As_2O_3 in the treatment of acute promyelocytic leukemia: As_2O_3 induces NB4 cell apoptosis with downregulation of Bci-2 expression and modulation of PML-RAR alpha/PML proteins, *Blood* 88(3):1052, 1996.
51. Chlebowski RT et al: Influence of hydrazine sulfate on abnormal carbohydrate metabolism in cancer patients with weight loss, *Cancer Res* 44:857, 1984.
52. Chlebowski RT et al: Hydrazine sulfate in cancer patients with weight loss, *Cancer* 59:406, 1987.
53. Chlebowski RT et al: Hydrazine sulfate influence on nutritional status and survival in non–small-cell lung cancer, *J Clin Oncol* 8:9, 1990.
54. Chlebowski RT, Grosvenor M: The scope of nutrition intervention with cancer-related endpoints, *Cancer* 74(suppl 9l):273, 1994.
55. Chou CK et al: Electrochemical treatment of mouse and rat fibrosarcoma with direct current, *Bioelectromagnets* 18:14, 1997.
56. Chung CH, Go P, Chang KH: PSK immunotherapy in cancer patients: a preliminary report, *Chung Hua Min Kuo Wei Sheng Wu Chi Mien I Hseuh Tsa Chih* 20(3):210, 1987.
57. Clark L, Combs GF Jr, Turnbull BW: The nutritional prevention of cancer with selenium: 1983 to 1993—a randomized clinical trial, *FESEB J* 10:A550, 1996 (abstract).
58. Cohen LA, Rose DP, Wynder EL: A rationale for dietary intervention in postmenopausal breast cancer patients: an update, *Nutr Cancer* 19:1, 1993.
59. Couet CE, Crews C, Hanley AB: Analysis, separation, and bioassay of pyrrholizidine alkaloids from comfrey *(Symphytum officinate)*, *Nat Toxins* 4(4):163, 1996.
60. Couldwell WT et al: Hypericin: a potential antiglioma therapy, *Neurosurgery* 35(4):705, 1994 (erratum appears in *Neurosurgery* 35[5]:993, 1994).
61. Criss WE et al: Inhibition of tumor growth with low dietary protein and dietary garlic extracts, *Fed Proc* 41:281, 1982.
62. D'Arcy PF: Adverse reactions and interactions with herbal medicines. I. Adverse reactions, *Adverse Drug React Toxicol Rev* 10:189, 1991.
63. Dady PJ: New Zealand cancer patients and alternative medicine, *N Z Med J* 100:110, 1987.
64. Das US, Prasad VV, Reddy DR: Local application of gamma-lineolenic acid in the treatment of human gliomas, *Cancer Lett* 94:147, 1995.

65. Dawson E, Nosovitch J, Hannigan E: Serum vitamin and selenium changes in cervical dysplasia, *Fed Proc* 46:612, 1984.

66. Dev SB, Hoffmann GA: Electrochemotherapy: a novel method of cancer treatment, *Cancer Treat Rev* 20(1):105, 1994.

67. Domenge C et al: Antitumor electrochemotherapy, *Cancer* 77:956, 1996.

68. Dossey L: *Healing Words,* San Francisco, 1993, Harper.

69. Downer SM et al: Pursuit and practice of complementary therapies by cancer patients receiving conventional treatment, *Br Med J* 309(6947):86, 1994.

70. Durie BG, Soehnlen B, Prudden JF: Antitumor activity of bovine cartilage extract (Catrix-S) in the human tumor stem cell assay, *J Biol Response Mod* 4(6):590, 1985.

71. Dwivedi C et al: Inhibitory effects of Maharishi-4 and Maharishi-5 on microsomal lipid peroxidation, *Pharmacol Biochem Behav* 39:649, 1991.

72. Early Breast Cancer Trialists' Collaborative Group: Systemic treatment of early breast cancer by hormonal, cytotoxic, or immune therapy—133 randomized trials involving 31,000 recurrences and 24,000 deaths among 75,000 women, *Lancet* 339:71, 1992.

73. Ernst E: Complementary medicine: changing attitudes, *Complement Ther Med* 2:121, 1994.

74. Ernst E: Complementary medicine: common misconceptions, *J R Soc Med* 88(5):244, 1995 (editorial).

75. Ernst, E: Complementary cancer treatments: hope or hazard? *Clin Oncol (R Coll Radiol)* 7(4):259, 1995.

76. Ferley IP et al: A controlled evaluation of a homeopathic preparation in the treatment of influenza-like syndomes, *Br J Clin Pharmacol* 27:329, 1989.

77. Fields J et al: Oxygen free radical (OFR) scavenging effects of an anti-carcinogenic natural product, Maharishi Amrit Kalask (MAK), *Pharmacologist* 32:A155, 1990 (abstract).

78. Filiaci F et al: Local treatment of nasal polyposis with capsaicin: preliminary findings, *Allergol Immunopathol (Madr)* 24(1):13, 1996.

79. Filov VA et al: Hydrazine sulfate: experimental and clinical results, mechanisms of action. In Filov VA et al., editors: *Medical therapy of tumors*, Leningrad, USSR, 1983, USSR Ministry of Health, p 92.

80. Filov VA et al: Results of clinical evaluation of hydrazine sulfate, *Vopr Onkol* 36:721, 1990.

81. Filov VA et al: Experience of the treatment with Sehydrin (hydrazine sulfate, HS) in the advanced cancer patients, *Invest New Drugs* 13(1):89, 1995.

82. Filshi J et al: Acupuncture for the relief of cancer-related breathlessness, *Palliat Med* 10(2):145, 1996.

83. Fisher P, Ward A: Complementary medicine in Europe, *Br Med J* 309:107, 1994.

84. Fotsis T et al: Genistein, a dietary ingested isoflavinoid, inhibits cell proliferation and in vitro angiogenesis, *J Nutr* 1995 125(suppl 3):790s, 1995.

85. Frame B et al: Hypercalcemia and skeletal effects in chronic hypervitaminosis A, *Ann Intern Med* 80:44, 1974.

86. Freedman LS et al: Dietary fat and breast cancer: where we are, *J Natl Cancer Inst* 85:764, 1994.

87. Friess H et al: Treatment of advanced pancreatic cancer with mistletoe: results of a pilot trial, *Anticancer Res* 16(2):915, 1996.

88. Fukushima M: Adjuvant therapy of gastric cancer: the Japanese experience, *Semin Oncol* 23(3):369, 1996.

89. Gabius HJ et al: The mistletoe myth: claims, reality, and provable perspectives, *Z Arztl Fortbild (Jena)* 90(2):103, 1996.

90. Garewal HS, Diplock AT: How safe are antioxidant vitamins? *Drug Saf* 13(1):8, 1995.

91. Gellert GA et al: Survival of breast cancer patients receiving adjunct psychosocial support therapy: a 10-year follow-up study, *J Clin Oncol* 11:66, 1993.

92. Genuis ML: The use of hypnosis in helping cancer patients control anxiety, pain, and emesis: a review of recent empirical studies, *Am J Clin Hypn* 37(4):316, 1995.

93. Gershanovich ML et al: Results of clinical study of antitumor action of hydrazine sulfate, *Nutr Cancer* 3:7, 1981.

94. Giovannucci E et al: A prospective study of dietary fat and risk of prostate cancer, *J Natl Cancer Inst* 85:1571, 1993.

95. Glass LF et al: Bleomycin-mediated electrochemotherapy of basal cell carcinoma, *J Am Acad Dermatol* 34(1):82, 1996.

96. Gold J: The use of hydrazine sulfate in terminal and preterminal cancer patients: results of investigational new drug (IND) study in 84 evaluable patients, *Oncology* 32:1, 1975.

97. Gold J: Anabolic profiles in late-stage cancer patients responsive to hydrazine sulfate, *Cancer* 3:13, 1981.

98. Gold J: Hydrazine sulfate: a current perspective, *Nutr Cancer* 9:59, 1987.

99. Goldin BR et al: The effect of dietary fat and fiber on serum estrogen concentrations in premenopausal women under controlled dietary conditions, *Cancer* 74:1125, 1994.

100. Gomes EM, Souto PR, Felzenszwalb I: Shark-cartilage–containing preparation protects cells against hydrogen peroxide–induced damage and mutagenesis, *Mutat Res* 367(4):204, 1996.

101. Goodwin WJ Jr, Lane HW, Bradford K: Selenium and glutathione peroxidase levels in patients with epidermoid carcinoma of the oral cavity and oropharynx, *Cancer* 51:110, 1983.

102. Gordon DW et al: Chaparral ingestion: the broadening spectrum of liver injury caused by herbal medications, *JAMA* 273(6):489, 1995.

103. Greenberg ER, Sporn MB: Antioxidant vitamins, cancer, and cardiovascular disease, *N Engl J Med* 334(18):1145, 1150, 1189, 1996.

104. Greenberg ER et al: A clinical trial of beta carotene to prevent basal-cell and squamous-cell cancers of the skin: the Skin Cancer Prevention Study Group, *N Engl J Med* 323(12):825, 1990.

105. Greenwald P: Preventive clinical trials: an overview, *Ann N Y Acad Sci* 768:129, 1995.

106. Greewald P: The potential of dietary modification to prevent cancer, *Prev Med* 25(1):41, 1996.

107. Gregerson (Jasnoski) MB, Roberts I, Amiri M: Absorption and imagery locate immune responses in the body, *Biofeedback Self-Regul* 21(2):149, 1996.

108. Grobstein C, Chairman, Committee on Diet, Nutrition and Cancer: *Assembly of Life Sciences, National Academy of Sciences*, Washington, DC, 1982, National Academy Press.

109. Grossgebauer K: The "cancell" theory of carcinogenesis: re-evolution of an ancient holistic neoplastic unicellular concept of cancer, *Med Hypotheses* 45(6):545, 1995.

110. Guengerich FP: Influence of nutrients and other dietary materials on cytochrome P-450 enzymes, *Am J Clin Nutr* 61(suppl 3):651s, 1995.

111. Gupta S et al: Plasma selenium level in cancer patients, *Indian J Cancer* 31(3):192, 1994.

112. Halicka HD et al: Apoptosis and cell cycle effects induced by extracts of the Chinese herbal preparation PC SPES (submitted for publication).

113. Hall CL et al: Overexpression of the hyaluron receptor RHAMM is transforming and is also required for H-ras transformation, *Cell* 82:19, 1995.

114. Harada M et al: Oral administration of PSK can improve the impaired anti-tumor CD4+ T-cell response in gut-associated lymphoid tissue (GALT) of specific-pathogen-free mice, *Int J Cancer* 70(3):362, 1997.

115. Hauser SP: Unproven methods in cancer treatment, *Curr Opin Oncol* 5(4):646, 1993.

116. Hawrylewica EJ, Zapata JJ, Blair WH: Soy and experimental cancer: animal studies, *J Nutr* 125(suppl 3l):698s, 1995.

117. Hayakawa K et al: Effect of krestin (PSK) as adjuvant treatment on the prognosis after radical radiotherapy in patients with non-small cell lung cancer, *Anticancer Res* 13(5C):1815, 1993.

118. Heinonen OP et al: Prostate cancer and supplementation with alpha-tocopherol and beta-carotene: incidence and mortality in a controlled trial, *J Natl Cancer Inst* 90(6):440, 1998.

119. Helary SS: Unproven treatments in cancerology, *Bull Cancer (Paris)* 78(10):915, 1991.

120. Heller R: Treatment of cutaneous nodules using electrochemotherapy, *J Fla Med Assoc* 82(2):147, 1995.

121. Heller R et al: Phase I/II trial for the treatment of cutaneous and subcutaneous tumors using electrochemotherapy, *Cancer* 77(5):964, 1996.

122. Henneckens CH et al: Lack of effect of long-term supplementation with beta carotene on the incidence of malignant neoplasms and cardiovascular disease, *N Engl J Med* 334(18):1146, 1189, 1996.

123. Herbert V: *Nutrition cultism: facts and fictions*, Phiadelphia, 1981, Stickley.

124. Herbert V: The antioxidant supplement myth, *Am J Clin Nutr* 60(2):157, 1994.

125. Hijikata Y et al: Traditional Chinese medicines improve the course of refractory leukemic lymphoblastic lymphoma and acute lymphocytic leukemia: two case reports, *Am J Chin Med* 23(2):195, 1995.

126. Horie Y et al: Bu ji (hozai) for treatment of postoperative gastric cancer patients, *Am J Chin Med* 22(3-4):300, 1994.

127. Horowitz RS et al: The clinical spectrum of Jin Bu Huan toxicity, *Arch Intern Med* 156(8):899, 1996.

128. Hrushesky WMJ: Circadian timing of cancer chemotherapy, *Science* 228:73, 1985.

129. Hsieh T et al: Regulation of androgen receptor (AR) and prostate specific antigen (PSA) expression in the androgen-responsive prostate LNCaP cells by ethanolic extract of the Chinese herbal preparation, PC SPES *Biochem Mol Biol Int* 42(3):535, 1997.

130. Hua-ling W: Electrochemical therapy of 74 cases of liver cancer, *Eur J Surg* (suppl 574):55, 1994.

131. Hunt TJ, Connelly JF: Shark cartilage for cancer treatment, *Am J Health Syst Pharm* 52(16):1756, 1760, 1995.

132. Iino Y et al: Immunochemotherapies versus chemotherapy as adjuvant treatment after curative resection of operable breast cancer, *Anticancer Res* 15(6B):2907, 1995.

133. Iino Y et al: Eight-year results of adjuvant immunochemotherapies vs. chemotherapy in the treatment of operable breast cancer. *18th International Congress of Chemotherapy.* June 27–July 2, 1993, Stockholm, Sweden, p. 162.

134. Jacknow DS et al: Hypnosis in the prevention of chemotherapy-related nausea and vomiting in children: a prospective study, *J Dev Behav Pediatr* 15:258, 1994.

135. Jackson J: Unproven treatment in childhood oncology: how far should paediatricians co-operate? *J Med Ethics* 20(2):77, 1994.

136. Jacob RA, Burri BJ: Oxidative damage and defense, *Am J Clin Nutr* 63(6):985s, 1996.

137. Jordan KS, Mackey D, Garvey E: A 39-year-old man with acute hemolytic crisis secondary to intravenous injection of hydrogen peroxide, *J Emerg Nurs* 17:8, 1991.

138. Joyce CRB: Placebo and complementary medicine, *Lancet* 344:1279, 1994.

139. Jurkowski JJ, Cave WB: Dietary effects of menhaden oil on the growth and membrane lipids of rat mammary tumors, *J Natl Cancer Inst* 74(5):1145, 1985.

140. Kaizer L et al: Fish consumption and breast cancer risk: an ecological study, *Nutr Cancer* 12:61, 1989.

141. Kalble T, Otto T: Unconventional methods in superficial bladder cancer, *Urologe A* 33(6):553, 1994.

142. Keller VE: Management of nausea and vomiting in children, *J Pediatr Nurs* 10(5):280, 1995.

143. Kelloff GJ et al: Mechanistic considerations in chemopreventive drug development, *J Cell Biochem Suppl* 20:1, 1994.

144. Kennedy AR: The evidence for soybean products as cancer preventive agents, *J Nutr* 126(2):582, 1996.

145. Kennedy CW, Donohue JJ, Wan XS: Effects of the Bowman-Birk protease inhibitor on survival of fibroblasts and cancer cells exposed to radiation and cis-platinum, *Nutr Cancer* 26(2):209, 1996.

146. Key TJA et al: Sex hormones in women in rural China and in Britain, *Br J Cancer* 62:631, 1990.

147. Kilcoyne RF et al: Minimal spinal hyperostosis with low-dose isotretinoin therapy, *Invest Radiol* 21:41, 1986.

148. Konishi F et al: Antitumor effect induced by a hot water extract of chlorella vulgaris (CE): resistant to meth-A tumor growth mediated by CE-induced polymorphonuclear leukocytes, *Cancer Immunol Immunother* 19:73, 1985.

149. Kosty MP et al: Cisplatin, vinblastine, and hydrazine sulfate in advanced non–small cell lung cancer: a randomized placebo-controlled, double-blind Phase III study of the cancer and leukemia group B, *J Clin Oncol* 12:1113, 1994.

150. Kroesen AJ et al: Incontinence after ileo-anal pouch anastamosis: diagnostic criteria and therapeutic sequelae, *Chirurg* 66(4):385, 1995.

151. Kuanhong Q: Analysis of the clinical effectiveness of 144 cases of soft tissue and superficial malignant tumors treated with electrochemical therapy, *Eur J Surg* (suppl 574):37, 1994.

152. Kushi M: *The macrobiotic approach to cancer*, Wayne, NJ, 1982, Avery.

153. Kuttan G et al: Prevention of 20-methylcholanthrene-induced sarcoma by a mistletoe extract, Iscador, *Carcinogenesis* 17(5):1107, 1996.

154. Ladermann JP: Accidents of spinal manipulation, *Ann Swiss Chiropractors Assoc* 7:161, 1981.

155. Lai SS: Clinical observations: a Chinese herbal formula for the treatment of pain and associated symptoms of cancer. Conference of the World Association of Chinese Medicine, Toronto, Ontario, Canada, 1995.

156. Lamm DL et al: Megadose vitamins in bladder cancer: a double-blind clinical trial, *J Urol* 151:21, 1994.

157. Lavie G et al: Hypericin as an inactivator of infectious viruses in blood components, *Transfusion* 35(5):392, 1995.

158. Lavie G et al: The chemical and biological properties of hypericin: a compound with a broad spectrum of biological activities, *Med Res Rev* 15(2):111, 1995.

159. Lee A, Langer R: Shark cartilage contains inhibitors of angiogenesis, *Science* 221:1185, 1983.

160. Lerner HJ, Regelson W: Clinical trial of hydrazine sulfate in solid tumors, *Cancer Treat Rep* 60:959, 1976.

161. Lerner IJ: The physician and cancer quackery: the physician's role in promoting the scientific treatment of cancer and discouraging questionable treatment methods, *N Y State J Med* 93(2):96, 1993.

162. Lerner IJ, Kennedy BJ: The prevalence of questionable methods of cancer treatment in the United States, *CA Cancer J Clin* 42:181, 1992.

163. Light SE et al: Phase II trial of ALL-trans retinoic acid (ATRA) in acute promyelocytic leukemia (APL), *Proc Am Soc Clin Oncol* 11:263, 1992 (abstract 861).

164. Lipp FJ: The efficacy, history, and politics of medicinal plants, *Alternat Ther Health Med* 2(4):36, 1996.

165. Lippman SM et al: Retinoid chemoprevention studies in upper aerodigestive tract and lung carcinogenesis, *Cancer Res* 54(suppl 7):2025s, 1994.

166. Lissoni P et al: A randomized study with the pineal hormone melatonin versus supportive care alone in patients with brain metastases due to solid neoplasms, *Cancer* 73:699, 1994.

167. Lissoni P et al: A randomized study with subcutaneous low-dose interleukin-2 alone vs interleukin 2 plus the pineal neurohormone melatonin in advanced solid neoplasms other than renal cancer and melanoma, *Br J Cancer* 69(1):196, 1994.

168. Lissoni P et al: A biological study on the efficacy of low-dose subcutaneous interleukin 2 plus melatonin, *Oncology* 52(5):360, 1995.

169. Lissoni P et al: A randomized study of neuroimmunotherapy with low-dose subcutaneous interleukin-2 plus melatonin, *Support Care Cancer* 3(3):194, 1995.

170. Long K, Long R: Diet and development of cancer, *Nurse Pract Forum* 6(4):183, 1995.

171. Lopez-Carillo L, Hernandez Avila M, Dubrow R: Chili pepper consumption and gastric cancer in Mexico: a case-control study, *Am J Epidemiol* 139(3):263, 1994.

172. Loprinzi ChL et al: Randomized placebo-controlled evaluation of hydrazine sulfate in patients with advanced colorectal cancer, *J Clin Oncol* 12:1121, 1992.

173. Loprinzi Ch L et al: Placebo-controlled trial of hydrazine sulfate in patients with newly diagnosed non-small-cell lung cancer, *J Clin Oncol* 12:1126, 1994.

174. Lowenthal RM: On eye of newt and bone of shark, *Med J Aust* 160(6):323, 1994.

175. Lowenthal RM: Alternative cancer treatments, *Med J Aust* 165(10):536, 1996.

176. MacGregor et al: Hepatotoxicity of herbal remedies, *Br Med J* 299:1156, 1989.

177. Maestroni GJ, Conti A: Melatonin in human breast cancer tissue: association with nuclear grade and estrogen receptor status, *Lab Invest* 75(4):557, 1996.

178. Maione TE, Sharpe RJ: Development of angiogenesis inhibitors for clinical applications, *Trends Pharmacol Sci* 11:457, 1990.

179. Malpas JS: Oncology, *Postgrad Med J* 69 (808):85, 1993.

180. Markman M: Shark cartilage: the Laetrile of the 1990s, *Cleve Clin J Med* 63(3):179, 1996.

181. Marnett LJ, Honn KV: Overview of articles on eicosanoids and cancer, *Cancer Metastasis Rev* 13(3-4):237, 1994.

182. Massion AO et al: Meditation, melatonin and breast/prostate cancer: hypothesis and preliminary data, *Med Hypotheses* 44(1):39, 1995.

183. Matsushima Y et al: Clinical and experimental studies of anti-tumoral effects of electrochemical therapy (ECT) alone or in combination with chemotherapy, *Eur J Surg Suppl* 574:59, 1994.

184. Matthew B: Evaluation of chemoprevention of oral cancer with *Spirulina fusiformis*, *Nutr Cancer* 24:197, 1995.

185. McCarthy MF: Fish oil may impede tumor angiogenesis and invasiveness by down-regulating protein kinase C and modulating eicosanoid production, *Med Hypotheses* 46(2):107, 1996.

186. McGinnis LS: Alternative therapies: 1990—an overview, *Cancer* 67(suppl 6):1788, 1991.

187. McGuire TR et al: Antiproliferative activity of shark cartilage with and without tumor necrosis factor-alpha in human umbilical vein endothelium, *Pharmacotherapy* 16(2):237, 1996.

188. McLarty JW et al: Beta-carotene, vitamin A, and lung cancer chemoprevention: results of an intermediate endpoint study, *Am J Clin Nutr* 62(suppl 6):1431s, 1995.

189. Merchant RE, Rice CD, Young HF: Dietary chlorella pyrenoidosa for patients with malignant glioma: effects on immunocompetence, quality of life, and survival, *Phytother Res* 4:220, 1990.

190. Messina MJ et al: Soy intake and cancer risk: a review of the in vitro and in vivo data, *Nutr Cancer* 2(2):113, 1994.

191. Milas L, Hanson WR: Eicosanoids and radiation, *Eur J Cancer* 31A(10):1580, 1995.

192. Mir LM et al: Electrochemotherapy, a novel antitumor treatment: first clinical trial, *C R Acad Sci Paris* 313:613, 1991.

193. Mir LM et al: Systemic antitumor effects of electrochemotherapy combined with histocompatible cells secreting interleukin-2, *J Immunother Emphasis Tumor Immunol* 17(1):30, 1995.

194. Miyazawa Y et al: Immunomodulation by a unicellular green algae (chlorella pyrenoidosa) in tumor-bearing mice, *J Ethnopharmacol* 24:135, 1994.

195. Moertel CG et al: A clinical trial of amygdalin (Laetrile) in the treatment of human cancer, *N Engl J Med* 306:201, 1982.

196. Molteni A, Brizio-Molteni L, Persky V: In vitro hormonal effects of soybean isoflavones, *J Nutr* 125(suppl 3):751s, 1995.

197. Monaco GP, Green S: Recognizing deception in the promotion of untested and unproven medical treatments, *N Y State J Med* 93(2):88, 1993.

198. Montbriand MJ: *Decision heuristics and patients with cancer: alternate and biomedical choices.* Unpublished doctoral dissertation, College of Medicine, University of Saskatchewan, Saskatoon, Saskatchewan, Canada, 1993.

199. Montbriand MJ: An overview of alternative therapies chosen by patients with cancer, *Oncol Nurs Forum* 21(9):1547, 1994.

200. Moon RC: Vitamin A, retinoids and breast cancer, *Adv Exp Med Biol* 364:101, 1994.

201. Morant R, et al: Warum Benutzen Tumorpatienten alternativemedizin? *Schweiz Med Wochenschr* 121:1029, 1991.

202. Morimoto T et al: Anti-tumor–promoting glyceroglycolipids from the green alga, Chlorella vulgaris, *Phytochemistry* 40:1433, 1995.

203. Morimoto T et al: Postoperative adjuvant randomized trial comparing chemoendocrine therapy, chemotherapy, and immunotherapy for patients with stage II breast cancer: 5-year results from the Nishinihon Cooperative Study Group of Adjuvant Chemoendorine Therapy for Breast Cancer (ACETBC) of Japan, *Eur J Cancer* 32A(2):235, 1996.

204. Morre DJ et al: Capsaicin inhibits plasma membrane NADH oxidase and growth of human and mouse melanoma lines, *Eur J Cancer* 32A(11):1995, 1996.

205. Munstedt K et al: Unconventional cancer therapy: survey of patients with gynecological malignancy, *Arch Gynecol Obstet* 258(2):81, 1996.

206. Naidu MRS, Das UN, Kishan A: Intratumoral gamma-linolenic acid therapy of human gliomas, *Prostagland Leukot Essent Fatty Acids* 45:181, 1992.

207. Nakadaira H et al: Distribution of selenium and molybdenum and cancer mortality in Niigata, Japan, *Arch Environ Health* 50(5):374, 1995.

208. Nakazato H et al: Efficacy of immunochemotherapy as adjuvant treatment after curative resection of gastric cancer: Study Group of Immunochemotherapy with PSK for Gastric Cancer, *Lancet* 343(8906):1122, 1994.

209. Nanji AA, et al: Dietary saturated fatty acids down-regulate cyclooxygenase-2 and tumor necrosis factor alfa and reverse fibrosis in alcohol-induced liver disease in the rat, *Hepatology* 26(6):1538, 1997.

210. National Research Council: *Diet and health: implications for reducing chronic disease risk,* 1989, Washington, DC, National Academy Press.

211. Nesher G, Zuckner J: Rheumatologic complications of vitamin A and retinoids, *Semin Arthritis Rheum* 24(4):291, 1995.

212. Niekerk Van W: Cervical cytological abnormalities caused by folic acid deficiency, *Acta Cytol* 10:67, 1966.

213. Nio Y et al: Immunomodulation by orally administered protein-bound PSK in patients with gastrointestinal cancer, *Biotherapy* 4(2):117, 1992.

214. Nishino H et al: Anti-tumor promoting activity of garlic extracts, *Oncology* 46:277, 1989.
215. Niwa Y: Effect of Maharishi-4 and Maharishi-5 on inflammatory mediators with special reference to their free radical scavenging effect, *Indian J Clin Pract* 1:23, 1991.
216. Nomura AMY et al: The effect of dietary fat on breast cancer survival among Caucasian and Japanese women in Hawaii, *Breast Cancer Res Treat* 18:8135, 1991.
217. Nordenstom BE: Electrostatic field interference with cellular and tissue function, leading to dissolution of metastases that enhances the effect of chemotherapy, *Eur J Surg Suppl* 574:121, 1994.
218. Nordenstrom BE: Survey of mechanisms in electrochemical treatment (ECT) of cancer, *Eur J Surg Suppl* 574:93, 1994.
219. Nordenstrom BE: The paradigm of biologically closed electric curcuits (BCEC) and the formation of an International Association (IABC) for BCEC systems, *Eur J Surg Suppl* 574:7, 1994.
220. Ochua Jr M et al: Trial of hydrazine sulfate (NSC-150014) in patients with cancer, *Cancer Chemother Rep* 59:1151, 1975.
221. Ogoshi K et al: Immunotherapy for esophageal cancer: a randomized trial in combination with radio-therapy and radiochemotherapy, *Am J Clin Oncol* 18(3):216, 1995.
222. Olson JA: Adverse effects of large doses of vitamin A and retinoids, *Semin Oncol* 10:290, 1983.
223. Omenn GS: What accounts for the association of vegetables and fruits with lower incidence of cancers and coronary heart disease? *Ann Epidemiol* 5(4):333, 1995.
224. Orr J et al: Nutritional status of patients with untreated cervical cancer, *Am J Obstet Gynecol*; 151:632, 1985.
225. Pandey DK et al: Dietary vitamin C and beta-carotene and risk of death in middle-aged men: the Western Electric Study, *Am J Epidemiol* 142(12):1269, 1995.
226. Parkin DM: Cancer in developing countries, *Cancer Surv* 19-20:519, 1994.
227. Pastorino U et al: Adjuvant treatment of state I lung cancer with high-dose vitamin A, *J Clin Oncol* 11:1216, 1993.
228. Patel VK et al: Reduction of metastases of Lewis lung carcinoma by an Ayurvedic food supplement in mice, *Nutr Res* 12: 667, 1992.
229. Pawlicki M et al: Results of delayed treatment of patients with malignant tumors of the lymphatic system, *Pol Tyg Lek* 46(48-49):922, 1991.
230. Pennes DR et al: Evolution of skeletal hyperostoses caused by 13-cis-retinoic acid therapy, *Am J Roentgenol* 151:967, 1988.
231. Petterson M: The camptothecin tree: harvesting a Chinese anticancer compound, *Alternat Ther Health Med* 2(2):23, 1996.
232. Piantadosi S: Hazards of small clinical trials, *J Clin Oncol* 8:1, 1990.
233. Pisani P, Parkin DM, Ferlay J: Estimates of the worldwide mortality from eighteen major cancers in 1985: implications for prevention and projections of future burden, *Int J Cancer*; 5:891, 1993.
234. Piscitelli SC et al: Disposition of phenylbutyrates and its metabolites, phenylacetate and phenylgluta-mine, *J Clin Pharmacol* 35(4):368, 1995.
235. Pittsley RA, Yoder FW: Retinoid hyperostosis: skeletal toxicity associated with long-term administration of 13-cis-retinoic acid for refractory ichthyosis, *N Engl J Med* 308:1012, 1983.
236. Prasad KN et al: Ayurvedic agents induce differentiation in murine neuroblastoma cells in culture, *Neuropharmacology* 31:599, 1992.
237. Prentice RL et al: Dietary fat reduction and plasma estradiol concentration in healthy postmenopausal women, *J Natl Cancer Inst* 82:129, 1990.
238. Primack A, Spencer J: *The collection and evaluation of clinical research data relevant to alternative medicine and cancer*, Bethesda, Md, April 1996, Office of Alternative Medicine, National Institutes of Health.
239. Prudden JF: The treatment of human cancer with agents prepared from bovine cartilage, *J Biol Response Mod* 4(6):551, 1985.
240. Puccio C et al: Treatment of metastatic renal cell carcinoma with Catrix, *Proc Annu Meet Am Soc Clin Oncol* 13:A769, 1994.
241. Pyrhonen S et al: Randomized comparison of fluorouracil, epidoxorubicin and methotrexate (FEMTX) plus supportive care with supportive care alone in patients with non-resectable gastric cancer, *Br J Cancer* 71(3):587, 1995.

242. Recchia F et al: Beta-interferon, retinoids and tamoxifen as maintenance therapy in metastatic breast cancer: a pilot study, *Clin Ther* 146(10):603, 1995.
243. Reizenstein P, Modan B, Kuller LH: The quandary of cancer prevention, *J Clin Epidemiol* 47(6):575, 1994.
244. Rexnu G, Yuanming G: The treatment of pain in bone metastases of cancer with the analgesic decoction of cancer and the acupoint therapeutic approach, *J Tradit Chin Med* 15(4):262, 1995.
245. Revici E: *Research in physiopathology as the basis of guided chemotherapy with special application to cancer*, Princeton, NJ, 1961, Van Nostrand.
246. Reynolds T: News, *J Natl Cancer Inst* 83:594, 1991.
247. Risberg T et al: The use of non-proven therapy among patients treated in Norwegian oncological departments: a cross-sectional national multicenter study, *Eur J Cancer* 31A(11):1785, 1995.
248. Risberg T et al: Spiritual healing among Norwegian hospitalised cancer patients and patients' religious needs and preferences, *Eur J Cancer* 32A(2):274, 1996.
249. Romney SL et al: Nutrient antioxidants in the pathogenesis and prevention of cervical dysplasias and cancer, *J Cell Biochem Suppl* 23:96, 1995.
250. Ronco AL, Halberg F: The pineal gland and cancer, *Anticancer Res* 16(4A):2033, 1996.
251. Rose DP et al: Effect of a low-fat diet on hormone levels in women with cystic breast disease. I. Serum steroids and gonadotropins, *J Natl Cancer Inst* 78:623, 1987.
252. Rose DP et al: The effects of a low-fat dietary intervention and tamoxifen adjuvant therapy on the serum estrogen and sex hormone-binding globulin concentrations of post-menopausal breast cancer patients, *Breast Cancer Res Treat* 27:253, 1993.
253. Rose DP: Dietary fat and breast cancer: controversy and biological plausibility. In Weisburger EK, editor: *Diet and breast cancer*, New York, 1994, Plenum, p 1.
254. Rose DP: The mechanistic rationale in support of dietary cancer prevention, *Prev Med* 25(1):34, 1996.
255. Sabo CE, Michael SR: The influence of personal massage with music on anxiety and side effects associated with chemotherapy, *Cancer Nurs* 9(4):283, 1996.
256. Sadoff L, Fuchs K, Hollander J: Rapid death associated with laetrile ingestion, *JAMA* 239:1532, 1978.
257. Sancier KM, Hu B: Medical applications of Qigong and emitted qi on humans, animals, cell cultures, and plants, *Am J Acupunct* 19:376, 1991.
258. Sawyer MG et al: The use of alternative therapies by children with cancer, *Med J Aust* 160:320, 1994.
259. Schumacher U et al: Biochemical, histochemical and cell biological investigations on the actions of mistletoe lectins I, II and III with human breast cancer cell lines, *Glycoconj J* 12(3):250, 1995.
260. Scotia Pharmaceuticals: Dose/survival relationship in 48 patients with non-resectable pancreatic carcinoma treated with a single 10-day treatment course of IV LiGLA, Clinical Study Protocol ISN 930095, January 31, 1994, Scotia Pharmaceuticals, Ltd. (appendix I).
261. Selvam R et al: The anti-oxidant activity of turmeric (*Curcuma longa*), *J Ethnopharmacol* 47(2):59, 1995.
262. Settheetham W, Ishida T: Study of genotoxic effects of antidiarrheal medicinal herbs on human cells in vitro, *Southeast Asian J Trop Med Public Health* 26(suppl 1):306, 1995.
263. Shafir Y, Kaufman BA: Quadriplegia after chiropractic manipulation in an infant with congenital torticollis caused by a spinal astrocytoma, *J Pediatr* 120:266, 1992.
264. Shamberger RC et al: Anorectal function in children after ileoanal pull-through, *J Pediatr Surg* 29(2):329 (discussion, 332), 1994.
265. Sharma HM, Dwivedi C, Satter BC: Antineoplastic properties of Maharishi-4 against DMBA-induced mammary tumors in rats, *Pharmacol Biochem Behav* 35:767, 1991.
266. Shekelle, PG, Adam AH: Spinal Manipulation, *Ann Intern Med* 117:590, 1992.
267. Shimizu H et al: Serum oestrogen levels in postmenopausal women: comparison of American whites and Japanese in Japan, *Br J Cancer* 62:451, 1990.
268. Shinke SP, Moncher MS, Singer BR: Native American youths and cancer risk reduction, *J Adolesc Health* 15(2):105, 1994.
269. Simonton OC, Matthews-Simonton S, Creighton J: *Getting well again*, Los Angeles, 1978, JP Tarcher.
270. Simopoulos AP, Herbert V, Jacobson B: *Genetic nutrition: designing a diet based on your family medical history*, New York, 1993, MacMillan.
271. Sipos EP et al: Inhibition of tumor angiogenesis, *Ann N Y Acad Sci* 732:263, 1994.

272. Slevin ML: Quality of life: philosophical question or clinical reality? *Br Med J* 305(6851):466, 1992.
273. Smit HF et al: Ayurvedic herbal drugs with possible cytostatic activity, *J Ethnopharmacol* 47(2):75, 1995.
274. Smith AY et al: Cystic renal cell carcinoma and acquired renal cystic disease associated with consumption of chaparral tea: a case report, *J Urol* 152(1):2089, 1994.
275. Salerno JW, Smith DE: Selective growth inhibition of a human malignant melanoma cell line by sesame oil in vitro, *Prostagland Leukot Essent Fatty Acids* 46:145, 1992.
276. Soltysiak-Pawluczuk D, Burzynski SR: Cellular accumulation of antineoplaston AS21 in human hepatoma cells, *Cancer Lett* 88(1):107, 1995.
277. Spiegel D et al: Effect of psychosocial treatment on survival of patients with metastatic breast cancer, *Lancet* 2:888, 1989.
278. Spigelblatt LS: Alternative medicine: should it be used by children? *Curr Probl Pediatr* 25(6):180, 1995.
279. Spigelblatt L: The use of alternative medicine by children, *Pediatrics* 94:811, 1994.
280. Spiller HA et al: Retrospective study of mistletoe ingestion, *J Toxicol Clin Toxicol* 34(4):405, 1996.
281. Spremulli E et al: Clinical study of hydrazine sulfate in advance cancer patients, *Cancer Chemother Pharmacol* 3:121, 1979.
282. Stal P: Iron as a hepatotoxin, *Dig Dis* 13(4):205, 1995.
283. Steenblock D: *Chlorella*, El Toro, Calif, 1987, Aging Research Institute, p 7.
284. Stemmermann GN et al: Breast cancer in women of Japanese and Caucasian ancestry in Hawaii, *Cancer* 56:206, 1985.
285. Stich HF et al: Mutagenic action of ascorbic acid, *Nature* 260:722, 1976.
286. Stich HF, Wei L, Whiting RF: Enhancement of the chromosome-demagascorbate by transition metals, *Cancer Res* 39:4145, 1979.
287. Strain JJ: Putative role of dietary trace elements in coronary heart disease and cancer, *Br J Biomed Sci* 51(3):241, 1994.
288. Sugita Y et al: The effect of antineoplaston: a new antitumor agent on malignant brain tumors, *Kurume Med J* 42(3):133, 1995.
289. Sun HD et al: Ai-Lin I treated 32 cases of acute promyelocytic leukemia, *Chin J Integrat Chin Western Med* 12:170, 1992.
290. Surh YJ, Lee SS: Capsaicin, a double-edged sword: toxicity, metabolism, and chemopreventive potential, *Life Sci* 56(22):1845, 1995.
291. Suto T et al: Clinical Study of biological response modifiers as maintenance therapy for hepatocellular carcinoma, *Cancer Chemother Pharmacol* 33(suppl):S145, 1994.
292. Syrjala KL et al: Relaxation and imagery and cognitive behavior training reduce pain during cancer treatment: a controlled clinical trial, *Pain* 189, 1995.
293. Takeda T et al: Bryonolic acid production in hairy roots of Trichosanthes kirilowii Max. Var Japonica Kitam. Transformed with Agrobacterium rhizogenes and its cytotoxic activity, *Chem Pharm Bull (Tokyo)* 42(3):730, 1994.
294. Tanaka K et al: Oral administration of chlorella vulgaris augments concomitant antitumor immunity, *Immunopharmacol Immunotoxicol* 12:277, 1990.
295. Tellegen A, Atkinson G: Openness to absorbing the self-altering experiences ("absorption"), a trait related to hypnotic susceptibility, *J Abn Psych* 83:268, 1974.
296. Thibault A et al: Phase I study of phenylacetate administered twice daily to patients with cancer, *Cancer* 75(12):2932, 1995.
297. Torisu M et al: Significant prolongation of disease-free period gained by oral polysaccharide K (PSK) administration after curative surgical operation of colorectal cancer, *Cancer Immunol Immunother* 31:261, 1990.
298. Torun M, Yardim S, Gonenc A, Sargin H, et al: Serum beta-carotene, vitamin E, vitamin C, and malondialdehyde levels in several types of cancer, *J Clin Pharm Ther* 20(5):259, 1995.
299. Trawick W: An Ayurvedic theory of cancer, *Med Anthropol* 13(1-2):121, 1991.
300. Tsuda H et al: Inhibitory effect of antineoplaston A10 and AS2-1 on human hepatocellular carcinoma, *Kurume Med J* 43(2):137, 1996.

301. Tsuda H et al: Toxicological study on antineoplaston A-10 and AS2-1 in cancer patients, *Kurume Med J* 42(4):241, 1995.
302. Tsukagoshi S et al: Krestin (PSK), *Cancer Treat Rev* 11(2):131, 1984.
303. Tsur M: Inadvertent child health neglect by preference of homeopathy to conventional medicine, *Harefuah* 122:137, 1992.
304. Tyler VE: *The new honest herbal: a sensible guide to herbs and related remedies*, Philadelphia, 1987, Stickley.
305. Tyson JE: Use of unproven therapies in clinical practice and research: how can we better serve our patients and their families? *Semin Perinatol* 19(2):98, 1995.
306. Ulett GA: Conditioned healing with electroacupuncture, *Altern Ther Health Med* 2(5):56, 1996.
307. Umezawa I et al: An acidic polysaccharide, chlon A, from chlorella pyrenoidosa, *Chemotherapy* 30(9):1041, 1982.
308. US Congress Office of Technology Assessment: *Immuno-augmentative therapy: unconventional cancer treatments*, Washington, DC, 1990, US Government Printing Office, pub. no. OTA-H-405, pp. 129-147.
309. US Congress Office of Technology Assessment: *Unconventional cancer treatments*, Washington, DC, 1990, US Government Printing Office, pub. no. OTA-H-405, pp. 75-81.
310. U.S. Department of Health and Human Services Public Health Service: *The Surgeon General's report on nutrition and health*, Washington, DC, 1988, US Govt. Printing Office, pub. no. NIH-88- 50210.
311. Van der Merwe CF, Booyens J: Oral gamma-linolenic acid in 21 patients with untreatable malignancy: an ongoing pilot open clinical trial, *Br J Clin Pract* 41:907, 1987.
312. van der Zouwe N, van Dam FS, Aaronson NK, Hanewald GJ: Alternative treatments in cancer: extent and background of utilization, *Ned Tijdschr Geneeskd* 138(6):300, 1994.
313. van Zandwijk: N-acetylcysteine (NAC) and glutathione (GSH): antioxidant and chemopreventive properties, with special reference to lung cancer, *J Cell Biochem Suppl* 22:24, 1995.
314. Vermeil C, Morin O: Role experimental des algues unicellulaires Protheca et Chlorella (Chorellaceae) dans l'immunogenese anticancereuse (sarcome murin BP 8), Societe de Biologie de Rennes, Seance du 21, 1976 Avril.
315. Wang XM, Yu RC, Wang YT: Study on advanced non-small cell lung cancer patients with Qi deficiency and blood stasis syndrome, *Chung Kuo Chung Hsi I Chieh Tsa Chih* 14(12):724, 1994.
316. Wargovich MJ: Diallyl sulfide, a flavor component of garlic (*Allium sativum*), inhibits dimethyl-hydrazine-induced colon cancer, *Carcinogenesis* 8:487, 1987.
317. Warpeha A, Harris J: Combining traditional and nontraditional approaches to nutrition counseling, *J Am Diet Assoc* 93(7):797, 1993.
318. West DW et al: Adult dietary intake and prostate cancer risk in Utah: a case-control study with special emphasis on aggressive tumors, *Cancer Causes Control* 2:85, 1991.
319. Wilkinson S: Aromatherapy and massage in palliative care, *Int J Palliative Nurs* 1(1):21, 1995.
320. Willett WC: Diet and health: what should we eat? *Science* 264(5158):532, 1994.
321. Willey LB et al: Valerian overdose: a case report, *Vet Hum Toxicol* 37(4):364, 1995.
322. Wilson DJ et al: Skeletal hyperostosis and extraosseous calcification in patients receiving long term etretinate (Tigason), *Br J Dermatol* 119:597, 1988.
323. Woerdenbag HJ et al: Isolation of two cytotoxic dipertenes from the fern Pteris multifada, *Z Naturforsch* [C] 51(9-10):635, 1996.
324. Wong GH, Kaspar RL, Zweiger G, Carlson C, et al: Strategies for manipulating apoptosis, *J Cell Biochem* 60(1):56, 1996.
325. Woolf GM et al: Acute hepatitis associated with the Chinese herbal product Jin Bu Huan, *Ann Intern Med* 121(10):729, 1994.
326. World Health Organization: *Prevention of cancer*, Geneva, 1964, Technical report series 276, World Health Organization.
327. Wynder EL: Cancer prevention: optimizing life-styles with special reference to nutritional carcinogenesis, *Monogr Natl Cancer Inst* 12:87, 1992.
328. Wynder EL, Rose DP, Cohen LA: Diet and breast cancer in causation and therapy, *Cancer* 58:1804, 1986.
329. Wynder EL et al: Comparative epidemiology of cancer between the United States and Japan: a second look, *Cancer* 67:746, 1991.

330. Ye WC et al: Triterpenoids from Pulsatilla chinensis, *Phytochemistry* 42(3):799, 1996.
331. Yeoh C, Kiely E, Davies H: Unproven treatments, *J Med Ethics* 20(2):75, 1994.
332. Yi-hong et al: Electrochemical therapy for intermediate and advanced liver cancer: a report of 50 cases, *Eur J Surg* (suppl 574):51, 1994.
333. Yonish-Rouach E et al: Wild-type p53 induces apoptosis of myeloid leukemic cells that is inhibited by interleukin-6, *Nature* 352:345, 1991.
334. Yoon TJ et al: Inhibitory effect of Korean mistletoe (Viscum album coloratum) extract on tumor angiogenesis and metastasis of haematogenous and non-haematogenous tumour cells in mice, *Cancer Lett* 20:97(1):83, 1995.
335. You W-C et al: Allium vegetables and reduced risk of stomach cancer, *J Natl Cancer Inst* 81:162, 1989.
336. Yu-ling X, Deruo L: Electrostatic therapy (EST) of lung cancer and pulmonary metastasis: report of 15 cases, *Eur J Surg* (suppl 574):91, 1994.
337. Yun T-K, Choi SY: Preventive effect of ginseng intake against various human cancers: a case-control study on 1987 pairs, *Cancer Epidemiol, Biomarkers, Prevention* 4(4):401, 1995.
338. Yunqin S et al: Electrochemical therapy in the treatment of malignant tumors on the body surface, *Eur J Surg* (suppl 574):41, 1994.

SUGGESTED READINGS

Kroesen AJ et al: Incontinence after ileo-anal pouch anastamosis — diagnostic criteria and therapeutic sequelae, *Chirurg* 66(4):385, 1995.
Parkin DM: Cancer in developing countries, *Cancer Surv* 19-20:519, 1994.
Reizenstein P, Modan B: Kuller LH: The quandary of cancer prevention, *J Clin Epidemiol* 47(6):575, 1994.
Rose DP: Dietary fat and breast cancer: controversy and biological plausibility. In Weisburger EK, editor *Diet and breast cancer*, New York, Plenum, 1994.
US Congress, Office of Technology Assessment: *Unconventional cancer treatments*, OTA-H-405, Washington, DC, September 1990, US Government Printing Office, pp. 75-81.

CHAPTER 7

Complementary/Alternative Therapies in the Treatment of Neurologic Disorders

Bruce J. Diamond, Samuel C. Shiflett, Nancy E. Schoenberger, Sangeetha Nayak, Ann C. Cotter, and Diane Zeitlin

Disorders of the central nervous system (CNS) affect the lives of hundreds of thousands of individuals each year, resulting in impairments in areas such as memory, attention, movement, sensation, mood, personality, and physiologic regulation. Neurologic disorders may become evident as acute, nonprogressive events or may follow a progressive, insidious course, inflicting an uncertain future on the lives of patients and families. Although modern medicine has made great strides in the management of acute trauma to the CNS, its success with the chronic aftermath is sometimes less impressive. Consequently, there are increasing numbers of individuals who survive neurologic disorders only to find themselves with enduring and sometimes profoundly debilitating impairments. For this reason, patients with neurologic disorders increasingly look to complementary/alternative medicine (CAM) in the hopes of finding relief for their conditions.

The number of CAM therapies that have been used to treat CNS disorders is quite large, yet the amount of research validating their effectiveness is often limited or nonexistent. The purpose of this chapter is to identify CAM techniques that are commonly used or suggested in treating neurologic sequelae and to summarize the adequacy of the research evidence for their effectiveness. Following a brief description of some of the most common CAM therapies used, etiology and sequelae of particular neurologic disorders will be described, along with evidence for the effectiveness of CAM treatments.

CAM THERAPIES

There are literally hundreds of CAM therapies used today in the treatment of every imaginable abnormal condition of the physical body. In an effort to narrow and focus

The authors wish to thank Jason Lerner, Olga Noskin, Gem Lucas, and Raluka Vlad for their contributions.

the field, the treatments of relevance to CNS disorders have been roughly categorized according to their mechanism of application and are summarized in Table 7-1, along with an indication of the medical condition for which they have been used. Included in Table 7-1 are a few techniques that represent "alternative" uses of techniques or medications already used in conventional medicine. These may not fit conventional concepts of alternative medicine, but we believe the techniques are important to mention. Also in Table 7-1 is a summary of the state of the research evidence ascertained at this time.

A few words of caution regarding the state of scientific evidence are warranted. Although a number of techniques have scientific evidence for effectiveness, lack of scientific evidence does not mean that the technique is not effective. Rather, it simply indicates that (1) no research has been conducted and/or published on a particular technique as applied to a particular medical condition, or it could indicate that (2) research articles have not been located in the highly diverse, often diffuse, and difficult-to-access alternative medicine literature. In many cases the lack of evidence may be the result of our attempt to include only those articles which are peer reviewed and have at least a minimally adequate research design, consisting of an experimental and control group, objective and valid outcome measures, a well-defined sample, and evidence of randomization and blinding. With a few notable exceptions, however, strict application of these criteria results in the elimination of whatever research evidence there is for most of the techniques. On the other hand, even those techniques which have been subjected to substantial amounts of research still lack the definitive degree of confidence that only large, multisite, double-blind studies bring to bear. Two CAM therapies, acupuncture and *Ginkgo biloba,* have received the greatest amount of research scrutiny and are discussed in detail below.

The following descriptions of CAM methods are not meant to provide a comprehensive list of definitions of all therapies used for neurologic conditions; such definitions are provided elsewhere in this textbook. Rather, therapies discussed in more detail here are used most frequently to treat neurologic conditions or have the most substantive research support.

Alternative Systems of Medical Practice

All of the "traditional" medical practices of varying cultures fall in the category of alternative systems of medical practice. These traditions include such systems as Ayurveda, traditional Chinese medicine, and shamanism, as well as several of the Western systems such as naturopathy and homeopathy. Alternative healing systems usually involve a large set of diverse practices and remedies that involve a number of different methods and are based on an underlying model of the healing process which may or may not correspond to conventional medical models. Consequently, it is difficult to evaluate the entire system in a single study or even a large research program. Specific aspects of tra-

Text continued on p. 176.

TABLE 7-1	CAM Therapy for Neurologic Disorders	
CAM Therapy	**Research Literature on Neurologic Disorders**	**Uses**

Alternative Systems of Medical Practice

Homeopathy	• Two meta-analyses across diagnoses with encouraging findings[72,80] • Two controlled studies for stroke [27,128] • One preliminary study for traumatic brain injury[178]	Research articles report some use for stroke, traumatic brain injury
Ayurvedic medicine	One uncontrolled study of hemiplegia showed decreased cholesterol levels and improved motor functioning[149]	System of medicine designed to treat a wide spectrum of physical and psychologic disorders

Non-Conventional Bodywork

Acupressure (shiatsu)	• One uncontrolled study regarding use as adjunct to stroke rehabilitation showed improvement[57] • One clinical observation in cerebral birth injury reported improvement in 89% of children treated[168]	Some applications to stroke, traumatic brain injury
Acupuncture*	Large literature of variable quality; less than 20 well-controlled studies on neurologic disorders, of which many showed positive effects	Among neurologic disorders, majority of research is on stroke
Alexander technique	One uncontrolled pilot study for Parkinson's disease showed improvement in motor functioning, daily activities, and depression[136]	Primarily used for postural difficulties and back and neck pain
Chiropractic*	• One controlled study of "whiplash" [43] • One case study on SCI with recovery of function[177] • One uncontrolled study of post–traumatic brain injury headache[64]	Most frequently used for musculoskeletal problems. Limited application to neurologic disorders
Craniosacral therapy*	• A few case reports of efficacy in treatment of cerebral palsy and Erb's palsy[170] • Anecdotal reports of good effects in traumatic brain injury and spinal cord injury	Used to treat pain conditions and a variety of functional problems. Potential applicability to central nervous system trauma
Massage therapy*	• Two controlled studies on spinal cord injury with encouraging findings[46,157] • One case series showed improvement in pressure ulcers[22]	Often used for musculoskeletal or stress-related conditions. Applicability as an adjunctive treatment for neurologic disorders

*See text for additional information.

TABLE 7-1	CAM Therapy for Neurologic Disorders—cont'd	
CAM Therapy	**Research Literature on Neurologic Disorders**	**Uses**
Reflexology	• One case series of stroke patients[181] • Three case reports on spinal cord injury[74] All with positive outcomes	Has been applied to stroke, brain injury, spinal cord injury, and childhood developmental disorders, including cerebral palsy
Feldenkrais method	Anecdotal information only	Has been applied to cerebral palsy, hemiplegia, and multiple sclerosis
Pilates method	Anecdotal information only	Has been applied to spinal cord injury, multiple sclerosis, and arthritis
Trager psychophysical integration	• Case reports for multiple sclerosis note improved strength, flexibility, balance, energy and morale • Controlled study for multiple sclerosis currently under way	Most often used for painful musculoskeletal conditions. Has been applied to Parkinson's disease, multiple sclerosis
Therapeutic riding	One case series of paraplegia/tetraplegia reports decreased spasticity, easier catheterization, improved bowel functioning, more balanced mood, and improved sleep[42]	Used to improve physical and emotional functioning of children and adults with disabilities, including cerebral palsy, multiple sclerosis, spinal deformities, paraplegia, muscular dystrophy, and lumbago

Mind-Body Interventions

Hypnosis*	Case reports on the treatment of stroke, spinal cord injury and traumatic brain injury note improvement in physical and emotional functioning[32,58,81,84,139]	Often used for pain reduction and behavior modification. Has been applied as adjunctive treatment for neurologic disorders
Meditation*	• Several studies have relevance to stroke prevention[11,31,52,130,163] • One anecdotal report of physical improvement following stroke[180] • One study for relaxation in spinal cord injury, equivalent to control group[164]	Used for stress management, health promotion, reduction of hypertension, which may have application for stroke prevention
Music therapy	• Three controlled trials[34,79,148] • Seven pre/post studies with objective outcome measures and numerous anecdotal and case reports When used as adjunct in rehabilitation for neurologic disorders, findings are encouraging for improved motor, speech, and emotional functioning	Used following stroke and brain injury to encourage verbal and nonverbal communication, to improve muscular coordination, and to minimize stress and anxiety

*See text for additional information.   *Continued.*

TABLE 7-1	CAM Therapy for Neurologic Disorders—cont'd	
CAM Therapy	**Research Literature on Neurologic Disorders**	**Uses**
T'ai Chi*	Two controlled studies show improved cardiorespiratory function, psychologic function, strength and balance, and reduced number of falls in healthy elderly[175,176]	Used to improve strength, balance, coordination, and concentration. Applicability to neurologic disorders
Yoga*	Little controlled research, but reports of use in multiple sclerosis with symptom improvement[38]	Used for stress management and health promotion, which may have applications for stroke prevention
Energy Healing Techniques		
Qi Gong*	Animal studies of paralysis, done in China, report positive findings[165] Small study in U.S. showed no effect in hemiplegia[20]	Substantial use in China for paralysis
Reiki	Anecdotal information. Controlled study on treatment of stroke is currently under way	Used as an adjunctive healing technique with a range of diagnoses
Therapeutic touch	• No controlled studies on neurologic disorders • Controlled studies on wound healing with mixed results (see Wirth[173] for review) may be applicable to pressure ulcers in spinal cord injury	Easily used as an adjunctive technique in rehabilitation settings. Taught at more than 30 nursing schools in the U.S.
Phytotherapies		
*Ginkgo biloba**	More than 20 controlled trials with humans; more than 20 animal or in vitro studies. Results are encouraging for treatment of cognitive deficits common to stroke and traumatic brain injury	Used for 20 to 30 years in Europe for impairments in memory and attention, edema, cerebral ischemia, vascular insufficiency, sequelae of stroke, and tinnitus
Hydergine	Three controlled studies of stroke with mixed results[6,15,126]	Approved by FDA for age-related cognitive decline; may have applicability for stroke prevention
Asian herbs	Large body of literature, most of it in Chinese, with very few controlled studies of individual herbs	Different combinations of herbs prescribed by practitioners, based on presenting symptoms and traditional Chinese medicine diagnostic procedures. Used for many neurologic disorders

*See text for additional information.

TABLE 7-1	CAM Therapy for Neurologic Disorders—cont'd	
CAM Therapy	**Research Literature on Neurologic Disorders**	**Uses**

Pharmacologic and Biologic Therapies

CAM Therapy	Research Literature on Neurologic Disorders	Uses
Bee venom therapy	Case reports of relief of multiple sclerosis symptoms. Studies in treatment of multiple sclerosis are under way	Used in the treatment of arthritis and multiple sclerosis
Dimethyl amino ethanol (DMAE)	• One pilot study showed elimination of Parkinson-related dyskinesia in 8 of 11 patients[93] • One pilot study on Huntington's chorea showed improvement in 5 of 7 people[161]	Available in health food stores as a nutritional supplement. Used to enhance cognitive functioning (e.g., memory, concentration). May have application for epilepsy
Dimethyl sulfoxide (DMSO)*	Substantial research in the 1970s and 1980s, with some encouraging findings for stroke and other brain injury, but less research now	Used following stroke and head injury. Appears to lower intracranial pressure, stabilize blood pressure, and increase blood flow to areas of injury
EDTA chelation*	• One uncontrolled study of stroke showed decrease in cerebral artery stenosis[88] • One case series without objective outcome measures reported "good recovery" from stroke for 60% of sample[108] • Because multiple sclerosis and Parkinson's disease are believed by some to be caused by heavy metal intoxication, chelation therapy has been recommended. However, no research evidence has shown that this technique is effective, or even that heavy metals are implicated, in these conditions	Conventionally used to treat lead poisoning. Use for cardiovascular disease is controversial
Hyperbaric oxygen*	• One controlled[106] and several uncontrolled[61,104] studies of stroke show some positive outcomes • One study of stroke discontinued[4] • Two controlled studies of traumatic brain injury[119,120] with mixed results • More than 10 animal studies with suggestive findings	Conventionally used to treat decompression sickness and air embolism. Use for cerebrovascular accident is controversial
Melatonin*	Research suggests role in stroke, Parkinson's, multiple sclerosis, and epilepsy but no controlled studies	Available in health food stores. Used in the treatment of sleep disturbance, depression

*See text for additional information.   *Continued.*

TABLE 7-1	CAM Therapy for Neurologic Disorders—cont'd	
CAM Therapy	**Research Literature on Neurologic Disorders**	**Uses**
Pharmacologic and Biologic Therapies—cont'd		
Piracetam	Of four double-blind, placebo-controlled studies of dementia, two showed significant improvement in memory and cognition[42a,134a] and two showed no difference[33,117]	Reported to enhance integrative brain mechanisms (e.g., memory, learning, problem solving)
Electrotherapy		
Bioelectromagnetics	• Functional electric stimulation[24] and electromagnetic biofeedback[9] are used conventionally in the treatment of neurologic disorders • Several studies report positive findings for wound healing including pressure sores in spinal cord injury[122] (see Vodovnik, Karba, 1992[159] for review)	Used to treat skin lesions, edema, muscle weakness, pain, and spasticity, and to accelerate wound healing
Magnetic stimulation	• Animal studies suggest applicability of pulsed electromagnetic fields to the treatment of stroke[49] • Most controlled studies for diagnosis rather than treatment	Used as a diagnostic and treatment tool for evaluating activity in corticospinal tracts in various neurologic disorders including multiple sclerosis, Parkinson's disease, and stroke.

*See text for additional information.

ditional Chinese medicine (TCM), for example, are discussed in this chapter within sections on bodywork (acupuncture and massage), bioenergy (Qi Gong), and phytotherapies (*Ginkgo biloba*).

Nonconventional Bodywork

Research involving the use of manipulative techniques to influence neurologic conditions has focused more on soft tissue than on articulatory techniques. This is reasonable, since dysfunction in CNS conditions stems from abnormal muscle tonus and motor control, not vertebral malalignment and peripheral nerve compression. Of the neuromuscular soft tissue techniques, proprioceptive neural facilitation (PNF) is the most commonly investigated. Although PNF is well reported in the physical therapy literature (and thus not regarded as "complementary" by some rehabilitation practitioners), it is included here because it serves as a model that may elucidate the underlying mechanism of other soft tissue neuromuscular techniques which have been less thoroughly researched.

There are very few articles in the chiropractic literature regarding treatment of traumatic brain injury.[35] Research on osteopathic manipulation and craniosacral therapy is sparse. There are a few case studies involving other neurologic conditions, such as cerebral palsy, Erb's palsy, and learning disorders, but none for spinal cord injury, stroke, brain injury, or multiple sclerosis (MS). Craniosacral therapy is sometimes used as part of a multidisciplinary treatment approach for spinal cord and brain injuries. Although no scientific studies have been conducted on this multidisciplinary approach, there is some anecdotal evidence from the Upledger Institute's Brain and Spinal Cord Dysfunction Program indicating its effectiveness with these conditions.[155] However, when craniosacral therapy is used in combination with other therapies, it is difficult to isolate its specific action and efficacy. Anecdotal evidence also exists for the effectiveness of craniosacral therapy in treating symptoms of a concussion, including loss of clarity of thinking, loss of equilibrium, and eye pain.[29]

A number of case reports of injuries attributed to chiropractic manipulation have been reported in the medical literature. Certain types of manipulation may produce greater risk than others. Among 49 cases of stroke following chiropractic manipulation in which the technique was described,[85] rotational manipulation of the upper cervical spine had been performed in 45 cases. It should be pointed out, however, that complications arising from chiropractic manipulation are less frequent than those observed in more commonly used interventions.[48,90,169]

While craniosacral therapy is asserted to be virtually risk free,[156] adverse effects have been reported in a small number of individuals with traumatic brain injury (TBI). In a study using craniosacral manipulation (i.e., the cranial osteopathy approach) with 55 TBI patients,[50] mild headaches following treatment were reported by a number of subjects. More severe reactions, however, were exhibited by three subjects, including an exacerbation of vertiginous symptoms; visceral symptoms involving the cardiac, respiratory, and gastrointestinal systems; psychologic disturbances necessitating psychiatric institutional care; and severe total body spasticity. It should be noted that such reactions are rare, occurring in only 5% of the subjects in the above study. Practitioners, particularly those treating TBI in their patients, are advised to be prepared to deal with this small but potential risk.

Acupuncture. Acupuncture is not a unitary method, and techniques are quite varied. For example, some involve the use of low-voltage electric current across the needles to strengthen the effects of the needles, and laser acupuncture uses a high-wavelength, low-energy laser.[100] Other forms include TCM, five elements, scalp, Korean hand, and auricular acupuncture. The use of burning herbs (moxa) on acupoints and cupping (creation of a vacuum over a small section of the skin) are integral parts of many forms of acupuncture, both Eastern and Western.

Research on the effectiveness of acupuncture is abundant, although many of the reports involve case studies rather than controlled research protocols, and much of the literature is in Chinese. A number of systematic reviews of acupuncture research involving pain management exist, but quality evidence regarding treatment of neurologic disorders is still sparse. Nevertheless, several reasonably well-controlled studies have reported that acupuncture has shown efficacy in the treatment of some neurologic conditions.

Evidence is clearly encouraging in the use of acupuncture in the treatment of stroke; however, the evidence is currently so limited that it can only be considered as suggestive. The research of Naeser et al.[99,100] is important because it suggests that major limiting factors in acupuncture effectiveness are the nature and extent of cerebral damage. Although treatment of TBI is common among acupuncturists trained in traditional Oriental methods and the limited evidence for the treatment of stroke is encouraging with respect to treatment of cerebral trauma, there are no reports of controlled research involving acupuncture in TBI. Similarly, except for a few research projects involving animal models, there is no evidence for the utility of acupuncture in the treatment of spinal cord injury (SCI). Acupuncture has shown potential for managing some symptoms in MS, epilepsy, and Parkinson's disease, but the research methodology is so poor that no firm conclusions can be drawn.

Phytotherapy

Herbal medicine involves the use of whole plant material, such as the root, stem, flower, or extract. Plant materials are by far the oldest form of medication and are part of virtually all indigenous medical traditions. Plant materials can be directly ingested, inhaled, or applied topically. Herbal medicine, like conventional pharmaceutic drugs, is believed to work either because of the action of a specific chemical in the herb or because of the synergistic interaction between various components of the plants. In fact, numerous medications and pharmaceutic compounds have their origin in substances originally isolated from plants. Some herbs and plant materials appear to have useful medicinal effects that may be of relevance to rehabilitation. For example, herbs have been reported to exert effects on vascular elasticity, act as antiplatelet activating factors, exhibit antiedemic properties, and improve cognitive functioning. Despite being "natural," not all plants and herbs are safe for human consumption, and such medicines should only be used with full knowledge of the nature and effects of the plant component in question and their possible interactions with a patient's medications.

Chinese herbs and other plants have been used in medical treatments for thousands of years. There are currently hundreds of natural substances available for use, and most TCM herbal prescriptions contain upwards of 15 ingredients, which makes it difficult to identify the specific components that exert a treatment effect. A number of botanic extracts have been identified as beneficial in the treatment of cerebral ischemia, cerebral thrombosis, and stroke. These substances are generally used as elements of complex decoctions. No controlled clinical trials of their efficacy have been located; however, some may exist in Chinese or Japanese scientific literature not yet translated in English. For further discussion of Chinese herbs applied to CNS trauma, see Shiflett et al.[134]

Ginkgo biloba. The leaf of the ginkgo tree has been part of the traditional Chinese pharmacopoeia for 5000 years. Standardized extracts of the ginkgo leaf are widely used in Asia, Germany, and France and are increasingly being used in the United States. Ginkgo shows promise in the treatment of some of the most salient and debilitating symptoms associated with stroke, TBI, cerebral vascular insufficiency, senile dementia, and normal and pathologic aging. For example, *Ginkgo biloba* extract (GBE) has been used in the treatment of stroke,[83] ischemia (i.e., inadequate oxygenation/reperfusion),[18] impairments in memory/information processing (i.e., observed in older people and in patients with Alzheimer's disease and other types of dementia),[54,71,115,144,160] vestibular disorders,[53] and tinnitus.[91]

A recent placebo-controlled study of GBE (EGb 761, the extract produced by Dr. Wilmar P. Schwabe Co., Gmb, Germany) examined efficacy in a sample of 202 patients with Alzheimer's disease or multiinfarct dementia.[76] Patients treated with GBE showed modest but significantly greater improvements on the cognitive subscale of the Alzheimer's Disease Assessment Scale (ADAS-COG) and on a geriatric assessment scale completed by relatives (Fig. 7-1). There were no differences between groups in the incidence or severity of adverse events.

While the duration of treatment and the window of time required to demonstrate efficacy have varied across studies, improvement generally has been observed within 4 to 12 weeks.[96,174] No serious side effects have been observed in clinical trials; however, in rare cases patients have shown allergic skin reactions, headache, and mild gastrointestinal tract upset.[70] Despite the fact that patients taking GBE are often receiving a variety of medications, there are no known drug interactions.[70]

Overall, GBE (most notably, EGb 761), has been cited in at least 130 publications, with approximately one third of the reports published in non-English journals. An analysis derived from a subset of 65 studies using experimental, quasi-experimental, or observational methods showed that 16 studies used in vitro methods, 14 involved animal models, and 35 reports were based on human models. The animal models that have been used to assess the activity of GBE have used rigorous laboratory-based techniques. For example, animal models of ischemia (i.e., using carotid artery clamping procedures)[107] have been used to examine the mechanisms underlying GBE's purported antiplatelet activat-

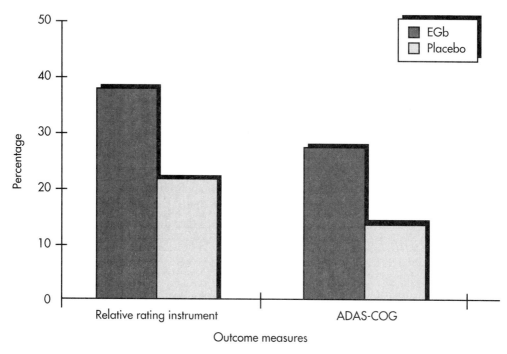

FIG. 7-1 Percentage of patients with dementia receiving *Ginkgo biloba* extract (EGb) or placebo who demonstrated statistically significant improvement on two outcome measures. (Data from Le Bars PL et al: *JAMA* 278[16]:1327, 1997.)

ing factor properties and its ability to confer protection against ischemia/reperfusion damage. Animal models (using both histologic and behavioral delayed-spatial alternation paradigms)[137] have also examined the effectiveness of GBE in treating brain injury and cerebral edema commonly observed in the acute stages of TBI.

Nearly 75% of the evaluated studies were based on experimental or quasi-experimental/observational methods. In 94% of the human studies, subjects were randomly assigned and control groups were used. A review of representative clinical studies published in peer-reviewed journals since 1990 shows that most of these studies employed randomized, placebo-controlled, double-blind procedures. Almost 97% of the studies involving humans used objective or standardized outcome measures. Many of the studies that were reviewed used universally recognized tests of neurobehavioral function, although in some instances descriptions of the outcomes measures lacked sufficient detail to enable adequate evaluation. Many of the outcome studies that evaluated activities of daily living were administered to geriatric patients and were largely based on self-report measures.

One of the major weaknesses or ambiguities in some of the studies (particularly those found in the German literature) is the vaguely defined diagnostic category "vascular insufficiency." Although patients included in this category tend to be geriatric and display slower processing and memory impairments, the precise correspondence of this diagnostic category to diagnostic categories used in the United States is uncertain. While most of the published studies on *Ginkgo biloba* have reported positive effects, not all studies have confirmed such efficacy. For example, Hartmann and Frick[54] evaluated 52 ambulatory patients with a diagnosis of vascular dementia. GBE was administered over a period of 3 months (20 ml three times daily of a drinking solution, equivalent to 150 mg daily dosage). Because of an unexpectedly strong placebo effect, patients treated with GBE displayed marginally but not significantly better results than placebo on psychometric performance.

Nonconventional Uses of Pharmacologic and Conventional Therapies

The category discussed in this section refers to a broad group of drugs and conventional treatments approved for one type of medical condition, but which are believed to have beneficial effects on other conditions for which they are not U.S Food and Drug Administration (FDA) approved (e.g., the common use of anticonvulsants for the treatment of pain or depression). Even though these alternative uses of conventional medical treatments are available under a doctor's supervision, they are sometimes difficult to obtain because so few physicians know about them or are willing to prescribe them.

Melatonin. Melatonin is a hormone produced continuously throughout the life cycle by the pineal gland. However, its production continuously declines with age. Melatonin secretion exhibits cyclic variation, with humans producing 5 to 10 times more melatonin at night than during the day. Melatonin has been reported to exert an inhibitory effect on the production of free radicals and/or to limit the damage they cause, thus exhibiting antioxidant effects. In one experiment in which a dilute solution of hydrogen peroxide was exposed to ultraviolet light, it was reported that melatonin was effective in reducing the number of free radicals.[51] The pineal gland, whose activity is mediated by melatonin, appears to exert a depressive influence on CNS excitability. There is evidence supporting a role for melatonin in the regulation of the gamma-aminobutyric acid (GABA) or benzodiazepine receptor complex, as a potentiator of this inhibitory neurotransmitter system.

Safety. Melatonin may play a role in a number of other conditions, including sleep disorders, chronic fatigue syndrome, fibromyalgia, depression, and Alzheimer's disease. Because of its apparent role in a number of medical conditions, there is a popular movement to self-administer melatonin in a "hormone replacement" or "hormone supplementation" program, since melatonin levels are generally believed to decline with age. This raises the urgent issue of safety, and several studies have addressed this concern. In a 1960 study 200 mg of melatonin was injected into human subjects with skin disorders, and no negative side effects were reported.[77] In healthy volunteers who were injected with a synthetic version of melatonin of varying doses the hormone was found to have tranquilizing properties.[5] Subjects injected with 75 mg of melatonin showed slower brain wave patterns, lower heart rates, and muscle relaxation, with no carryover fatigue or negative effects on memory performance, with a similar pattern of response observed in elderly subjects administered 50 mg per day. Despite the apparent safety of the use of melatonin over a short period, there is no evidence regarding the long-term effects of melatonin supplementation, so caution is necessary in its use. At least, melatonin should be administered under the supervision of a physician.

Electromagnetic Therapies

A number of electromagnetic therapies that might be considered alternative in many medical fields are used conventionally in rehabilitation. These include functional neuromuscular stimulation (FNS) and biofeedback. FNS is a form of electrical stimulation in which muscles are activated sequentially to allow performance of motor tasks. See Chae et al.[24] for a discussion of FNS as applied to SCI, stroke-related hemiplegia, and other types of paralysis. Biofeedback generally involves the use of equipment to measure internal physiologic events, make people aware of their occurrence, and teach people to manipulate them.[9] In the treatment of neurologic disorders the most frequently used form of biofeedback is myoelectric (or electromyogram [EMG]), which is based on myoelectric signals from muscles and can be used to regulate body positions, movement, blood pressure, and sphincter control. EMG biofeedback is used in the treatment of stroke, SCI, cerebral palsy, TBI, MS, and dyskinesias. See Basmajian[9] for a discussion of EMG biofeedback in the treatment of neurologic disorders.

SPECIFIC NEUROLOGIC DISORDERS

In the following section, six specific neurologic disorders are discussed: stroke, brain injury, SCI, MS, Parkinson's disease, and epilepsy. Following a brief description of the etiology and symptomatology of each condition, the research evidence for the use of CAM therapies is discussed.

Stroke

Stroke is associated with an interruption of blood flow to some portion of the brain or brainstem as a result of hemorrhage or arterial blockage by thrombi or emboli. The immediate results are the classic symptoms of a stroke, which include numbness, weakness, or paralysis of face, arm, or leg, especially on one side of the body. There may be difficulty speaking or understanding simple statements. An individual may experience sudden or decreased vision in one or both eyes, dizziness, loss of balance, or loss of coordination. Other symptoms may include sudden, unexplainable, and intense headache; sudden nausea, fever, and vomiting; and brief loss of consciousness or period of decreased consciousness such as fainting, confusion, convulsions, or coma.[125] Because cerebral metabolism depends on a fairly constant supply of blood and oxygen, deprivation of oxygen in the brain can result in extensive damage within 10 to 20 seconds and irreversible damage after 3 to 10 minutes.[131] There are four major types of stroke: (1) cerebral occlusion or *thrombotic* (i.e., when a clot forms in an artery supplying blood to the brain, totally obstructing blood flow) and cerebral stenosis (partial obstruction of an artery); (2) *embolic* stroke, which occurs when a clot from a nonbrain region breaks loose and is carried in the bloodstream to an artery in the brain, plugging a blood vessel and cutting off the brain's blood supply; (3) *lacunar* stroke, which involves multiple, small cerebral infarcts affecting subcortical regions; and (4) *hemorrhagic* stroke, which occurs when a hemorrhage results in blood spilling into brain tissue or into the area surrounding the brain. Stroke ranks third among all causes of death in the United States, and over the course of a lifetime, four of five families will be touched by stroke. Stroke is a major cause of long-term disability, with 550,000 Americans annually suffering a stroke and nearly two thirds of the survivors having impairments.[86]

Several well-recognized deficit patterns are associated with lesion site. Anterior cerebral artery stroke is associated with contralateral lower- and sometimes upper-extremity paresis and hypesthesia as well as impaired judgment; middle cerebral artery infarct may be accompanied by contralateral upper- and lower-extremity paresis and hypesthesia, visual field deficits, agnosia, and aphasias. Posterior cerebral artery lesions may result in visual deficits, deficits in memory and cognition, alexia, agraphia, and balance problems. Cerebellar infarcts involve coordination and motor planning and execution. Brainstem lesions may involve any of the above, as well as vegetative functions such as respiration and autonomic regulation. More detailed descriptions of anatomic localization of deficits may be found elsewhere.[121] Any of the above lesions may be accompanied by long-term sequelae of seizures, spasticity, dysphagia, incontinence, depression, memory and learning impairments, peripheral nerve injuries, reflex sympathetic dystrophy, and sexual impairments.[45]

Acupuncture. In general, acupuncture has been reported to work best when used as early as possible on stroke patients, and it appears to be more effective with stroke patients if their lesions are singular, shallow, and with a small focus, instead of large, bilateral lesions with deep multiple foci.[27] In research based at the University of Lund, Sweden, it was hypothesized that the sensory stimulation of traditional acupuncture points with needles and electrostimulation may promote the restructuring and consolidation of coordinated motor function of affected limbs in the stroke patient, thus serving to enhance the recovery of postural control.[82] In a well-controlled study 40 hemiparetic male and female patients who received 10 weeks of acupuncture along with standard physical therapy (PT) and occupational therapy (OT) beginning 10 days after stroke recovered faster and had significant improvements in activities of daily living (Barthel index), quality of life (Nottingham Health Profile), and balance and mobility (measured by an idiosyncratic motor function assessment scale), in contrast to a control group of 38 patients who received only the standard physical and occupational therapy[65] (Fig. 7-2). A drawback to this study is the lack of a sham acupuncture condition; positive results could also be attributable to general sensory stimulation of the muscles surrounding the acupuncture point rather than "acupuncture" per se. In a follow-up of the 48 survivors in this study, conducted approximately 3 years after original treatment,[82] subjects received perturbations (vibratory stimulation to the calf muscle or galvanic stimulation of the vestibular nerves) in three different tests, each with the patients' eyes open and closed. Sig-

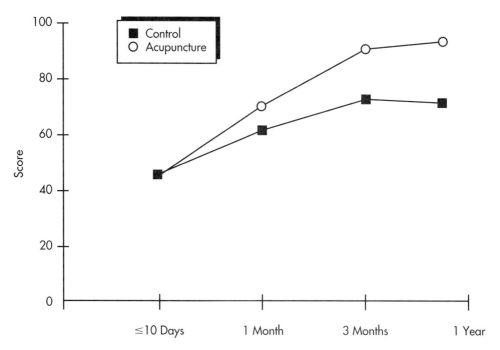

FIG. 7-2 Functional outcome on Barthel's index of activities of daily living for stroke patients with severe hemiparesis receiving acupuncture plus standard therapy or standard therapy alone. (From Johansson BB: *Scand J Rehabil Med* 29:87, 1993.)

nificantly more of the treatment group (17 of 21) than of the control group (9 of 25) could maintain stance on all six tests ($p < 0.0025$).

A research program directed by Margaret Naeser and colleagues at the Boston University Medical Center and Boston VA provides some evidence for the efficacy of acupuncture in the treatment of stroke under certain limiting conditions. In a study comparing real versus sham acupuncture in the treatment of paralysis in acute stroke patients,[99] 16 patients with right-side paralysis who had suffered left-hemisphere ischemic infarction were randomly assigned to receive either 20 real acupuncture treatments (11 points, some with electrical stimulation) or 20 sham acupuncture treatments (nonacupoints with no electrical stimulation) over a 1-month period beginning 1 to 3 months after stroke onset. The outcome measure was "good" versus "poor" response on the Boston Motor Inventory for upper and lower extremities. Results indicated that significantly more patients had a good response following real acupuncture than sham acupuncture when a computed tomography (CT) scan indicated that there was lesion in half or less than half of the motor pathways involving the periventricular white matter ($p < 0.013$). In a follow-up study, Naeser et al.[100] demonstrated similar results with laser acupuncture; however, five of the seven patients in this study had been subjects in the 1992 acupuncture study.[99] In a study of both chronic and acute stroke patients,[101] eight chronic stroke patients were treated with acupuncture beginning after 6 months to 8 years following stroke, and three acute stroke patients were treated with acupuncture beginning 2 months after stroke onset. Patients received 20 or 40 acupuncture treatments over a 2- to 3-month period. All patients had good response, defined as improvement on at least four of six hand tests, and this improvement was sustained for at least 2 months after completion of the acupuncture treatments. The researchers concluded that acupuncture may be an additional beneficial treatment method for stroke patients with hand paresis, even when started as late as 5 to 8 years after stroke. There was no control condition in this study; however, chronic patients were their own controls in the sense that their condition had been stable for 6 months or more before treatment. This same study also reported that patients exhibiting a beneficial response to treatment had damage to less than half of the motor pathway areas, as seen on CT scans.

Two other randomized, controlled trials of acupuncture treatment of stroke support the previously described findings. In a study of ischemic stroke conducted in Taiwan, when compared to subjects receiving standard rehabilitation only, subjects receiving acupuncture in addition to standard care had significantly better functional outcomes as measured by the Barthel Index at 1 month and 3 months after stroke.[58a] Subjects began receiving treatment within 36 hours after stroke and received 12 treatments over a 4-week period. Subjects with poor neurologic scores responded better to acupuncture than did controls, whereas there was no difference for subjects with good neurologic scores, suggesting that acupuncture has an incrementally helpful effect only when the condition is serious enough that full recovery is not likely through spontaneous recovery or standard rehabilitation. In a Norwegian study, 45 patients with cerebral infarctions or cerebral hemorrhages were randomly entered into either a standard rehabilitation condition or the acupuncture plus standard rehabilitation condition[121a]. Six weeks after treatment, individuals receiving acupuncture had significantly better outcomes in activities of daily living and on the Motor Assessment Scale and Nottingham Health Profile.

Ginkgo biloba. Research into the mechanisms of action of *Ginkgo biloba* suggests that it may improve cognitive function by altering arterial and vascular elasticity.[28] In addition, evidence derived from animal models and clinical studies supports the idea that *Ginkgo biloba* acts as an antiplatelet activating factor.[18] Taken together, these findings suggest that *Ginkgo biloba* can play a role in treating the symptoms of cerebrovascular disease during both the acute and chronic stages. Ginkgo has shown efficacy in the treatment of stroke in clinical investigations. For example, Maier-Hauff[83] reported that in 50 subarachnoid hemorrhage patients who had been administered GBE (L1 1370) in a placebo-controlled, double-blind study, GBE was effective in countering the effects of cerebral insufficiency with significant improvements noted in attention and verbal short-term memory. These results may argue in favor of early initiation of ginkgo therapy to treat the varied metabolic changes that may accompany cerebral ischemia, such as free-radical production and electrolyte shifts (e.g., increases in extracellular K^+ and intracellular Ca^{2+}, lactic acidosis), as well as increased release of free fatty acids, prostaglandins, and excitatory neurotransmitters.[36]

Hofferberth[56] conducted a double-blind, placebo-controlled trial to examine the effects of EGb 761 on neurophysiologic and psychometric parameters in patients with cerebrovascular disease. Thirty-six patients took part in the study, half of whom received EGb 761 at a dosage of 120 mg per day for 8 weeks; the other half were given a placebo. A high proportion of slow-wave activity in the electroencephalogram (EEG) spectrum generally indicates neurologic damage. After 4 to 8 weeks of therapy the proportion of theta waves (i.e., slow-wave activity) in the EEG spectrum was reduced in the patients given treatment with EGb 761. The neurophysiologic changes were evident as an increase in the relative power of the alpha component of the cortical EEG, which suggests that EGb 761 may be able to play a therapeutic role in treating cerebrovascular disease (i.e., stroke).[36]

Homeopathy. The research evidence on the use of homeopathic remedies for neurologic conditions is sparse. *Arnica montana* is an herb that is popular in the mountainous areas of Europe for the treatment of acute traumatic injuries, and it is a frequently used homeopathic remedy. Savage and Roe[127] studied 40 inpatients within 7 days after a stroke in a double-blind study with random assignment to either treatment or control group. Twenty of the patients received *A. montana,* and the 20 patients in the control condition received an equivalent dose of an unmedicated lactose powder similar in appearance to *A. montana*. The authors found no differences between the groups in mortality, survival, and functioning over a 3-month period. The investigators conducted a second study in 1978 with *A. montana* of a different dilution. Results replicated the early study, where no beneficial effect of the herb was found after stroke. Several case studies exist involving stroke, each using a different homeopathic remedy and, not surprisingly, report improvements in the patient's condition.[37,132]

Massage. Massage has been suggested to be a valuable adjunct in treatment regimens for hemiplegia.[172] Soothing massage before performing exercises can help reduce spasticity, and in cases of flaccid paralysis a more stimulating massage can help stimulate nerves and increase circulation.

Other Manual Manipulation. Investigators of PNF have studied both laboratory measures of nervous system excitability and clinically relevant parameters, such as hemiplegia. It is thought that contraction of antagonist muscle groups invokes a neurally mediated decrease in tone by way of inhibition of motoneurons via centrally mediated reflexes.[145] Entyre and Abraham[41] found that use of the contract-relax-antagonist-contract (CRAC) technique significantly decreased motor pool excitability during performance of the maneuver. Wang[166] found that in patients with hemiplegia of both long and short duration, gait speed and cadence improved in a cumulative manner after 12 sessions of PNF. On the other hand, when PNF used alone was compared with electromyographic muscle stimulation in hemiplegic patients, PNF produced less improvement than electrical stimulation.[73]

Hypnosis. In case reports of patients treated with hypnosis following a stroke, it has been reported that patients have shown increased movement in hemiplegic limbs, improved ambulation,[32,58,84] and the return of normal speech.[32,84] However, findings from these case studies are confounded because they occurred during the first year after the accident, a period during which spontaneous recovery is still probable.

Meditation. With regard to stroke prevention, the most robust finding is the success of meditation for reducing hypertension,[11,52,130,163] and there is also evidence of reduction in cholesterol level.[31] Given the success of meditation for reducing hypertension and the fact that hypertension is a predisposing factor for stroke and recurrence of stroke, it seems reasonable to conclude that meditation may be effective in reduction of risk for stroke. Although no studies were located that address specifically the issue of stroke prevention, in a well-controlled, randomized study comparing several relaxation techniques, regular practice of transcendental meditation (TM) by elderly nursing home residents was associated with (1) significantly reduced systolic blood pressure and (2) significantly increased 3-year survival rate, when compared with the simple relaxation and no-treatment conditions.[3] After 3 years, 100% of the TM group were alive in contrast to 68% of the no-treatment group.

Botanicals. Ischemia reoxygenation plays an important role in the pathogenesis of stroke and brain trauma. Some non-Chinese herbs can exert a protective effect shielding cells from the pathologic effects of ischemic reoxygenation. This protective effect may be mediated by antioxidant and free-radical scavenging properties, which suggests a role for herbal therapies in the treatment of stroke and neurotrauma.[140] Uchida et al.[153] reported that in stroke-prone, spontaneously hypertensive rats, the herb *Persimmon tannin* appeared to have helped increase the rat's life span, in addition to reducing the severity of damage resulting from brain hemorrhage and infarction. Kampo herbal formulations, which contain several ingredients and are available in various forms, have been reported to reduce the complications resulting from ischemia.[44] Through in vitro experimentation (i.e., via an electron spin resonance technique) Kampo formulations and components have shown radical scavenging activity, which suggests that Kampo, when used in treatment of brain damage, could play a preventive role in reducing the ischemic complications following brain trauma. In a similar way, the extract *Kava (Piper methysticum)* and its constituents have also displayed antiischemic properties in rodent models. The kava constituents were found to display protective and anticonvulsive effects in two models of focal ischemia.[8]

Energy Healing. McGee and Chow[89] relate a number of case studies on the success of Qi Gong for many different medical conditions, including stroke, paralysis, and cerebral palsy. However, truly rigorous research is sparse.

Diet and Nutrition. Epidemiologic studies have suggested that a daily diet of fruits and vegetables has a protective effect against stroke. Ness and Powles[102] conducted a review of studies published between 1966 and 1995 on the protective action of fruits and vegetables against cardiovascular disease. Nine of 14 studies on stroke showed that the consumption of fruits and vegetables had a significant protective association with stroke. Similar results were found in a 17-year follow-up of 11,000 subjects who consumed a vegetarian diet.[69] The authors found that daily consumption of fresh fruit was associated with significantly reduced mortality from cerebrovascular disease and ischemic heart disease.

The protective action of fruits and vegetables is attributed to dietary antioxidant vitamins (beta-carotene and vitamin C) and flavonoids. This hypothesis was examined in a 15-year follow-up of 552 males.[68] The investigators found an inverse relation between the intake of dietary antioxidants and stroke incidence. Antioxidants prevent low-density lipoprotein (LDL) oxidation and therefore reduce its absorption by macrophages and the subsequent formation of atherosclerotic plaques. Support for the protective antioxidant action of vitamin C was found in a review of the research literature between 1966 and 1996.[103] The review indicated a protective association of measures of vitamin C intake or blood levels of vitamin C and cardiovascular disease. Although evidence was limited, there was support for the premise that vitamin C had a protective effect against stroke. Research suggests that garlic has the ability to provide some protection against atherosclerosis, coronary thrombosis, and stroke, effects that are believed to be directly related to its ability to inhibit aggregation of blood platelets.[151]

Nutritional supplementation has been suggested to reduce the risk of a subsequent occurrence of cerebrovascular accident. Although these recommendations are often based on a presumed protective mechanism of action within the body based on the biochemistry of the substance, little research directly relating these substances to effective treatment of neurologic conditions exists, and when the limited studies are examined closely, there is often contradictory information. For example, the belief that fish consumption reduces risk of stroke is supported by several retrospective studies,[62,67] but a recent population-based retrospective study not only failed to support these earlier findings, but tended to contradict them, finding a slightly higher level of stroke in men with the highest level of reported fish consumption.[109]

Melatonin. It has been proposed that the nocturnal rise in melatonin level that is observed in humans may mediate the lower nocturnal risks for heart attack and stroke. When human blood platelets are incubated in a melatonin solution, the hormone reduces their tendency to clump by as much as 85%.[97] Some research also suggests a link between melatonin and cholesterol. That is, melatonin has been shown to partially block cholesterol production resulting in a reduction in LDL accumulation.[98]

Chelation. Although chelation therapy is recommended for the treatment and prevention of cerebrovascular disorders, there are no controlled trials to substantiate its use. In one uncontrolled trial cerebral arterial occlusion was measured in 57 patients before and after treatment with 10 to 46 sessions of chelation therapy. Eighty-eight percent of the patients improved (criteria for improvement not stated), and cerebral arterial stenosis was reported to be reduced from a mean 28% to 10%.[88] A retrospective analysis was conducted in Brazil of 2870 patients who were treated with chelation therapy between 1983 and 1985.[108] These patients had a variety of vascular and degenerative diseases, with about 18% of the patients (504) diagnosed with cerebrovascular disease or degenerative CNS disease. The investigators reported "marked recovery" in 24% of the patients and "good recovery" in 60%. Animal studies with another chelating agent, deferoxamine, showed that the hypoxic-ischemic injury is reduced if deferoxamine is administered soon after the injury.[7,60,111]

Hyperbaric Oxygen. A problem for stroke patients is the deprivation of oxygen in key brain areas resulting from an interruption of blood flow. Hyperbaric oxygen (HBO) therapy has been advocated in these circumstances, since it may enhance neuronal viability by its ability to increase the amount of dissolved oxygen in the blood without changing blood viscosity.[95] In a large study by Neubauer and End,[104] 122 patients with thrombotic stroke were treated with HBO in addition to standard treatment. In the bedridden group 64% of the patients improved by showing ability to use a wheelchair or to walk with or without aids. In the wheelchair group 71% of the patients showed improved ambulation. In the group categorized as walking with aids, 56% of the patients improved enough to walk independently. However, in a study of HBO therapy for the treatment of acute ischemic stroke in patients who had had middle cerebral artery occlusion, the results were mixed.[106] In addition, while there have been a number of animal studies and isolated small clinical/case-based studies, there has been no major study showing the benefit of this treatment for wide-scale application. In general, existing research suggests that HBO therapy in patients with stroke may be beneficial, but additional research is clearly needed.

Safety. Issues of safety and toxicity have been a major concern surrounding HBO therapy. Adverse effects such as increased free-radical production and peroxidation have been reported.[120] However, serious side effects have been virtually eliminated by keeping pressures at 1.5 to 2 atmospheres (atm), limiting exposure time, and following more rigorous procedures during compression and decompression.[105]

Brain Injury

Brain injury refers to damage to the brain caused by either external trauma (motor vehicle accidents, gunshot wounds) or internal lesions (tumor, anoxic injury). Traumatic brain injury is of two major types: the more common, closed-head injuries in which rapid movement of the brain within the skull results in global deficits and open-head injuries, which involve penetration of the skull and localized damage. Mild TBI refers to brain injury that may produce no obvious problems, signs, or symptoms and may go unexamined and untreated. However, increasing evidence suggests that mild brain injury (i.e., incurred in a single episode or in repeated episodes in contact sports such as football) can result in permanent damage.

There are numerous causes of TBI; the most common are motor vehicle accidents, which account for 50% of all injuries. Falls account for 21% of injuries, firearms for 12%, and sports/recreational accidents for 10%. Each year, 373,000 Americans are hospitalized as a result of TBI. Of these, 99,000 have severe lifelong disabilities. Males in the 14- to 24-year-old age-group are at the greatest risk for TBI, and more than 30,000 children are permanently disabled each year as a result of brain injuries.[17]

The effects of TBI vary widely, ranging from mild concussive syndromes that may result in little to mild loss of function, to moderate and severe head injuries that may leave people with long-term impairments and disabilities. After acute effects of TBI are stabilized, patients with moderate and severe injuries usually require long-term care for treatment and rehabilitation of conditions such as seizures, spasticity, movement disorders, neuroendocrine dysfunction, cranial and sensory nerve impairments, and significant cognitive deficits and mood disturbances.

Ginkgo biloba. *Ginkgo biloba* extract has reportedly shown efficacy in improving outcomes in animal models of TBI. For example, EGb 761 has been found to enhance recovery in rats with bilateral frontal damage following 30 days of treatment. Rats have shown decreased activity and sensitivity to light and noxious stimuli, along with improved performance on a delayed spatial-alternation learning task, when administered GBE before injury.[137] Improved motor function was also found in an experimental model of cortical hemiplegia.[16] Brailowsky et al.[16] administered EGb 761 using two rat models of hemiplegia, one induced by aspiration and a second group subjected to reversible inactivation of motor cortex (i.e., via GABA infusion). Rats given the GBE exhibited a faster, more complete recovery from motor deficits, with histologic analysis also showing that EGb 761–treated rats had significantly smaller ventricular diameters than untreated animals (i.e., rats to which only saccharin solutions were given).

Homeopathy. In a study funded by the Office of Alternative Medicine at the National Institutes of Health, Woo et al.[178] investigated the efficacy of *Hellaeborous niger* with mild TBI. They found that 10 patients with mild TBI showed a significant reduction in symptoms of fatigue, anxiety, and depression following treatment with *H. niger*.

Hypnosis. In a study without a control condition, hypnosis was used in the treatment of headache or vertigo following brain injury in a sample of 155 patients. Almost half of the patients reported resolution of symptoms, and another 20% had significant symptom reduction.[23] Outcome was best for those who had been injured less than 6 months before treatment. In two case reports of young people with TBIs, hypnotic treatment was followed by increased social interaction, improved mood, increased participation in treatment, and substantial gains in physical therapy.[32]

Hyperbaric Oxygen. Research on the use of hyperbaric oxygen in brain injury is less encouraging than in stroke. Hyperbaric oxygen therapy may have beneficial effects for reducing brain edema after head injury without impairing tissue oxygen delivery.[141] In general, the limited research suggests that HBO therapy may speed up the healing process and lower the mortality rate, but may not substantially improve functioning.[30,105,119,120]

Spinal Cord Injury

Spinal cord injury refers to the loss of neurologic function following traumatic injury to the spinal cord. There are approximately 250,000 spinal cord–injured individuals living in the United States today with, on average, 11,000 new injuries reported each year. Traumatic motor vehicle accidents cause 48% of SCIs; falls constitute 21%, violence 15%, and sports 14% of SCIs. The location and severity of injury determine how the individual with SCI is affected. Fifty-five percent of SCIs result in tetraplegia, with the remaining 45% resulting in paraplegia.[135] If the spinal cord is only partially transected (as in approximately 54% of cases), some nerve impulses will be transmitted accompanied by incomplete loss of function. However, total transection of the spinal cord results in complete loss of function below the level of the lesion (i.e., complete injury). Level of injury corresponds with severity of neurologic deficit. Patients usually require surgical spinal stabilization followed by long-term intensive rehabilitation by a team of professionals. Depending on the level of injury, patients may exhibit need for respiratory support, chronic pulmonary conditions, cardiac and autonomic abnormalities, loss of bowel and bladder control, muscle weakness, spasticity, changes in body composition and regulation, sexual dysfunction, and skin breakdown. Persons who survive SCI frequently have chronic medical problems that may be amenable to CAM interventions.

Acupuncture. Research using animal models has suggested that acupuncture may be effective in inducing regeneration in nerve tissue. Rats given treatment with electroacupuncture exhibited spontaneous sprouting of severed sciatic nerve tissue with a 14% to 30% increase in regeneration rate compared with the no-treatment group.[12] Additional results from animal models in which spinal cord contusion was induced suggest that electroacupuncture applied 1 hour after SCI decreased posttraumatic sequelae.[114] One uncontrolled study of the use of acupuncture in the treatment of persons with SCI reported improvements in functioning and decrease in parasthesias.[171] However, the study did not report results on any quantifiable outcomes or involve comparisons with a control group. Therefore, because of the absence of comparison controls and quantifiable measures of pain or mobility, it is difficult to draw any definite conclusions about the efficacy of treatment.

Massage. There appear to be a modest number of studies on the use of massage therapy in the treatment of CNS problems, with the majority of the published articles in Russian or German. Of the small number of English-language studies reviewed to date, the majority pertain to the use of massage therapy in the treatment of SCI (i.e., reflex responses and circulatory difficulties). In one study the effect of a 3-minute therapeutic massage of the triceps surae muscle group was examined for its effect on the H-reflex amplitude in 10 individuals with SCI.[46] Although a decrease in mean peak-to-peak amplitude in the H-reflex occurred during massage, no long-term effects were noted. In another study massage therapy, along with elastic stocking compression, was used to treat thrombophlebitis in individuals with SCI.[157] Twenty-six subjects with complete paraplegia or tetraplegia were given massage and permanent elastic stocking compression, in addition to active and passive mobilization of the extremities. A control group of 15 paraplegics and tetraplegics was given treatment with only mobilization of the extremities. No evidence of thrombophlebitis or pulmonary embolism was observed in any of the massage/compression subjects as compared with a 40% incidence of thrombophlebitis and a 13% incidence of pulmonary embolism in the control group.

Casady and Curry[22] discussed the benefits of light sacral massage for pressure ulcer prevention in spinal cord–injured individuals, if used in the immediate postinjury period. In a retrospective review of medical records of 49 acutely injured SCI patients the authors found that length of immobilization was significantly associated with subsequent decubitus ulcer formation and therefore suggested that the use of pressure-relieving therapies such as massage should be used in the early stages of acute SCI. A description of the proper application of massage to pressure areas can be found in Tappan.[146] For the immobilized patient massage therapy can be useful in alleviating muscular tightness in the back or neck caused by the long-term maintenance of a particular body position. It can also facilitate relaxation and/or sleep for a patient who may be tense or in an uncomfortable position. Since massage has been suggested for spastic and flaccid paralysis following stroke,[172] it could be used to treat paralysis in the SCI population as well.

Chiropractic. There are a few studies regarding chiropractic manipulation for SCI. In a randomized, double-blind study of 30 patients who experienced pain 12 weeks after "whiplash" trauma sustained in motor vehicle accidents, it was reported that chiropractic therapy that included "phasic neck exercises" to treat eye-head-neck-arm coordinated movements produced significant reduction in neck pain.[43] In a case study an 11-year-old boy who had a diagnosis of incomplete tetraplegia below C7[177] experienced little change during 3 months of conventional treatment but demonstrated substantial improvement in motor functioning following 2 weeks of spinal manipulation (in addition to a rehabilitation program that continued for 2 months). In another case study a man who sought medical attention with complete paralysis of both arms and legs following a motor vehicle accident caused by a dislocation of C5 was given a relaxant, anesthesia, and treatment with closed manipulation, which was reported to have resulted in a rapid and full recovery.[40]

Hypnosis. Following hypnosis and self-hypnosis a spinal cord–injured patient reported decreased "phantom pain" in his paralyzed arm, allowing a return to work,[139] and another showed improved strength, decreased pain, and increased functional use of his arms.[81] Attempts to treat spasticity have apparently been less successful.[25]

Energy Healing. Two studies from China pertained to paralysis and SCI. In one study 43 paralysis patients (19, hemiplegia; 24, paraplegia) were treated with emitted Qi from several Qi Gong masters.[59] Treatment also included massage of certain acupoints and performance of Qi Gong exercises that had been adjusted for physical limitations attributable to the paralysis. Results indicated that there were improvements in various functional indicators, including range of motion, walking, and activities of daily living, and in various psychosomatic symptoms. In an animal study, young pigs with surgically induced SCI received either Qi Gong or no treatment.[165] After 3 months, 91% of the pigs receiving Qi Gong could walk, whereas 0% of pigs in the control group could walk. The quality of these two studies is not known, since the information is based only on brief abstracts of conference presentations. In addition to the limited research evidence, there are a number of practitioners and at least one hospital in China which specialize in the use of Qi Gong to treat paralysis and other neurologic disorders. Walker[162] claimed that thousands of paralysis patients have been treated at the Army General Qi Gong Hospital in Beijing, China, with 90% showing some improvement and 46% experiencing complete recovery from their paralysis. On the other hand, Brown[20] reported that a well-known Qi Gong master from China was unable to improve functioning in post-stroke hemiplegia patients in a controlled demonstration study conducted in the United States.

Multiple Sclerosis

Multiple sclerosis is a chronic disease of the CNS white matter, the cause of which is unknown, that is characterized by diffuse lesions or plaques, with the highest incidence of lesions occurring in the periventricular white matter. This degeneration is primarily due to scattered neuronal demyelination and oligodendrocyte loss throughout the CNS.[92,121] Recent clinical data implicate autoimmune mechanisms, perhaps triggered by an unknown infectious agent or environmental factors encountered early in life.[147] The disruption in neurotransmission is mainly due to the destruction and scarring of myelin.[154] Recent magnetic resonance imaging (MRI) studies involving MS have reported breakdowns in the blood-brain barrier and abnormal autoimmune response, possibly of viral cause. In addition to producing a marked decrease in life expectancy (i.e., 9.5 years in men and 14 years in women), MS can produce profound and adverse effects on an individual's physical, mental, and social well-being.[147] MS is the third most common cause of significant disability in young to middle-aged adults, exceeded only by trauma and arthritis.[129]

The earliest symptoms of MS are usually somatosensory, including tingling and burning sensations, tightness of the extremities, and, less often, severe neuralgic pains. Numbness or absence of sensory symptoms occurs less often. Vision is often impaired in MS because of the optic nerve's susceptibility to MS plaques, and symptoms include nystagmus, impairment in ocular motility, blurred or double vision, and optic neuritis involving unilateral dimming of vision, accompanied by photophobia and pain accompanying eye movement. Motor symptoms include stiffness and heaviness in the extremities (usually lower) and cramps, spasms, or pain, with patients often having tonic "seizures" or dystonic posturing of parts of the body.*

These may evolve into an abnormal reflex activity and tremors, which then progress to severe spastic paraparesis. It is now well known that cognitive impairments exist in individuals with MS, with prevalence rates ranging from 43% to 65%.[113] MS is a disease that is characterized most commonly by exacerbation and remission of symptoms, with each period of remission ending with a lower level of functional status. The other most common course is that of steady progression of symptoms.

The age of onset of MS ranges from 15 to 50 years. It is most often seen in young adults, with one third of all cases occurring before age 20 years.[2] The prevalence of MS is reported to be 6 to 14 per 100,000 in the southern United States and southern Europe, increasing in the more temperate latitudes to 30 to 80 per 100,000 in Canada, northern Europe, and the northern United States.[2] Immigration studies suggest that predisposing conditions for MS may be critical before age 15 years.

At present, there are no specific treatments that can prevent or reverse the course of demyelination during MS progression.[154] The focus of current major treatment procedures is primarily symptomatic, with the goal of alleviating the associated complications as well as lessening the length and severity of exacerbations. Similarly, most rehabilitative procedures have not been very successful at significantly altering the course of MS. Thus MS patients often have long-term deficits and may benefit from interventions that support overall health and well-being to offset a usually progressive condition.

Acupuncture. Acupuncture shows promise as a diagnostic tool for detecting MS before its clinical manifestations are expressed.[138] For example, even early in the course of the disease, it has been reported that in individuals with MS, acupuncture points show heightened sensitivity. Furthermore, MS patients who were administered a combination of traditional acupuncture (i.e., "Tien-Hsin Twelve Points" or "Ma Dan Yang's Points") and cerebral acupuncture showed more rapid improvement, which may suggest that combination acupuncture may be more effective than traditional acupuncture alone. In a case report Rampes[116] found symptomatic improvement from the pain associated with trigeminal neuralgia, and Miller,[94] in a small study, reported that acupuncture was effective in reducing spasticity.

Botanicals. Evening primrose oil has been reported to slow the progression of MS.[151] However, it should not be assumed that botanicals are harmless simply because they are natural, or that they have positive effects in some conditions. Tyler,[152] for example,

---

*References 13, 55, 66, 87, 110, 150.

indicated that echinacea, a popular "immune enhancer," should not be used by persons with systemic disorders, including MS.

Diet and Nutrition. Several diets, high in vegetable-cereal and low in animal and butter fat, are recommended to prevent MS and prevent relapses in patients with MS. One of the most consistent epidemiologic findings in MS is the higher prevalence of MS in populations that consumed diets rich in animal fats.[10] Swank and Dugan[142] reviewed several surveys conducted in different parts of the world and found a significant correlation between dietary fats of animal origin and incidence of MS. A case-controlled, matched study of 155 patients with MS and 155 healthy control subjects showed that of several environmental risk factors considered, the MS group had a predominantly meat (vs. vegetable) diet during childhood. Swank and Dugan[143] looked at the effect of low-fat diet on patients with MS with various degrees of disease severity (minimum, moderate and severe). They followed patients for 34 years and found that the greatest benefit (i.e., survival rate and activity level) was seen in those with minimum disability at the onset of the trial.

Melatonin. The pineal gland has been implicated in the pathogenesis of MS. Researchers studied nocturnal plasma melatonin levels and the presence of pineal calcification (PC) on CT scan in a cohort of 25 patients (age range, 27 to 72 years) admitted to a hospital for exacerbation of symptoms. There was a positive correlation between melatonin levels and age of onset of symptoms and an inverse correlation with the duration of illness. Abnormal alpha–melatonin stimulating hormone (MSH) levels were found in more than 70% of patients. These findings support the hypothesis that MS may be associated with pineal dysfunction and suggest that alterations in the secretion of alpha-MSH may occur during exacerbation of symptoms.[21,125]

The fall of melatonin secretion during the prepubertal period (which may disrupt pineal-mediated immunomodulation) may either stimulate the reactivation of the infective agent or increase the susceptibility to infection during the pubertal period. Similarly, the rapid fall in melatonin secretion just before delivery may account for the frequent occurrence or relapse in MS patients during the postpartum period. In contrast, pregnancy (which is associated with high melatonin concentrations) is often accompanied by remission of symptoms. Thus the presence of high melatonin levels may provide a protective effect, whereas a decline in melatonin secretion may increase the risk for the development and exacerbation of MS.[124]

Parkinson's Disease

Parkinson's disease (PD) is a neurodegenerative movement disorder affecting approximately 1% of the population, mostly 65 years of age and older.[19] The likelihood of developing PD increases with age, a history of depression, or severe extrapyramidal manifestations. The average age of onset is around 55 years of age in both sexes with the range of onset showing a wide distribution of 20 to 80 years of age.[121] Men appear to be more susceptible than women, with a male/female ratio of 3/2. The mean prevalence rate of PD is approximately 160 per 100,000 people; however, by age 70 years the rate has increased to 550 per 100,000.

The etiology of this disorder is believed to be based on a combination of factors, such as accelerated aging, toxin exposure, genetic predisposition, and oxidative stress,[63] although the cause of PD is still a matter of speculation. The most prominent symptoms of PD are tremors, bradykinesia, rigidity, and postural instability. Another common characteristic feature of PD is "freezing," a transient inability to perform active movement, especially affecting the legs, but also the eyelids, arms, and facial muscles.[39,121] Other prominent symptoms include hypokinesia and difficulty in changing direction, as well as disorders in swallowing, speech, and writing.[39] Fatigue and dementia are also commonly observed in parkinsonism. Tremor is one of the first symptoms to appear and is recognized in 70% of patients.[121] Most symptoms begin unilaterally but often become bilateral as the disease progresses. Many of these impairments are probably attributable to basal ganglia involvement, which plays an important role in motor planning and programing.[39]

Acupuncture. Electroacupuncture stimulation of the fibula at low frequencies of 4 to 8 Hz reportedly resulted in reduced tremor and muscle tone in PD patients.[78] Furthermore, a complete or partial resolution of muscle rigidity or tremor was noted in 94% of 63 patients after a combination treatment involving acupuncture and herbs, with the goal of enhancing the regenerative process in the disease site at the substantia nigra–corpus striatum tract.[167]

Melatonin. MIF-1, a synthetic tripeptide with MSH-release inhibitory properties, has been reported to improve symptoms of PD, attenuate levodopa-related dyskinesias, and diminish the dyskinetic movement of tardive dyskinesia. There is evidence to suggest that MIF-1 increases nigrostriatal dopaminergic activity, but its ability to improve these symptoms cannot be explained solely on the basis of the drug's effect on striatal dopaminergic neurons. MIF-1 has been reported to potentiate the melanocyte-whitening effect of melatonin in rats, and it produces mood elevation in patients with PD and tardive dyskinesia. Therefore it is possible that the effects of MIF-1 in movement disorders are associated with increased melatonin secretion. Thus hypothalamic MIF may modulate nigrostriatal dopaminergic functions in part via pineal melatonin, which would constitute a novel mechanism by which hypothalamic peptides act to modulate the expression of movement disorders.[123]

Epilepsy

Epilepsy affects about 40 million people worldwide. Epileptic seizures are the result of a temporary dysfunction of the brain caused by an abnormal hypersynchronous electrical discharge of neurons in the cortex. Currently, no medical treatments are able to cure or induce permanent remission of epileptic symptoms. Treatment has designated three main goals: elimination of seizures or reduction of their frequency; avoidance of side effects associated with long-term treatments; and prediction and eventual prevention of epileptogenesis.

A typical epileptic syndrome is characterized by a cluster of signs and symptoms occurring at the same time.[121] Syndromes are characterized by type, family history, the presence of abnormal neurologic findings, age of onset, and the patient's response to medication. Epilepsy can be categorized as arising from a known versus an idiopathic or cryptogenic origin. The classification of epilepsies is largely empiric and is usually not based on pathologic or etiologic origin. The most prominent forms of epilepsy involving complex partial seizures are (1) *temporal lobe epilepsy*, the most commonly observed syndrome in adults, which mainly involves the hippocampus, amygdala, and parahippocampal gyrus; (2) *frontal lobe epilepsy*, characterized by bizarre motor and vocal manifestations and showing almost no abnormality on EEG recordings; (3) *epilepsia partialis continua (EPC)*, involving unremitting motor seizures that may involve part or all of the body; and (4) *posttraumatic epilepsy*, which occurs after brain injury and is usually observed in the first year after the accident. Seizures in generalized epilepsies are subdivided to include such general types as "absence" seizures, "tonic-clonic" seizures, and "benign convulsions" and "neonatal seizures" (mostly occurring in children and infants).[121]

Acupuncture. Acupuncture has been used to treat epilepsy both during an acute attack and after the attack, during remission. When applied during an attack, it has been used to stop the convulsions, clear the phlegm, and open the orifices.[179] In a study using scalp acupuncture involving 24 acupuncture points with electrical stimulation durations of 0.2 seconds at 6 Hz, 90% of the 98 subjects showed improvement.[133] On the other hand, in an animal model of epilepsy, Chen and Huang[26] concluded that acupuncture had no therapeutic effects on experimentally induced epilepsy and may even aggravate the condition.

Yoga. Panjwani et al.[112] reported that, based on assessments made of seizure control and electroencephalographic alterations in 32 patients with idiopathic epilepsy, yoga meditation could play a beneficial role in the management of patients with epilepsy.

Melatonin. Researchers have found that melatonin lowers the excitability of individual neurons and acts as a mild anticonvulsant. Patients with epilepsy whose brain wave patterns were evaluated both before and after the injection of melatonin displayed normalized brain waves following melatonin injection. Recent data from biochemical and electrophysiologic studies support the idea that the anticonvulsant and depressive effects of melatonin on neuron activity may depend on its antioxidant and antiexcitotoxic roles (i.e., acting as a free-radical scavenger and brain glutamate receptor regulator).[1,118]

SUMMARY

Alternative treatments used as complementary tools show promise in helping to treat a variety of the signs and symptoms of neurologic disorders. Impairments resulting from neurologic injury can become evident across multiple functional domains and affect such diverse areas as cognition, affect, sensation, motor activity/control, proprioception, and the regulation of autonomic, autoimmune, and vascular function. Thus, given the complexity of the systemic dysregulation that may follow neurologic injury, it is not surprising that functional activities are affected in an equally variable manner. CAM therapies provide an equally diverse spectrum of techniques that may expand the range of options that clinicians may use.

Neurologic disorders, however, do not merely represent clusters of signs and symptoms, but are manifested in the struggles and challenges faced by patients, families, and society. These patients reflect a growing cultural, religious, and ethnic diversity—a diversity that embraces many of the concepts and practices of CAM. It is from this social context that alternative therapies may represent socially, medically, and economically viable complementary options for treating acute and chronic neurologic impairments. For example, depressed mood, motivation, and feelings of self-efficacy, which may influence the course and effectiveness of mainstream medicine, may be treated with hypnotherapy. Craniosacral therapy may be a useful supplemental approach in multidisciplinary programs for the treatment of spinal cord and brain injuries. The emotional and psychologic impact of neurologic disorders can be devastating to patients and families. Thus the integration of religion and spirituality treatment methods into mainstream medicine may offer a solace that could be beneficial to them. Massage therapy has reportedly shown efficacy in the prevention of thrombophlebitis and pulmonary embolism in SCI patients with paraplegia, as well as in the treatment of symptoms arising from stroke. Acupuncture has been used to treat pain, dysphasia, and disorders of motor control, sensation, and cognition. Bioelectromagnetic techniques have shown promise in treating skin wounds, pain, depression, and cognitive impairments, in addition to finding applications in the diagnosis and assessment of motor/nerve pathway function. Herbal and pharmacologic treatments have been used to treat a variety of neurologic signs and symptoms. For instance, GBE has shown antiplatelet properties and vascular regulatory activity and has also been used to treat disorders of memory, affect, and information processing.

If the efficacy of various CAM therapies is validated in well-designed clinical trials, will mainstream medicine use them? In surveys evaluating the attitudes of North American physicians toward "alternative" therapies, it has been reported that 50% to 70% of physicians have recommended that their patients see a specialist in some form of CAM.[14,47,158] However, many physicians have reported little understanding of alternative techniques.[47,75] In a Canadian study, 56% of general practitioners surveyed thought that concepts and methods of CAM could be of benefit in conventional medical practice,[158] and in a survey of physicians in the United States, 70% of the respondents expressed an interest in training in various areas of CAM.[14] Overall, it would appear that a growing number of physicians view CAM as offering potential treatment benefits that could enrich mainstream medicine and the health and well-being of this nation.

REFERENCES

1. Acuna-Castroviejo D, et al: Cell protective role of melatonin in the brain, *J Pineal Res* 19(2):57, 1995.
2. Adams RD, Victor M: *Principles of neurology*, ed 5, New York, 1993, McGraw-Hill.
3. Alexander CN et al: Transcendental meditation, mindfulness, and longevity: an experimental study with the elderly, *J Personality Social Psychol* 57(6):950, 1989.
4. Anderson DC et al: A pilot study of hyperbaric oxygen in the treatment of human stroke, *Stroke* 22(9):1137, 1991.
5. Anton-Tay F, Diaz JL, Fernandez-Guardiola A: On the effect of melatonin upon human brain: its possible therapeutic implications, *Life Sciences* 10(15):841, 1971.
6. Arrigo A et al: Effects of intravenous high dose co-dergocrine mesylate ('Hydergine') in elderly patients with severe multi-infarct dementia: a double-blind, placebo-controlled trial, *Curr Med Res Opin* 11(8):491, 1989.
7. Babbs CF: Role of iron ions in the genesis of reperfusion injury following successful cardiopulmonary resuscitation: preliminary data and a biochemical hypothesis, *Ann Emerg Med* 14(8):777, 1985.
8. Backhaub C, Krieglstein J: Extract of kava (*Piper methysticum*) and its methysticin constituents protect brain tissue against ischemic damage in rodents, *Eur J Pharmacol* 215(2-3):265, 1992.
9. Basmajian JV: Biofeedback in physical medicine rehabilitation. In DeLisa JA, Gans BM, editors: *Rehabilitation medicine: principles and practice*, ed 3, Philadelphia, 1998, Lippincott-Raven.
10. Bates D: Dietary lipids and multiple sclerosis, *Upsala J Med Sci (supplement)* 48(suppl):173, 1990.
11. Benson H: Systemic hypertension and the relaxation response, *N Engl J Med* 296:1152, 1977.
12. Bensoussan A: Does acupuncture therapy resemble a process of physiological relearning? *Am J Acupunct* 22:137, 1994.
13. Berger JR, Sherematat WA, Melamed E: Paroxysmal dystonia as the initial manifestation of multiple sclerosis, *Arch Neurol* 41:747, 1984.
14. Berman BM et al: Physicians' attitudes toward complementary or alternative medicine: a regional survey, *J Am Board Fam Pract* 8:361, 1995.
15. Bochner F, Eadie MJ, Tyrer JH: Use of an ergot preparation (hydergine) in the convalescent phase of stroke, *J Am Geriatr Soc* 21(1):10, 1973.
16. Brailowsky S et al: Effects of Ginkgo biloba extract on cortical hemiplegia in the rat. In Christen Y, Costentin J, Lacour M, editors: *Effects of Ginkgo biloba extract (EGb 761) on the central nervous system*, Paris, 1992, Elsevier, pp. 95-103.

17. Brain Injury Association: *Fact sheet: traumatic brain injury,* Washington, DC, 1995, Brain Injury Association, Inc.
18. Braquet P et al: Is there a case for PAF antagonists in the treatment of ischemic disease?, *Trends Pharmacol Stud* 10:23, 1989.
19. Broe GA et al: Neurological disorders in the elderly at home, *J Neurol Neurosurg Psychiatr* 39(4):362, 1976.
20. Brown DA: Qigong master fails to substantiate claims during demonstration project, *MISAHA Newslett* 14-15:7, 1997.
21. Cahill GM, Grace MS, Besharce JC: Rhythmic regulation of retinal melatonin: metabolic pathways, neurochemical mechanisms, and the ocular circadian clock, *Cell Molecular Neurobiol* 11(5):529, 1991.
22. Casady L, Curry K: The relationship between extended periods of immobility and decubitus ulcer formation in the acutely spinal cord-injured individual, *J Neurosci Nurs* 24(4):185, 1992.
23. Cedercreutz C, Lahteenmaki R, Tulikoura J: Hypnotic treatment of headache and vertigo in skull injured patients, *Int J Clin Experiment Hypnosis* 24(3):195, 1976.
24. Chae J et al: Functional neuromuscular stimulation. In DeLisa JA, Gans BM, editors: *Rehabilitation medicine: principles and practice,* ed 3, Philadelphia, 1998, Lippincott-Raven.
25. Chappell DT: Hypnosis and spasticity in paraplegia, *Am J Clin Hypnosis* 7(1):33, 1964.
26. Chen R-C, Huang Y-H: Acupuncture on experimental epilepsies, *Proc Natl Sci Council* 8(1):72, 1984.
27. Chen Y-M, Fang Y-A: 108 cases of hemiplegia caused by stroke: the relationship between CT scan results, clinical findings and the effect of acupuncture in treatment, *Acupunct Electro-Therapeutics Res* 15:9, 1990.
28. Christen Y, Costentin J, Lacour M: Effects of ginkgo biloba extract (Egb 761) on the central nervous system, *IPSEN Institute International Symposium,* Montreaux, Switzerland, 1991.
29. Churchill PS, Dail NW: Massage/bodywork. Paper presented at *Alternative medicine: implications for clinical practice,* Harvard Medical School, Boston, MA, 1996.
30. Clifton GL: Hypothermia and hyperbaric oxygen as treatment modalities for severe head injury, *New Horizons* 3(3):474, 1995.
31. Cooper MJ, Aygen MM: A relaxation technique in the management of hypercholesterolemia, *J Human Stress* 5:24, 1979.
32. Crasilneck HB, Hall JA: The use of hypnosis in the rehabilitation of complicated vascular and post-traumatic neurological patients, *Int J Clin Experiment Hypnosis* 18(3):145, 1970.
33. Croisile B et al: Long-term and high-dose piracetam treatment of Alzheimer's disease, *Neurology* 43(2):301, 1993.
34. Cross P et al: Observations on the use of music in rehabilitation of stroke patients, *Physiother Can* 36(4):197, 1984.
35. Dalby BJ: Chiropractic diagnosis and treatment of closed head trauma, *J Manipulative Physiol Ther* 19(6):392, 1993.
36. DeFeudis FV: *Ginkgo biloba extract (EGb 761): pharmacological activities and clinical applications,* Paris, 1991, Elsevier.
37. Desai M: Paralysis, *Indian J Homeopathic Med* 23(2):109, 1988.
38. Despres L: Yoga and MS, *Yoga J* 135:94, 1997.
39. Dombovy ML: Rehabilitation concerns in degenerative movement disorders of the central nervous system. In Brandom RL, editor: *Physical medicine and rehabilitation,* Philadephia, 1996, WB Saunders.
40. Duke RF, Spreadbury TH: Closed manipulation leading to immediate recovery from cervical spine dislocation with paraplegia [letter], *Lancet* 2(8246):577, 1981.
41. Entyre BR, Abraham LD: H-reflex changes during static stretching and two variations of proprioceptive neuromuscular facilitation techniques, *Electroencephalogr Clin Neurophysiol* 63:174, 1986.
42. Exner G et al: Basic principles and effects of hippotherapy within the comprehensive treatment of paraplegic patients, *Rehabilitation* 33(1):39, 1994.
42a. Ferris SH et al: Combination choline/piracetam treatment of senile dementia, *Psychopharmacol Bull* 18:84, 1982
43. Fitz-Ritson D: Phasic exercises for cervical rehabilitation after "whiplash" trauma, *J Manipulative Physiol Ther* 18(1):21, 1995.

44. Fushitani S et al: [Studies on attenuation of post-ischemic brain injury by kampo medicines-inhibitory effects of free radical production. I.], *Yakugaku Zasshi* 114(6):388, 1994.

45. Garrison SJ, Rolak LA: Rehabilitation of the stroke patient. In DeLisa JA, Gans BM, editors: *Rehabilitation medicine: principles and practice,* ed 2, Philadelphia, 1993, JB Lippincott, pp. 801-824.

46. Goldberg J et al: The effect of therapeutic massage on H-reflex amplitude in persons with a spinal cord injury, *Phys Ther* 74(8):728, 1994.

47. Goldszmidt M et al: Complementary health care services: a survey of general practitioners' views, *Can Med Assoc J* 153(1):29, 1995.

48. Gorman RF: Vertebral artery occlusion following manipulation of the neck [letter], *NZ Med J* 90(640):76, 1979.

49. Grant G, Cadossi R, Steinberg G: Protection against focal cerebral ischemia following exposure to a pulsed electromagnetic field, *Bioelectromagnetics* 15:205, 1994.

50. Greenman PE, McPartland JM: Cranial findings and iatrogenesis from craniosacral manipulation in patients with traumatic brain syndrome, *J Am Osteopath Assoc* 95(3):182, 191, 1995.

51. Gutteridge JM: Ageing and free radicals, *Med Lab Sci* 49(4):313, 1992.

52. Hafner RJ: Psychological treatment of essential hypertension: a controlled comparison of meditation and meditation plus biofeedback, *Biofeedback Self Regulation* 7:305, 1982.

53. Hamann KF: Physikalische Therapie des vestibulären Schwindels in Verbindung mit Ginkgo-biloba-Extrakt, *Therapiewoche* 35:4586, 1985.

54. Hartmann A, Frick M: Wirkung eines Ginkgo-Spezialextraktes auf psychometrische Parameter bei Patienten mit vaskulär bedingter Demenz, *Munchener Medizinische Wochenschrift* 133(suppl 1):S23, 1991.

55. Heath PD, Nightingale S: Clusters of tonic spasms as an initial manifestation of multiple sclerosis, *Ann Neurol* 12:494, 1986.

56. Hofferberth B: Einfluß von Ginkgo biloba-Extrakt auf neurophysiologische und psychometrische Meßergebnisse bei Patienten mit hirnorganischem Psychosyndrom, *Arzneimittel-Forschung* 39(8):918, 1989.

57. Hogg PK: The effects of acupressure on the psychological and physiological rehabilitation of the stroke patient, *Dissertation Abstracts Int* 47(2-B):841, 1986.

58. Holroyd J, Hill A: Pushing the limits of recovery: hypnotherapy with a stroke patient, *Int J Clin Experiment Hypnosis* 37(2):120, 1989.

58a. Hu HH et al: A randomized controlled trial on the treatment for acute partial ischemic stroke with acupuncture, *Neuroepidemiology* 12:106, 1993.

59. Huang M: Effect of emitted qi combined with self-practice of qigong in treating paralysis. (Abstract), *First World Conference for Academic Exchange of Medical Qigong,* Beijing, China, 1988.

60. Hurn PD et al: Deferoxamine reduces early metabolic failure associated with severe cerebral ischemic acidosis in dogs, *Stroke* 26(4):688, 1995.

61. Jain KK: Effect of hyperbaric oxygenation on spasticity in stroke patients, *J Hyperbaric Med* 4(2):55, 1989.

62. Jamrozik E et al: The role of lifestyle factors in the etiology of stroke. A population-based case-control study in Perth, Western Australia, *Stroke* 25(1):51, 1994.

63. Jankovic J: Theories on the etiology and pathogenesis of Parkinson's disease, *Neurology* 43(suppl 1):29, 1993.

64. Jensen OK, Nielsen FF, Vosmar L: An open study comparing manual therapy with the use of cold packs in the treatment of post-traumatic headache, *Cephalalgia* 10(5):241, 1990.

65. Johansson K, et al: Can sensory stimulation improve the functional outcome in stroke patients? *Neurology* 43:2189, 1993.

66. Joynt RJ, Green D: Tonic seizures as a manifestation of multiple sclerosis, *Arch Neurol* 6:293, 1962.

67. Keli SO, Feskens EJM, Kromhout D: Fish consumption and risk of stoke: the Zutphen study, *Stroke* 25(2):328, 1994.

68. Keli SO, et al: Dietary flavonoids, antioxidant vitamins, and incidence of stroke: the Zutphen study, *Arch Intern Med* 156:637, 1996.

69. Key TJ et al: Dietary habits and mortality in 11,000 vegetarians and health conscious people: results of a 17 year follow up, *Br Med J* 313(7060):775, 1996.

70. Kleijnen J, Knipschild P: Ginkgo biloba, *Lancet* 340:1136, 1992.
71. Kleijnen J, Knipschild P: Ginkgo biloba for cerebral insufficiency, *Br J Clin Pharmacol* 34:352, 1992.
72. Kleijnen J, Knipschild P, ter Riet G: Clinical trials of homeopathy, *Br Med J* 302:316, 1991.
73. Kraft GH, Fitts SS, Hammond MC: Techniques to improve function of the arm and hand in chronic hemiplegia, *Arch Phys Med Rehabil* 73:220, 1992.
74. Kunz K, Kunz B: The paralysis report, *J Reflexol Res Rep* 8:1,1987.
75. LaValley JW, Verhoef MJ: Integrating complementary medicine and health care services into practice, *Can Med Assoc J* 153(1):45, 1995.
76. Le Bars PL et al: A placebo-controlled, double-blind, randomized trial of an extract of Gingko biloba for dementia, *JAMA* 278(16):1327, 1997.
77. Lerner AB, Case JD: Melatonin, *Federation Proceedings* 19(2):590, 1960.
78. Li S: A new method of acupuncture in treatment of Parkinson's syndrome, *Int J Clin Acupunct* 6(2):193, 1995.
79. Li S-J, et al: Music and medicine in China: The effects of music electro-acupuncture on cerebral hemiplegia. In Maranto CD, editor: *Applications of Music in Medicine*, Washington, DC, 1991, National Association for Music Therapy, Inc, pp. 191-199.
80. Linde K et al: Are the clinical effects of homeopathy placebo effects? A meta-analysis of placebo-controlled trials, *Lancet* 350(9081):834, 1997.
81. Lucas D, Stratis DJ, Deniz S: From the clinic: hypnosis in conjunction with corrective therapy in a quadriplegic patient: a case report, *Am Corrective Ther J* 35(5):116, 1981.
82. Magnusson M, Johansson K, Johansson BB: Sensory stimulation promotes normalization of postural control after stroke, *Stroke* 25(6):1176, 1994.
83. Maier-Hauff K: LI 1370 nach zerebraler Aneurysma-Operation, *Munchener Medizinishe Wochenschrift* 133(suppl 1):S34, 1991.
84. Manganiello AJ: Hypnotherapy in the rehabilitation of a stroke victim: a case study, *Am J Clin Hypnosis* 29(1):64, 1986.
85. Martiensen J, Nilsson N: Cerebrovascular accidents following upper cervical manipulation: the importance of age, gender and technique, *Am J Chiropractic Med* 2(4):160, 1989.
86. Matchar DB, et al: The stroke prevention patient outcomes research team: goals and methods, *Stroke* 24(12):2135, 1993.
87. Matthews WB: Tonic seizures in disseminated sclerosis, *Brain* 81:193, 1958.
88. McDonagh EW, Rudolph CJ, Cheraskin E: An oculocerebrovasculometric analysis of the improvement in arterial stenosis following EDTA chelation therapy. In Cranton EM, editor: *A textbook on EDTA chelation therapy*, New York, 1989, Human Sciences Press, pp. 155-166.
89. McGee CT, Chow EPY: *Miracle healing from China...qigong*, Coeur d'Alene, ID, 1994, MediPress.
90. McGregor M, Haldeman S, Kohlbeck FJ: Vertibrobasilar compromise associated with cervical manipulation, *Top Clin Chiropractics* 2(3):63, 1995.
91. Meyer B: A multicenter randomized double-blind study of Ginkgo biloba extract versus placebo in the treatment of tinnitus. In Fünfgeld EW, editor: *Rökan, Ginkgo biloba: recent results in pharmacology and clinic*, Berlin, 1988, Springer-Verlag, pp. 245-250.
92. Miller AE: Clinical features. In Cook SD, editor: *Handbook of multiple sclerosis*, New York, 1990, Marcel Dekker, pp. 169-186.
93. Miller E: Deanol in the treatment of levodopa-induced dyskinesias, *Neurology* 24:116, 1974.
94. Miller RE: An investigation into the management of the spasticity experienced by some patients with multiple sclerosis using acupuncture based on traditional Chinese medicine, *Complement Ther Med* 4:58, 1996.
95. Mink RB, Dutka AJ: Hyperbaric oxygen after global cerebral ischemia in rabbits does not promote brain lipid peroxidation, *Crit Care Med* 23(8):1398, 1995.
96. Mouren X, Caillard P, Schwartz F: Study of the anti-ischemic action of Egb 761 in the treatment of peripheral arterial occlusive disease by TcPo2 determination, *Angiology* 45:13, 1994.
97. Muller JE, et al: Circadian variation in the frequency of onset of acute myocardial infarction, *N Engl J Med* 313(21):1315, 1985.

98. Muller-Wieland D, et al: Melatonin inhibits LDL receptor activity and cholesterol synthesis in freshly isolated mononuclear leukocytes, *Biochem Biophys Res Comm* 203(1):416, 1994.

99. Naeser MA, et al: Real versus sham acupuncture in the treatment of paralysis in acute stroke patients: a CT scan lesion site study, *J Neurol Rehabil* 6:163, 1992.

100. Naeser MA et al: Laser acupuncture in the treatment of paralysis in stroke patients: a CT scan lesion site study, *Am J Acupuncture* 23(1):13, 1995.

101. Naeser MA et al: Acupuncture in the treatment of hand paresis in chronic and acute stroke patients - improvement observed in all cases, *Clin Rehabil* 8:127, 1994.

102. Ness AR, Powles JW: Fruit and vegetables, and cardiovascular disease: a review, *Int J Epidemiol* 26(1):1, 1997.

103. Ness AR, Powles JW, Khaw KT: Vitamin C and cardiovascular disease: a systematic review, *J Cardiovasc Risk* 3(6):513, 1996.

104. Neubauer RA, End E: Hyperbaric oxygenation as an adjunct therapy in strokes due to thrombosis: a review of 122 patients, *Stroke* 11(3):297, 1980.

105. Neubauer RA, Gottlieb SF, Pevsner H: Hyperbaric oxygen for treatment of closed head injury, *South Med J* 87(9):933, 1994.

106. Nighoghossian N et al: Hyperbaric oxygen in the treatment of acute ischemic stroke, *Stroke* 26(8):1369, 1995.

107. Oberpichler H, et al: PAF antagonist ginkgolide B reduces postischemic neuronal damage in rat brain hippocampus, *J Cerebral Blood Flow Metab* 10(1):133, 1990.

108. Olszewer E, Carter JP: EDTA chelation therapy in chronic degenerative disease, *Med Hypotheses* 27(1):41, 1988.

109. Orencia AJ et al: Fish consumption and stroke in men: 30-year findings of the Chicago Western Electric Study, *Stroke* 27(2):204, 1996.

110. Osterman PO, Westerberg CE: Paroxysmal dysarthria and other transient neurological disturbances in disseminated sclerosis, *J Neurol Neurosurg Psychiatry* 29:323, 1966.

111. Palmer C, Roberts RL, Bero C: Deferoxamine posttreatment reduces ischemic brain injury in neonatal rats, *Stroke* 25(5):1039, 1994.

112. Panjwani U et al: Effect of sahaja yoga practice on seizure control and EEG changes in patients of epilepsy, *Indian J Med Res* 103:165, 1996.

113. Peyser JM et al: Guidelines for neuropsychological research in multiple sclerosis, *Arch Neurol* 47(1):94, 1990.

114. Politis MJ, Korchinski MA: Beneficial effects of acupuncture treatment following experimental spinal cord injury: a behavioral morphological and biochemical study, *Acupuncture Electro-Therapeutics Res* 15(1):37, 1990.

115. Rai GS, Shovlin C, Wesnes KA: A double-blind, placebo controlled study of Ginkgo biloba extract ('Tanakan') in elderly outpatients with mild to moderate memory impairment, *Curr Med Res Opin* 12:350, 1991.

116. Rampes H: Treatment of trigeminal neuralgia with electro-acupuncture in a case of multiple sclerosis, *Acupuncture Med* 12(1):45, 1994.

117. Reisberg B et al: Piracetam in the treatment of cognitive impairment in the elderly, *Drug Devel Res* 2:475, 1982.

118. Reiter RJ et al: A review of the evidence supporting melatonin's role as an antioxidant, *J Pineal Res* 18(1):1, 1995.

119. Rockswold GL, Ford SE: Preliminary results of a prospective randomized trial for treatment of severely brain-injured patients with hyperbaric oxygen, *Minnesota Med* 68:533, 1985.

120. Rockswold GL et al: Results of a prospective randomized trial for treatment of severely brain-injured patients with hyperbaric oxygen, *J Neurosurg* 76:929, 1992.

121. Rowland LP: *Merritt's textbook of neurology*, ed 9, Baltimore, 1995, Williams & Wilkins.

121a. Sallstrom S: Acupuncture in the treatment of stroke patients in the subacute stage: a randomized, controlled study, *Complement Ther Med* 4:193, 1996.

122. Salzberg CA et al: The effects of non-thermal pulsed electromagnetic energy (Diapulse) on wound healing of pressure ulcers in spinal cord-injured patients: A randomized, double-blind study, *Wounds: A Compendium of Clinical Research and Practice* 7(1):11, 1995.

123. Sandyk R: MIF induced augmentation of melatonin function: possible relevance to mechanisms of action of MIF-1 in movement disorders, *Int J Neurosci* 52(1-2):79, 1990.

124. Sandyk R: Multiple sclerosis: the role of puberty and the pineal gland in its pathogenesis, *Int J Neurosci* 68(3-4):209, 1993.

125. Sandyk R, Awerbuch GI: Nocturnal plasma melatonin and alpha-melanocyte stimulating hormone levels during exacerbation of multiple sclerosis, *Int J Neurosci* 67(1-2):173, 1992.

126. Santambrogio S et al: Is there a real treatment for stroke? Clinical and statistical comparison of different treatments in 300 patients, *Stroke* 9(2):130, 1978.

127. Savage RH, Roe PF: A double blind trial to assess the benefit of Arnica montana in acute stroke illness, *Br Homeopathic J* 66:207, 1977.

128. Savage RH, Roe PF: A further double blind trial to assess the benefit of Arnica montana in acute stroke illness, *Br Homeopathic J* 67:210, 1978.

129. Scheinberg L, Smith CR: Rehabilitation of patients with multiple sclerosis, *Neurol Clin* 5(4):585, 1987.

130. Schneider RH, Alexander CN, Wallace RK: In search of an optimal behavioral treatment for hypertension: a review and focus on transcendental meditation. In Gentry WD, Julius S, editors: *Personality, elevated blood pressure, and essential hypertension*, Washington, DC, 1992, Hemisphere.

131. Sessler GJ: *Stroke: how to prevent it/how to survive it*, Englewood Cliffs, NJ, 1981, Prentice-Hall.

132. Sherr J: A case of hemiplegia, *Homeopathy Links* 7(1):27, 1994.

133. Shi Z et al: The efficacy of electro-acupuncture on 98 cases of epilepsy, *J Tradit Chin Med* 7(1):21, 1987.

134. Shiflett SC et al: Complementary and alternative medicine. In DeLisa JA, Gans BM, editors: *Rehabilitation medicine: principles and practice*, ed 3, Philadelphia, 1998, JB Lippincott.

134a. Smith RC et al: Pharmacologic treatment of Alzheimer's-type dementia: new approaches, *Psychopharmacol Bull* 20:542, 1984.

135. Staas WE et al: Rehabilitation of the spinal cord-injured patient. In DeLisa JA, Gans BM, Editors: *Rehabilitation medicine: principles and practice*, ed 2, Philadelphia, 1993, JB Lippincott, pp. 886-915.

136. Stallibrass C: An evaluation of the Alexander technique for the management of disability in Parkinson's disease—a preliminary study, *Clin Rehabil* 11:8, 1997.

137. Stein DG, Hoffman SW: Chronic administration of Ginkgo biloba extract (EGb 761) can enhance recovery from traumatic brain injury. In Christen Y, Costentin J, Lacour M, editors: *Effects of Ginkgo biloba extract (EGb 761) on the central nervous system*, Paris, 1992, Elsevier, pp. 95-103.

138. Steinberger A: Specific irritability of acupuncture points as an early symptom of multiple sclerosis, *Am J Chin Med* 14(3-4):175, 1986.

139. Sthalekar HA: Hypnosis for relief of chronic phantom pain in a paralysed limb: a case study, *Austral J Clin Hypnother Hypnosis* 14(2):75, 1993.

140. Stolc S: [Hypoxia-reoxygenation damage to the nervous system: Perspectives in pharmacotherapy], *Ceskoslovenska Fystologie* 44(1):8, 1995.

141. Sukoff MH, Ragatz RE: Hyperbaric oxygenation for the treatment of acute cerebral edema, *Neurosurgery* 10(1):29, 1982.

142. Swank RL, Dugan BB: *The multiple sclerosis diet book: a low-fat diet for the treatment of MS*, New York, 1987, Doubleday.

143. Swank RL, Dugan BB: Effect of low saturated fat diet in early and late case of multiple sclerosis, *Lancet* 336(8706):37, 1990.

144. Taillandier J et al: Ginkgo biloba extract in the treatment of cerebral disorders due to aging: longitudinal, multicenter, double-blind study versus placebo. In Fünfgeld EW, editor: *Rökan, Ginkgo biloba: recent results in pharmacology and clinic*, Berlin, 1988, Springer-Verlag, pp. 291-301.

145. Tanigawa MC: Comparison of the hold-relax procedure and passive mobilization on increasing muscle length, *Phys Ther* 52:725, 1972.

146. Tappan FM: *Healing massage techniques: holistic, classic, and emerging methods*, Norwalk, Conn, 1988, Appleton & Lange.

147. Taylor RS: Rehabilitation of persons with multiple sclerosis. In Brandom RL, editor: *Physical medicine and rehabilitation,* Philadelphia, 1996, WB Saunders.
148. Thaut MH et al: Effect of rhythmic auditory cueing on temporal stride parameters and EMG patterns in hemiplegic gait of stroke patients, *J Neurol Rehabil* 7:9, 1993.
149. Tripathi SN, Upadhyaya BN, Dwivedi LD: Management of hemiplegia with gum guggulu, *Rheumatism* 25(3):155, 1990.
150. Twomey JA, Espir MLE: Paroxysmal symptoms as the first manifestations of multiple sclerosis, *J Neurology, Neurosurg Psychiatry* 43:296, 1980.
151. Tyler VE: *The honest herbal,* ed 3, New York, 1993, Pharmaceutical Products Press.
152. Tyler VE: *Herbs of choice,* New York, 1994, Pharmaceutical Products Press.
153. Uchida S et al: Prolongation of life span of stroke-prone spontaneously hypertensive rats (SHRSP) ingesting persimmon tannin, *Chem Pharm Bull* 38(4):1049, 1990.
154. Umphred DA: *Neurological rehabilitation,* ed 2, St Louis, 1990, Mosby.
155. Upledger JE: *Your inner physician and you,* Berkeley, Calif, 1991, North Atlantic Books.
156. Upledger JE: Craniosacral therapy [letter], *Phys Ther* 75(4):328, 1995.
157. van Hove E: Prevention of thrombophlebitis in spinal injury patients, *Paraplegia* 16:332, 1978-1979.
158. Verhoef MJ, Sutherland LR: Alternative medicine and general practitioners: opinions and behaviour, *Can Fam Physician* 41:1005, 1995.
159. Vodovnik L, Karba R: Treatment of chronic wounds by means of electric and electromagnetic fields. Part 1. Literature review, *Med Biol Engineering Computing* 30(3):257, 1992.
160. Vorberg G: Ginkgo biloba extract (GBE): A long-term study of chronic cerebral insufficiency in geriatric patients, *Clin Trials J* 22(2):149, 1985.
161. Walker JE, et al: Dimethylaminoethanol in Huntington's chorea, *Lancet* 1(7818):1512, 1973.
162. Walker M: The healing powers of qigong (chi kung), *Towsend Letter for Doctors,* 1994.
163. Wallace RK, et al: Systolic blood pressure and long-term practice of the Transcendental Meditation and TM-Sidhi program: effects of TM on systolic blood pressure, *Psychosomatic Med* 45:41, 1983.
164. Walter A: An evaluation of meditation as a stress reduction technique for persons with spinal cord injury, *Dissertation Abstracts Int* 46(11):3251, 1986.
165. Wan S et al: Repeated experiments by using the emitted qi in treatment of spinal cord injury (Abstract), Second World Conference on Academic Exchange of Medical Qigong, San Clemente, Calif, 1994, China Healthways Institute.
166. Wang RY: Effect of proprioceptive neuromuscular facilitation on the gait of patients with hemiplegia of long and short duration, *Phys Ther* 74:1108, 1994.
167. Wang X: Combination of acupuncture, qigong and herbs in the treatment of Parkinsonism, *Int J Clin Acupuncture* 4(1):1, 1993.
168. Wang Z: Sequelae of cerebral birth injury in infants treated by acupressure, *J Tradit Chin Med* 8(1):19, 1988.
169. Watson NA: Acute brain stem stroke during neck manipulation, *Br Med J* 288:641, 1984.
170. Weiselfish S: An overview of Erb's Palsy with case history documenting treatment with manual and craniosacral therapy, *Phys Ther Forum* 9:12, 1990.
171. Wen HL: Acute central cervical spinal cord syndrome treated by acupuncture and electrical stimulation (AES), *Compar Med East West* 6(2):131, 1978.
172. Westcott EJ: Traditional exercise regimens for the hemiplegic patient, *Am J Phys Med* 46(1):1012, 1967.
173. Wirth DP: Complementary healing intervention and dermal wound reepithelialization: an overview, *Int J Psychosomatics* 42(1-4):48, 1995.
174. Witte S, Anadere I, Walitza E: Improvement of hemorheology with ginkgo biloba extract: decreasing a cardiovascular risk factor, *Fortschritte Der Medizin* 110:247, 1992.
175. Wolf SL et al: The effect of tai chi and computerized balance training on postural stability in older subjects, *Phys Ther* 77(4):371, 1997.
176. Wolfson LW, Whipple R, Derby C: Balance and strength training in older adults: intervention gain and t'ai chi maintenance, *J Am Geriatr Soc* 44:498, 1996.

177. Woo C-C: Post-traumatic myelopathy following flopping high jump: a pilot case of spinal manipulation, *J Manipulative Physiol Ther* 16(5):336, 1993.
178. Woo E et al: Homeopathic treatment of mild traumatic brain injury, *Grant Application Submitted to the Office of Alternative Medicine at the National Institutes of Health*, 1993.
179. Yang J: Treatment of status epilepticus with acupuncture, *J Tradit Chin Med* 10(2):101, 1990.
180. Yoffe E: Meditate away paralysis, *Natural Health* 50, 1995.
181. Zhao Z: Effect of foot reflexology on the hemiplegia by cerebral vascular thrombosis. In China Reflexology Association, *China Reflexology Symposium Report*, 1994.

SUGGESTED READINGS

Basmajian JV, Nyberg R, editors: *Rational manual therapies*, Baltimore, 1993, Williams & Wilkins.
Christen Y, Costentin J, Lacour M, editors: Effects of ginkgo biloba extract (Egb 761) on the cental nervous system, *IPSEN Institute International Symposium*, Montreaux, Switzerland, 1991, Elsevier.
DeLisa JA, Gans BM et al, editors: *Rehabilitation medicine: principles and practice*, ed 3, Philadelphia, 1998, Lippincott-Raven.
Pomeranz B, Stux G: *Scientific bases of acupuncture*, New York, 1989, Springer.
Funfgeld EW, editor: *Rokan, Ginko biloba: recent results in pharmacology and clinic*, Berlin, 1988, Springer Verlag.

CHAPTER 8

Complementary/Alternative Therapies in the Treatment of Psychiatric Illnesses

James A. Peightel, Thomas L. Hardie, and David A. Baron

This chapter examines the scientific support for several complementary/alternative medicine (CAM) treatment strategies in a selected group of psychiatric illnesses. Database materials and methods commonly available to practitioners and one specialty database for CAM have been used in this review. Our intent is to provide a literature review for the reader and an overview of potentially clinically significant complementary medical treatments in psychiatry. Some portions of the CAM literature are not yet included in electronic databases; therefore the review presented does not comprise an exhaustive treatise on the subject. It is hoped that the reader of this chapter will gain an initial insight into the breadth of CAM practices that many patients are seeking for their mental health concerns.

The chapter has several subsections. First is an overview of study selection method and findings obtained in current database material available to practitioners. Second, a brief overview is presented of the epidemiology and clinical characteristics of the disorders reviewed. Third, findings are summarized and areas of promise that would benefit from further study are discussed.

Psychiatry shares much with the alternative medical community. Both fields have treatments that are historically better studied using qualitative methods and single-case designs rather than double-blind crossover methods. For a number of years psychiatry rejected the scientific method as an ineffective method of exploration, believing that the detailed description and analysis of an individual case provided a more appropriate source of clinical data. Psychiatry has changed, and continues to change, from these early perceptions and now embraces controlled trials with statistical analysis. It has improved the taxonomy of psychopathology, focused on the outcome of treatments, and demanded strict scientific rigor. The psychiatric literature continues to support case reports and small pilot studies that spark theory formation. "Alternative medicine" faces many of the same challenges that psychiatry had to overcome. For alternative practitioners to champion their efforts in the mainstream of care, they must embrace scientific rigor, when possible, and openly challenge their own assertions.[7]

Psychiatry is an area of medicine in which there is significant overlap between CAM interventions and conventional psychiatric treatments. For example, use of relaxation techniques adapted from hypnosis, previously considered solely an alternative therapy, is an accepted treatment recommendation for stress reduction in both fields. Also shared with CAM are low levels of research support for the psychotherapies delivered as a standard of care. Thus reviewing CAM interventions in psychiatry provides definition challenges from the start. The psychiatric illnesses chosen are those having the greatest impact on society; the CAM treatments reviewed are those with the greatest number of published reports.

SCIENTIFIC EVALUATION

In this chapter the studies reviewed are considered to have met the standard of scientific merit if they satisfy the following conditions[135]:

- The disease or syndrome of interest should be clearly (operationally) defined.
- Studies should include controls consistent with the intention and design.
- Where possible, there should be placebo controls (or positive control should be used).
- There should be random sampling and random allocation.
- Where possible, blinding techniques should be used.
- Sample size should be adequate to control for both type 1 and type 2 errors and must be appropriate for the statistics presented.
- Studies, where possible, should be prospective and have crossover conditions.

(Other studies are reviewed based on their availability or in circumstances in which few studies meet the established standard.)

Psychiatric Illnesses Deemed Worthy of Interest

The chapter is limited to disorders of major clinical importance. The importance of a psychiatric disorder is derived from the following characteristics: significant prevalence (number of people affected), severity (impact on daily functioning), and cost (to the individual or society). Four psychiatric disorders (major depression, anxiety disorders, primary insomnia, and schizophrenia) and one psychiatric-related condition (stress) have been chosen. Each satisfies one or more of the three characteristics and is commonly seen in clinical practice. Depression and anxiety are common, disabling conditions that generate significant costs to society. Schizophrenia, with its lifelong course and negative impact on daily functioning, is one of the most expensive illnesses to treat, despite its low incidence. Stress is pervasive in today's society and is a common mood state. It is often confused with syndromal anxiety disorders. These disorders all demonstrate the severity and social cost for inclusion. Sleep disturbance is a common complaint in most health care settings and, when persistent (i.e., primary insomnia), its severity can be disabling and extremely costly to society as well.

Procedures Considered to Be CAM

The alternative medical literature reviewed include Ayurvedic, acupuncture, Qi Gong, chelation, chiropractic, craniosacral, nutritional, homeopathic, hypnosis, massage, naturopathic, herbal, prayer, and yogic therapies. Studies from other methods were evaluated if determined to be of potential impact.

Methodology for Identifying Research Studies of CAM Procedures

For practitioners to consider the use of CAM procedures or to respond to questions about the practices of alternative therapy providers, they are, first, faced with how to obtain reliable information about these treatments and their effectiveness. The normal routes of professional peer-reviewed journals, U.S. Food and Drug Administration (FDA) information, and referenced scientific publications provide, at best, limited information for those seeking to evaluate the CAM literature. The second most commonly available source of citations is the electronic database. The starting point chosen for this chapter was the National Medical Library's MEDLARS, the most accessible and comprehensive medical database.

A MEDLARS search (January 1993 to May 1997) was conducted to identify articles for review and to determine the volume of research available. Each alternative form of treatment was entered, along with the word "research" and the specific disorder (e.g., "Ayurveda" and "research" and "anxiety"). All identified abstracts were reviewed. The abstracts generated from this search were evaluated using inclusion-exclusion criteria. The inclusion-exclusion criteria were designed to remove articles not related to the diagnostic category (e.g., anxiety related to medical illness would not be counted) and those having total sample sizes less than 10. This method of searching resulted in 11 articles that satisfied these criteria, highlighting the difficulties encountered by nonalternative health care providers in obtaining and evaluating the scientific merit of CAM treatments.

Looking at the material from another perspective, a search on "depression" and "research" identified 3225 citations, but when "acupuncture" (the most prevalent of the alternative methods identified) was added, the result was 3 citations.

To provide a more informative review, the search was expanded back in time and Psychlit indices were also searched for relevant material. In addition, a DataStars Allied and Alternative Medicine (AMED) database covering CAM from 1985 to the present was searched.[93] These sources were further complemented by discussion with practitioners in CAM. The material presented represents the sum efforts of these searches.

DEPRESSION

Depression is a psychopathologic condition whose hallmark is a disturbance in mood. Being "depressed" can be a symptom of a transient mood state, a character trait, or a major mood disorder. As a transient mood state, depression presents as a time-limited, subjective sense of feeling "low" or "blue." These feelings are often associated with real or perceived loss. A depressed personality style is characterized as the person who always "sees the glass half empty" (i.e., is overly pessimistic, with a limited capacity to experience joy). Major depressive disorder (MDD), as defined by the *Diagnostic and Statistical Manual of Mental Disorders, Fourth Edition (DSM-IV)*, is one of the mood disorders and is operationally defined as the experiencing of at least five of the following symptoms or conditions:

- Feeling sad or "blue" most of the day, nearly every day for at least 2 weeks
- Losing interest in past pleasurable activities
- Experiencing changes in weight and sleep patterns
- Experiencing loss of energy
- Feeling worthless, hopeless, and helpless
- Having poor concentration
- Having thoughts of not wanting to go on living

Major depressive disorder is only one of the *DSM-IV* depressive disorders. The others are dysthymic disorder (DD, a condition similar to MDD but with less intense symptoms, no suicidal ideation, and a duration of at least 2 years) and depressive disorder not otherwise specified (which includes disorders with depressive symptoms that do not meet criteria for MDD). Also included in the mood disorders are the bipolar disorders (bipolar I and bipolar II disorders, cyclothymic disorder, and bipolar disorder not otherwise specified) and other mood disorders (mood disorder attributable to medical condition, substance-induced mood disorder, and mood disorder not otherwise specified). The reader unfamiliar with these conditions may consult the *DSM-IV* or a recent basic psychiatric textbook for additional information. Mood disorders may co-occur with other psychiatric disorders or with nonpsychiatric medical disorders, or they may occur as a side effect of medications or illegal drug use. Major depressive disorder may begin at any age; however, it most commonly presents in the mid-20s through the 40s. Symptoms tend to develop gradually over days to weeks and are often attributed to stressful life events. Although some patients suffer only a single episode that may remit without treatment, more than half of patients will have another depressive episode and may be at risk to develop bipolar disorder. The course of recurrent major depression is highly variable and is virtually impossible to predict. The more depressive episodes a patient has, the greater the likelihood of additional episodes and the greater the chance of a suicide attempt.

Prevalence and Economic Impact

The lifetime risk for experiencing a major depressive disorder is 7% to 12% for men and 20% to 25% for women; the increased incidence in women is not a function of more frequent help-seeking behavior.[121] Apart from gender differences, prevalence rates are unrelated to race, education level, income, or civil status. Recent data have demonstrated that the age at onset has decreased in many Western cultures. Post et al.[118] reported that psychosocial stressors may play little or no role in the onset of subsequent depressive episodes. A series of reports issued jointly by the Harvard School of Public Health and the World Health Organization entitled "The Global Burden of Disease and Injury Series" provided a comprehensive picture of recent (1996) and projected (2020) health in eight worldwide demographic regions.[66] The results included the following conclusions:

- In both developing and developed regions worldwide, depression is the leading cause of disease burden for women.
- In 1990, MDD was responsible for the fourth highest disease burden worldwide, and by 2020 it is expected to be second only to ischemic heart disease.
- Major depressive disorder was the No. 1 cause of disability in the world in 1990. In the United States, the estimated cost of depression annually is 43.7 billion dollars.

Etiology of Depressive Disorders

To date, no single etiologic agent has been identified as the cause of depression. Given the fact that there are a number of depressive disorders with varying clinical presentations, it is highly unlikely that a sole causative factor will be determined. Depression is a biopsychosocial phenomenon with a number of causative factors including biochemical, genetic, and psychologic. Medical illnesses, including stroke, thyroid disease, cancer, heart disease, and hepatitis, along with a long list of medications, have been associated with the development of depression. Theories of etiology are often developed after a reported successful treatment strategy is discovered. Given the current popularity of biologic intervention for the treatment of depression, it is of no surprise that genetic predisposition, monoamine synaptic transmission abnormalities, and psychologic trauma are viewed as the bases of these disorders in the United States. Cultural variations in etiologic theory are often based on basic religious or cultural tenets, such as yin and yang in the Asian culture and Pratyaksha-Gyan, Anuman, Yukti, and Sakhya in Indian Ayurveda.

Current conventional treatment strategies vary with the form of depression being treated. Diagnostic specificity is of utmost importance in determining appropriate treatment selection. Major depressive disorder is most commonly treated with a combination of pharmacotherapy and psychotherapy (talk therapy). For severe, treatment-refractory depression, electroconvulsive therapy (ECT) may be used. Dysthymic disorder (DD) is usually treated with psychotherapy. ECT is not indicated for DD, although antidepressant medication may be effective. Bipolar disorder is most commonly treated in the United States with a mood stabilizer such as lithium, valproic acid, or carbamazepine. Treatment for depression resulting from a medical disease is by treating the underlying medical condition. For a review of current conventional treatments, the reader may refer to a standard psychiatric textbook (see Suggested Readings).

Review of CAM Treatment Strategies

The following literature review is not intended to be an endorsement or an indictment of CAM treatments for depression. The standard used to evaluate the published studies reviewed is from a Western cultural perspective. Study designs that are flawed from this perspective do not necessarily invalidate the technique or procedure, but they do not confirm claims of efficacy. With a placebo response rate as high as 50% in persons with depression, open-label trials, no matter how large, are at best suspect and difficult to generalize to a patient population.

In a number of areas alternative and conventional treatment strategies overlap. Establishing and maintaining a healthful lifestyle and reducing psychologic stress are viewed as important adjuncts to treatment in both schools of thought.

Orthomolecular Therapy

Orthomolecular psychiatric therapy as defined by Linus Pauling[115,116] is the treatment of mental disease by providing the optimal molecular environment for the brain, especially the optimal concentrations of substances normally present in the human body. Pauling asserted that mental disease results from low concentrations in the brain of any one of the following vitamins: thiamine (B_1), nicotinic acid (B_3), pyridoxine (B_6), cyanocobalamin (B_{12}), biotin (H), ascorbic acid (C), and folic acid. In addition to vitamin deficiency, deficient molecular concentrations of essential fatty acids may also cause psychiatric symptoms.

Bell et al. [11] studied 16 nonalcoholic inpatient volunteers who met *Diagnostic and Statistical Manual of Mental Disorders, Third Edition, Revised (DSM-IIIR)* criteria for major depression (N = 14) or bipolar disorder (N = 2) to evaluate the effect of vitamins B_1, B_2, and B_6 augmentation of tricyclic antidepressant treatment in geriatric depression with cognitive dysfunction. The results, although statistically nonsignificant, did suggest a trend in improvement in affective and cognitive symptoms in the active treatment group compared with those receiving placebo. The proposed theory for the mechanism of action is that vitamin B augmentation stimulates synthesis of neurotransmitters[15] and that B complex vitamins act synergistically with tricyclics to produce enhanced clinical improvement.[31,60] The data presented in this small pilot study warrant additional, larger-scale trials to determine potential efficacy in this (geriatric) and other depressed patient populations.

Based on Pauling's hypotheses that mental disease is caused by abnormal reaction rates, as determined by genetic makeup and diet and by abnormal molecular concentrations or imbalances of essential substances, 5-hydroxytryptophan (5-HT), an endogenous serotonin precursor, has been studied to assess its potential antidepressant properties. Byerley et al.[19] published an extensive review of the antidepressant efficacy and adverse effects of 5-HT. In addition to providing an overview of serotonergic brain mechanisms, the study reviewed seven open-label studies of 5-HT in the treatment of depression.* Sano[132] studied 107 patients with endogenous depression and reported that 74 (6%) were either cured or showed dramatic improvement. Fujiwara and Otsuki,[53] following a similar design, reported marked improvement in 4 and improvement in 6 of 20 endogenously depressed patients. Matussek et al.[104] found that 7 of 24 depressed study subjects were either symptom free or had a "good improvement" with 5-HT supplementation. Similarly, Takahashi et al.[145] reported that 7 of 24 moderately to severely depressed inpatients had a "clear-cut" recovery when treated with 5-HT. Nakajima et al.[110] reported a favorable response in 40 of 59 (67.8%) depressed patients, while Kaneko et al.[76] reported improvement in 10 of 18 patients with endogenous depression. In all, 148 of 251 (59%) patients given treatment with 5-HT were reported as improved. All of these trials were open-label trials, lacked diagnostic rigor in identifying their study populations, and were limited by a study period of only 3 to 4 weeks. In addition to the open-label trials, five double-blind, controlled studies were reported.[3,98,106,151,153] The results of the double-blind trials revealed an initial efficacy but a reduction of effectiveness over time, possibly reflecting a placebo effect. Lopez-Ibor and Almo[98] indicated that 5-HT may potentiate the effectiveness of monoamine oxidase inhibitors (MAOIs). The study of Mendlewicz and Youdin[106] was the only one that did not demonstrate 5-HT to be more effective than placebo. The conclusion of Byerley et al.[19] after reviewing all of the studies was that 5-HT has antidepressant properties; however, double-blind, placebo-controlled investigations with large sample sizes of well-defined patients are clearly indicated to definitively assess effectiveness. Final conclusions should be reserved until data from the larger, better-controlled trials are analyzed.

Rosenbaum et al.[127] conducted an open-label pilot study of oral s-adenosyl-L-methionine (SAM) in the treatment of major depression.[127] SAM is made from L-methionine and adenosine triphosphate by methionine-adenosyl-transferase.[21,59] Reynolds and Stramentinoli[122] demonstrated that SAM is directly involved in the metabolism of folate. This compound is widely marketed in Europe for the treatment of osteoarthritis and a number of hepatic conditions.[101,107] It is also reported to have potent antiinflammatory properties, with fewer side effects than ibuprofen.[101] Fazio et al.[45] tested the efficacy of SAM in treating schizophrenia and noted an improvement in

---

*References 19, 53, 76, 104, 110,132, 145, 152.

mood only. In a follow-up open trial with depressed patients, they reported remission in 14 of 35 patients. In a series of clinical trials by independent investigators Angoli et al.[2] and Lipinski et al.[96] using intravenous (IV) SAM in single-blind studies, the compound was reported to be an effective antidepressant with a more rapid onset of action and far fewer side effects than tricyclic antidepressants. Rosenbaum[127] reviewed six double-blind, placebo-controlled studies that demonstrated increased effectiveness when compared with placebo. Consistent study design flaws were a lack of diagnostic homogeneity, varying degrees of symptom severity in the study population, and small sample size. Carney et al. [22] reported that 3 of 12 (25%) positive responders to IV SAM had a "switch state" to mania or hypomania. SAM does appear to have putative antidepressant effects. Its possible mechanism of action is unknown but may be related to an increase in serotonin turnover,[2] inhibition of norepinephrine reuptake, or increase in folate activity. Despite the promising preliminary results and the call for additional large-scale efficacy trials, the authors were unable to identify any recent research with this compound. Additional studies exploring its effectiveness as a sole antidepressant and a potential adjunctive agent are indicated.

Alpha-methyltryptophan (AMPT), a precursor of alpha-methylserotonin (AM5HT), is a synthetic analog of the endogenous amino acid tryptophan.[124] Sourkes[142] has described AM5HT as a "substitute neurotransmitter" that is metabolized slowly and is present in the system for long periods (no actual time was reported) after a single dose. In that 1991 concept report, Sourkes proposed that AMTP may be effective in treating depression and sleep disorders. No clinical trial data were presented.

Zimilacher et al.[163] reported on the use of L-5-hydroxy-tryptophan alone and in combination with a peripheral decarboxylase inhibitor in the treatment of depression. In an open study of 25 depressed patients, therapeutic efficacy was found to be equal to that of traditional antidepressants, with a more rapid onset of action. It should be noted that this study suffers from serious methodologic flaws. In 18 of the 25 patients there were no fixed trial conditions, and clinical evaluations were determined from a retrospective analysis of case records.

Boman[14] published an excellent review of the use of L-tryptophan as an antidepressant and hypnotic. In addition to an adequate review of the metabolic activity of L-tryptophan, Boman provided an extensive review of the published clinical trials on its use for depression and sleep disorders. He pointed out the frequent flaws in methodology but was able to identify a large (N = 115), 12-week, double-blind, placebo-comparison study.[149] The findings were that L-tryptophan and amitriptyline were of equal antidepressant potency and that the combination of the two compounds was superior to either drug used alone. All active medication groups were significantly more effective than placebo. Although the research design was acceptable, the identification of depressed study subjects was poorly defined and the issue of diagnostic homogeneity was not addressed. Also, no mention was made of attempts to control for other clinical variables. Better-controlled trials are warranted, particularly in the use of L-tryptophan as an augmentation agent with an MAOI.

Botanic Therapies

Plant extracts have been used for centuries to treat a wide variety of illnesses. *Hypericum perforatum*, a member of the Hypericaceae family, commonly known as St. John's wort, is a botanical indicated for the treatment of anxiety, depression, and insomnia. This compound has been licensed in Germany since 1984 and is reported to be a popular remedy for mood symptoms. In an overview and meta-analysis of randomized clinical trials of St. John's wort for depression, Linde et al. [95] reported that the *Hypericum* extracts contain at least 10 active components that may contribute to its pharmacologic effects. They include flavonoids, naphthodianthrons, xanthones, and bioflavonoids. Holzl[70] claimed that the mechanism of action as an antidepressant is unclear; however, Bisset[12] reported that hypericin, one of the active constituents, is an experimental MAOI and claimed that an average daily dose of 2 to 4 g (equal to 0.2 to 1.0 mg of hypericin) may be effective in treating psychogenic disturbances, depressive states, anxiety, or nervous excitement. Wagner and Bladt[155a] challenged this assertion on the basis that it has not been confirmed in adequately controlled trials.

Linde et al.[95] in their meta-analysis searched Medline Silver Platter CD-ROM (1983 to 1994), Psychlit and PsychIndex (1987 to 1994), Medline (1966 to 1996), and Phytodok and Embase (1974 to 1996) with no language restrictions. They identified 23 randomized trials, which included 1757 outpatients with mild to moderately severe depression. Fifteen trials were placebo controlled, and eight compared *Hypericum* with another drug treatment. All of the trials, which were conducted outside the United States, were assessed by at least two reviewers. Had the search been restricted to English-language publications, no studies would have been identified. Their results were that *Hypericum* extracts were significantly superior to placebo and comparably effective to standard antidepressants. Their primary criticisms were the lack of well-defined groups of patients, varying of extract concentrations, and use of doses ranging from 300 to 1000 mg per day. Linde et al. also pointed out that unpublished trials and multiple publications from the same data set could have led to an artificially inflated number of subjects who participated in published trials. Concerning adverse side effects, their review found a low incidence of reported problems with tolerance. Phototoxicity was reported in animals taking high doses of *Hypericum*. No data were provided regarding long-term safety in humans.

Gelenberg[56] reviewed the literature on St. John's wort. In addition to clarifying that the word "wort" is Old English for "plant," Gelenberg reviewed Ernst's literature search on *Hypericum*.[42] He identified 14 studies comparing *Hypericum* with placebo and 4 comparing it with conventional antidepressant medications. The majority of the studies were conducted within the last few years, were written in German, and were published in journals unfamiliar to an international audience. He reported that eight of the trials were placebo controlled and met conventional methodologic standards. All eight studies concluded that St. John's wort produced minimal adverse side effects and was superior to placebo. Gelenberg concluded, "The fact that a product is natural does not mean that it is either safe or efficacious. By the same token, there is no reason why an herb or other plant product cannot have healing powers."

Hubner, Lande, and Podzuweit[74] conducted a randomized, placebo-controlled, double-blind trial on the effects of *Hypericum* treatment on mild depression with somatic symptoms. Thirty-nine patients were included in the study. Study subjects' symptoms were monitored using the Hamilton Depression (HAMD) scale, the von Zerssen Health Complaint Survey, the Clinical Global Impressions (CGI) scale, and questions on somatic symptoms. They reported that 70% of those treated with *Hypericum* were symptom free at 4 weeks of treatment and their HAMD scores were significantly improved ($p < 0.05$) when compared with placebo (Fig. 8-1).

These results support the effectiveness of *Hypericum* in mild depression. Additional studies are warranted to confirm these findings.

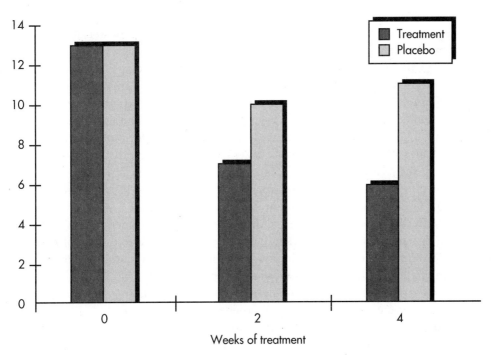

FIG. 8-1 Improvement after 4 weeks of *Hypericum* treatment as compared to placebo. (Modified from Hubner WD, Lande S, Podzuweit H, *J Geriatr Psychiatr Neurol* 7(suppl 1):S12, 1994.)

Woelk, Burkard, and Grunwald[159] conducted a drug-monitoring survey study of 663 private practitioners on the effectiveness of *Hypericum* extract LI 160 in 3250 patients. Their results suggested effectiveness and tolerability of the substance. The reductions of physical symptoms associated with mild and moderate depression (as measured by the Depression Scale of von Zerssen) are presented in Fig. 8-2. Adverse side effects were reported by 79 patients (2.4% of the sample), and 48 (1.5% of the sample) discontinued the treatment during the trial. The authors concluded that 30% of the study patients "normalized or improved" during *Hypericum* treatment. The large sample size of this study suggests safety. However, conclusions supporting effectiveness are questionable because of the lack of randomization of subjects and absence of placebo controls.

Medicine is an empiric science, and while some purported remedies have been found to be ineffective or even hazardous when subjected to systematic study, others have "stood the test of time and science."[56] Despite preliminary results warranting larger trials, because of an absence of data regarding long-term safety, efficacy, and product purity of non–FDA regulated nutritional supplements, he recommended against the use of St. John's wort for now. Interestingly, none of the other single or multicenter trials reviewed by Schmidt and Sommer,[137] Martinez et al.,[102] Witte et al.,[158] or Hansgen and Vesper[63] reported on the possible use of St. John's wort as an adjunctive agent with standard antidepressant treatments. Given the supplement's well-documented lack of side effects, this may be a reasonable area for future clinical trials. One methodologic problem that appeared in all the studies reviewed was the lack of diagnostic rigor used to identify a homogeneous depressed patient population. The operational definition of depression varies greatly in the studies; some used highly reliable measures and others appeared to allow for the inclusion of patients with other forms of psychopathology. To accurately compare results in depression treatment studies, it is important for the study design to control for patient variables such as age, sex, and most important, type of depression. The OAM, as well as the NIMH and several of its funded clinical centers, are now testing and comparing the effectiveness of St. John's wort in major depressive disorders using comparator groups receiving an anti-depressant drug and placebo.

Saki, [131] reporting on the use of herbal drugs to treat resistant depression, claimed that Saiko-ka-ryukotsu-borei-to, an Oriental compound, can be used in patients unable to tolerate conventional anxiolytics and antidepressants. He advocated the use of this agent in combination with low doses of standard medications. That study presented data on the biochemical properties of a number of herbal preparations. The author concluded that the efficacy of herbal medicines has not yet been demonstrated in double-blind, controlled studies and that the effective components are still unknown. He pointed out that the same plant might contain varying levels of bioactive components depending on the stage of plant growth, plant location, and environmental conditions in different years.

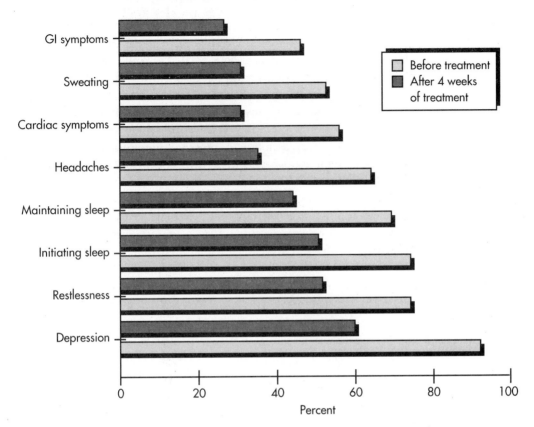

FIG. 8-2 Percentage of 3250 patients displaying symptoms before and after treatment with *Hypericum* extract. (Modified from Woelk H, Burkard G, Grunwald J, *J Geriatr Psychiatr Neurol* 7(suppl 1):S34, 1994.

Although weak with regard to clinical application, the previously cited study demonstrated that accurate analysis of herbal compounds is attainable and is an important first step in assessing the role of these compounds in treating depression.

Kampo, traditional Asian medicine, is a combination compound used to treat physical and psychiatric disorders. Saiko-ka-ryukotsu-borei-to is reported to be effective in treating anxiety and depression.[133] Tanra et al.[146] described a new compound, TJS-010, as having possible antidepressant or anxiolytic effects. This compound is composed of seven herbal ingredients. No human trials were cited; however, animal (rat) laboratory data were presented. The animal experiments were well controlled and demonstrated biologic activity. Before making assumptions about efficacy in humans, Phase I (clinical safety in normal control subjects), Phase II (effectiveness in identified patients), and Phase III (multicenter trials with large numbers of patients) clinical trials are needed.

Acupuncture

Acupuncture has been used for centuries to treat virtually all forms of pain and disease. Xiujuan[160] reported on 20 cases of "mental depression" treated at the Institute of Mental Health at Beijing Medical University by inserting needles into extrachannel points. Study subjects were compared with 21 control cases medicated with amitriptyline. Results, as measured by HAMD scale ratings, revealed no significant differences in therapeutic effects. A detailed description is provided on how and where the needles were applied. Study patients were described as manic depressive, involutional depressive, and depressive neurotic. How the diagnosis was made was not described, nor was the control (or lack of) of other clinical variables. Our literature search revealed two other published clinical trials, those of Romoli[125] and Chen,[27] confirming Xiujuan's results.

Kurland,[86] an associate professor of neurology at Northwestern University Medical School, published a series of three case reports utilizing acupuncture augmented by electrical stimulation of the needles (Acu-EST). He concluded that Acu-EST was less effective than ECT but did assist in reducing symptoms of depression without producing memory impairment. He asserts that "Acu-EST was a reasonable alternative to ECT." This statement cannot be supported by a case series of three but does warrant a well-controlled clinical trial.

Homeopathy

Reilly et al.[119] claimed homeopathic treatment may be used as primary therapy in combination with conventional interventions. Davidson et al.,[33] reporting on homeopathic treatment of depression and anxiety, described a case of a 47-year-old woman whose depressive and anxious symptoms improved on fluoxetine (Prozac) and calcarea carbonica (a homeopathic remedy). It is difficult to evaluate efficacy based on single case reports, and we were unable to identify any other controlled trials. Larger, well-controlled trials are warranted.

Ayurveda

Ayurveda is the medicine of the gods, according to Hindu mythology. This ancient Indian treatment has its roots in religion and metaphysics. Ayurvedic treatment of mental illness includes herbal preparations and various forms of psychotherapy. We were unable to identify any clinical trials using Ayurveda for the treatment of depression. Dube[40] has written on the nosology and therapy of mental illness in Ayurveda in descriptive terms. Obyesekere[113] and Dube et al.[41] have written comprehensive overviews of psychiatric training, therapies, and theory in the Ayurvedic tradition for the interested reader.

T'ai Chi Chuan

An ancient Chinese proverb, "Stagnant water is putrid," is interpreted to emphasize the importance of regular exercise in promoting good physical and mental health.[83] Specific forms of sitting, stretching, and squatting to promote health date back to 770 B.C. in China. T'ai chi chuan is traditional Chinese shadow boxing and is now commonly used to promote health. A review of the literature on exercise in the treatment of depression concluded that regular exercise reduces stress often associated with depression and the intensity of mood symptoms.[103,123]

Aromatherapy

Aromatherapy is the use of distinct fragrances to treat disease. Rovesti and Colombo[128] have divided several fragrances with proposed psychotropic effects into two categories, nerve sedative and nerve stimulant. Komori et al.[84] published an original report on the effects of citrus fragrance on immune function and depressive states. They studied 20 depressed male inpatients. All subjects met *DSM-IIIR* criteria for major depressive disorder.[4] Twenty age-matched normal controls also participated in the trial. In addition to monitoring depression ratings, extensive neuroimmunologic parameters were followed. This study had an open-label design. Results revealed that depressed patients improved with citrus fragrance and tricyclic antidepressant. Immunologic measures showed a dramatic improvement with citrus therapy. In addition, citrus fragrance made it possible to reduce the doses of antidepressants. However, the initial dose that was reduced with citrus fragrance was below the normal therapeutic range initially. No serum level determinations of tricyclic antidepressants were reported, making this reported finding difficult to interpret. Komori et al.[84] concluded that the use of citrus fragrance in treating depressed patients could be of psychoneuroimmunologic benefit. The data presented would appear to confirm their claim. However, as the authors accurately point out, caution must be exercised in interpreting the findings because of a small sample size, lack of blinding in the study design, and very low dosing with tricyclic antidepressants in the active control group. Stimulation of the olfactory system can trigger a wide range of emotional responses through paired association as well as trigger cravings in patients with a substance abuse disorder. Despite the lack of well-controlled data, exploration into the role of aromatherapy in treating depression is warranted.

Prayer

There are few outcome studies reviewing the effects of prayer in the treatment of mental illness. This is somewhat curious, as the therapeutic role of hopefulness is well known and prayer is intuitively correlated to hopefulness. Larson[87] has provided a comprehensive review of the effects of religiosity on several psychiatric conditions. His review of the psychiatric literature reveals 87% of the research reports that have examined religious involvement as a variable report a positive therapeutic effect, with the remaining 13% reporting a negative impact on mental health. Galanter et al.[54] surveyed 193 psychiatrists who were members of the Christian Medical and Dental Society.

Respondents rated the Bible and prayer as potential interventions for those with suicidal intent, grief reaction, sociopathy, and alcoholism. The results of the survey suggested that for prayer to be an effective therapeutic modality, the patient needed to have strong religious beliefs.[54]

Despite limited research in this area, it appears that religious conviction may improve mental health. Controlled trials of the therapeutic effect of prayer as a treatment modality are warranted. Caution should be taken to avoid overestimation of the positive effects of prayer independent of other components of living a religious life.

Advances in Neuroscience

Recent advances in neuroscience in general and, specifically, neuroimaging have for the first time provided a technology to observe changes in brain function in patients with depression. Computer-analyzed electroencephalogram (CEEG), single photon emission computed tomography (SPECT), and magnetic resonance imaging (MRI) are proving to be valuable tools in identifying the neuroanatomy and neurophysiology of depression.[57] In addition to providing a better understanding of the etiology of the mood disorders, this technology may assist in monitoring the impact of current treatments and provide valuable information needed to develop and refine new, therapeutic interventions. Any treatment that results in a sustained improvement in mood and behavior should be considered biologic. As George et al.[58] pointed out, "The outdated and false distinction between organic and functional psychiatric diseases (and treatments) may ultimately be abandoned." Similarly, as current CAM treatments demonstrate efficacy in large, well-designed clinical trials, their distinction from conventional treatment will become blurred. Many of the antidepressant therapies reviewed, although currently considered alternative, may, in fact, prove to be primary treatments or augmentation to existing mainstream interventions.

A common flaw in all of the studies reviewed was the relative lack of diagnostic rigor employed in the study design. Not identifying a homogeneous patient population when studying an illness with a variety of clinical presentations is problematic.

INSOMNIA

Insomnia, as described by the *DSM-IV*, is difficulty initiating or maintaining sleep or nonrestorative sleep that lasts at least 1 month. This lack of sleep results in clinically significant distress, which impairs social and/or occupational functioning.[5] Insomnia is one of the dyssomnias, a group of disorders characterized by difficulty in initiating or maintaining sleep or by excessive sleepiness. A hallmark of these disorders is a core disturbance in the quality, amount, or timing of sleep with a marked preoccupation with the inability to attain restful sleep. Chronic insomnia can have a marked negative impact on mood, motivation, attention, energy levels, and concentration.[5] Chronically disturbed sleep can also be a symptom of mood disorders (major depression or mania), anxiety disorders, substance abuse, or chronic pain. Occasionally, sleep problems may result from situational anxiety, excessive physiologic stimulation (caffeine, strenuous exercise just prior to bed, or the like), or environmental factors (noise, temperature, lack of comfort with the bed). Complaints of sleep disturbance increase with age and among women. This finding may be related to the decreased need for sleep and lack of exercise in elderly individuals and perimenopausal symptoms, such as hot flashes, which affect some middle-aged women. The actual prevalence of primary insomnia is unknown. However, population surveys conducted in the United States report a 1-year prevalence rate of complaints of insomnia to be 30% to 40% in adults.[5]

Secondary insomnia, sleep disorders that are the result of a known underlying cause, are treated by attending to the primary etiologic factor (i.e., treating the depressive or anxiety disorder or relieving physical pain). The sleep disorder associated with drug abuse, particularly of heroin and cocaine, will often last for months after stopping abuse. A recent National Institutes of Health (NIH) conference exploring the integration of behavioral and relaxation techniques in the treatment of chronic pain and insomnia concluded that behavioral interventions such as relaxation training and biofeedback may produce improvement in some aspects of sleep but questioned whether the magnitude of improvement in sleep onset and total sleep time was clinically significant.[112] The CAM literature is replete with reports on the treatment of insomnia.

Acupuncture

Acupuncture has been used for thousands of years by practitioners of traditional Chinese medicine (TCM) to treat insomnia. Yi[161] reported on 86 cases of insomnia treated by double-point needle insertion. The author reported "fairly satisfactory results in the treatment of insomnia" in all 86 cases. Clinical data were for the most part limited to a discussion of the needle insertion technique. Any large trial that reports an improvement in 100% of the study subjects must be viewed with some level of skepticism.

Changlxin,[26] reporting in a published lecture on acupuncture treatment of insomnia, offers a poetic and philosophic description of insomnia from the Chinese perspective. However, no data or clinical cases are reported. Cangliang[20] published a synopsis of 62 cases of insomnia treated by auricular point embedding therapy. This form of acupuncture uses the embedding of Compositus Semen Vaccariae (a traditional Chinese medicine) at specific auricular points. Of the 62 cases in the therapeutic group, 39 were rated as markedly improved, 30 as improved, 3 as with no effect. A few cases were listed as both markedly improved and improved. This study is virtually impossible to assess from a Western perspective. Patient classification was based on the following: (1) liver and kidney yin deficiency, (2) heart and spleen deficiency, (3) disturbance of the heart by phlegm-fire, and (4) yin deficiency leading to hyperactivity of fire. Although meaningful to the practitioner trained in these concepts, they might be uninterpretable to Western scientists. This study offered no references. Leye et al.[92] reported a large series of 124 cases of dyssomnia treated with acupuncture at Sishencong points. Results were as follows: 73 cases (59%) cured, 26 cases (21%) markedly improved, 10 cases (8%) improved, and 15 cases (12%) unimproved. Only one case was presented, and no references were listed. Nan and Qingming[111] compared auricular pressing therapy to a Western medicine control group. In the Western medicine control group, subjects were administered 10 mg diazepam orally before sleep for 30 days. Results were as follows: in the auricular pressing (AP) group 30 cases were cured, 35 cases improved, and 15 cases were considered ineffective, and in the Western (diazepam) group 11 cases were improved and 69 cases were designated ineffective. In the discussion the authors concluded the AP group was "better than the Western medicine group." However, they did report that diazepam was more effective initially, but lost effectiveness over time, while AP improved with time. The study sample included 80 cases of neurosis, 31 cases of neurasthenia, and 7 cases of cerebral trauma. This study offered no references and an inadequate description of methodology.

Yukang[162] published a "short paper" on the therapeutic effect of acupuncture in treating 50 cases of insomnia. Results were that all but two cases reported improvement. One case was presented as being representative of the entire sample. This report had no references, and content was very limited. All of the reviewed reports on the use of acupuncture followed the same pattern of no references, scant description of methodology, and remarkably high response rates. Montakab and Langel[108] in a review of acupuncture treatment of insomnia concluded that polysomnographic studies are needed to verify the effectiveness of acupuncture. To date, no such data are available.

Suanzaorentang

Chen and Hsieh[29] reported on the use of suanzaorentang, an ancient Chinese remedy, in the treatment of insomnia. Sixty patients with poorly defined sleep disorders were treated with 1 g suanzaorentang 30 minutes before bedtime for 2 weeks. A 1-week placebo washout preceded active treatment. Results reported were that during active treatment all sleep measures were significantly improved with no side effects observed. Having reported these remarkable, albeit unbelievable, results, the authors concluded that the compound merits further extensive investigation.

Cranial Electrostimulation

Cranial electrostimulation (CES) is a therapeutic technique that uses low-level electrical signals applied to the eyelids and mastoid process to induce calming and, ultimately, sleep. In 1953, Gilyarovski et al.[59] coined the term "electrosleep" and applied the technique for the treatment of insomnia. The procedure was used almost exclusively in eastern Europe until the first International Symposium for Electrosleep was held in 1966.[109] Despite numerous reports[10,30] of clinical effectiveness, inadequacies in research design have resulted in skepticism in the West.[148]

Klawansky et al.[80] conducted a meta-analysis of randomized, controlled trials of CES. They identified 18 randomized, controlled trials of CES versus sham treatment. They uncovered significant methodologic flaws in the study designs and a failure to report the data needed to conduct a meta-analysis in reviewed studies. Although improvement was noted in treating anxious mood, no definite data were available on efficacy for insomnia.

Four studies have examined electrosleep, resulting in differing conclusions. Frankel et al.[51] reviewed the effectiveness of electrosleep in treating chronic primary insomnia. This study identified many of the flaws in the clinical trials that reported efficacy and concluded that electrosleep is not an effective treatment for insomnia. Cartwright and Weiss[24] reported on a 2-year follow-up of 10 subjects with primary insomnia treated in a double-blind study of electrosleep. Results were a modest improvement in the active treatment group and no residual therapeutic effects in the sham control group. The authors concluded that clear-cut improvements resulting from active treatment with electrosleep remained in doubt. Levitt et al.[91] conducted a clinical trial of 13 subjects to assess the effectiveness of electrosleep. The design was double-blind and placebo controlled. The results were that electrosleep was no better than placebo in improving sleep. Nagata et al.,[109] reporting on electrosleep in normal adults, insomniacs, and hypertensive patients, concluded that the procedure produced significant improvement in sleep latency, soundness of sleep, and mood at morning awakening. Four prominent U.S. studies were cited (Feighner et al.,[46] Hearst et al.,[67] Rosenthal and Masserman,[126] and Weiss[156]), which all concluded that electrosleep improved sleep and anxiety. Despite the apparent controversy concerning effectiveness, no recent articles were identified in the literature.

Low-Energy Emission Therapy

Low-energy emission therapy (LEET) was developed as a treatment for chronic insomnia. This procedure consists of low-amplitude–modulated electromagnetic fields delivered by means of a mouthpiece in direct contact with the oral mucosa.[114] LEET was reported as safe, well tolerated, and effective in improving sleep in patients with chronic insomnia.[114] This was a large, well-designed study that clearly demonstrated a reduction of insomnia.

Reite et al.[120] demonstrated that LEET was effective in inducing sleep in healthy volunteers. This was a scientifically sound clinical trial. The literature reviewed suggests the clinical efficacy of LEET in the treatment of insomnia.

Valerian

Valerian is an ancient herbal remedy used to treat anxiety and insomnia. Lindahl and Lindwall[94] reported it to be safe and effective in treating insomnia in 21 of 27 study subjects. The authors pointed out that their results cannot be extrapolated to long-term use but believe long-term follow-up trials are indicated. This would appear to be indicated based on the positive pilot data presented.

Tryptophan

Tryptophan, the metabolic precursor of serotonin, is one of the eight essential amino acids. This compound has been reported to have therapeutic effectiveness in the treatment of insomnia.[14] In a comprehensive review of the literature, Schneider-Helmert and Spinweber[138] reported that L-tryptophan may be effective in alleviating disorders of initiating and maintaining sleep (DIMS) but concluded that, despite some sedative properties, the clinical utility, optimal dose, and mechanism of action remain to be determined. Demisch et al.[38] conducted the first reported double-blind, placebo crossover study. However, all of the study findings were based on subjective ratings only. The results did suggest a positive effect in selected patient groups. The authors concluded that successful treatment with L-tryptophan is possible only if patients are carefully selected.

Despite its reported safety, a batch of contaminated tryptophan from Japan was discovered in the United States. A number of serious adverse events were reported to the FDA, which resulted in its being banned from sale in America.

Melatonin

Melatonin is one of the most intensely advertised sleep aid "health" products sold in the United States. Melatonin's physiologic functions include regulation of sleep and synchronization of circadian rhythms, yet the significance of melatonin secretion in patients who complain of insomnia is unknown.[75] Butler[18] warned that no studies have determined the recommended dose, timing, duration of use, side effects, long-term effects, or interactions with other medications: "If melatonin does reset the body's clock, it may reset it wrong" to worsen insomnia.

SCHIZOPHRENIA AND PSYCHOTIC DISORDERS

The illness that we now call schizophrenia has been recognized in most cultures and described throughout much of recorded history. The process of diagnosis in the West has evolved from descriptive and theoretic to criteria based, as in the recently published *DSM-IV*.[5] Characteristic symptoms of schizophrenia involve severe disturbance in several areas including language and communication, content of thought, perception, affect, sense of self, volition, relationship to the outside world, and motor behavior. Disturbances in language and communication include looseness of association, derailment, circumstantiality, tangentiality, neologisms, and word salad. Disturbances of thought content are characterized by delusions or false fixed beliefs and ideas of reference. Disturbances of perception include auditory, visual, tactile, and olfactory hallucinations. Disturbances of affect may take a variety of qualities including lability and oddity, but most commonly there is a blunting or flattening of affect with little intensity or range. Disturbances in sense of self may include losing touch with who one is or an overwhelming perplexity, doubt, or confusion about the meaning of one's life and illness. Disturbances in volition involve a decrease in self-initiated and goal-directed activity and invariably affect work performance and functioning in other roles. Disturbance in relationship to the outside world is demonstrated by withdrawal from involvement with other people and attention directed inward toward self-absorbed, illogical ideas and fantasies. Disturbances in motor behavior ranges from markedly decreased reaction to the environment, as in catatonic stupor, to repetitive, ritualistic, or aggressive agitation.[61] The disorder of schizophrenia is conceptualized as a syndrome that is heterogeneous in its cause, presenting picture, course, response to treatment, and outcome. Nevertheless, the syndrome is assumed to be an illness rather than merely a socially unacceptable or odd and eccentric set of behaviors.[77] Subtypes of schizophrenia include paranoid, disorganized, catatonic, undifferentiated, and residual.

In terms of both personal and societal costs, schizophrenia is one of the most devastating illnesses. An estimated 0.5% to 1% of the population suffers from schizophrenia. The incidence and prevalence rates of any psychiatric disorder, however, are a function of diagnostic criteria, and not all methods or studies reviewed here have similar diagnostic definitions. Schizophrenia commonly strikes at an early age so, unlike patients with heart disease or cancer, schizophrenic patients usually live long after onset and continue to suffer from the typical stepwise deterioration of cognitive and emotional functioning.[150] Schizophrenia also creates an enormous financial burden on individuals, families, and society. Recent estimates of the direct and indirect costs of schizophrenia to society were between $10 and $20 billion with approximately two thirds of the costs being a consequence of the relative lack of productive employment. However, human suffering and the social and psychologic costs for patients and families cannot be measured monetarily.[77]

Currently there is no established scientific cure for schizophrenia, but treatments have been identified that affect symptoms and level of functioning in patients. Antipsychotic medications have been rigorously studied and are not reviewed here. Some treatment approaches complement psychopharmacology or address the living environment stressors that can exacerbate psychotic symptoms. For example, inpatient "milieu therapy" has a long history as a treatment plan component,[78] and family "expressed emotion" has been identified as a factor in the severity and course of schizophrenic symptoms.[43] CAM therapy studies will be reviewed by method where studies were identified in our search. It is, at times, difficult to define what is "alternative."

Other psychotic disorders mentioned in this section are schizoaffective disorder and mania. Schizoaffective disorder is essentially a diagnosis of both schizophrenia and an affective disorder, usually major depression or bipolar (manic depressive) disorder. Mania is characterized by a distinct period of abnormally or persistently elevated, expansive, or irritable mood for more than 1 week. Other symptoms common but not required for a diagnosis of mania include the following[5]:

- Inflated self-esteem or feelings of grandiosity
- Decreased need for sleep
- Rambling or pressured speech
- Racing thoughts
- Distractibility
- Increased risk-taking behavior
- Increased goal-directed behavior

Hypnosis

Hypnosis as a treatment method has historically been accepted as useful and safe for neurotic disorders and personality disorders since the early work done by Freud and his contemporaries. It is not generally considered an alternative or complementary treatment. However, hypnotherapy used with schizophrenic and psychotic patients has been doubted and debated for the past 100 years. The controversy surrounding the use of hypnosis with psychotic individuals centers around four main concerns. First, it was argued that psychotic patients were incapable of being hypnotized; second, it was feared that hypnosis might worsen psychotic symptoms; third, some authorities feared the patient might enter and prefer the fantasy of hypnotic imagery; and fourth, it was feared that hypnosis would induce excessive dependency in the psychotic individual.[134] A review of the literature revealed evidence for and against this hypothesis. Scagnelli-Jobsis[134] reviewed a variety of clinical studies and case reports that call into question all four tenets previously described. Baker[9] also identified potential benefits and focused on techniques that increase relaxation and improve ego strengths and self-image. Both authors emphasized that hypnotherapy is not a substitute for chemotherapy or other treatment modalities. However, heated debate continues among hypnotherapists, with Spiegel[143] calling into question the validity of Scagnelli-Jobsis'[134] hypothesis of lowered hypnotic responsivity in psychotic patients.[9,68,]

The nature of hypnosis makes it difficult to complete controlled, blinded studies. The therapeutic relationship, induction techniques, and interventions in hypnotherapy are highly dependent on the style of the practitioner. Psychotherapy research and many CAM therapies wrestle with similar problems.

Movement Therapy

Inpatient psychiatric units regularly use recreational, art, music, occupational, relaxation, dance, and movement therapies in the milieu treatment of schizophrenic and psychotic patients. To evaluate the effect of movement therapies the Volwiler Body Movement Analysis (VBMA) scale was developed. The scale provides a quantitative measure of 19 aspects of body movement, and data indicate that psychotic children were significantly different from control children in most categories of body movement.[155] This scale has been used by others in an attempt to confirm the effectiveness of movement and dance therapies, but rigorous controlled studies were not found in the literature.[6]

Acupuncture

Few clinical studies using acupuncture in psychotic disorders were found in our search. Keys[79] suggested that one reason is the diagnostic system differences between TCM and the Western approach.[5] Chronic pain, migraine, headache, anxiety, and other physical conditions may have an impact on the severity and course of psychotic disorders. For example, stress, physical pain, and irritability can exacerbate psychotic symptoms. Reducing these aggravating factors using acupuncture may improve the overall clinical picture.[32]

Shi and Tan[141] investigated the therapeutic effects of acupuncture treatment in 500 cases of schizophrenia. However, this study clearly exemplifies diagnostic criteria translation difficulties. According to TCM differentiations, the patients in the study were grouped by the following types: "Manic type" schizophrenics (181 cases) were afflicted with an excited state of mania based on the theory that the etiologic factor was "double yang." Depressive type schizophrenics (140 cases) were characterized by melancholy and tension and were thought to have "double yin." "Paranoid" type schizophrenics (179 cases) were exemplified by terror and worry and are thought to be related to the spleen. The specific subtype of schizophrenia directed the point locations of the acupuncture performed. The results cited were that 55% were cured, 16.8% had remarkable improvement, and 16.6% had no effect. These results appear impressive, but the broad range of the diagnosis of schizophrenia and the variety of different acupuncture interventions performed render these results questionable.[157]

Herbal and Chinese Medicine

There was little research identified on the use of botanic extracts, homeopathic agents, or traditional Chinese medicines in the treatment of psychotic disorders. However, the use of these methods may be more widespread then this paucity of studies implies. Despite rigorous efforts, articles were not identified in the literature.

Ma et al.[100] reported on 30 cases of chronic schizophrenics who received treatment with a variety of neuroleptic medications and were considered nonresponders. The study reported that seven immunologic functioning markers were measured and six of the seven were significantly different as compared with a control group. In an attempt to regulate proportion and function of immune cells, 30 patients were given the immunomodulating herb xin shen ling. The brief psychosis rating scale (BPRS) and the nurses' observation scale for inpatient evaluation (NOSIE) were used to assess changes in clinical symptoms before and after treatment. The results showed that BPRS and

NOSIE ratings before treatment were significantly higher than after treatment ($p < 0.05$). The clinical efficacy rate was 67%. The authors reported up to 3 years of follow-up in some cases with better than expected relapse rates. This study used standard rating tools, tested for result significance, and presented interesting possibilities, but lacked a control group and clear diagnostic and dosing details.

Ma and colleagues[100] (1995) reported on the use of acupuncture combined with a medicinal concoction of several herbs called Ding Jing Hong Pill, a secret recipe handed down from the author's father. He reported on 53 schizophrenic patients given treatment (21 males and 32 females ranging from 17 to 50 years of age). He reported that the length of treatment varied from 1 week to 30 days and claimed all were cured. The author provided few details of his treatment or research methodology. The results seem highly questionable.

Carod and Vazquez-Cabrera[23] presented a case report of a 34-year-old female schizophrenic patient who experienced significant reduction in presenting symptoms using herbal therapy in combination with neuroleptic medication and suggested a possible complementary nature of the treatment.

Dietary Therapy

A review of the literature found a number of studies suggesting that dietary control or supplementation may have a complementary role in the current treatment of psychosis. Aschheim[8] proposed dietary interventions derived from established animal studies. He proposed diets in which essential amino acid composition has been modified to produce a defined imbalance of dopamine and norepinephrine precursors. The author suggested that decreasing the amount of available dopamine complements the dopamine blockade by neuroleptic drugs and potentiates antipsychotic effects. This in turn might allow for lower neuroleptic doses and diminish drug-related side effects and tardive dyskinesia (TD) risk. However, the report is primarily hypothetical and suggests further animal and human studies.

Bruinvels and Pepplinkhuizen[16] studied a group of schizoaffective patients with episodic psychosis and speculated that a disturbance in serine metabolism may be related to their psychotic symptoms. This group of patients was characterized by the occurrence of generalized sensory perceptual distortions of light, sound, shapes, and distances, especially at the onset of the psychosis. It was postulated that in this group an increased demand for glycine, as in porphyria, may be the trigger for an increased production of 1-carbon units resulting in greater endogenous production of beta-carotenes and/or isoquinolines, which may act as "psychotic" substances.[17] After recovery of the patients, serine, glycine, or glucose was administered orally to find out whether an enhancement of serine conversion would reintroduce psychotic symptoms. The authors suggested their results imply that a subgroup of schizoaffective patients may suffer from a metabolic disturbance in the 1-carbon transfer system and reported evidence that psychotic symptoms may improve on a carbohydrate-rich, low-protein diet.[17,117] However, only 25 subjects were studied, and many other variables were not identified. Metabolic differences in psychotic patients merit further study.

Older studies looked at the use of L-tryptophan in mania. Van Praag et al.[151] studied five manic patients in a double-blind, placebo-controlled crossover study using chlorpromazine and L-tryptophan and found L-tryptophan slightly superior in all parameters studied. Chambers and Naylor[25] completed a similar study with 10 female patients and found L-tryptophan no better than placebo. These conflicting conclusions illustrate the limitations of small numbers even in well-designed and controlled studies and the need to replicate results.

Rubin[129] discussed the possible clinical and etiologic overlap of psychotic disorders and pellagra (characterized by the three Ds—dementia, diarrhea, and dermatitis—and caused by a niacin deficiency). He discussed a newly discovered trace-3 essential fatty acid that provides the substrate upon which niacin and other B vitamins act to form prostaglandins, and postulated a common deficit in both disorders. Rubin reported on symptom improvement in 12 psychiatric patients with a variety of diagnoses, including schizophrenia, that were treated with linseed oil, a substance rich in the identified fatty acid. The study raises some interesting metabolic questions about diet and illness, but a clear limitation of the study method is that patients remained on their standard regimen of antipsychotic or antianxiety medication.[71-73,130]

Vlissides et al.[154] completed a double-blind, controlled trial of gluten-free versus gluten-containing diet on an inpatient ward with 24 patients for 14 weeks using the Psychotic In-Patient profile (PIP). Most suffered from psychotic disorders, especially schizophrenia. There were beneficial changes in the study patients between pretrial and gluten-free periods in five dimensions of the PIP. This improvement continued during the gluten challenge period, but the authors attributed these changes to the increased attention the subjects received (Hawthorne effect). Two patients improved during the gluten-free period and relapsed when the gluten diet was reintroduced. The study concluded that the majority of psychotic patients are not affected by the elimination of gluten from the diet, but readily acknowledged the difficulties and limitations in the study design. Freed et al.[52] and Harper et al.[64] explored the interesting possibility that gluten impedes absorption of haloperidol. Diet-related absorption effects of medication are an area worthy of additional study.

Culture

Cultural and religious beliefs have been shown to have a significant effect on an individual's mental and physical health. There is a large and growing body of ethnographic research and literature devoted to studying this premise that is not reviewed here.[85] However, many medical and mental health practitioners increasingly view illness from a perspective that takes the patient's cultural or religious beliefs into account.[99]

Although not typically thought of as "alternative," to do this, we reviewed a few case examples of treatment interventions for psychotic disorders where the cultural context was crucial in bringing about clinical improvements.[50,65,85]

Farmer and Falkowski[44] described psychotic illness in a Nigerian woman born in London who grew up in a family and community highly influenced by traditional Nigerian culture. She developed a brief postpartum psychotic episode that partially responded to chlorpromazine but worsened over the next few weeks. The quality of her psychosis became dominated by "delusional" beliefs about her ancestors, feeling she had spells placed on her, and hearing voices of people she knew in Africa. She believed her illness was the result of "bewitchment"; that psychiatric medication could only calm, not cure her; and that "strong medicine men from home" were needed to deal with "ju-ju" and break the spell on her. Her continued disturbed behavior remained resistant to both neuroleptic medication and ECT. The case report stated that her husband was able to return with her to Nigeria for intervention by native healers and, soon after, a complete recovery occurred. A letter received from her husband 2 years later confirmed that she remained well.

STRESS

Stress is a common experience in the world around us. Its purpose is presumed to be rooted in our primary survival instincts.[34] It allows us to attend to potentially threatening situations and muster mental and physical resources to cope with them. Many researchers have examined the effects of long-term arousal on both the psychologic and physical systems of the body. A simple review of a commonly used stress reduction handbook or medical or nursing textbook will reveal references on hypnosis, dietary modification, exercise, components of yoga (breathing and stretching), relaxation, meditation, herbal and homeopathic remedies, and encouragement to lead a more spiritual life as potential treatments.[34,139] These practices might now be considered more mainstream than alternative. Stress is an inherently difficult area to study. Quantifying stress levels is problematic. If it is situational and thus changes with the passage of time, evaluating the effects of a treatment is difficult. Evaluating potent treatments that work quickly (like a drug) is much easier than evaluation of subtle interventions. Think of the effects of exercise for someone under stress at work. The full benefit of their exercise efforts may not be effective for weeks. Will the patient's work stress and coping remain constant? These questions are offered to illustrate the difficulty in evaluating these treatments. Failure to address these issues allows skeptics to reject treatments as ineffective and others to endorse natural remedies that are largely unproved. This is clearly the case in stress. Inconsistent operational definitions and measurement tools result in problematic analysis. The studies below suffer from some methodologic problems but point to areas for future research.

Yoga and Meditation

Dostalek[39] explored the effectiveness of yoga in disease prevention and the reduction of stress. The study included 40 yoga practitioners and 40 non–yoga practitioners, each group divided equally based on sex. Participants were measured using the PGI (Perceived Guilt Index) Attitude Scale, PGI Health Questionnaire N-2, State-Trait Anxiety Inventory, Presumptive Stressful Life Events Scale, and Jenkins Activity Survey. The findings indicated significant differences between male yoga and non–yoga practitioners in attitude toward yoga, neuroticism, state and trait anxiety, and stressful life events during the past year. Significant differences for females were found for attitude toward yoga, social desirability, and stressful life event scores during the past year. Yoga practitioners had significantly higher mean scores on yoga attitude and social desirability than did non–yoga practitioners.[39]

Schell et al.[136] examined the effects of hatha yoga exercise in 25 healthy women. The authors examined a number of physiologic and psychologic measures in a non-randomly assigned study comparing those experienced in yoga to a similar nonpracticing group. The endocrine measures proved to be nonsignificant between the groups with significant findings in pulse, life satisfaction, excitability, aggressiveness, emotionality, and somatic complaints. The authors suggested that yoga groups have improved coping. The study's nonrandom assignment and small sample size make it difficult to agree with the author's claims but do point to suggestive evidence for the impact of yoga on stress. These studies suggest that yoga has a positive effect on stress as measured. The studies suffer from methodologic flaws including nonrandom selection and assignment to treatment; these flaws limit the scientific credibility of their findings.

Qi Gong

Qi Gong training and meditation have been studied by Ryu et al.[130] to determine effects on stress hormone levels. Twenty subjects who were engaged in Qi training for at least 4 months were enrolled in the study. Blood was drawn before, during, and after training to examine beta-endorphin, adrenocorticotropic hormone (ACTH), and dehydroepiandrosterone sulfate (DHEA-S). The findings indicate significant ($p < 0.05$) increased levels of beta-endorphin at both midtraining and posttraining draws. There were no significant differences for ACTH and DHEA-S.

The study points to hormonal changes that are related to stress reduction. The sample suffers from lack of a control group within the design and random selection. The findings are suggestive and consistent with many of the studies relating to transcendental and other meditation, Buddhist meditation, and T'ai chi, all pointing to the stress-relieving benefits of these activities.[97] Most of these studies suffer from similar problems when looked at in aggregate.

Dance

Lest'e and Rust[90] examined the effects of dance on anxiety in a 2 × 2 design, the two factors being physical exercise and aesthetic appreciation. One hundred fourteen college students were divided into four conditions: dance class, sports class, music class, and mathematics. The subjects did not suffer from any psychopathologic conditions; stress or anxiety was measured using the State Trait Anxiety Inventory, and Likert self-reports assessed previous experience and level of interest. The results demonstrated significant decrease in anxiety for the students in the dance classes. This effect was more pronounced than for those in sports classes. The other classes showed no effect. The data indicated an effect beyond that of exercise in the reduction of state anxiety scores. The authors have provided appropriate cautions about the use of their findings and their lack of generalizablity.[47] The findings provide an interesting twist on the use of dance to expand stress reduction or anxiolytic qualities of general exercise. This area seems to warrant further study.

Herbal Treatments

A number of herbal treatments have been anecdotally recommended for the treatment of anxiety or stress, including kava, valerian, hops, gingko, peppermint, and chamomile. Many of these herbal compounds have been extensively studied from a biochemical perspective.[69] When reviewing the evidence for valerian root as an example for herbal treatments, the clinical trials were limited to two studies. Further searches failed to identify additional reports.[81,88] The extensive basic scientific work reflects the continuing search for effective herbal medicine treatments. Despite the broad use of these compounds by the public, there appears to be limited research to support or deny their efficacy in stress reduction. This is especially true when evaluating either duration of treatment effects or long-term safety.

Many of the areas reviewed in this section offer significant scientific support for their use as treatments. This is consistent with what is seen in clinical practice. CAM methods are common interventions in the treatment of stress in a primary care practice. Despite the strength of the work that has been reviewed, several general issues merit discussion. The definition of what defines stress or being stressed remains elusive. The lack of a discrete clinical entity weakens all the research in this area. Comparison of the effectiveness of treatment between studies cannot be made with objectivity. Studies could be improved by employing double-blind placebo studies where feasible.

ANXIETY

Pathologic anxiety is different from stress in its intensity and effects on functioning. *DSM-IV* anxiety disorders include panic disorder, specific and social phobias, obsessive compulsive disorders, posttraumatic stress disorders, acute stress disorders, generalized anxiety disorders, and anxieties related to other conditions and substance abuse.

The cost of anxiety disorders is unclear, but "more than 23 million Americans with anxiety disorders face much more than just normal stress."[1]

The lifetime prevalence of panic disorder (with or without agoraphobia) is between 1.5% and 3.5%. The 1-year prevalence rates are between 1% and 2%. Panic displays a bimodal distribution, with peaks in late adolescence and in the mid-30s. Close biologic family members of individuals with panic disorder have a four to seven times greater chance of suffering from this disorder.[5] Panic is an intense fear or discomfort in which four (or more) of the following symptoms have a rapid onset and crescendo in 10 minutes: palpitations, sweating, shaking, shortness of breath, choking, chest pain, nausea, feeling faint, derealization or depersonalization, fear of going crazy, fear of dying, tingling sensations, and chills or hot flushes in the absence of a disease causing these symptoms.

The estimated lifetime prevalence of obsessive compulsive disorder is 2.5%, and 1-year prevalence is 1.5% to 2.1%, making it a fairly rare disorder.[5] The disorder usually becomes evident first in adolescence or early adulthood, although it may begin in childhood. Age of onset is earlier in males than in females. Those with the disorder have waxing and waning courses, with flares that are related to stress.[5] Obsessive compulsive disorder presents either of the following symptoms: obsessions or compulsions. Obsessions are defined as recurrent and persistent thoughts, impulses, or images that are intrusive and inappropriate and result in distress. Thoughts are not simply worries. The patient attempts through either active or passive means to relieve the thoughts, and the person understands that the thoughts are from his or her mind. Compulsions are defined as repetitive behaviors or mental activities driven to reduce obsessions and distress. The obsessions or compulsions result in distress, are time-consuming, and interfere with daily functioning.

Reports that anxiety runs in families have been inconsistent for generalized anxiety disorder, with most failing to find a cluster. Individuals with the disorder describe feeling anxious and nervous all their lives. Onset in childhood or adolescence and after age 20 years are both common, with more cases starting early. The course is chronic and variable and may intensify with stress.[5] Generalized anxiety disorder becomes evident with the following symptoms: excessive worry lasting for more days than not for at least 6 months, about a number of events. The person's worry is beyond his or her control, and three (or more) of the following six symptoms are present: restlessness, tires easily, problems concentrating, irritability, muscle tension, sleep problems; in addition, these symptoms have affected daily functioning.

Music

The use of music to alter mood and anxiety dates back to the Greeks. Springe[144] explored the anxiolytic effect of music on anxious mood generated by dental surgery procedures. Subjects were divided into two groups of 50, with one group choosing to listen to music of their selection. The other group was exposed to white noise preoperatively until sedated. The subjects' anxiety was measured using a variety of physiologic measurements. Significance findings included pulse rate, mean arterial blood pressure, and plasma ACTH value. The findings indicated the effectiveness of music in reducing acute anxiety.[144]

The selection and assignment process were not discussed, and the study would be improved if it had included a psychometric measure of anxiety. However, the size of the study and power of physiologic data indicate the effectiveness of music. Other areas to develop include the strength of this treatment over time and realistic limits for its use. Although effective in an anxiety-provoking situation, it may be ineffective in panic.

Massage

Filed et al.[48] have studied massage for the reduction of diagnosable anxiety in a child psychiatry inpatient setting. They exposed 72 adolescents and children with depression and adjustment disorder to daily, 30-minute back massage for 5 days. The patients were randomly stratified to either the massage group or a group watching a restful video. Patient responses to treatment were measured using State Anxiety Inventory for Children (STAIC), Profile of Mood States (POMS), behavior and activity observation ratings, pulse rate, saliva cortisol and 24-hour urine cortisol values, and nighttime sleep recording. The findings reported a reduction of anxiety and fidgeting ratings, decrease in saliva cortisol temporal to the massage, improvements in sleep, and reduction in STAIC values for those children with depression during the treatment phase. Longer-term effects were reduced depression for both depressed and adjustment-disordered children and improved anxiety and fidgeting ratings for both groups. The biochemical effects of treatment diminished over the 5-day period.[48]

The findings provide evidence for the effect of massage in reducing anxiety and improving depression. This study suffers from self-stated problems in examining a "mixed bag" of conditions under the name of adjustment disorder, and from being a small, single-site study. Even with these limitations, the study provides support and direction for continued investigation in this area.

Ferrell-Torry and Glick[47] examined the effects of 2 days of 30-minute massage on cancer pain and anxiety. They used a convenience sample of nine patients, examining pain and anxiety with visual analog scales and anxiety using the State-Trait Anxiety Inventory (STAI-Y-1). Pulse and respiratory rates and blood pressure were also obtained before and after each session of massage. The findings were significant for reduction of pain and anxiety, increased relaxation, and changes in many of the physiologic measures obtained. The findings suggest that massage modified both anxiety and pain.

The study is exploratory by the author's admission and the sample selection and size do not allow for generalization. Further, the nature of anxiety associated with pain and/or chronic illness such as cancer may be distinct from the psychiatric anxiety disorders that are the focus of this chapter.

Acupuncture

Tao[147] examined the use of acupuncture to reduce depression and anxiety in patients with chronic physical diseases. Of the 68 subjects, 11 suffered from anxiety, 8 from depression, and 49 from both. They were assigned in a single-blind, premeasure and postmeasure, noncontrolled study design. Changes in depression and anxiety were assessed using the Hospital Anxiety and Depression scale. The study reported that 70% of the patients with anxiety and 90% of patients with depression returned to normal levels as measured by the instruments used.[147]

The use of this work in treating anxiety and depression in the medically ill is a significant confounding variable in considering the pure anxiolytic effect of this treatment. The strength of these findings is limited by the lack of a control group. The study does support the need for further work in this area.

Yoga and Meditation

Shannahoff-Khalsa and Beckett[140] examined the effect of Kundalini yoga versus a combination of relaxation-response techniques and mindfulness meditation as a control group. A total of 25 subjects were randomly assigned to the groups after matching for age, sex, and "meditation status." Five measures were obtained, including the Yale-Brown Obsessive Compulsive Scale, Symptoms Checklist-90-R, Profile of Mood States, Perceived Stress Scales, and the Purpose in Life test. Brain imaging using 37-channel magnetometers was used in nonmeditating patients before and after treatment. Significant differences were reported at 3 months on all scales for those using Kundalini yoga, and none for those receiving relaxation-response techniques and mindfulness meditation.

The findings suggest significant impact for a specific form of yoga and little response to other forms of meditation. The small study size suggests that the negative finding for the control treatment should be viewed with caution, as the risk of a type 2 error is high. The study builds on the common use of yoga techniques in stress reduction and points to treatments that may be more effective in a severe anxiety disorder. This area merits further exploration with larger sample size and more sophisticated designs.

In other work the effect of meditation-based stress reduction programs was compared with a relaxation program in addressing anxiety disorders.[82] The program was based on mindfulness meditation and involved 22 subjects prescreened with the Symptom Checklist-90-Revised and the Medical Symptom Checklist and then screened with a structured clinical interview meeting the *DSM-IIIR* criteria for generalized anxiety disorder or panic disorder (with or without agoraphobia).[4] Anxiety was measured using self-ratings, therapist ratings, HAMD scales, and Beck anxiety and depression scales before treatment and weekly throughout the treatment protocol, then after treatment monthly for 3 months. Patients taking medication were not excluded from the study because of small sample size. Subjects were assigned to one of two treatment groups: meditation or relaxation group without a control group. The report does not state whether subjects were randomly assigned to these groups. The descriptive data reported use the patients as their own control. Statistics reported for each group did not show statistical significance on the SCL-90 anxiety scales. Both the relaxation and mindfulness meditation groups demonstrated a significant ($p > 0.001$) level on the HAMD rating, the Beck anxiety and depression scales, and the Fear survey scheduled between their pretreatment and posttreatment results.[82] This study is consistent with the earlier findings of Lehrer and colleagues[89] in detecting only limited differences between similar treatment methods in 16 anxious subjects as determined by the IPAT anxiety inventory.

This study attempted to isolate the effects of these treatments in patients with anxiety disorders and identify longer-term effectiveness of these treatments. The small size of the study and lack of control group limit the use of the findings to encouraging future research. The current understanding of panic disorder's etiology suggests a biologic connection, and its relationship to generalized anxiety disorder is arguable. This weakens the findings by further limiting the sample for diagnosis. DeBerry et al.[37] studied 32 geriatric subjects randomly assigned to one of three conditions: meditation-relaxation (MR), cognitive restructuring, and pseudotreatment control. The subjects were measured using the State-Trait Anxiety Inventory and the Beck Depression Inventory. The authors reported that MR was a modality for reducing state anxiety in anxious elderly individuals. They also reported that to maintain reduction of anxiety, constant practice of MR was required. These findings are consistent with earlier findings from these authors.[35-37] The small cell size for each of the treatment conditions makes full endorsement of the findings risky, as it is difficult to eliminate significant type 2 error in the treatment conditions for which no significant difference was found.

Herbal Products

Suanzaoretang, an ancient Chinese remedy used for weakness, irritability, and insomnia, has been tested in double-blind, controlled conditions against diazepam.[28] Ninety patients with Morbid Anxiety Inventory scores between 14 and 30 were recruited from an anxiety clinic. The patients were divided into three conditions: suanzaoretang 250 mg three times daily, diazepam 2 mg three times daily, and placebo. The subjects were all given a 1-week placebo washout. Treatments were evaluated using the Morbid Anxiety Inventory, Hamilton Anxiety Scale, the Digital Symbol Substitution Test, and self-rating of functioning (five-point Likert). Patients were also monitored for a variety of blood chemistry values. The patients were treated for 3 weeks on a regimen of active compounds. The findings indicated that suanzaoretang is an effective anxiolytic lacking the muscular tension–relieving and insomnia-relieving qualities of diazepam. This is consistent with the reports that suanzaoetang improved "psychomotor performance."[28]

This study is consistent with the standard expected of a drug trial. The single site and the size of the trial are all that keep this from meeting the standards required of studies examining medications for clinical use. The authors of this study recommended further investigation of this compound. It is disheartening to see that this was written a number of years ago, and no follow-up work is found in the literature search of the MEDLARS.

Electrosleep

Moore and colleagues[108a] have reported a double-blind study with a crossover structure design. They recruited 17 subjects with persistent anxiety and insomnia. The method of diagnosis is not discussed, and using a crossover design exposed the patient to electrosleep or a sham version of the treatment. There were 5 nights of treatment in each condition. Patients were assessed using the Likert self-rating scale for anxiety, insomnia, and depression, Taylor's Manifest Anxiety scale, the Beck depression inventory, and Eysenck's personality inventory.

No significant results were demonstrated between groups. The study's failure of diagnostic accuracy for inclusion and small sample size place it at risk for type 2 error. It should be viewed with caution. Flemenbaum[49] reported significantly positive results in a less rigorous, open-label clinical study with a 6-month follow-up. His study was uncontrolled and also was weakened by the use of patients from a number of outdated diagnostic categories.

Homeopathy

The effectiveness of homeopathic treatment in patients with depression and anxiety was studied in 12 adults using individually selected homeopathic remedies. Subjects had major depression, social phobia, or panic disorder. The patients either self-selected or were referred to this treatment after poor response to other treatments. Treatment length varied from 7 to 80 weeks. Outcomes were measured by a clinical global scale (N = 12), the self-rated SCL-90 scale (N = 8), and the Brief Social Phobia Scale (N = 4). The research reports response rates were 58% on the clinical global improvement scale and 50% on the SCL-90 or the Brief Social Phobia Scale.[55] Despite noble attempts, the study is examining different patient populations over differing time spans using different compounds. This study does not build a strong base for recommending treatment.

McCutcheon[105] examined 72 adults with above-average anxiety scores who were randomly assigned to either antianxiety homeopathic treatment or a placebo for 15 days. A "four-measures," double-blind format was used, and determinations of pulse rate, sleep quality, and state and trait anxiety were obtained. Posttest comparisons were nonsignificant except for a small reduction in amount of sleep loss for those receiving homeopathic treatment. In further analyses noted, subjects were unable to successfully predict their group assignment. The researcher noted that a homeopathic remedy aids in reducing the sleep loss often associated with anxiety.[105]

TABLE 8-1	Meta-Analysis and Summaries of Complementary/Alternative Therapies Used in Psychiatry		
Psychiatric Diagnosis	CAM Therapy	Result	Reference
Depression	Herbal (*Hypericum*)	Superior to placebo (N = 1757) (meta-analysis)	1. Linde (1996)
		8/14 studies, + effect	2. Gelenberg (1997)
		Patient surveys report + effects (N = 3250)	3. Woelk (1994)
Depression	Cognitive-behavioral	Both using meta-analysis Multiple studies, + effect	1. Wexler (1991)
		>65 studies, + effects pharmacotherapy	2. Gaffan (1995)
Insomnia	Cognitive-behavioral	Sleep improvement (? clinically significant)	1. NIH (1996)
		66 studies, greater magnitude and enhancement (meta-analysis)	2. Murtagh and Greenwood (1995)
		Sleep latency decrease; greater sleep maintenence (meta-analysis)	3. Morin et al. (1994)
Anxiety	Cranioelectrostimulation	8 studies report + effects (meta-analysis)	Klawansky et al. (1995)
Anxiety, panic disorders, posttraumatic stress	Cognitive-behavioral	Multiple studies show + effects	Barlow and Cassandra (1996)
Panic disorder	Cognitive-behavioral	More than 20 studies, + effect (meta-analysis)	Clum et al. (1993)

References: Barlow DH, Cassandra LL: Advances in the psychosocial treatment of anxiety disorders: implications for national health care, *Arch Gen Psychiatry* 53:727, 1996; Clum GA et al: A meta-analysis of treatments for panic disorder, *J Consult Clin Psychol* 61(2):317, 1993; Gaffan EA et al: Research allegiance and meta-analysis: the case of cognitive therapy for depression, *J Consult Clin Psychol* 63(6):966, 1995; Klawansky S et al: Meta-analysis of randomized controlled trials of cranial electrostimulation, *J Nerv Ment Dis* 183(7):478, 1995; Morin CM et al: Nonpharmacological interventions for insomnia: a meta-analysis of treatment efficacy, *Am J Psychiatry* 151(8):1172, 1994; Murtagh DR, Greenwood KM: Identifying effective psychological treatments for insomnia: a meta-analysis, *J Consult Clin Psychol* 63(1):79, 1995; National Institutes of Health: Integration of behavioral and relaxation approaches into the treatment of chronic pain and insomnia, *JAMA* 276(4):313, 1996; Wexler BE, Cicchetti DV: The outpatient treatment of depression: implications of outcome research for clinical practice, *J Nerv Ment Dis* 180(5):277, 1991.
+, Positive.

SUMMARY

We have come to several conclusions from our exploration of research material in CAM medicine and psychiatric illness. The review presented in this chapter identifies areas for potential future research in CAM and mental illness; however, the research literature remains sparse in numbers and weak in scientific validation for many, if not most, of the treatments reviewed. There are few valid replication studies of work with positive findings and few challenges of the studies with design weaknesses by CAM researchers.

Table 8-1 presents a summary and meta-analysis of several CAM therapies in psychiatry. Cognitive-behavioral therapies (CBTs), which contain components of relaxation, visual imagery, flooding, and other conditioning parameters, although not explicitly discussed in the text, demonstrate that positive research evidence exists regarding their singular or combined usage (with medication), especially in the mildly depressed patient. As mentioned earlier, although CBTs have been considered an accepted, conventional treatment for depression, insomnia, and anxiety, they, along with herbal treatment, can also represent—under certain protocols—alternatives to antidepressant drug treatments, for which there are strong meta-analysis reports for efficacy. (To more completely integrate research information, the *Journal of Consulting and Clinical Psychology* (August 1996) has published studies dealing with antidepressant drug therapies and the *Archives of General Psychiatry* (August 1996) has published reports on behavioral therapies.)

Areas such as herbal medicine and bioelectric magnetic treatments offer the most promise. These areas show the most vigorous studies and support from basic science. Improving clinical trials may lead to more effective and efficient treatments. Indeed, some of yesterday's natural or alternative cures are today's mainstream insurance-reimbursable medicine.

REFERENCES

1. Adler N, Cave L: NIMH launches anxiety disorders education program. In NIH Web page www.nih.gov//news/pr/oct96/nimh-22.htm, Washington, DC, 1996, National Institutes of Health.
2. Angoli A, Angreoli V, Cassacchia M: Effect of s-adenosyl-L-methionin (SAM) upon depressive symptoms, *J Psychiatr Res* 13:43, 1976.
3. Angst J, Woggond FJ, Schoefi KR: Treatment of depression: L-5HT vs. imipramine—results of two open and one double-blind clinical trial, *Arch Psychiatr Nerve Kr* 224(Oct. 11):775, 1997.
4. American Psychological Association: *Diagnostic and statistical manual of mental disorders, third edition, revised (DSM-IIIR)*, Washington, DC, 1987, American Psychiatric Press.
5. American Psychological Association: *Diagnostic and statistical manual of mental disorders, fourth edition (DSM-IV)*, Washington, DC, 1994, American Psychiatric Press.
6. Apter A et al: Movement therapy with psychotic adolescents, *Br J Med Psychol* 51:155, 1978.
7. Arnold LE: Screening and evaluating alternative and innovative psychiatric treatments: a contextual framework. *Psychopharmacol Bull* 30(1):61, 1994.

8. Ascheim E: Dietary control of psychosis, *Med Hypn* 41:327, 1993.

9. Baker L: The use of hypnotic techniques with psychotics, *Am J Clin Hypn* 25(4):283, 1983.

10. Banshchikov VM et al: Current status of the problem of electric sleep, *Vopr Kurortol Fizioter Lech Fiz Kult* 31(3):215, 1966.

11. Bell I et al: Brief communication: vitamin B_1, B_2, and B_6 augmentation of tricyclic antidepressant treatment in geriatric depression with cognitive dysfunction, *J Am Coll Nutr* 11(2):159, 1992.

12. Bisset NG et al: *Herbal drugs and phytopharmaceuticals: a handbook for practice on a scientific basis,* Stuttgart, 1994, Medpharm Scientific, p 273.

13. Deleted in proofs.

14. Boman B: L-Tryptophan: a rational anti-depressant and a natural hypnotic? *Aust N Z J Psychiatry* 22:83, 1988.

15. Bradford HF: *Chemical neurobiology: an introduction to neurochemistry,* 1986, New York, WM Freeman.

16. Bruinvels J, Pepplinkhuizen L: Serine, glycine and carbohydrates in schizoaffective disorders, *Bibl Nutr Dicta* 38:168, 1986.

17. Bruinvels J et al: *Role of serine, glycine, and tetrahydrofolic P acid cycle in schizo-affective psychosis,* Chicester, 1980, Wiley.

18. Butler R: Warnings about melatonin, *Geriatrics* 51(2):16, 1996.

19. Byerley W et al: 5-Hydroxytryptophan: a review of its antidepressant efficacy and adverse effects, *J Clin Psychopharmacol* 7(3):127, 1987.

20. Cangliang Y: Clinical observations of 62 cases of insomnia treated by auricular point imbedding therapy, *J Tradit Chin Med* 8(3):190, 1988.

21. Cantoni GL: S-adenosylmethionine: a new intermediate formed enzymatically from L-methionine and adenosine triphosphate, *J Biol Chem* 204:403, 1953.

22. Carney MWP, Chary TNK, Bottiglieri T: Switch mechanisms in affective illness and oral s-adenosylmethionine (SAM), *Br J Psychiatry* 150:43, 1987.

23. Carod FJ, Vazquez-Cabrera C: [A transcultural view of neurological and mental pathology in a Tzeltal Maya community of the Altos Chiapas], *Rev Neurol* 24(131):848, 1996.

24. Cartwright RD, Weiss M: The effects of Electrosleep on insomnia revisited, *J Nerv Ment Dis* 161(5):134, 1975.

25. Chambers CA, Naylor GJ: L-Tryptophan in mania, *Br J Psychiatry* 132:555, 1978.

26. Changlxin X: Lectures on formulating acupuncture prescriptions: selection and matching of acupoints—acupuncture treatment of insomnia, *J Tradit Chin Med* 7(2):151, 1987.

27. Chen A: An introduction to sequential electric acupuncture (SEA) in the treatment of stress related physical and mental disorders, *Acupunct Electrother Res* 17(4):273, 1992.

28. Chen H, Hsiem MT, Shibuya TK: Suanzaorentang versus diazepam: a controlled double-blind study in anxiety, *Int J Clin Pharmacol Ther Toxicol* 24(12):646, 1986.

29. Chen HC, Hsich MT: Clinical trial of suanzaoretang in the treatment of insomnia, *Clin Ther* 7(3):334,1985.

30. Chumakova LT, Kirllova ZA: Effectiveness of Electosleep, *Excerp Med* 128:20, 1966.

31. Coppen A, Chaudhry S, Swade C: Folic acid enhances lithium prophylaxis, *J Affect Disord* 10:9, 1986.

32. Das A: Schizophrenia and complementary treatments including acupuncture. *Towsen Lett* (April) 105:250, 1992.

33. Davidson J et al: Homeopathic treatment of depression and anxiety, *Alternat Ther* 3(1):46, 1997.

34. Davis M, Eshelman R, McKay M: *The relaxation and stress reduction workbook,* ed 4, Oakland, 1995, New Harbinger.

35. DeBerry S: An evaluation of progressive muscle relaxation on stress related symptoms in a geriatric population, *Int J Aging Hum Devel* 14(4):255, 1981.

36. DeBerry S: The effects of meditation-relaxation on anxiety and depression in a geriatric population, *Psychother Theory Res Pract* 19(4):512, 1982.

37. DeBerry S, Davis S, Reinhard KE: A comparison of meditation-relaxation and cognitive/behavioral techniques for reducing anxiety and depression in a geriatric population, *J Geriatr Psychiatry* 22(2):231, 1989.

38. Demisch K et al: Treatment of severe chronic insomnia with L-tryptophan: results of double-blind cross-over study, *Pharmacopsychiatr* 20:242, 1987.

39. Dostalek C: Physiologic bases of yoga techniques in the prevention of diseases: CIANS-ISBM Satellite Conference Symposium—lifestyle changes in the prevention and treatment of disease, Hannover, Germany, 1992, *Homeostasis Health Dis* 35(4-5):205, 1994.
40. Dube KC: Nosology and therapy of mental illness in ayurveda, *Comparat Med East West* 4(3):209, 1978.
41. Dube KC, Kumar A, Dube S: Psychiatric training and therapies in ayurved, *Am J Chin Med* 13(1-4):13, 1985.
42. Ernst E: [St. John's wort as antidepressive therapy], *Fortschr Med* 113(25):354, 1995.
43. Falloon IRH et al: Family management in the prevention of exacerbation of schizophrenia, *N Engl J Med* 306:1447, 1982.
44. Farmer AE, Falkowski WF: Maggot in the salt, snake factor and the treatment of atypical psychosis in West African women, *Br J Psychiatry* 146:446, 1985.
45. Fazio C et al: Effetti terapeutici e meccanismo d'azlone della S-adenosil-metionina (SAMe) nelle sindrml depressive, *Minerva Med* 64(29):1515, 1973.
46. Feighner JP, Braun SL, Oliver JE: Electrosleep treatment: double-blind study, *J Nerv Ment Disord* 157:121, 1973.
47. Ferrell-Torry A, Glick O: The use of therapeutic massage as a nursing intervention to modify anxiety and the perception of cancer pain, *Cancer Nurs* 16(2):93, 1993.
48. Filed T et al: Massage reduces anxiety in child and adolescent psychiatric patients, *J Am Acad Child Adolesc Psychiatry* 31(1):125, 1992.
49. Flemenbaum A: Cerebral electrotherapy (electrosleep): an open-clinical study with a six month follow-up, *Psychosomatics* 15:20, 1974.
50. Forsheim P: Cross-cultural views of self in the treatment of mental illness: disentangling the curative aspects of myth from the mythic aspects of cure, *Psychiatry* 53:304, 1990.
51. Frankel BL, Buchbinder R, Synger F: Ineffectiveness of electrosleep in chronic primary insomnia, *Arch Gen Psychiatry* 29:563, 1973.
52. Freed WJ et al: Wheat gluten impedes absorption of haloperidol, *Biol Psychiatry* 13:769, 1978.
53. Fujiwara J, Otsuki S: Subtype of affective psychosis classified by response on amine precursors and monoamine metabolism, *Folia Psychiatr Neurol* 28:94, 1974.
54. Galanter M, Larson D, Rubenstone E: Christian psychiatry: the impact of evangelical belief on clinical practice [see comments], *Am J Psychiatry* 148(1):90, 1991.
55. Gaus W, Hogel J: Studies on the efficacy of unconventional therapies: problems and designs, *Arzneimittelforschung* 45(1):88, 1995.
56. Gelenberg AJ: St. John's wort: nostrum for depression, *Biol Ther Psychiatry Newslett*: 8:15, 1997.
57. George M et al: Daily repetitive transcranial magnetic stimulation (rTMS) improves mood in depression, *Neuro Report* 6:1853, 1995.
58. George MS, Keller TA, Post RM: Activation studies in mood disorders, *Psychiat Ann* 24(12):648, 1994.
59. Gilyarovski VA et al: A's Electroson, *Medguaz* 6:10, 1953.
60. Godfrey PSA et al: Enhancement of recovery from psychiatric illness by methylfolate, *Lancet* 336:392, 1990.
61. Goldman HH: *Review of general psychiatry*, ed 2, New York, 1988, Appleton and Lange.
62. Haidvogl M: Clinical Studies of homeopathy: the problem of a useful design. In Endler PC, Schulte J, editors: *Ultra high dilution physiology and physics*, Boston, 1994, Kluwer Academic, p 221.
63. Hansgen KD, Vesper J: Antidepressive Wirksamkeit eines hochdosierten hypericum-extracktes, *Munch Med Wschr* 138:35, 1996.
64. Harper, EH et al: Is schizophrenia rare if grain is rare? *Biol Psychiatry* 19:385, 1984.
65. Harrell S: Pluralism, performance and meaning in Taiwanese healing: a case study, *Culture Med Psychiatry* 15:45, 1991.
66. Harvard School of Public Health: Global health statistics, vol 2. In Murray CJL, Lopez AD, editors: *Global burden of disease and injury* series, 1996, Cambridge, Mass, Harvard University.
67. Hearst ED et al: Electrosleep therapy: a double-blind trial, *Arch Gen Psychiatry* 30(4):463, 1974.
68. Hodge JR: Can hypnosis help psychosis? *Am J Clin Hypnosis* 30(4):248, 1988.
69. Hoffman D: *The herbalist*, Hopkins, Minn, 1994, Hopkins Technology.

70. Holzl J: Zeitschrift fur Phytotherapie, *Inhaltsstoffe und wirkmechanismen des johannishrauts*14:255, 1993.

71. Horrobin DF: Prostaglandin deficiency and endorphin excess in schizophrenia: the case for treatment with penicillin, zinc and evening primrose oil, *J Orthomol Psychiatr* 8:13, 1979.

72. Horrobin, DF: Niacin flushing, prostaglandin E and evening primrose oil: a possible objective test for schizophrenia, *J Orthomolecular Psychiatr* 9:33, 1980.

73. Horton EW: Prostaglandin E and schizophrenia, *Lancet* 1:313, 1980.

74. Hubner WD, Lande S, Podzuweit H: Hypericum treatment of mild depressions with somatic symptoms, *J Geriatr Psychiatr Neurol* 7(suppl 1):S12, 1994.

75. James S et al: Melatonin administration in insomnia, *Neuropsychopharmacol* 3(1):19, 1990.

76. Kaneko M et al: L-5-HTP treatment and serum 5-HT level after L-5-HTP loading on depressed patients, *Neuropsychobiol* 5:232, 1979.

77. Kaplan HI, Sadock BJ: *Textbook of psychiatry*, New York, 1985, Williams & Wilkins.

78. Keith SJ, Matthew SM: Group, family, and milieu therapies and psychosocial rehabilitation in the treatment of the schizophrenic disorders. In Grinspoon L, editor: *Psychiatry 1982 Annual Review*, Washington, DC, 1982, American Psychiatric Press.

79. Keys S: Attitudes towards the use of acupuncture in the treatment of the elderly mentally ill, *Complement Ther Med* 3:242, 1995.

80. Klawansky S et al: Meta-analysis of randomized controlled trials of cranial electrostimulation, *J Nerv Ment Dis* 183(7):478, 1995.

81. Klich R: Verhaltenstorungen im Kindesaler und deren Therapie, *Med Welt* 26(25):1251, 1975.

82. Kobat-Zinn J et al: Effectiveness of meditation-based stress reduction programs in the treatment of anxiety disorders, *Am J Psychiatr* 149:936, 1992.

83. Koh TC: T'ai chi chuan, *Am J Chin Med* IX(1):15, 1981.

84. Komori T et al: Effects of citrus fragrance on immune function and depressive states, *Neuroimmunomodulation* 2:174, 1995.

85. Krieger MJ, Zussman M: The importance of cultural factors in a brief reactive psychosis, *J Clin Psychiatr* 42(6):248, 1981.

86. Kurland HD: ECT and Acu-EST in the treatment of depression, *Am J Chin Med* 4(3):289, 1976.

87. Larson D: Role of prayer in mental health, *Alternat Complement Ther* March/April:91, 1996.

88. Leathwood PD, Chauffard F: Quantifying the effect of mild sedatives, *J Psychiatr Res* 17(2):115, 1982-1983.

89. Lehrer PM et al: Progressive relaxation and medication: a study of the psychophysiological and therapeutic differences between the two techniques, *Behav Res Ther* 21(4): 651, 1983.

90. Lest'e A, Rust J: Effects of dance on anxiety, *Perception Motor Skills* 58(3):767, 1984.

91. Levitt E, James N: A clinical trial of electrosleep therapy with a psychiatric inpatient sample, *Austral N Z J Psychiatr* 9:287, 1975.

92. Leye X, Leqing X, Xiufeng Y: 124 cases of dyssomnia treated with acupuncture at sishencong points, *J Tradition Chin Med* 14(3):171, 1994.

93. Library, M.ICB, AMED-Allied and alternative medicine, 1985 to date, Knight-Ridder Information (DataStar): Yorkshire, UK, Boston Spa West.

94. Lindahl O, Lindwall L: Double blind study of a valerian preparation, *Pharmacol Biochem Behav* 32:1065, 1988.

95. Linde K et al: St John's wort for depression—an overview and meta-analysis of randomized clinical trials [see comments], *Br J Med* 313(7052):253, 1996.

96. Lipinski JF et al: An open trial of S-adenosylmethionine for the treatment of depression, *Am J Psychiatr* 141:448, 1984.

97. Liu G et al: Changes in brain stem and cortical auditory potentials during Qi-gong meditation, *Am J Chin Med* XVIII:95, 1990.

98. Lopez-Ibor Almo JJ: Depressive AquaValenta Undaraskiete Depressionen, *Psychiatr* 152:35, 1976.

99. Lukoff D, Lu FG, Turner R: Cultural considerations in the assessment and treatment of religious and spiritual problems, *Psychiatr Clin North Am* 18(3):467, 1995.

100. Ma QH, Ju YL, Zhang ZL: [Immunological study of inefficiency schizophrenics with deficiency syndrome treated with xin shen ling], *Chung Hsi I Chieh Ho Tsa Chih* 11(4):215, 197, 1991.
101. Marcolongo R et al: Double-blind multicentre study of the activity of S-adenosyl-methionine in hip and knee osteoarthritis, *Curr Ther Res* 37:82, 1985.
102. Martinez B et al: Hypericum in the treatment of seasonal affective disorder, *J Geriatr Psychiatr Neurol* 7(suppl 1): S29, 1994.
103. Martinsen EW, Hoffart A, Solberg O: Comparing aerobic with nonaerobic forms of exercise in the treatment of clinical depression: a randomized trial, *Compr Psychiatr* 30(4):324, 1989.
104. Matussek N et al: The effect of L-5-hydroxytryptophan alone and in combination with a decarboxylase inhibitor in depressive patients, *Adv Biochem Psychopharmacol* 11:399, 1974.
105. McCutcheon LE: Treatment of anxiety with a homeopathic remedy, *J Appl Nutr* 48(1-2):2, 1996.
106. Mendlewicz J, Youdin MBH: Antidepressant potentiation of 5-hydroxytryptophan by L-deprenyl in affective illness, *J Affect Dis* 2:137, 1980.
107. Micali M, Chiti D, Balestra V: Double blind controlled clinical trial of SAMe administered orally in chronic liver disease, *Curr Ther Res* 33:1004, 1983.
108. Montakab H, Langel G: The effect of acupuncture in the treatment of insomnia: clinical study of subjective and objective evaluation, *Schweiz-Med-Wochenschr-Supplement* 62:49, 1994.
108a. Moore JA, Mellor CS, Standage KF, Strong H: A double-blind study of electrosleep for anxiety and insomnia, *Biol Psychiatr* 10(1):59, 1975.
109. Nagata K et al: Studies of electrosleep on normal adults, insomniacs, and hypertensive patients, *Tokushima J Experiment Med* 28:69, 1981.
110. Nakajima T, Kudo Y, Kaneko Z: Clinical evaluation of 5-hydroxytryptophan as an antidepressant drug, *Folia Psychiatr Neurol* 32:223, 1978.
111. Nan L, Qingming Y: Insomnia treated by auricular pressing therapy. *J Tradition Chin Med* 10(3):174, 1990.
112. National Institutes of Health: Integration of behavioral and relaxation approaches into the treatment of chronic pain and insomnia, *JAMA* 276(4):313, 1996.
113. Obeyesekere G: The theory and practice of psychological medicine in the ayurvedic tradition, *Culture Med Psychiatr* 1:155, 1977.
114. Pasche B et al: Effects of low energy emission therapy in chronic psychophysiological insomnia, *Sleep* 19(4):327, 1996.
115. Pauling L: On the orthomolecular environment of the mind: orthomolecular therapy, *Am J Psychiatr* 131(11):1251, 1974.
116. Pauling L: Orthomolecular psychiatry, *Science* 19:265, 1986.
117. Pepplinhwaizen L et al: Schizophrenia-like psychosis caused by a metabolic disorder, *Lancet* 1(8166):454, 1980.
118. Post, RM, Weiss RB, Ketter TA: The temporal lobes and affective disorders: basic and clinical perspective. In Bolwig T: *The temporal lobes and the limbic system*, London, 1992, Wrightson Biomedical.
119. Reilly D et al: Is evidence for homeopathic treatment reproducible? *Lancet* 344:1601, 1994.
120. Reite M et al: Sleep inducing effect of low energy emission therapy, *Bioeletromagnetics* 15:67, 1994.
121. Research: Agency for Health Care Policy and Research: Clinical Practice Guideline no. 5, Depression in primary care, Rockville, Md, 1993, US Department of Health and Human Services.
122. Reynolds EH, Stramentinoli G: Folic acid S-adenosyl-l-methionine and affective disorders, *Psychologic Med* 13:705, 1983.
123. Rief W, Hermanutz M: Responses to activation and rest in patients with panic disorder and major depression, *Br J Clin Psychol* 35(4):605, 1996.
124. Roberge AC, Missala K, Sourkes TL: Alpha-methyltryptophan: effects on synthesis and degradation of serotonin in the brain, *Neuropharmacol* 11:197, 1972.
125. Romoli A: Ear acupuncture in psychosomatic medicine, *Acupunct Electrother Res* 18(3-4):185, 1993.
126. Rosenthal SH, Masserman JH: *Current psychiatric therapies*, vol. 12, New York, 1972, Grune & Stratton.
127. Rosenbaum JF et al: An open-label pilot study of oral S-adenosyl-L-methionine in major depression: interim results, *Psychopharmacol Bull* 1:189, 1988.

128. Rovesti P, Colombo E: Aromatherapy and aerosol, *SPC* 19(1-4):475, 1973.
129. Rubin DO: The major psychoses and neuroses as omega-3 essential fatty acid deficiency syndrome: substrate pellagra, *Biol Psychiatr* 16(9):837, 1981.
130. Ryu H et al: Acute effect of qigong training on stress hormonal levels in man, *Am J Chin Med* XXIV(2):193, 1996.
131. Saki M, Pogady J: [Newest advances in clinical phytotherapy in Chinese psychiatry], *Cesk Psychiatr* 90(1):48, 1994.
132. Sano I: L-5-hydroxytryptophan (L-5HTP) therapie, *Folia Psychiatr Neurol* 26:7, 1972.
133. Sarai K: Oriental medicine as therapy for resistant depression: use of some herbal drugs in the Far East (Japan), *Prog Neuropsychopharmacol Biol Psychiatr* 16(2):171, 1992.
134. Scagnelli-Jobsis J: Hypnosis with psychotic patients: a review of the literature and presentation of theoretical framework, *Am J Clin Hypn* 25(1):22, 1983.
135. Scavone JM: *Essentials of clinical research,* Boston, 1991, Healthways Communications.
136. Schell EJ, Allolio B, Schonecke W: Physiological and psychological effects of Hatha-yoga exercise in healthy women, *Int J Psychosom* 41(1-4):46, 1994.
137. Schmidt U, Sommer H: St. John's wort extract in the ambulatory therapy of depression: attention and reaction ability are preserved, *Fortschr Med* 11(19):339, 1993.
138. Schnieder-Helmert D, Spinweber C: Evaluation of L-tryptophan for treatment of insomnia: a review, *Psychopharmacol* 89:1, 1986.
139. Schoen Johnson B: *Psychiatric-mental health nursing,* ed 4, New York, 1997, Lippincott.
140. Shannahoff-Khalsa DS, Beckett LR: Clinical case report: efficacy of yogic techniques in the treatment of obsessive compulsive disorders, *Int J Neurosci* (March) 85(1-2):1, 1996.
141. Shi Z, Tan M: An analysis of the therapeutic effect of acupuncture treatment in 500 cases of schizophrenia, *J Tradition Chin Med* 6(2):99, 1986.
142. Sourkes T: Alpha-methyltryptophan as a therapeutic agent, *Neuropsychopharmacol Biol Psychiatr* 15:935, 1991.
143. Spiegel D: Hypnosis with psychotic patients: comment on Scagnelli-Jobsis, *Am J Clin Hypnosis* 25(4):289, 1983.
144. Springe R: Some neuroendocrinologic effects of so-called anxiolytic music, *Int J Neurol* 19-20:186, 1986.
145. Takahashi S, Kondo H, Kato N: Effects of 5-hydroxytryptophan on brain monoamine metabolism and evaluation of its clinical effect in depressive patients, *J Psychiatr Res* 12:177, 1975.
146. Tanra AJ et al: TJS-010: a new prescription of kampo medicine with putative antidepressive and anxiolytic properties: a behavioral study using experimental models for depression and anxiety, *Hiroshimal J Med Sci* 43(4):145, 1995.
147. Tao DJ: Research on the reduction of anxiety and depression with acupuncture, *Am J Acupunct* 21(4):327, 1993.
148. Templer DI: The efficacy of electrosleep therapy, *Can Psychiatr Assoc J* 20(8):607, 1975.
149. Thomson J et al: The treatment of depression in general practice: a comparison of L-tryptophan, amitriptyline, and a combination of L-tryptophan and amitriptyline with placebo, *Psychol Med* 12:741, 1982.
150. Tolbott JA, Hales RE, Yudofsky SC: *Textbook of psychiatry,* Washington, DC, 1988, American Psychiatric Press.
151. Van Praag AJ et al: Tryphophan in mania, *Arch Gen Psychiatr* 30:56-62. 1974.
152. VanHiele LJ: 5-Hydroxytriptophan in depression: the first substitution therapy in psychiatry, *Neuropsychobiol* 6:230, 1980.
153. VanPraag HM: Management of depression with serotonin precursors, *Biol Psychiatr* 16:291, 1981.
154. Vlissides DN, Venulet A, Jenner FA: Gluten free/gluten load controlled trial in a secure ward population, *Br J Psychiatr* 148:447, 1986.
155. Volwiler-Gunning S, Holmes TH: Dance therapy with psychotic children: definition and quantitative evaluation, *Arch Gen Psychiatr* 28:707, 1973.
155a. Wagner H, Bladt S: Inhibition of MAO by fractions and constituents of hypericum extract, *J Geriatr Psychiatr Neurol* 7(suppl 1):S65, Oct 1994.

156. Weiss MF: The treatment of insomnia through the use of electrosleep: an EEG study, *J Ment Dis* 157(2):108, 1973.
157. Wen ST: The development of psychiatric concepts in traditional Chinese medicine, *Arch Gen Psychiatr* 29:569, 1973.
158. Witte B et al: Treatment of depressive symptoms with a high concentration hypericum preparation: a multicenter placebo-controlled double-bind study, *Fortschr Med* 113(28):404, 1995.
159. Woelk H, Burkard G, Grunwald J: Benefits and risks of the hypericum extract LI 160: drug monitoring study with 3250 patients, *J Geriatr Psychiatr Neurol* 7(suppl 1):S34, 1994.
160. Xiujuan Y: Clinical observation on needling extrachannel points in treating mental depression, *J Tradition Chin Med* 14(1):14, 1994.
161. Yi R: Eighty-six cases of insomnia treated by double point needling—Dailing through to waiguan, *J Tradition Chin Med* 5(1):22, 1985.
162. Yukang W: An observation on the therapeutic effect of acupuncture in threating 50 cases of insomnia, *Int J Clin Acupunct* 3(1):91, 1992.
163. Zimilacher K, Battegay R, Gastpar M: L-5-hydroxytryptophan alone and in combination with a peripheral decarboxylase inhibitor in the treatment of depression, *Neuropsychobiol* 20:28, 1988.

SUGGESTED READINGS

Brodie HK, Brodie SM: An overview of trends in psychiatry research, *Am J Psychiatry* 130:1309, 1973.

Daniel W: *Biostatistics: A foundation for analysis in the health sciences,* New York, 1995, Wiley.

Goleman D, Gurin J: *Mind body medicine: how to use your mind for better health,* Yonkers, 1993, Consumer Reports Books.

Maxmen JS, Ward NG: *Essential psychopathology and its treatment,* ed 2 (rev. for DSM-IV), New York, 1995, WW Norton.

CHAPTER 9

Complementary/Alternative Therapies in the Treatment of Alcohol and Other Addictions

Patricia D. Culliton, Tacey Ann Boucher, and Milton L. Bullock

Despite recent attention in the media as a new phenomenon, the integration of the complementary/alternative medicine (CAM) and substance abuse treatment fields has an extensive past. For example, the use of herbs to treat the effects of alcohol consumption dates back hundreds of years. Sanitariums for people with drug and alcohol disorders used saline and electric baths in treatment in the late 1800s, and early in the twentieth century, street peddlers sold remedies for substance abuse even though the remedies themselves frequently contained morphine or cocaine in substantial doses.[134] Spirituality and prayer were introduced into mainstream addiction medicine in the 1900s and provide the foundation for the most commonly used intervention for alcoholism in the United States.[27,129] Today, other methods such as acupuncture and nutrition are gaining popularity for the treatment of substance use disorders.

The progressive integration of CAM methods into addiction medicine has been bolstered by growing popular sentiment toward CAM and the desire of treatment counselors and physicians to broaden their treatment arsenals. The development of drug courts in numerous states, which often mandate offenders to acupuncture treatment programs, also has contributed to the merger of these treatment fields. Although research lags behind integration efforts, during the last three decades scientists and clinicians have generated useful preliminary data regarding treatment efficacy.

We have three goals in writing this chapter. First, we present the reader with useful information on the various forms of CAM therapies used to treat addictions. Second, we provide an overview of empiric findings relevant to the efficacy of CAM for the treatment of substance abuse. Third, we propose potential models for the integration of CAM with conventional or biomedicine and offer predictions concerning the future of CAM for the treatment of substance abuse.

EPIDEMIOLOGY OF SUBSTANCE ABUSE

The extraordinary prevalence of substance abuse in the United States and the attendant human and economic costs of this disease have been amply documented in the academic and popular literature.[77,193] The consequences of misuse vary widely depending on the user's social environment, substance of choice, and pattern of use, but may result in hundreds of physiologic ailments and include any number of social costs. Figures released by the American Medical Association (AMA) indicate that 25% to 40% of general hospital inpatients are receiving treatment for complications resulting from alcoholism.[19] Substance abuse is one of the most prevalent and costly diseases in the United States, and a leading preventable cause of death.

Substance abuse and treatment are complex issues and are of great importance in the United States and around the world. The negative impact of misuse can be seen in every social institution, including the community, the workplace, the criminal justice system, the schools, and the family. In 1993, approximately 30% of both lung disease and cancer deaths and 21% of cardiovascular deaths were caused by tobacco.[123] The latest figures, for the first 6 months of 1995, show an increase of 10% in drug-related hospital emergency department episodes—from 252,600 to 279,100. Cocaine-related episodes rose by 21%, heroin-related episodes by 27%, and methamphetamine-related episodes by 35%.[123] All of this means a significant increase in health care costs.

BRIEF SUMMARY OF EFFICACY

Despite the widespread use of drugs and its staggering costs to society, surprisingly little is known about rates of treatment success. Dropout rates from clinical programs are acknowledged to be high and vary between 50% and 85%.[27,115,211] Treatment centers do not always consider dropouts when reporting their outcomes, instead focusing on the abstinence rates of treatment completers. Based on the findings of controlled clinical trials, an overall rate of abstinence of 20% to 25% seems typical. However, evidence for the efficacy of clinical models of treatment and their component parts is largely unavailable.[61] Alcoholism is a heterogeneous disorder, numerous combinations of factors satisfy the diagnostic criteria for alcoholism, and it has recently been acknowledged that no single model or standardized package of care will suffice.[2,40,79,163] The same is true for a number of other drugs including cocaine, opiates, and nicotine.[10,58] Dreams of finding a "magic bullet" to prevent or treat drug misuse are fading, leading researchers and treatment professionals to suggest increasing the frequency, intensity, and/or types of treatment services offered. According to one theory, increased treatment services should result in increased rates of abstinence. Some research has contradicted this and shown that for most persons with alcohol dependence there is little difference in outcome between longer, more intensive treatment programs and shorter, less intensive approaches.[4,131,132,165] However, research generally has not focused on the combination of treatment methods.[145]

CAM approaches offer treatment providers the opportunity to improve overall treatment outcomes by expanding and enhancing the treatment continuum. Treatment programs increasingly combine methods from both CAM and conventional frameworks to such an extent that therapies like acupuncture and hypnosis are almost commonplace.

THEORIES ON DEPENDENCE

Although we know that the majority of humans use drugs such as nicotine and alcohol, we also know that the majority of users rarely misuse the substances.[81] Whereas some individuals with addiction move in and out of treatment programs for years, or even a lifetime, others have been known to have spontaneous remission.[93,209] Genetics provides one method of explaining the etiology or epidemiology of addictive behaviors, but exceptions abound. At present, no one theory has been able to explain the phenomenon known as addiction, or dependence. Researchers do agree that the causes of addiction are complex and probably varied.

During a period of the early 1900s it became fashionable to view addiction as a moral failing or character flaw. Treatment suggestions included church attendance, prayer, and hard work. Today, moral explanations have given way to the disease models, although remnants of the former view remain.

Sociologists have typically focused on the environment or social interactions.[81] Social change, cultural expectations, inequalities in the social system, and the impact of labeling have all been cited as causal factors.[9,61] Psychologic traditions differ as their models of substance abuse typically implicate mental or behavioral disorders that arise out of physical and environmental factors. Substance abuse may provide relief from suffering or provide a stimulating distraction.[9,230] Recently psychiatry has branched toward physiologic approaches and turned its attention to the role of neurotransmitters in the etiology and maintenance of addiction.[81]

PHYSIOLOGIC EXPLANATIONS: GENETICS AND NEUROCHEMISTRY

Despite cultural differences in the behavior manifestations of substance use, recent neurochemical and molecular findings provide strong evidence for physiologic models of dependence.[72] Research has shown that there are genetic influences related to characteristics of alcohol and drug abuse such as alcohol-metabolizing enzymes, personality traits, and related neurochemical receptors.[50,63,86,95] Although alcoholism has been the focus of research efforts, there is evidence to suggest that genetic explanations may be applicable to other substances.[232]

Numerous advances have been made in neurochemistry and molecular biology, with profound implications for addictions research.*

Knowledge about the molecular pharmacology of most drugs of abuse has led researchers to examine the roles of neurotransmitters in addiction. Findings have impli-

---

*References 5, 55, 60, 108, 109, 141, 185, 212.

cated serotonin, dopamine, and endogenous opioid activity in the brain in many aspects of drug use and abuse.[141,175] While links to other neurotransmitters will certainly be identified in the next decade, serotonin, dopamine, norepinephrine, and endogenous opioids provide the basis for current theories.

OVERVIEW OF STANDARD TREATMENTS
Behavioral Treatment

"Standard treatment" is somewhat of a misnomer when used to describe the behavioral and social approaches of contemporary chemical dependency treatment programs. Treatment has become highly specialized, with a variety of approaches and options available including inpatient, residential, day-care, and outpatient programs. The most frequently encountered behavioral techniques and components include comprehensive assessment, medical services, sociotherapies, psychosocial education, 12-step work, relapse prevention, cognitive therapies, psychotherapies, behavioral therapies, family therapy, occupational therapy, and brief interventions. Variations in the interpretation and application of each of these components contribute to program diversity. In recent years a wide variety of procedures, both psychologic and somatic, have been tried in the treatment of alcoholism. No one therapy has been proved definitely superior to another.[4,64,131,132,165]

Pharmacologic Treatments

Alcohol. Currently, only two pharmaceuticals have been approved in the United States for the treatment of alcoholism: disulfiram and naltrexone. Disulfiram is a commonly used aversive agent that has shown positive outcomes in clinical trials when used as an adjunct to psychosocial treatments. However, dropout rates of patients using disulfiram have been exceptionally high.[52] Naltrexone is an opiate antagonist that has had good results in early clinical trials.[144,145,213] However, definitive judgment awaits the results of additional trials currently in progress. Other opiate antagonists are being tested, but of these, naltrexone has shown the most promise.

A third drug, calcium acetylhomotaurinate (Acamprosate), has shown promise in European trials for the treatment of alcoholism. Extensive testing in Europe has shown a dose-response and placebo-relative effectiveness in the achievement of abstinence, maintenance of sobriety, and treatment retention.[1,6,28,110,194] Trials of efficacy are currently under way in the United States. Selective serotonin reuptake inhibitors (SSRIs), gamma-aminobutyric acid (GABA)-ergic and dopaminergic agents, and calcium channel agonists are also being explored for their usefulness in treating alcoholism.

Opiates. Three approaches have been taken toward the treatment of opiate dependence. The first involves opiate agonists such as methadone and L-alpha-acetylmethadol (LAAM). The second uses partial opiate agonists such as buprenorphine, and the third uses opiate antagonists such as naltrexone.[79]

Cocaine. No pharmaceutical has been identified yet for the treatment of cocaine dependence. Several have shown a subjective impact on craving, although none directly impact dependence or use. The dopaminergic system has been the target of the majority of agents (dopamine agonists), because of its relationship to reinforcement. Serotonergic systems have also been targeted with agents such as fluoxetine, ritanserin, and sertraline. Classic tricyclic antidepressants have also been used commonly in treatment.[59,60]

Marijuana. Although the cause and effect are difficult to determine, dependence on marijuana appears to be driven by psychopathology rather than psychopharmacology. At this time, psychosocial interventions are used to treat cannabis dependence, rather than medication.[66]

Stimulants. Other dopamine agonists (bromocriptine) and tricyclic antidepressants (desipramine) have been used; however, controlled research regarding treatment of amphetamine abuse is scarce.[92]

Sedative-Hypnotics (Benzodiazepines). The pharmacologic treatment of benzodiazepine withdrawal typically involves the substitution of a less addictive barbiturate, such as phenobarbital. Anticonvulsants such as carbamazepine or valproate may also be substituted, although they do not fully evaluate subsequent issues of craving.[229]

Hallucinogens. Despite their abuse potential, benzodiazepines may be used to treat negative reactions to hallucinogens. Medication is not used for the treatment of chronic abuse of hallucinogens; if treatment is necessary, psychotherapy or 12-step programs are recommended.[153]

Nicotine. Ironically, nicotine is the only pharmacologic agent approved by the U.S. Food and Drug Administration (FDA) for the treatment of smoking cessation. Rather than being smoked, nicotine replacement therapy is administered using transdermal systems (patch), gum, spray, or inhaler. The results of nonnicotine medications such as clonidine (nonreceptor antagonist), anxiolytic (buspirone), and antidepressant medications (doxepine, bupropion, fluoxetine) are indeterminate.[173]

CAM AND THE TREATMENT OF CHEMICAL DEPENDENCY

This section focuses on the literature surrounding chemical dependency treatment and CAM. We have decided to review several substances based on the prevalence and/or severity of use and, in the following cases, because of the prevalence of CAM literature: heroin and opiates, alcohol, cocaine, nicotine, and hallucinogens. We also discuss briefly amphetamine and benzodiazepine abuse. The CAM methods selected for discussion were determined by the extent and quality of available literature and research; acupuncture is a focal point because of the large volume of literature (see following discussion).

Acupuncture

Acupuncture is highlighted in this chapter for two principal reasons. First, literature on the use of acupuncture for the overall treatment of substance abuse is more prevalent than for any other CAM method. In particular, a greater number of descriptive and controlled studies have been published regarding the efficacy of acupuncture. Second, acupuncture is the most widely used CAM method for the treatment of substance abuse (excluding spirituality or prayer in conventional 12-step programs). Acupuncture is even mandated for the treatment of offenders by many drug courts.

In the 1980s, crack cocaine, high rates of recidivism, and the lack of a magic bullet to treat substance use disorders provided the opportunity for acupuncture to enter the mainstream. Acupuncture had been growing in popularity for treating alcoholism, and data had been published indicating that acupuncture increases treatment retention.[26] The National Acupuncture Detoxification Association (NADA) was formed in 1985 as a membership and training organization with references to "barrier-free treatment."[36] The sudden influx of a new treatment population of young crack-smoking men and women who either were not receiving successful treatment or were in urban areas that could not serve the dramatic increase in treatment requests opened the way for acupuncture. It was believed that acupuncture would provide inexpensive and effective treatment for large numbers of individuals.

At present, NADA trainers have taught more than 4000 acupuncturists, counselors, nurses, and physicians how to perform acupuncture for substance abuse in the United States, and almost that many in Europe. It is estimated that 700 to 1000 chemical dependency programs are offering acupuncture for the treatment of addictions in the United States, and new programs are implemented regularly.[188]

A list of studies conducted on the use of acupuncture is summarized in Table 9-1. A list of review articles is given in Table 9-2. Despite the large number of studies, treatment protocols often lack standardization and the majority lack methodologic rigor. Some of these studies are reviewed in more detail later in this section.

The Treatment Experience. NADA regards acupuncture as an adjunctive treatment for addictions. However, depending on location and the local policy of treatment admissions, entry into acupuncture for addictive disorders can occur by several different methods. Individuals can walk in to a freestanding acupuncture clinic or program, be mandated by a "drug court" to a particular acupuncture program, be incarcerated in a jail or prison that offers acupuncture, or be a client of a hospital-based, outpatient or residential facility that offers acupuncture as part of its treatment regimen. Once admis-

TABLE 9-1 Studies of Acupuncture and the Addictions

Author, Year	Substance	Number	Design	Methods	Journal
Avants et al., 1995	Cocaine	40	s,b,r,p	Z,H,O,i	*J Subst Abuse Treat*
Bullock, ongoing	Alcohol	—	s,b,r,l,p,c,f	—	*(Ongoing)*
Bullock et al., 1997	Cocaine	438	s,b,r,l,p,c,f	Z,H,O,I	*J Subst Abuse Treat*
Bullock et al., 1989	Alcohol	80	s,b,l,p,c,f	Z,H,O,I	*Lancet*
Bullock et al., 1987	Alcohol	54	s,b,l,c	Z,H,O,I	*Alcohol Clin Exp Res*
Choy et al., 1983	Smoking	514	l,f	—,—,—,—	*Am J Med*
Choy et al., 1978	Morphine	84	a,w,m,s,c	—,H,O,na	*Biochem Biophys Res Comm*
Clavel and Benhamou, 1985	Nicotine	651	s,r,l,c,f	Z,H,o,I	*Br Med J*
Clement-Jones et al., 1979	Heroin	12 + 50 control	w,m,s,c	—,H,O,—	*Lancet*
Cottraux et al., 1983	Smoking	558	s,r,l,c,f	Z,H,O,I	*Behav Res Ther*
Facchinetti et al., 1985	Alcohol	14	m,s,c	—,H,O,i	*Subst Alcohol Actions Misuse*
Fuller, 1982	Smoking	194	s,l,f	—,—,—,—	*Med J Aust*
Gillams et al., 1984	Smoking	81	s,b,r,l,p,c,f	—,—,O,I	*Practitioner*
Gurevich et al., 1996	Dual diagnosis	77	l,c,f	—,o,—	*J Subst Abuse Treat*
Hackett et al., 1984	Nicotine	72	s,l,c,f	—,o,—	*Practitioner*
Ho et al., 1979	Morphine	74/121	a,w,s,c	—,H,O,na	*Neuropharmacology*
Kao and Lu, 1974	Multiple	23	w,l,p	—,—,—,—	*Am J Acupunct*
Karrell, 1990	Polydrug	60	w,s,l,c,f	—,—,—,—	*Addiction Recovery*
Konefal et al., 1994	Multiple	568	s,r,l,c	—,H,O,—	*J Addict Dis*
Kroenig and Oleson, 1985	Narcotic/ methadone	14	w,l	—,O,—	*Int J Addictions*
Lamontagne et al., 1980	Smoking	75	s,r,l,c	—,H,O,I	*Can Med Assoc J*
Lao, 1995	Alcohol	30	l,c	—,H,O,I	*Am J Acupunct*
Leung, 1977	Opiates	17	w,l,p	—,—,—,—	*Am J Acupunct*
Lewenberg, 1985	Alcohol	50/76	l,f	—,o,—	*Clin Ther*
Lipton et al., 1994	Cocaine	192	s,b,r,l,p,f	Z,H,O,I	*J Subst Abuse Treat*
Low, 1977	Smoking	150+	w,l,f	—,—,—,—	*Med J Aust* (letter)
Machovec and Man, 1978	Nicotine	58	s,b,l,c,p,f	—,—,—,I	*Am J Clin Hypnosis*
Malin et al., 1988	Opiates	56	a,w,s,c	—,H,O,na	*Biol Psychiatry*

Reference	Drug	N	Design	Methods	Journal
Man and Chuang, 1980	Methadone	35	w,s,l,c	—,—,O,—	Int J Addictions
Margolin et al., 1993	Cocaine	48	s,b,l,p	—,H,O,—	Am J Chin Med
Margolin et al., 1995	Cocaine/opiate	12	s,b,l, p	—,H,O,—	Am J Chin Med
Margolin et al., 1993	Cocaine	32	s,l,f	—,H,O,I	NIDA Res Monogr (abstract)
Martinand Waite, 1981	Nicotine	405	s,b,r,l,p,c	—,H,O,I	N Z Med J
Milanov and Toteva, 1993	Alcohol	25	w,s,l	—,H,—,I	Am J Acupunct
Newmeyer et al., 1984	Opiates	460/297	s,l,c,f	—,—,O,—	J Psychoactive Drugs
Ng et al., 1975	Morphine	36	a,w,s,c	—,H,O,N/A	Am J Chin Med
Olms, 1984	Alcohol	34 cases	w,l	—,—,—,—	Am J Acupunct
Parker and Mok, 1977	Smoking	41	w,b,l,p,c,f	—,—,—,—	Am J Acupunct
Patterson, 1974	Multiple	40	w,l,f	—,—,—,—	Clin Med
Sacks, 1975	Multiple	187/642/150	Multiple case	—,—,—,—	Am J Acupunct
Sainsbury, 1974	Heroin	1	w, case	—,—,—,—	Med J Aust
Severson et al., 1977	Heroin	8	s,l,f	—,—,—,I	Int J Addictions
Shakur and Smith, 1979	Multiple	6	w, case	—,—,—,—	Am J Acupunct
Shuaib, 1976	Opium +	19	w, case	—,—,—,—	Am J Chin Med
Smith, 1988	Crack	1500	L	—,—,—,I	Am J Acupunct
Steiner et al., 1982	Nicotine	32	s,b,r,l,p	—,H,O,I	Am J Chin Med
Sween et al., 1996	Multiple	106	s,l,c	—,H,O,—	Presented at NADA Conference, May 24
Tan et al., 1987	Smoking	418	s,b,l,p,c	—,—,o,—	Am J Acupunct
Thorer and Volf, 1996	Alcohol	35	s,b,r,c	—,H,O,—	Presented at conference
Timofeev, 1994	Alcohol	48	s,l,f	—,—,—,—	Bull Exp Biol Med
Toteva and Milanov, 1996	Alcohol	118	w,s,r,l,c,f	—,H,O,I	Am J Acupunct
Washburn et al., 1993	Opiates/heroin	100	s,b,r,l,p	—,H,O,i	J Subst Abuse Treat
Washburn et al., 1990	Opiates	100	w,s,b,r,l,p	—,h,O,—	Multicultural Inquiry
	(3 studies)	123	demographic	—,—,O,—	Res Aids
		63	w,s,l,c,f	—,—,O,—	
Wells et al., 1995	Heroin/cocaine	60	w,s b,r,l,p,f	—,H,O,I	Am J Addictions
Wen and Cheung, 1973	Opiates	40	w,l,f	—,—,o,—	Asian J Med

Design key: a, Animal study; b, single blind; c, control group (other than placebo); f, follow-up; l, clinical; m, mechanism; p, placebo control; r, randomized; s, prospective; w, addresses active withdrawal.

Methods key: H, same type of statistic used with Ho; I, inclusion/exclusion criteria addressed; O, outcome measurements valid; Z, sample size appropriate (power calculated); N/A, not applicable; *lower case z, h, o, i*, same criteria but incomplete or inadequate.

Continued

TABLE 9-1	Studies of Acupuncture and the Addictions—cont'd				
Author, Year	Substance	Number	Design	Methods	Journal
Wen and Teo, 1975	Opiates	70 (f)	w,s,l,c,f	—,—,O,—	Modern Med Asia
Wen, 1977	Opiates	6	w,s,l	—,—,o,—	Modern Med Asia
Wen et al., 1978	Opiates	71	m,s,l,c	—,H,O,— -	Compar Med East West
Wen et al., 1978	Opiates	8 (f)	m,s,l	—,H,O,—	Bull Narc
Wen et al., 1979	Morphine	14	a, m,s,c	—,H,O,N/A	Am J Chin Med
Wen, 1980	Opiates	300	w,s,l,c,f	—,—,o,—	Am J Chin Med
Wen et al., 1980	Heroin	37	m,s,l,c	—,H,O,—	Am J Chin Med
Worner et al., 1992	Alcohol	56	s,r,l,c	—,H,O,I	Drug Alcohol Depend
Yang and Kwok, 1986	Morphine	119	a,w,s,c	—,H,O,N/A	Am J Chin Med
Zalessky et al., 1983	Nicotine	85	s,l,f	—,—,O,—	Int J Acupunct
					Electrotherapeutics Res

Design key: *a,* Animal study; *b,* single blind; *c,* control group (other than placebo); *f,* follow-up; *l,* clinical; *m,* mechanism; *p,* placebo control; *r,* randomized; *s,* prospective; *w,* addresses active withdrawal.
Methods key: *H,* same type of statistic used with Ho; *I,* inclusion/exclusion criteria addressed; *O,* outcome measurements valid; *Z,* sample size appropriate (power calculated); *N/A,* not applicable; *lower case z, h, o, i,* same criteria but incomplete or inadequate.

TABLE 9-2	Reviews of Acupuncture Studies	
Author, Year	**Topic**	**Substance**
Blum et al., 1978	Neurochemical mechanism	Opiates
Brewington et al., 1994	Review of efficacy	Multiple drugs
Brumbaugh, 1993	History and protocol	Multiple drugs
Brumbaugh, 1994	Summary of practice	Multiple drugs
Culliton and Kiresuk, 1996	General review; review of efficacy	Multiple drugs
Lipton and Maranda, 1983	Review of finding	Heroin
McLellan et al., 1993*	Research methodology	Multiple drugs
Mendelson, 1978	Hypothesis of mechanism	Alcohol and heroin
Ng, 1996	Review of 5 studies	Opiate
Omura, 1975	Presentation	Multiple drugs
Schwartz, 1988	Review of studies	Smoking
Sharps, 1977	Overview of history	Multiple drugs
Smith et al., 1982	Descriptive, Lincoln hospital acupuncture/addiction therapy program	
Smith and Kahn, 1988	General review	Multiple drugs
Ter Riet, et al., 1990†	Review of efficacy	Multiple drugs
Whitehead, 1978	Review of efficacy	Multiple drugs

Al studies are nonsystematic except the following: *Meeting summary and †Systematic.

sion criteria have been met, however, the process for NADA-style acupuncture is relatively uniform. Patients receive treatment in a group setting, seated in large chairs with arms and high backs to provide support if they fall asleep during the treatment. Subdued lighting, soft music, and caffeine-free herbal tea usually accompany the process. Both ears are swabbed with alcohol; then five half-inch, presterilized, disposable needles are placed in each ear. The NADA protocol uses the points Shen Men, sympathetic, kidney, liver, and lung (Fig. 9-1). For 40 minutes the participants sit back and relax while the treatment takes place. Eating, talking, and walking around are discouraged, and the acupuncturist keeps watch over the room to promote a state of safety and comfort. At the end of the session the needles are removed and placed in a biohazard container for proper disposal, and the ears are wiped with a dry cotton ball to protect against the rare occurrence of a drop or two of blood. Again varying from program to program, patient data collection may include an extensive history, various research instruments, and objective physiologic measures, but the standard requirement consists of a consent-to-treatment form and a precise record of date and number of treatments, symptoms, points used, and the response to the treatment. An acupuncturist or acupuncture detoxification specialist can treat several people within a short time, thereby creating a cost-efficient delivery system.

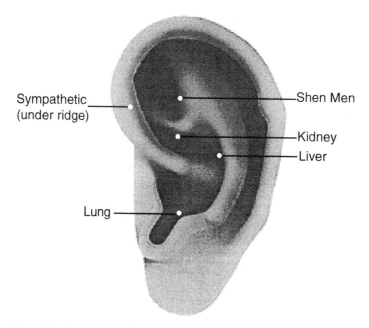

Fig. 9-1   The five points often used in ear acupuncture for the treatment of substance abuse. The points are bilateral, and variations can exist in either number or placement.

Key Concepts and Debates. The administration of acupuncture for the treatment of substance abuse has been standardized in the United States through the efforts of Michael Smith at Lincoln Hospital in New York City and, eventually, NADA. Acupuncture typically refers to five-point, bilateral acupuncture, in which five tiny needles are placed in the cartilage ridge and concha of each ear at the five points mentioned earlier. However, variations exist within practice and research and are discussed below.

Points Used. Although the number of points used in addiction treatment has been standardized in clinical practice, this has not always been the case in the research setting. Although popular among practitioners, the five-point, bilateral auricular protocol has typically been modified for research. The Bullock studies[24-26] have traditionally used a three-point protocol, and the Yale model incorporates four points. Ulett has advocated one-point protocols, claiming that multiple points complicate interpretation.[126] Although body points are often used in clinical practice, they are rarely used in research. The appropriate points to insert the needle may be located using a galvanometer, a machine that measures skin conductivity, but these devices have been criticized as inaccurate.[126] Practitioners typically locate points visually or by patient reaction such as sensitivity to pressure.

Stages of Intervention. In biomedicine, substance abuse intervention occurs in stages. The medications offered to help patients through the primary stages of withdrawal are not necessarily the same ones offered during rehabilitation or for relapse prevention. Acupuncture was initially applied during the detoxification stage to help patients through withdrawal. In the United States during the 1980s the use extended to rehabilitation and relapse prevention. However, research has not clearly demonstrated the effectiveness of acupuncture as defined by these stages of treatment.

Treatment Goals. Goals for acupuncture intervention may include decreased symptoms of withdrawal, relief from somatic symptoms, prevention of craving, increased treatment retention, hastened treatment readiness, improved quality of life, decreased substance use, and abstinence. These concepts may be measured in research using a variety of standardized instruments and laboratory testing.

Key Research Issues. A number of weaknesses frequently arise in substance abuse research,[36] particularly in studies employing acupuncture or other CAM methods. When designing a study, researchers often fail to differentiate between acceptable use and misuse of various substances. Although several standardized measurement tools exist, they are used infrequently or erratically in CAM research. In addition, the failure to recognize degrees of misuse often results in the inability to control for the "severity" of the addiction.

Comparison and control groups have often been inappropriate or absent from substance abuse and CAM research.[36] In acupuncture research there has been considerable debate over the use of sham or placebo treatments as controls. The five-point auricular acupuncture protocol generally has not been used in research because of the controversy over identifying an inactive placebo. Most acupuncturists believe that the puncturing of the ears by 10 or more needles could cause a generalized treatment effect by virtue of neurotransmitter mediation, regardless of their specific location. As stated earlier, the Minneapolis group has typically used three points, while the Yale group has settled on four in their acupuncture controlled studies. Whether auricular sham points constitute an adequate placebo is unknown, although preliminary research has been conducted.[7]

Success for the treatment of substance abuse has been measured using a variety of measures including abstinence, decreased use, decreased cravings, diminished withdrawal symptoms, improved outlook, and increased productivity. These variations often make studies difficult to evaluate or compare. One research group may report its intervention as successful because consumption was significantly reduced even though the majority of subjects relapsed, while another group may evaluate similar findings as a treatment failure. Data may actually be misleading if subjects who dropped out of treatment prematurely were excluded from the analysis.

Acupuncture research, in particular, has been criticized for its lack of clinical relevancy. The number and placement of needles used in research may differ from those used in a clinical setting, as may the environment and the therapist interaction with the subject. Critics suggest that findings from this sort of research cannot be generalized to the clinical setting.

Heroin and Opiates

Acupuncture. Early research applying acupuncture for the treatment of substance use disorders was conducted in China on patients going through opiate withdrawal. In 1973, Wen and Cheung[222] noticed that opium-addicted patients receiving ear accupuncture (EA) as a presurgical analgesic reported reduced withdrawal symptoms. Wen and others conducted a number of studies on humans and animals (Table 9-1) and, despite debatable methods, made important distinctions between craving and abstinence and between detoxification and subsequent rehabilitation.[220,222,223]

Animal studies have generally reported positive findings for the treatment of opiate withdrawal, usually morphine.[30,73,114,140] Treatment of animals has focused on EA. The administration of EA in female WHT mice and Sprauge-Dawley rats has been reported to reduce opiate withdrawal symptoms such as wet dog shakes, teeth chattering, diarrhea, and abnormal posturing. Furthermore, preliminary animal research indicates that increases in plasma ACTH during withdrawal may be reduced during EA. The majority of human studies regarding EA and opiate withdrawal suffer from inadequate methodology. Despite clinical reports and preliminary trials which suggest that EA decreases the symptoms and duration of withdrawal,[221-223] the efficacy of EA for the treatment of opiate withdrawal remains unknown. Studies focused on opiate addictions that claim stronger research designs have used standardized auricular acupuncture rather than EA.[216,218] Furthermore, these studies have focused on relapse prevention rather than withdrawal. At this time, there is no evidence that acupuncture is effective in the prevention of relapse for the treatment of opiates.[20]

Other CAM Therapies. Other CAM therapies (Table 9-3) have been used for the treatment of opiates, although in most cases efficacy has not been consistently shown. Therapies include biofeedback,[4,21] yoga,[178] neuroelectric transcranial stimulation (NET),* transcendental meditation (TM),[56,142,147] nutrition,[12,133] and hallucinogens.[70,125,162,183]

Alcohol

Alcohol addiction has been treated by means of a wide variety of CAM therapies. However, two therapies stand out in both popular and academic literature. Acupuncture and nutrition therapies both have received a significant amount of attention. Nutrition programs have not attained the same level of standardization as acupuncture programs, nor is there a governing body comparable to NADA. However, the American Dietetic Association has issued a position statement that nutritional supplements, mod-

---

*References 3, 44, 45, 54, 62, 65, 80, 151, 152.

TABLE 9-3	CAM Therapies for the Treatment of Opiate Misuse
Therapy and Reference(s)	**Conclusion**
Biofeedback	
Brinkman, 1978	Positive
Fahrion, 1995	Positive
Yoga	
Shaffer, Lasalvia, 1997	Negative
Neuroelectric Therapy	
Alling et al., 1990	Inconclusive
Ellision et al., 1987	Positive
Elmoghazy et al., 1989	Positive
Gariti et al., 1992	Negative
Gomez and Mikhail, 1978	Positive
Gossop et al., 1984	Negative
Jarzembski, 1985	Inconclusive
Patterson et al., 1993	Positive
Patterson et al., 1994	Positive
Transcendental Meditation	
Gelderloos et al., 1991	Positive
O'Connell and Alexander, 1995	Positive
Orme-Johnson and Farrow, 1977	Positive
Nutrition	
Beckley-Barrett, Mutch, 1990	Positive
Mohs et al., 1990	N/A
Hallucinogens	
Halpern 1996	Inconclusive
McKenna 1996	Inconclusive
Popik et al., 1995	Inconclusive
Sheppard 1994	Positive

ified diets, and nutritional education can improve the efficacy of chemical dependency treatment.[12]

Acupuncture. Alcohol addiction was first treated with EA at Lincoln Hospital in New York. However, EA was replaced by auricular acupuncture when clinicians observed no difference between the two methods. Treatment standardization was motivated by early clinical findings,[179,186,189,190] resulting in the four- to five-point protocols discussed earlier. Research has predominantly focused on human populations.

Although several controlled studies have been published, few meet the standards of methodologic rigor. To date, the studies of Bullock et al.[24,26] have been the most rigorous and most frequently cited. In both studies persons with chronic alcoholism were assigned to either true or sham acupuncture. The true-acupuncture group showed significantly decreased drinking episodes and desire to drink and fewer treatment readmissions than placebo controls. In the second study significant effects were maintained through the 6-month follow-up: the placebo control group had more than twice the number of drinking episodes and readmissions to detoxification centers (Tables 9-4 and 9-5).

Two controlled studies (Worner et al.[233] and Toteva and Milanov[208]) have been touted as replications of the studies of Bullock et al. cited earlier. However, numerous differences in both protocol and methodology make comparison difficult. Toteva and Milanov reported statistically significant differences in the treatment group compared with controls on some measures, including an increased rate of treatment retention and increased abstinence. However, Worner et al. reported no statistically significant differences in rates of relapse or treatment retention between the groups.[36]

The first large-scale, randomized, controlled trial for the treatment of alcoholism is ongoing by our group at Hennepin County Medical Center in Minneapolis and funded by the National Institute of Alcohol Abuse and Alcoholism. This trial is also concerned with clinically relevant models of delivery. In addition to a standardized four-point research protocol, other therapeutic elements are introduced into one of the study arms, including body points based on individual symptoms, music, dim lighting, and conversation.

Nutrition. More than 20 studies have been published on the efficacy of nutrition therapies for the treatment of alcoholism.[11,67,122,228] Poor methodology and the lack of a standardized treatment protocol make evaluation of these studies difficult. We have singled out seven studies (five in animals and two in humans) for inclusion in this chapter. Overall, despite difficulties in reporting, follow-up, or statistical power, the methodology of these studies is of higher quality.

An early study conducted by Rogers et al.[169] divided 50 Wistar rats into six groups. Each rat in five of the groups received 100 mg a day of either glutamine, glutamic acid, sodium glutamate, asparagine, or glycine. A sixth group received no supplements and served as control. The glutamine group significantly decreased their alcohol consumption. The other five groups increased their consumption but, when the supplemented groups were compared with controls, the increases were not significant.

Register et al.[167] compared the free-choice consumption of Sprague-Dawley rats that were fed six different diets designed to mimic human diets. A "teen-age" type of diet—with poor nutritional content—was administered to five groups. Some of the groups also received a spice mixture, a regular coffee mixture, decaffeinated coffee, a vitamin and mineral supplement, or a combination of these. The sixth group received an optimal diet. The rats fed the teen-age diet showed a progressive preference for

TABLE 9-4	Completion Rates for Each Treatment Phase	
	No. of Patients (%)	
Treatment Phase	Treatment Group (N = 40)	Control Group (N = 40)
I	37 (92.5)	21 (52.5)
II	26 (65.0)	3 (7.5)
III	21 (52.5)	1 (2.5)

From Bullock ML, Culliton PD, Olander RT: Controlled trial of acupuncture for severe recidivist alcoholism, *Lancet* 1(8652):1436, 1989.
$p < 0.001$ for the difference between the completion rate for each phase.

TABLE 9-5	Admissions to the Detoxification Center During Follow-Up Intervals			
	No. of Admissions*		Mean (SEM) No. of Admissions	
Follow-Up Interval	Treatment Group	Control Group	Treatment Group	Control Group
One month[†]	25	59	0.62 (0.20)	1.54 (0.32)
Three months[‡]	24	65	0.59 (0.17)	1.67 (0.42
Six months[‡]	26	62	0.69 (0.41)	1.56 (0.20)

From Bullock ML, Culliton PD, Olander RT: Controlled trial of acupuncture for severe recidivist alcoholism, *Lancet* 1(8652):1436, 1989.
*Total = 75 for treatment group and 186 for control group.
[†]$p < 0.01$.
[‡]$p < 0.05$.

drinking the alcohol solution. Caffeine also appeared to be a powerful inducer of free-choice consumption, whereas the spice mixture had no impact. Vitamin and mineral supplements did result in significantly reduced alcohol intake.

A link between thiamin deficiency and alcohol intake and metabolism was identified.[46,154] In a controlled trial, Eriksson et al.[46] noted that thiamin deficiency increased free-choice consumption in a mixed strain of rat derived from Wistar, Sprague-Dawley, and Long-Evans rats. High-thiamin, thiamin-deficient, and optimal-nutrition groups were given either water or ethanol during the first 4 weeks of research. During the last 3 weeks the alcohol-only group was given the choice between alcohol or water. Throughout the study the high-thiamin group drank significantly less alcohol than appropriate controls. However, the thiamin-deficient group did not clearly drink more alcohol unless consumption was related to the total energy or fluid intake during the free-choice period.

Pekkanen[154] induced thiamin deficiency in three ways: by means of diet or by the injection of one of two thiamin antagonists. Results of this controlled study indicated that the increase in ethanol intake is related to the roles of thiamin in the brain rather than a reduction in food intake.

Collipp et al.[33] reported on three experiments performed on zinc-deficient and pair-fed Sprague-Dawley rats. Zinc deficiency did increase the voluntary intake of ethanol, which was statistically significant in the first (body weight, 58 to 81 g) and third (body weight, 120 to 199 g) experiments. After 6 weeks of the deficient diet, the percentage of alcohol consumed declined when a normal diet was administered.

Blum et al.[16] have conducted a series of trials on amino acid supplements for a variety of substance use disorders. Supplements are designed to restore brain neurotransmitter balance, increasing the availability of enkaphalin in the brain, as well as levels of dopamine, norepinephine, serotonin, brain gamma-aminobutyric acid (GABA), and aminergic neurotransmitters. Results of a trial (N = 62) showed significant improvement in retention, stress reduction, and ease of detoxification compared with placebos.

Gallimberti et al.[53] studied the impact of gamma-hydroxybutyric acid (GHB) on ethanol withdrawal. Despite a limited number of subjects (N = 23), in this double-blind trial GHB was superior to placebo in reducing symptoms of alcohol withdrawal, such as tremors, sweating, nausea, depression, anxiety, and restlessness.

Studies indicate that a variety of nutritional supplements and programs hold promise for the treatment of alcohol addiction and withdrawal. However, for the most part research has been piecemeal and methodologically unsound. Strategic planning and some standardization of outcome measures are necessary if future research is to have a significant impact on the treatment of addictions.

Other complementary/alternative medicine therapies. Numerous CAM methods have been used for the treatment of alcohol abuse and dependence (Table 9-6). Available literature reveals that the majority of studies conducted on the use of other CAM therapies are preliminary, often with inadequate sample size, follow-up, measures, or controls. Despite the bulk of research conducted on some methods, treatment protocols vary to such a degree that results are not comparable. For example, more than 20 different protocols could be employed when treating addictive disorders with hypnosis, with therapists focusing on such features as reduced urge, symptom substitution, or cue sensitization.[84] Outcome measures may include abstinence, reduction in use, decreased cravings or symptoms of withdrawal, improved mood states or treatment retention, and increased productivity. Furthermore, the number of sessions and duration of treatment may vary, making it difficult to generalize findings even when the outcome measures are comparable. Therefore, whether the majority of studies report positive (biofeedback,* prayer,[129,130,135,158] light therapy,[42,124,160,172] and herbs†), negative (hypnosis‡), or inconclusive (hallucinogens§), outcomes, little can be said about the efficacy of these methods for the reasons listed above.

Methodologic problems such as inadequate statistical analysis, inclusion/exclusion criteria, handling of dropouts, and reliability and validity of measurement tools reduce our confidence in other findings (prayer,[129,130,135,158] yoga,[13,137] NET,[151,152,191] TM,[56,142,147] restricted environmental stimulation therapy [REST],[18,34,166] and relaxation[204]). Furthermore, despite clinical use, a few therapies have not been researched at all for the treatment of addictions (eye movement desensitization and reprocessing [EMDR[181]], homeopathy, and aromatherapy).

Cocaine

Acupuncture. Cocaine is included in this chapter because of its widespread use and abuse potential. At present there are no known, effective treatments for cocaine dependence. Although the crack cocaine epidemic helped open doorways to acupuncture as a treatment method, little has been done to study the application of acupuncture or other CAM methods to this disorder. While clinical and case reports have shown promise for the treatment of craving and depression and for promoting abstinence,[8,117,118] randomized, controlled trials have failed to replicate these positive findings.

Lipton et al.[106] randomly assigned 192 patients to true or sham four-point auricular treatment. Forty-two patients were excluded from analysis, and only 30 patients completed 2 or more weeks of treatment. Although there was a significant group by time in treatment interaction, there was no difference in treatment retention or self-report.

Recently Bullock et al.[25] conducted two linked but concurrent studies of three-point auricular acupuncture in the treatment of cocaine addiction. The first study (N = 236) randomly assigned residential clients to true, sham, or conventional treatment. The second (N = 202) applied true five-point acupuncture to randomly selected day-treatment clients at three dose levels (8, 16, or 28 treatments). The study failed to confirm the efficacy of acupuncture for the treatment of cocaine addiction. Overall, significant differences were not found between the true, sham, psychosocial, and dose-response groups on any outcomes, including retention, abstinence, and mood states. However, the authors suggested that the lack of a no-treatment control may have masked treatment effects. The standardized method of treatment, rather than an individualized approach, may also have influenced the results of the study.

---

*References 37, 38, 48, 49, 155, 156, 157, 204, and 217.
†References 87 to 91, 105, 148, 159, 180, and 235.
‡References 43, 84, 97, 102, 192, 197, and 214.
§References 70, 112, 125, 162, 168, and 183.

TABLE 9-6	CAM Therapies for Treatment of Alcohol Misuse
Therapy and Reference	**Conclusion**
Hypnosis	
Edwards, 1966	Negative
Jacobson et al., 1973	Negative
Katz, 1980	Inconclusive
Lenox and bonny, 1976	N/A
Smith-Moorhouse, 1969	Positive
Stoil, 1989	Inconclusive
Wadden, Penrod, 1981	Inconclusive
Biofeedback	
DeGood and Vallee, 1978	N/A
Denney et al., 1991	Positive
Fahrion et al., 1992	Positive
Fahrion, 1995	Positive
Peniston et al., 1993	Positive
Peniston, Kulkosky, 1990	Positive
Peniston, 1989	Positive
Taub et al., 1994	Positive
Weingarten et al., 1980	N/A
REST	
Borrie, 1990	Positive
Cooper et al., 1988	Positive
Rank, Suedfeld, 1978	Positive
Prayer	
Miller, 1990	Positive
Miller, 1997	Positive
Muffler et al., 1997	Positive
Peteet, 1993	Positive
Yoga	
Benson, 1969	Positive
Nespor and Cs-Emy, 1994	Positive
NET	
Patterson et al., 1993	Positive
Patterson et al., 1994	Positive
Smith, O'Neill, 1975	Inconclusive

EMDR, Eye movement desensitization and reprocessing; *NET,* neuroelectric therapy; *REST,* restricted environmental stimulation therapy.

TABLE 9-6	CAM Therapies for Treatment of Alcohol Misuse—cont'd
Therapy and Reference	**Conclusion**

Transcendental Meditation	
Gelderloos et al., 1991	Positive
O'Connell, Alexander, 1995	Positive
Orme-Johnson, Farrow, 1977	Positive
Herbs	
Keung, 1993	Positive
Keung, Vallee, 1993 (Part I)	Positive
Keung, Vallee, 1993 (Part II)	Positive
Keung, Vallee, 1994	Positive
Keung et al., 1995	Positive
Li-li et al., 1985	Positive
Overstreet et al., 1996	Positive
Petri and Takach, 1990	Positive
Shanmugasundaram et al., 1986	Positive
Xie et al., 1994	Positive
EMDR	
Shapiro et al., 1994	Positive
Light Therapy	
Eastwood, Stiasny, 1978	Inconclusive
Poikolainen, 1982	Inconclusive
McGrath, Yahia, 1993	Positive
Satel, Gawin, 1989	Positive
Hallucinogens	
Halpern, 1996	Positive
Ludwig et al., 1970	Negative
McKenna, 1996	Inconclusive
Popik et al., 1995	Inconclusive
Rezvani et al., 1995	Positive
Sheppard, 1994	Inconclusive
Relaxation	
Taub et al., 1994	Negative

Other CAM Therapies. A few other methods have been used in clinical settings for the treatment of cocaine abuse and addiction (Table 9-7). With the exception of hallucinogens, for which the literature is mostly inconclusive,[125,162,176] the findings of preliminary studies have been positive. However, methodologic problems including inadequate controls, a lack of statistical analysis, absence of follow-up data, and failure to use standardized measurement tools, along with variations in treatment protocol, reduce our confidence in the validity of these findings (TM,[56,142,147] NET,[54,151,152] nutrition,[12,17,76,133] herbs[210]).

Nicotine

Hypnosis. The American Medical Association has approved hypnosis as a valid medical treatment; thus clinicians have applied hypnosis for the treatment of numerous symptoms, including the treatment of nicotine addiction. Like nutrition therapies, hypnotic procedures have not been standardized for the treatment of addictions, and

TABLE 9-7	CAM Therapies for the Treatment of Cocaine Misuse
Therapy and Reference	**Author's Conclusion**
Transcendental Meditation	
O'Connell, Alexander, 1995	Positive
Gelderloos et al., 1991	Positive
Orme-Johnson, Farrow, 1977	Positive
Nutrition	
Beckley-Barrett, Mutch, 1990	Positive
Blum et al., 1988	Positive
Horne, 1988	Positive
Mohs et al., 1990	N/A
Herbs	
Upton, 1994	Positive
Hallucinogens	
McKenna, 1996	Inconclusive
Popik et al., 1995	Inconclusive
Sershen et al., 1994	Positive
Neuroelectric Therapy	
Gariti et al., 1992	Negative
Patterson et al., 1993	Positive
Patterson et al., 1994	Positive

patients may be exposed to any of 20 or more strategies.[84] Although the mechanism is unknown, a number of physiologic changes take place during hypnosis. Memory, cognition, perception, and physiology may be altered in susceptible subjects. Hypnosis may reduce sympathetic nervous system activity, oxygen consumption and carbon dioxide elimination; lower blood pressure and heart rate; and increase activity in certain kinds of brain waves.[195]

Although preliminary findings have been promising, studies have been repeatedly criticized for lack of commonality, insufficient data reporting, lack of proper control groups, and inadequate follow-up procedures.[75,84,98] Results of controlled trials vary significantly, with rates of abstinence ranging from 4% to 88%. Higher success rates seem linked to a number of factors, such as longer sessions, a greater number of sessions, the presence of adjunctive treatment, and suggestions tailored to patient goals and fears rather than standardized suggestions.[75]

Lambe et al.[99] conducted a randomized, controlled trial (N = 180) and reported a 21% abstinence rate for the treatment group compared with 6% of controls. At 6 months the rates were 21% and 22%, respectively. However, these statistics are inflated, since 50% of the hypnosis group dropped out of the study after randomization and were apparently excluded from the analysis rather than included as treatment failures.

Other CAM Therapies. Several other therapies have been used to treat addiction to nicotine (Table 9-8). The efficacy of acupuncture has been assessed in a number of trials*; however, reviews of this literature have evaluated findings as either negative or inconclusive.[20,205] REST also deserves mention. Numerous studies have reported reduction in use and improvements in mode states for chamber REST, although the methods used have not been ideal.[10,198-200] For cocaine, overall, the findings of preliminary studies have been positive, but small sample size, inadequate data handling and analysis, lack of follow-up, inadequate controls, failure to randomly select subjects or to report inclusion/exclusion criteria, and variations in treatment protocol reduce our confidence in the validity of these findings (nutrition,[12,41,133] massage,[71] light therapy,[39] TM,[56,142,147] biofeedback,[37,48] relaxation[207,234]).

Hallucinogens

As stated earlier, chronic abuse of hallucinogens is not typically treated by addiction medicine programs. Treatment for the abuse of hallucinogens has focused primarily on withdrawal. Overall, the abuse of hallucinogens has not been a focal point for CAM treatments. However, there is limited evidence that flotation REST may help alleviate the symptoms of withdrawal and diminish the psychotic-like symptoms of people who have taken phencyclidine (PCP) or lysergic acid diethylamide (LSD).[18]

---

*References 29, 31, 35, 57, 100, 111, 113, 121, 196.

TABLE 9-8	CAM Therapies for the Treatment of Nicotine Misuse	
Therapy and Reference(s)	**Conclusion**	

Acupuncture

Brewington et al., 1994	Negative
Choy et al., 1983	Positive
Clavel, Benhamon, 1985	Negative
Cottraux et al., 1983	Negative
Gillams et al., 1984	Negative
Lamontagne et al., 1980	Negative
Low, 1977	Positive
Machovec, Man, 1978	Negative
Martin, Waite, 1981	Negative
Steiner et al., 1982	Negative
Ter Reit et al., 1990	Negative

REST

Barabasz et al., 1986	Positive
Suedfeld, Ikard, 1974	Positive
Suedfeld et al., 1972	Positive
Suedfeld, 1990	Positive

Nutrition

Beckley-Barrett, Mutch, 1990	Positive
Douglass et al., 1985	Positive
Mohs et al., 1990	N/A

Massage

Hernandez-Reif et al., 1993*	Positive

Light therapy

Dilsaver et al., 1987	Positive

Transcendental meditation

Gelderloos et al., 1991	Positive
O'Connell, Alexander, 1995	Positive
Orme-Johnson, Farrow, 1977	Positive

Biofeedback

DeGood and Vallee, 1978	N/A
Fahrion, 1995	Positive

Relaxation

Surawy and Cox, 1986	N/A
Wynd, 1992	Positive

REST, Restricted environmental stimulation therapy.

Hallucinogens present a special case in the field of CAM, since attention has focused on these drugs as potential treatments for alcohol and drug disorders rather than as agents of abuse. The two drugs that have received the most attention are LSD and ibogaine. LSD affects serotonin receptors, and advocates believe it to be an effective anticraving agent. However, despite the positive findings of case studies, a review of controlled studies suggests that LSD is not an effective treatment for alcoholism.[112]

Ibogaine, a stimulant with hallucinogenic properties at high doses, is an N-methyl-D-aspartate (NMDA) antagonist. Preliminary data indicate efficacy in attenuating the development of tolerance and in decreasing the symptoms of dependence. Ibogaine is available at treatment centers in several European countries; however, no controlled clinical data are available on the use of ibogaine for the treatment of addictions. Ibogaine is listed as a Schedule I substance in the United States and therefore is not available for uses other than research.[162,168,183]

Benzodiazepines and Amphetamines

The only controlled trial that has been conducted using CAM for the treatment of benzodiazepine withdrawal studied relaxation and electromyogram biofeedback.[136] Although the trial was controlled, the sample size was seven. Findings were reportedly negative, although follow-up was only conducted for the relaxation group.

Acupuncture has been used for the treatment of both benzodiazepine and methamphetamine addictions. Although several clinical studies are under way, no solid data are available.

THE FUTURE OF CAM AND SUBSTANCE MISUSE

CAM seems destined to lose its distinct identity within the realm of behavioral interventions for the treatment of addictions. Although considered CAM in other fields of medicine, spirituality and prayer have become mainstream in the treatment of addictions as the foundation for the majority of 12-step programs. With the rise of drug courts throughout the United States and walk-in detoxification programs, acupuncture seems destined to take a similar path. Furthermore, consumer interest in CAM appears to be increasing the popularity of a number of methods such as nutrition.

Despite the increasing integration of CAM with behavioral treatments, the divide between pharmacologically based addiction medicine programs and psychosocial chemical dependency treatment programs is expanding. Researchers and clinicians have begun to encourage patients to use pharmacologic and behavioral treatments in conjunction with each other. Yet, methadone maintenance and other addiction medicine programs often provide limited psychosocial support, while psychosocial programs may not offer pharmacologic therapies. Insurance and consumer dollars have been targeted at psychosocial treatment, whereas research dollars have been filtered into drug trials, certainly reinforcing the division between addiction medicine programs and chemical dependency treatment programs.

SUMMARY

The lack of sound research hinders our ability to make clinical recommendations regarding CAM and substance misuse. However, at present it seems reasonable to say that acupuncture is safe and cost-effective, and may be helpful in the treatment of addictions. Several nutritional therapies, such as zinc supplements, glutamine, and healthful diets, have shown positive trends in preliminary laboratory tests, as have a number of other methods (Tables 9-3 and 9-6 to 9-8). High-quality research is needed to further our understanding both of CAM and of the physiology of addictions.

Because chemical dependency treatment centers and addiction medicine clinics have been unable to find reliable "magic bullet" treatments, new methods to help clients with detoxification, relapse prevention, symptom relief, treatment readiness, and retention are needed. The integration of CAM could potentially increase the treatment arsenal. Federal funding for CAM research has been increasingly available, and the recent creation of the Office of Alternative Medicine provides a central location for information and assistance. Thus opportunities for addiction researchers interested in CAM have increased. With the proper research and guidance, the future of CAM therapies for the treatment of addiction holds promise.

REFERENCES

1. Ades J, Lejoyeux M: Clinical evaluation of acamprosate to reduce alcohol intake, *Alcohol and Alcoholism Supplement* 2:275, 1993.
2. Allen J: Overview of alcoholism treatment: settings and approaches, *J Mental Health Admin* 16(2):5562, 1989.
3. Alling FA, Johnson BD, Elmoghazy E: Cranial electrostimulation (CES) use in the detoxification of opiate-dependent patients, *J Subst Abuse Treatment* 7:173, 1990.
4. Annis HM: Is inpatient rehabilitation of the alcoholic cost effective? con position, *Adv Alcohol Subst Abuse* 1-2:175, 1985.
5. Anton RF, Kranzler HR, Meyer RE: Neurobehavioral aspects of the pharmacotherapy of alcohol dependence, *Clin Neurosci* 3:145, 1995.
6. Aubin HJ, Soyka M: 1996. Acamprosate in clinical practice: the French experience. Acamprosate in relapse prevention of alcoholism: Proceedings of the First CAMPRAL Symposium ESBRA, Stuttgart, Germany, September 1995. Springer-Verlag Berlin Heidelberg, pp. 111-119.
7. Avants SK, Margolin A, Chang P et al: Acupuncture for the treatment of cocaine addiction, *J Subst Abuse Treatm* 12(3):195, 1995.
8. Avants SK, Margolin A, Kosten TR: Cocaine abuse in methadone maintenance programs: integrating pharmacotherapy with psychosocial interventions, *J Psychoactive Drugs* 26(2):137, 1994.
9. Babor T: Social, scientific and medical issues in the definition of alcohol and drug dependence. In Edwards G, Lader M: *The nature of drug dependence,* monograph (Society for the Study of Addictions), New York, 1990, Oxford University Press, pp. 19-40.
10. Barabasz AF, Baer L, Sheehan DV, Barabasz M: A three-year follow-up of hypnosis and restricted environmental stimulation therapy for smoking, *Int J Clin Exper Hypnosis* 34(3):169, 1986.
11. Beasley JD, Grimson RC, Bicker AA, et al: Follow-up of a cohort of alcoholic patients through 12 months of comprehensive biobehavioral treatment, *J Subst Abuse Treatm* 8(3):133, 1991.
12. Beckley-Barrett LM, Mutch PB: Position of the American Dietetic Association: nutrition intervention in treatment and recovery from chemical dependency, *ADA Reports* 90(9):1274, 1990.

13. Benson H: Yoga for drug abuse, *N Engl J Med* 281(20):1133, 1969.
14. Berg BJ, Volpicelli JR, Alterman AI, O'Brien C: The relationship between endogenous opioids and alcohol drinking: the opioid compensation hypothesis. In Naranjo CA, Sellars EM, editors: *Novel pharmacological interventions for alcoholism*, New York, 1991, Springer-Verlag.
15. Blum K, Newmeyer JA, Whitehead C: Acupuncture as a common mode of treatment for drug dependence: possible neurochemical mechanisms, *J Psychedelic Drugs* 10(2):105, 1978.
16. Blum K, Trachtenberg MC, Ramsay JC: Improvement of inpatient treatment of the alcoholic as a function of neurotransmitter restoration: a pilot study, *Int J Addictions* 23(9):991, 1988.
17. Blum K et al: Enkephalinase inhibition and precursor amino acid loading improves inpatient treatment of alcohol and polydrug abusers: double-blind placebo-controlled study of the nutritional adjunct SAAVE, *Alcohol* 5(6):481, 1988.
18. Borrie RA: The use of restricted environmental stimulation therapy in treating addictive behaviors, *Int J Addictions* 25(7A-8A):995, 1990.
19. Brady K: Prevalence, consequences and costs of tobacco, drug and alcohol use in the United States: training about alcohol and substance abuse for all primary care physicians. In Circa CM, editor: Proceedings of a Conference Sponsored by the Josiah Macy, Jr. Foundation, October 2-5, 1994, Phoenix.
20. Brewington V, Smith M, Lipton D: Acupuncture as a detoxification treatment: an analysis of controlled research, *J Subst Abuse Treatm* 11(4):289, 1994.
21. Brinkman DN: Biofeedback application to drug addiction in the University of Colorado drug rehabilitation program, *Int J Addictions* 13(5):817, 1978.
22. Brumbaugh AG: Acupuncture: new perspectives in chemical dependency treatment, *J Subst Abuse Treatm* 10(1):35, 1993.
23. Brumbaugh AG: Acupuncture. In Miller NS, editor: *Principles of Addiction Medicine*, Chevy Chase, Md, 1994, ASAM.
24. Bullock ML, Culliton PD, Olander RT: Controlled trial of acupuncture for severe recidivist alcoholism, *Lancet* 1(8652):1435, 1989.
25. Bullock ML, Kiresuk TJ, Pheley AM, et al: Auricular acupuncture in the treatment of cocaine abuse, *J Subst Abuse Treatm*, in press.
26. Bullock ML, Umen AJ, Culliton PD, Olander RT: Acupuncture treatment of alcoholic recidivism: a pilot study, *Alcoholism Clin Exper Res* 11(3):292, 1987.
27. Chappel J: Long-term recovery from alcoholism, *Rec Adv Addictive Disord* 16(1):177, 1993.
28. Chick J: Acamprosate as an aid in the treatment of alcoholism, *Alcohol Alcoholism* 30(6):785, 1995.
29. Choy DS, Lutzker L, Meltzer L: Effective treatment for smoking cessation, *Am J Med* 75(6):1033, 1983.
30. Choy YM, Tso WW, Fung KP, et al: Suppression of narcotic withdrawals and plasma ACTH by auricular electroacupuncture, *Biochem Biophys Res Comm* 82(1):305, 1978.
31. Clavel F, Benhamou S: Helping people to stop smoking: randomised comparison of groups being treated with acupuncture and nicotine gum with control group, *Br Med J* 291:1538, 1985.
32. Clement-Jones V, Mcloughlin L, Lowry PJ, et al: Acupuncture in heroin addicts: changes in met-enkephalin and β-endorphin in blood and cerebrospinal fluid, *Lancet* 2(8139):380, 1979.
33. Collipp PJ, Kris VK, Castro-Magana M, et al: The effects of dietary zinc deficiency on voluntary alcohol drinking in rats, *Alcoholism* 8(6):556, 1984.
34. Cooper GD, Adams HB, Scott JC: Studies in reduced environmental stimulation therapy (REST) and reduced alcohol consumption, *J Subst Abuse Treatm* 5(2):61, 1988.
35. Cottraux JA, Harf R, Boissel JP, et al: Smoking cessation with behaviour therapy or acupuncture: a controlled study, *Behav Res Ther* 21(4):417, 1983.
36. Culliton P, Kiresuk T: Overview of substance abuse acupuncture treatment research, *J Alternat Compl Med* 2(1):149, 1996.
37. Degood DE, Valle RS: Self-reported alcohol and nicotine use and the ability to control occipital EEG in a biofeedback situation, *Addictive Behav* 3:13, 1978.
38. Denney MR, Baugh JL, Hardt HD: Sobriety outcome after alcoholism treatment with biofeedback participation: a pilot inpatient study, *Int J Addict* 26(3):335, 1991.
39. Dilsaver SC, Majchrzak MJ: Bright artificial light produces subsensitivity to nicotine, *Life Sci* 42:225, 1988.

40. Donovan DM, Marlatt GA: Behavioral treatment. In Galanter M, editor: *Recent developments in alcoholism*, vol 11, Ten years of progress, New York, 1993, Plenum Press, pp. 397-411.

41. Douglass JM, Rasgon IM, Fleiss PM, et al: Effects of a raw food diet on hypertension and obesity, *South Med J* 78(7):841, 1985.

42. Eastwood MR, Stiasny LS: Psychiatric disorder, hospital admission and season, *Arch Gen Psychiatr* 35:769, 1978.

43. Edwards G: Hypnosis in treatment of alcohol addiction: controlled trial, with analysis of factors affecting outcome, *Q J Stud Alcohol* 27(2):221, 1966.

44. Ellison F, Ellison W, Daulonded JP, Daubech JF: Opiate withdrawal and electrostimulation: double blind experiment, *L'Encephale* 13:225, 1987.

45. Elmoghazy EE, Johnson BD, Alling FA: A pilot study of a neurostimulator device vs. methadone in alleviating opiate withdrawal symptoms: problems of drug dependence (NIDA Research Monograph No. 95) Rockville, Md, 1989, National Institute of Drug Abuse, pp. 388-389.

46. Eriksson K, Pekkanen L, Rusi M: The effects of dietary thiamin on voluntary ethanol drinking and ethanol metabolism in the rat, *Br J Nutr* 43(1):1, 1980.

47. Facchinetti F, Petraglia F, Nappi G, et al: Functional opioid activity varies according to the different fashion of alcohol abuse, *Substance Alcohol Actions Misuse* 5:6, 1985.

48. Fahrion SL: Human potential and personal transformation, *Subtle Energies* 6(1):55, 1995.

49. Fahrion SL, Walters ED, Coyne L, Allen T: Alterations in EEG amplitude, personality factors and brain electrical mapping after alpha-theta brainwave training: a controlled case study of an alcoholic in recovery, *Alcoholism Clin Exper Res* 16(3):547, 1992.

50. Froelich JC: Genetic factors in alcohol self-administration, *J Clin Psychiatr* 56(suppl 7):15, 1995.

51. Fuller JA: Smoking withdrawal and acupuncture, *Med J Austral* 1(1):28, 1982.

52. Fuller RK, Branchey L, Brightwell DR, et al: Disulfiram treatment of alcoholism: a VA cooperative study, *JAMA* 11:1449, 1986.

53. Gallimberti L, Canton G, Gentile N, et al: Gamma-hydroxybutyric acid for treatment of alcohol withdrawal syndrome, *Lancet* 2(8666):787, 1989.

54. Gariti P, Auriacombe M, Incmikoski R, et al: A randomized double-blind study of neuroelectric therapy in opiate and cocaine detoxification, *J Subst Abuse* 4(3):299, 1992.

55. Gawin FH: Chronic neuropharmacology of cocaine: progress in pharmacotherapy, *J Clin Psychiatr* 49(suppl):11, 1988.

56. Gelderloos P, Walton KG, Orme-Johnson D, Alexander CN: Effectiveness of the transcendental meditation program in preventing and treating substance misuse: a review, *Int J Addictions* 26(3):293, 1991.

57. Gillams J, Lewith GT, Machin D: Acupuncture and group therapy in stopping smoking, *Practitioner* 228:341, 1984.

58. Glynn TJ, Greenwald P, Mills SM, Manley MW: Youth tobacco use in the United States: problem, progress, goals and potential solutions, *Prev Med* 22(4):568, 1993.

59. Gold MS: Cocaine (and crack): clinical aspects. In Lowinson JH, Ruiz P, Millman RB, Langrod JG, editors: *Substance abuse: a comprehensive textbook*, ed 3, Baltimore, 1997, Williams & Wilkins, pp. 181-198.

60. Gold MS, Miller NS: Cocaine (and crack): neurobiology. In Lowinson JH, Ruiz P, Millman RB, Langrod JG, editors: *Substance abuse: a comprehensive textbook*, ed 3, Baltimore, 1997, Williams & Wilkins, pp. 166-180.

61. Goldstein A: Introduction. In Goldstein A, editor: *Molecular and cellular aspects of the drug addictions*, New York, 1989, Springer-Verlag, pp. xiii-xviii.

62. Gomez E, Mikhail AR: Treatment of methadone withdrawal with cerebral electrotherapy (electrosleep), *Br J Psychiatry* 134:111, 1978.

63. Goodwin DW: *Genetic influences in alcoholism*, Chicago, 1987, Year Book.

64. Goodwin DW, Gabrielli WF: Alcohol: clinical aspects. In Lowinson JH, Ruiz P, Millman RB, Langrod JG, editors: *Substance abuse: a comprehensive textbook*, ed 3, Baltimore, 1997, Williams & Wilkins, pp. 142-147.

65. Gossop M, Bradley B, Strang J, Connell P: The clinical effectiveness of electrostimulation vs. oral methadone in managing opiate withdrawal, *Br J Psychiatry* 144:203, 1984.

66. Grinspoon L, Bakalar JB: Marihuana. In Lowinson JH, Ruiz P, Millman RB, Langrod JG, editors: *Substance abuse: a comprehensive textbook,* ed 3, Baltimore, 1997, Williams & Wilkins, pp. 199-206.
67. Guenther RM: Nutrition and alcoholism, *J Appl Nutr* 35:44, 1983.
68. Gurevich MI, Duckworth D, Imhof JE, Katz JL: Is auricular acupuncture beneficial in the inpatient treatment of substance abusing patients? a pilot study, *J Subst Abuse Treatm* 13(2):165, 1996.
69. Hackett GI, Burke P, Harris I: An anti-smoking clinic in general practice, *Practitioner* 228:1079, 1984.
70. Halpern JH: The use of hallucinogens in the treatment of addiction, *Addict Res* 4(2):177, 1996.
71. Hernandez-Reif M, Field T, Hart S: Smoking cravings are reduced by self-massage, unpublished data.
72. Higgins ST: Comments. In Onken LS, Blaine JD, Boren JJ, editors: Integrating behavioral therapies with medications in the treatment of drug dependence, NIDA research monograph 150, Rockville, Md, 1995, U.S. Department of Health and Human Services, pp. 170-179.
73. Ho WK, Wong HK, Wen HL: The influence of electroacupuncture on naloxone-induced morphine withdrawal. III. The effect of cyclic-AMP, *Neuropharmacology* 18(11):865, 1979.
74. Ho WK et al: The influence of electroacupuncture on naloxone-induced morphine withdrawal in mice: elevation of brain opiate-like activity, *Eur J Pharmacol* 49:197, 1978.
75. Holroyd J: Hypnosis treatment for smoking: an evaluative review, *Int J Clin Exper Hypnosis* 28(4):341, 1980.
76. Horne DE. Clinical impressions of SAAVE and tropamine, *J Psychoactive Drugs* 20(3):333, 1988.
77. Institute for Health Policy: *Substance abuse: the nation's number one health problem: key indicators for policy,* Princeton, NJ, 1993, Brandeis University for Robert Wood Johnson Foundation.
78. Institute of Medicine: *Broadening the base of treatment for alcohol problems,* Washington, DC, 1990, National Academy Press.
79. Jaffe JH, Knapp CM: Opiates: clinical aspects. In Lowinson JH, Ruiz P, Millman RB, Langrod JG, editors: *Substance abuse: a comprehensive textbook,* ed 3, Baltimore, 1997, Williams & Wilkins, pp. 158-165.
80. Jarzembski WB: Electrical stimulation and substance abuse treatment, *Neurobehav Toxicol Teratol* 7:119, 1985.
81. Kalant H: The nature of addiction: an analysis of the problem. In Goldstein A, editor: *Molecular and cellular aspects of the drug addictions,* New York, 1989, Springer-Verlag, pp. 1-28.
82. Kao AH, Lu LYC: Acupuncture procedure for treating drug addiction, *Am J Acupuncture* 2:201, 1974.
83. Karrell R: Acupuncture in an adolescent treatment setting, *Addiction Recovery* 10:24, 1990.
84. Katz N: Hypnosis and the addictions: a critical review, *Addictive Behav* 5:41, 1980.
85. Kendler KS, Neale M, Heath A, et al: A twin-family study of alcoholism in women, *Am J Psychiatry* 151(5):707, 1994.
86. Kendler KS, Kessler RC: A population-based twin study of alcoholism in women, *JAMA* 268(14):1877, 1992.
87. Keung WM: Biochemical studies of a new class of alcohol dehydrogenase inhibitors from Radix Puerariae, *Alcoholism Clin Exper Res* 17(6):1254, 1993.
88. Keung WM, Vallee BL: Daidzin and daidzein suppress free-choice ethanol intake by Syrian golden hamsters, *Proc Nat Acad Sci USA* 90(21):10008, 1993.
89. Keung WM, Vallee BL: Daidzin: a potent, selective inhibitor of human mitochondrial aldehyde dehydrogenase, *Proc Nat Acad Sci USA* 90:1247, 1993.
90. Keung WM, Vallee BL: Therapeutic lessons from traditional Oriental medicine to contemporary occidental pharmacology. In Jansson B, Jornvall H, Rydberg U, et al, editors: *Toward a molecular basis of alcohol use and abuse,* Boston, 1994, Birkhauser Verlag, pp. 371-381.
91. Keung WM, Lazo O, Kunze L, Vallee BL: Daidzin suppresses ethanol consumption by Syrian golden hamsters without blocking acetaldehyde metabolism, *Proc Nat Acad Sci USA* 92(19):8990, 1995.
92. King GR, Ellinwood EH: Amphetamines and other stimulants. In Lowinson JH, Ruiz P, Millman RB, Langrod JG, editors: *Substance abuse: a comprehensive textbook,* ed 3, Baltimore, 1997, Williams & Wilkins, pp. 207-222.
93. Klingemann HK: Coping and maintenance strategies of spontaneous remitters from problem use of alcohol and heroin in Switzerland, *Int J Addictions* 27(12):1359, 1992.

94. Konefal J, Duncan R, Clemence C: The impact of the addition of an acupuncture treatment program to an existing Metro-Dade County outpatient substance abuse treatment facility, *J Addictive Dis* 13(3):71, 1994.
95. Kosten TR, Kreck MJ, Ragunath J, Kleber HB: A preliminary study of beta endorphin during chronic naltrexone maintenance treatment in ex-opiate addicts, *Life Sci* 31(1):55, 1986.
96. Kroenig RJ, Oleson TD: Rapid narcotic detoxification in chronic pain patients treated with auricular electroacupuncture and naloxone, *Int J Addiction* 20:1347, 1985.
97. Jacobson NO, Silfverskiold NA: Controlled study of a hypnotic method in the treatment of alcoholism, with evaluation by objective criteria, *Br J Addiction* 68:25, 1973.
98. Johnston EJ, Donoghue JR: Hypnosis and smoking: a review of the literature. *Am J Clin Hypnosis* 13(4):265, 1971.
99. Lambe R, Osier C, Franks P: A randomized controlled trial of hypnotherapy for smoking cessation, *J Fam Pract* 22(1):61, 1986.
100. Lamontagne Y, Annable L, Gagnon MA: Acupuncture for smokers: lack of long-term therapeutic effect in a controlled study, *Can Med Assoc J* 122(7):787, 1980.
101. Lao HH: A retrospective study on the use of acupuncture for the prevention of alcoholic recidivism, *Am J Acupuncture* 32(1):29, 1995.
102. Lenox JR, Bonny H: The hypnotizability of chronic alcoholics, *Int J Clin Exper Hypnosis* 24(4):419, 1976.
103. Leung A: Acupuncture treatment of withdrawal symptoms, *Am J Acupuncture* 5:43, 1977.
104. Lewenberg A: Electroacupuncture and antidepressant treatment of alcoholism in a private practice, *Clin Therap* 7(5):611, 1985.
105. Li-Li F, O'Keefe DD, Powell WJ: Pharmacologic studies on *Radix puerariae*: effect of puerarin on regional myocardial blood flow and cardiac hemodynamics in dogs with acute myocardial ischemia, *Chin Med J* 98(11):821, 1985.
106. Lipton DS, Brewington V, Smith M: Acupuncture for crack-cocaine detoxification: experimental evaluation of efficacy, *J Subst Abuse Treatm* 11(3):205, 1994.
107. Lipton DS, Maranda MJ: *Detoxification from heroin dependency: an overview of method and effectiveness: evaluation of drug treatment programs,* Adv Alcohol Subst Abuse 2(1):31, 1982.
108. Litten RZ, Allen JL: Pharmacotherapies for alcoholism: promising agents and clincial issues, *Alcoholism Clin Exper Res* 15(4):620, 1991.
109. Litten RZ, Allen J, Fertig J: Pharmacotherapies for alcohol problems: a review of research with focus on developments since 1991, *Alcoholism Clin Exper Res* 20(5):859, 1996.
110. Littleton J: Acamprosate in alcohol dependence: how does it work? *Addiction* 90:1179, 1995.
111. Low S: Acupuncture and nicotine withdrawal, Med J Austral 2:687, 1977.
112. Ludwig A, Levine J, Stark L: *LSD and alcoholism: a clinical study of treatment efficacy,* Springfield, Ill, 1970, Charles C Thomas.
113. Machovec FJ, Man SC: Acupuncture and hypnosis compared: 58 cases, *Am J Clin Hypnosis* 21(1):45, 1978.
114. Malin DH, Murray JB, Crucian GP, et al: Auricular microelectrostimulation: naloxone-reversible attenuation of opiate abstinence syndrome, *Biol Psychiatry* 24:886, 1988.
115. Mammo A, Weinbaum D: Some factors that influence dropping out from outpatient alcoholism treatment facilities, *J Stud Alcohol* 54(1):92, 1991.
116. Man PL, Chuang MY: Acupuncture in methadone withdrawal, *Int J Addictions* 15(6):921, 1980.
117. Margolin A, Avants SK, Kosten TR, Chang P: Acupuncture reduces cocaine abuse in methadone-maintained patients, NIDA research monograph no. 32, Washington, DC, 1993, DHHS.
118. Margolin A, Chang P, Avants SK, Kosten TR: Effects of sham and real auricular needling: implications for trials of acupuncture for cocaine addiction, *Am J Chin Med* 21(2):103, 1993.
119. Margolin A, Avants SK, Chang P, et al: A single-blind investigation of four auricular needle puncture configurations, *Am J Chin Med* 23(2):105, 1995.
120. Margolin A, Avants SK, Birch S, Kosten TR: Methodological investigations for a multisite trial of auricular acupuncture for cocaine addiction: a study of active and control auricular zones, *J Subst Abuse Treatm* 13(6):471, 1996.

121. Martin GP, Waite PM: The efficacy of acupuncture as an aid to stopping smoking, *NZ Med J* 93(686):421, 1981.

122. Mathews-Larson J, Parker RA: Alcoholism treatment with biochemical restoration as a major component, *Int J Biosocial Res* 9(1):92, 1987.

123. Mcginnis M, Foege WH: Actual causes of death in the United States, *JAMA* 270:2207, 1993.

124. Mcgrath RE, Yahia M: Preliminary data on seasonally related alcohol dependence, *J Clin Psychiatry* 54(7):260, 1993.

125. Mckenna DJ: Plant hallucinogens: springboards for psychotherapeutic drug discovery, *Behav Brain Res* 73:109, 1996.

126. Mclellan AT, Grossman DS, Blaine JD, Haverkos HW: Acupuncture treatment for drug abuse: a technical review, *J Subst Abuse Treatm* 10(6):569, 1993.

127. Mendelson G: Acupuncture and cholinergic suppression of withdrawal symptoms: a hypothesis, *Br J Addiction* 73:166, 1978.

128. Milanov I, Toteva S: Acupuncture treatment of tremor in alcohol withdrawal syndrome, *Am J Acupuncture* 21(4):319, 1993.

129. Miller WR: Spirituality: the silent dimension in addiction research: the 1990 Leonard Ball oration, *Drug Alcohol Rev* 9:259, 1990.

130. Miller WR: Spiritual aspects of addictions treatment and research, *Mind/Body Med* 2(1):37, 1997.

131. Miller WR, Hester RK: Inpatient alcoholism treatment: who benefits? *Am Psychologist* 41:794, 1986.

132. Miller WR, Rollnick S: *Motivational interviewing,* New York, 1991, Guilford Press.

133. Mohs ME, Watson RR, Leonard-Green T: Nutritional effects of marijuana, heroin, cocaine and nicotine, *J Am Dietetic Assoc* 90(9):1261, 1990.

134. Morgan HW, editor: *Drugs in America: a social history,* 1800-1980, Syracuse, NY, 1981, Syracuse University Press.

135. Muffler J, Langrod JG, Richardson JT, Ruiz P: Religion. In Lowinson JH, Ruiz P, Millman RB, Langrod JG, editors: *Substance abuse: a comprehensive textbook,* ed 3, Baltimore, 1997, Williams & Wilkins, pp. 492-499.

136. Nathan RG, Robinson D, Cherek DR: Alternative treatments for withdrawing the long-term benzodiazepine user: a pilot study, *Int J Addictions* 21(2):195, 1986.

137. Nespor K, Cs-Emy L: [Alcohol and drugs in Central Europe: problems and possible solutions], *Casopis Lekaru Ceskych* (Czech) 133(16):483, 1994.

138. Newmeyer T, Johnson G, Klot S: Acupuncture as a detoxification modality, *J Psychoactive Drugs* 16:241, 1984.

139. Ng L: Auricular acupuncture in animals: effects of opiate withdrawal and involvement of endorphins, *J Alternat Compl Med* 2(1):61, 1996.

140. Ng L et al: Modification of morphine withdrawal syndrome in rats following transauricular electrostimulation: an experimental paradigm for auricular electroacupuncture, *Biol Psychiatry* 10:575, 1975.

141. Nutt DJ: Addiction: brain mechanisms and their treatment implications, *Lancet* 347:31, 1996.

142. O'Connell DF, Alexander CN: Introduction: recovery from addictions using trancendental meditation and Maharishi Ayur-Veda. In O'Connell DF, Alexander CN, editors: *Self recovery: treating addictions using transcendental meditation and Maharishi Ayur-Veda,* New York, 1995, Harrington Park Press.

143. Olms JS: New: an effective alcohol abstinence acupuncture treatment, *Am J Acupuncture* 12(2):145, 1984.

144. O'Malley SS, Croop RS, Wroblewski JM, et al: Naltrexone in the treatment of alcohol dependence: a combined analysis of two trials, *Psychiatr Ann* 11:681, 1995.

145. O'Malley SS, Jaffe AJ, Chang G, et al: Naltrexone and coping skills therapy for alcohol dependence: a controlled study, *Arch Gen Psych* 49:881, 1992.

146. Omura Y: Electro-acupuncture for drug addiction withdrawal, *Acupuncture Electro-Therapeutics Res Int J* 1:231, 1975.

147. Orme-Johnson DW, Farrow JJ, editors: Scientific research on the transcendental meditation program: collected papers, vol 1, Rheinweiler, W. Germany, 1977, MERU Press.

148. Overstreet DH, Lee YW, Rezvani AH, et al: Suppression of alcohol intake after administration of the Chinese herbal medicine NPI-028 and its derivatives, *Alcoholism Clin Exper Res* 20(2):221, 1996.

149. Parker L, Mok M: The use of acupuncture for smoking withdrawal, *Am J Acupuncture* 5:363, 1977.
150. Patterson MA: Electro-acupuncture in alcohol and drug addictions, *Clin Med* 81:9, 1974.
151. Patterson MA, Patterson L, Flood NV, et al: Electrostimulation in drug and alcohol detoxification: significance of stimulation criteria in clinical success, *Addiction Res* 1:130, 1993.
152. Patterson MA, Krupitsky E, Flood N, et al: Amelioration of stress in chemical dependency detoxification by transcranial electrostimulation, *Stress Med* 10:115, 1994.
153. Pechnick RN, Ungerleider JT: Hallucinogens. In Lowinson JH, Ruiz P, Millman RB, Langrod JG, editors: *Substance abuse: a comprehensive textbook,* ed 3, Baltimore, 1997, Williams & Wilkins, pp. 230-237.
154. Pekkanen L: Effects of thiamin deprivation and antagonism on voluntary ethanol intake in rats, *J Nutrition* 110(5):937, 1980.
155. Peniston EG: Alpha-theta brainwave training and beta-endorphin levels in alcoholics, *Alcoholism Clin Exper Res* 13(2):271, 1989.
156. Peniston EG, Kulkosky PJ: Alcoholic personality and alpha-theta brainwave training, *Med Psychother* 3:37, 1990.
157. Peniston EG et al: EEG alpha-theta brainwave synchronization in Vietnam theater veterans with combat-related post-traumatic stress disorder and alcohol abuse, *Adv Med Psychother* 6:37, 1993.
158. Peteet JR: A closer look at the role of a spiritual approach in addictions treatment, *J Subst Abuse Treatm* 10(3):263, 1993.
159. Petri G, Takach G: Application of herbal mixtures in rehabilitation after alcoholism, *Planta Medica* 56(6):692, 1990.
160. Poikolainen K: Seasonality of alcohol-related hospital admissions has implications for prevention, *Drug Alcohol Dependence* 10:65, 1982.
161. Pomeranz B: Scientific basis of acupuncture. In Stux G, Pomeranz B: *Acupuncture: textbook and atlas,* Berlin, 1987, Springer-Verlag.
162. Popik P, Layer RT, Skolnick P: 100 years of ibogaine: neurochemical and pharmacological actions of a putative anti-addictive drug, *Pharmacol Rev* 47(2):235, 1995.
163. Powell BJ, Penick EC, Read MR, Ludwig AM: Comparison of three outpatient treatment interventions: a twelve-month follow-up of men alcoholics, *J Stud Alcohol* 46(4):309, 1985.
164. Preliminary estimates from the Drug Abuse Warning Network: advance report no 14, Office of Applied Studies (OAS), Rockville, Md, 1996, Substance Abuse and Mental Health Services Administration (SAMHSA).
165. Project MATCH Research Group matching alcoholism treatments to client heterogeneity: Project MATCH posttreatment drinking outcomes, *J Stud Alcohol* 58(1):7, 1997.
166. Rank D, Suedfeld P: Positive reactions of alcoholic men to sensory deprivation, *Int J Addiction* 13(5):807, 1978.
167. Register UD, Marsh SR, Thurston DT, et al: Influence of nutrients on intake of alcohol, *J Am Dietetic Assoc* 61:159, 1972.
168. Rezvani AH, Overstreet DH, Lee Y: Attenuation of alcohol intake by ibogaine in three strains of alcohol-preferring rats, *Pharmacol Biochem Behav* 52(3):615, 1995.
169. Rogers LL, Pelton RB, Williams RJ: Amino acid supplementation and voluntary alcohol consumption by rats, *J Biol Chem* 220(1):321, 1956.
170. Sacks L: Drug addiction, alcoholism, smoking, obesity, treated by auricular staplepuncture, *Am J Acupuncture* 3:147, 1975.
171. Sainsbury MJ: Acupuncture in heroin withdrawal, *Med J Austral* 2(3):102, 1974.
172. Satel SL, Gawin FH: Seasonal cocaine abuse, *Am J Psychiatry* 146:534, 1989.
173. Schmitz JM, Jarvik ME, Schneider NG: Nicotine. In Lowinson JH, Ruiz P, Millman RB, Langrod JG, editors: *Substance abuse: a comprehensive textbook,* ed 3, Baltimore, 1997, Williams & Wilkins, pp. 276-293.
174. Schwartz JL: Evaluation of acupuncture as a treatment for smoking, *Am J Acupuncture* 16:135, 1988.
175. Sellers EM, Higgins GA, Sobell MB: 5-HT and alcohol abuse, *Trends Pharmacol Sci* 13(2):69, 1992.
176. Sershen H, Hashim A, Lajtha A: Ibogaine reduces preference for cocaine consumption in C57BL/6 by mice, *Pharmacol Biochem Behav* 47:13, 1994.

177. Severson L, Markoff RA, Chin-Hoon A: Heroin detoxification with acupuncture and electrical stimulation, *Int J Addictions* 12(7):911, 1977.

178. Shaffer HJ, Lasalvia TA: Comparing Hatha yoga with dynamic group psychotherapy for enhancing methadone maintenance treatment: a randomized clinical trial, *Alternat Ther Health Med* 3(4):57, 1997.

179. Shakur M, Smith MO: The use of acupuncture in the treatment of drug addiction, *Am J Acupuncture* 7(3):223, 1979.

180. Shanmugasundaram E, Subramaniam U, Santhini R, Shanmugasundaram K: Studies on brain structure and neurological function in alcoholic rats controlled by an Indian medicinal formula (SKV), *J Ethnopharmacol* 17:225, 1986.

181. Shapiro F, Vogelmann-Sine S, Sine LF: Eye movement desensitization and reprocessing: treating trauma and substance abuse, *J Psychoactive Drugs* 26(4):379, 1994.

182. Sharps H: Acupuncture and the treatment of drug withdrawal symptoms, *Pharmchem Newslett* 1, 1977.

183. Sheppard SG: A preliminary investigation of ibogaine: case reports and recommendations for further study, *J Subst Abuse Treatm* 11(4):379, 1994.

184. Shuaib BM: Acupuncture treatment of drug dependence in Pakistan, *Am J Chin Med* 4(4):403, 1976.

185. Simon EJ: Opiates: neurobiology. In Lowinson JH, Ruiz P, Millman RB, Langrod JG, editors: *Substance abuse: a comprehensive textbook,* ed 3, Baltimore, 1997, Williams & Wilkins, pp. 148-157.

186. Smith MO: Chinese theory of acupuncture detoxification, *Am J Acupuncture* 12(4):386, 1985.

187. Smith MO: Acupuncture treatment for crack: clinical survey of 1500 patients treated, *Am J Acupuncture* 16(3):241, 1988.

188. Smith MO: *Lincoln hospital acupuncture detoxification: the early days,* Presented at NADA annual meeting, Chicago, 1997.

189. Smith MO, Khan I: An acupuncture programme for the treatment of drug-addicted persons, *Bull Narcotics* 40(1):35, 1988.

190. Smith MO et al: Acupuncture treatment of drug addiction and alcohol abuse, *Am J Acupuncture* 10(2):161, 1982.

191. Smith RB, O'Neill L: Electrosleep in the management of alcoholism, *Biol Psychiatry* 10(6):675, 1975.

192. Smith-Moorhouse PM: Hypnosis in the treatment of alcoholism, *Br J Addiction* 64:47, 1969.

193. Socioeconomic evaluations of addictions treatment: executive summary, Washington, DC, 1993, Center of Alcohol Studies, Rutgers University.

194. Soyka M, Soyka M:. Clinical efficacy of acamprosate in the treatment of alcoholism: acamprosate in relapse prevention of alcoholism: Proceedings of the 1st CAMPRAL-Symposium-ESBRA, Stuttgart, Germany, Sept 1995, Springer-Verlag, pp. 155-171.

195. Spiegel D, Bloom JR, Kraemer HC, Gottheil E: Effect of psychosocial treatment on survival of patients with metastatic breast cancer, *Lancet* 2(8668):888, 1989.

196. Steiner RP, Hay DL: Davis AW: Acupuncture therapy for the treatment of tobacco smoking addiction, *Am J Chin Med* 10(1-4):107, 1982.

197. Stoil M: Problems in the evaluation of hypnosis in the treatment of alcoholism, *J Subst Abuse Treatm* 6:31, 1989.

198. Suedfeld P: Restricted environmental stimulation and smoking cessation: a fifteen-year progress report, *Int J Addictions* 25:861, 1990.

199. Suedfeld P, Ikard F: The use of sensory deprivation in facilitating the reduction of cigarette smoking, *J Consult Clin Psychol* 42:888, 1974.

200. Suedfeld P et al: An experimental attack on smoking (attitude manipulation in restricted environments) III, *Int J Addictions* 7:721, 1972.

201. Surawy C, Cox T: Smoking behaviour under conditions of relaxation: a comparison between types of smokers, *Addictive Behav* 11(2):187, 1986.

202. Sween JA, Shabazz CD, Carter D: The short-term symptom-relief effect of acupuncture on men and women in a residential drug and alcohol treatment program: results of a pilot study, presented at the National Acupuncture Detoxification Association (NADA) Conference, Portland, Or, 1996.

203. Tan C, Sin T, Huang X: The use of laser on acupuncture points for smoking cessation, *Am J Acupuncture* 15:137, 1987.

204. Taub E, Steiner SS, Weingarten E, Walton KG: Effectiveness of broad spectrum approaches to relapse prevention in severe alcoholism: a long-term, randomized, controlled trial of transcendental meditation, EMG biofeedback and electronic neurotherapy, *Alcoholism Treatm Q* 11(1-2):187, 1994.

205. Ter Riet G, Kleijnen J, Knipschild A: Meta-analysis of studies into the effect of acupuncture on addiction, *Br J Gen Pract* 40(338):379, 1990.

206. Thorer H, Volf N: Acupuncture after alcohol consumption: a sham controlled assessment, paper presented to British Medical Acupuncture Society, London, October 1996.

207. Timofeev MF: Internal inhibition: a form of nonconflict breaking mental alcohol dependence in narcology, *Bull Exper Biol Med* 117(2):149, 1994.

208. Toteva S, Milanov I: The use of body acupuncture for treatment of alcohol dependence and withdrawal syndrome: a controlled study, *Am J Acupuncture* 24(1):19, 1996.

209. Tuchfield BS: Spontaneous remission in alcoholics: empirical observations and theoretical implications, *J Stud Alcohol* 42(7):626, 1981.

210. Upton R: *Minimizing the effects of addiction and withdrawal through herbal and nutritional support (alcohol and cocaine), herbal support for alcohol and cocaine withdrawal,* Anaheim, 1994, Expo West.

211. Vaillant G, Clark W, Cyrus C, et al: Prospective study of alcoholism treatment: eight year follow-up, *Am J Med* 75:455, 1993.

212. Valenzuela CF, Harris RA: Alcohol: neurobiology. In Lowinson JH, Ruiz P, Millman RB, Langrod JG, editors: *Substance abuse: a comprehensive textbook,* ed 3, Baltimore, 1997, Williams & Wilkins, pp. 119-141.

213. Volpicelli JR, Alterman AI, Hayashida M, O'Brien C: Naltrexone in the treatment of alcohol dependence, *Arch Gen Psychiatry* 49:876, 1992.

214. Wadden TA, Penrod JH: Hypnosis in the treatment of alcoholism: a review and appraisal, *Am J Clin Hypnosis* 24(1):41, 1981.

215. Washburn A, Keenan P, Nazareno J: Preliminary findings: study of acupuncture-assisted heroin detoxification, *Multicultural Inquiry Res AIDS Q Newslett* 4:3, 1990.

216. Washburn AM et al: Acupuncture heroin detoxification: a single-blind clinical trial, *J Subst Abuse Treatm* 10(4):345, 1993.

217. Weingarten E, Hartman L, Holcomb Z: Frontalis EMG of dropouts from inpatients treatment for alcoholism, *Int J Addictions* 15(7):1113, 1980.

218. Wells E, Jackson R, Diaz O, et al: Acupuncture as an adjunct to methadone treatment services, *Am J Addictions* 4(3):198, 1995.

219. Wen HL: Fast detoxification of drug abuse by acupuncture and electrical stimulation (AES) in combination with naloxone, *Mod Med Asia* 13:13, 1977.

220. Wen HL: Acupuncuture and electrical stimulations (AES) outpatient detoxification. *Mod Med Asia* 15:39, 1979.

221. Wen HL: Clinical experience and mechanism of acupuncture and electrical stimulation (AES) in the treatment of drug abuse, *Am J Chin Med* 8(4):349, 1980.

222. Wen HL, Cheung SYC: Treatment of drug addiction by acupuncture and electrical stimulation, *Asian J Med* 9:138, 1973.

223. Wen HL, Teo SW: Experience in the treatment of drug addiction by electro-acupuncture, *Mod Med Asia* 11:23, 1975.

224. Wen HL, HO WKK, Wong HK, et al: Reduction of adrenocorticotropic hormone (ACTH) and cortisol in drug addicts treated by acupuncture and electrical stimulation (AES), *Compar Med East West* 6(1):61, 1978.

225. Wen HL, HO WKK, Ling N, et al: The influence of electro-acupuncture on naloxone-induced morphine withdrawal. II. Elevation of immunoassayable beta-endorphin activity in the brain but not the blood, *Am J Chin Med* VII(3):237, 1979.

226. Wen HL, Ho WK, Ling N, et al: Immunoassayable beta-endorphin level in the plasma and CSF of heroin addicted and normal subjects before and after electroacupuncture, *Am J Chin Med* 8(1-2):154, 1980.

227. Wen HL, Ng TH, Ho WKK, et al: Acupuncture in narcotic withdrawal: a preliminary report on biochemical changes in the blood and urine of heroin addicts, *Bull Narcotics* 30(2):31, 1978.

228. Werbach MR: *Nutritional influences on mental illness: a sourcebook of clinical research,* Tarzana, Calif, 1991, Third Line Press.

229. Wesson DR, Smith DE, Ling W, Seymour RB: Sedative-hypnotics and tricyclics. In Lowinson JH, Ruiz P, Millman RB, Langrod JG, editors: *Substance abuse: a comprehensive textbook,* ed 3, Baltimore, 1997, Williams & Wilkins, pp. 223-229.

230. Westermeyer J, Lyfoung T, Westermeyer M, Neider J: Opium addiction among Indochinese refugees in the US: characteristics of addictions and their opium use, *Am J Drug Alcohol Abuse* 17(3):267, 1991.

231. Whitehead PC: Acupuncture in the treatment of addiction: a review and analysis, *Int J Addictions* 13(1):1, 1978.

232. Winger G, Hofmann FG, Woods JH: *A handbook on drug and alcohol abuse: the biomedical aspects,* ed 3, New York, 1992, Oxford University Press.

233. Worner TM, Zeller B, Schwarz H, et al: Acupuncture fails to improve treatment outcome in alcoholics, *Drug Alcohol Dependence* 30(2):169, 1992.

234. Wynd CA: Relaxation imagery used for stress reduction in the prevention of smoking relapse, *J Adv Nurs* 17(3):294, 1992.

235. Xie CI, Lin RC, Antony V, et al: Daidzin: an antioxidant isoflavonoid, decreases blood alcohol levels and shortens sleep time induced by ethanol intoxication, *Alcoholism Clin Exper Res* 18(6):1443, 1994.

236. Yang MMP, Kwok JSL: Evaluation on the treatment of morphine addiction by acupuncture: Chinese herbs and opioid peptides, *Am J Chin Med* 14(1-2):46, 1986.

237. Zalesskiy V, Belousova I, Flolov G: Laser-acupuncture reduces cigarette smoking: a preliminary report, *Acupuncture Electro-Therapeutics Res Int J* 8:297, 1983.

SUGGESTED READINGS

Babor T: Social, scientific, and medical issues in the definition of alcohol and drug dependence. In Griffith E, Malcom L, editors: *The nature of drug dependence,* monograph (Society for the Study of Addictions), New York, 1990, Oxford University Press pp. 19-40.

Brewington V, Smith M, Lipton D: Acupuncture as a detoxification treatment: an analysis of controlled research, *J Substance Abuse Treatment* 11(4):289, 1994.

Donovan DM, Marlatt GA: Behavioral treatment. In Galanter M, editor: *Recent developments in alcoholism,* vol 11, Ten years of progress. New York, 1993, Plenum, pp. 397-411.

Halpern JH: The use of hallucinogens in the treatment of addiction, *Addiction Res* 4(2):177, 1996.

Litten RZ, Allen J, Fertig J: Pharmacotherapies for alcohol problems: a review of research with focus on developments since 1991. *Alcoholism: Clin Exper Res* 20(5):859, 1996.

Lowinson JH, Ruiz P, Millman RB, Langrod JG, editors: *Substance abuse: a comprehensive textbook,* ed 3, Baltimore, 1997, Williams & Wilkins.

Nutt DJ: Addiction: brain mechanisms and their treatment implications, *Lancet.* 374:31, 1996.

Onken LS, Blaine JD, Boren JJ, editors: *Integrating behavioral therapies with medications in the treatment of drug dependence,* NIDA Research Monograph 150. Rockville, Md, 1995, US Department of Health and Human Services.

Popik P, Layer RT, Skolnick P: 100 Years of Ibogaine: neurochemical and pharmacological actions of a putative anti-addictive drug, *Pharmacol Rev* 47(2):235, 1995.

Stoil M: Problems in the evaluation of hypnosis in the treatment of alcoholism, *J Substance Abuse Treatment* 6:31, 1989.

Werbach MR: *Nutritional influences on illness: a sourcebook of clinical research,* ed 2, Tarzana, Calif, 1991, Third Line Press.

CHAPTER 10

Complementary/Alternative Therapies in the Treatment of Pain

Ann Gill Taylor

Prevalence and incidence data about pain reveal reasons for interest in CAM/alternative medicine (CAM) therapies by the public, some health care professionals, and some scientists. Pain sufferers are seeking multimodal approaches to pain management. Individuals with chronic pain and cancer pain often hear the message from their conventional health care providers that conventional medicine has no more to offer to reduce or relieve their pain. These messages may be overt or covert and lead the patient to seek CAM methods. Survey results indicate that almost 10% of the U.S. population, approximately 25 million people, saw a practitioner in 1994 for at least one of the following therapies: chiropractic, relaxation techniques, therapeutic massage, and acupuncture.[170]

Many health care professionals and researchers have overlooked the impact of pain on satisfaction with care, adherence to recommended care regimens, and use of health care services.[75] The philosophy of many CAM therapies is one that fosters a sense of well-being, human integrity, and healing the person rather than curing the disease. These factors have a potentially important role in relieving pain. Many CAM therapists, too, operate from a partnership perspective in which the patient is viewed as an active participant in the therapy, enhancing a sense of control and self-efficacy, factors shown to be important in the effective management of pain.[1,191] Popularity of CAM therapies may very well be sending the message that there are multiple factors of great importance to the patient.

This chapter is aimed at establishing a broader consensus than currently exists among many conventional practitioners about the therapeutic value of a range of therapies that can be used as adjunctive methods in the treatment of pain. Conventional clinicians promote an interdisciplinary approach to pain management, which is often limited to scientific findings derived from the disciplines of biology, physiology, medicine, nursing, psychology, and sociology.

The purpose of this chapter is to review studies testing the effects of CAM therapies and revealing efficacy for pain relief either as a single method or as an adjunctive therapy to pharmacologic intervention. A review of the literature revealed evidence to demonstrate the efficacy of a number of methods in the treatment of pain. Major databases (Medline, AIDSline, CancerLit, Current Contents, Health Star, Nursing & Allied Health, PsychLit) were searched from the date of origin of the databases to 1997 with additional hand searching to obtain the latest published materials. The selected reviews of pain outcomes research are guided by the state of the art in the field of CAM, and the primary criteria for inclusion of articles are the following: meta-analyses combining controlled clinical studies, systematic reviews of controlled studies, randomized controlled trials, or controlled studies.

CHARACTERISTICS AND PREVALENCE OF PAIN
Definition and Types of Pain

Pain is a ubiquitous feature of life and one of the primary reasons that individuals seek assistance within the health care system. Despite advances in the understanding of pain mechanisms and management, the cause of an individual's pain is frequently poorly understood, and if understood, the pain is often inadequately managed.[228] The inherent subjectivity of pain is an impediment to its understanding and treatment. Pain can persist without an identifiable injury or disorder; likewise, injury can occur without pain. Thus the relationship between tissue damage and pain is not isomorphic (one to one). In addition to biochemical and physiologic factors, a range of behavioral, affective, cognitive, and sociocultural factors influence an individual's experience of pain. These factors not only influence the subjectivity of the pain experience, but also may have implications for the efficacy and selection of treatment methods.

Pain is defined as an unpleasant sensory and emotional experience associated with actual or potential tissue damage or described in terms of such damage.[101] Pain is typically classified as one of three types: acute, chronic, or cancer-related pain. Acute pain is associated with tissue damage that results from surgery, trauma, or painful medical procedures. Acute pain generally serves a biologically useful function signaling an underlying pathologic condition that, once identified, can be treated.[230] Acute pain is expected to diminish with healing and time. In contrast, pain associated with trauma that persists beyond the "usual healing period" or pain that accompanies a disease process that persists for extended periods can be considered chronic pain.[228] Cancer-related pain has characteristics of both acute and chronic pain and can result from the disease process (e.g., bone metastases, nerve compression or infiltration) and from therapy (e.g., surgery, radiation treatments). Cancer patients often report suffering that is not directly related to their pain but results from psychologic issues (e.g., fear, worry associated with financial ruin) associated with the diagnosis of cancer.[192]

The Epidemiology of Pain

Pain is a high-priority symptom related to problems of cancer, heart disease and stroke, diabetes, acquired immunodeficiency syndrome (AIDS), trauma, and chronic disabling conditions for more than 120 million persons in the United States, costing more than $100 billion in lost productivity and health care.[69,228]

Data in the box on p. 285 reveal the eight general categories and specific types of painful conditions seen in family practices. Pain center/clinic populations reflect yet another perspective on pain prevalence. Represented in this population are conditions such as headache, reflex sympathetic dystrophy (complex regional syndrome), extremity pain, neuroma of the lower extremity, neuralgia or neuropathic pain, fibrous myositis, myalgia and myositis, musculoligamentous pain, neck pain, and multiple types of back-related conditions including lumbosacral radiculopathy–ligamentous pain, low back pain, herniated lumbar disk, postlaminectomy syndrome, lumbosacral spinal stenosis, lumbar strain or sprain, and sacroiliac strain.[120]

In a national survey of 1539 households in which respondents were asked to report any serious or bothersome medical conditions, back problems, arthritis, sprains or strains, and headache were cited among the 10 most frequently reported principal medical conditions.[68] Anxiety and depression, which often accompany painful conditions, were also cited among the top 10 conditions.

Prevalence of pain in the United States is further explicated in a number of other reports. "The Nuprin Pain Report"[224] focused on the recall of events in the previous year among adults 18 years of age and older and delineated headache, backaches, muscle pains, joint pains, and premenstrual or menstrual pains as being common painful problems. Most of the respondents reported that they had three to four physical pain problems every year.

The National Center for Health Statistics surveyed both physicians and patients about pain and other health issues.[5] Information obtained from household interviews revealed the frequency of painful conditions to be as follows: arthritis, back pain, lower-extremity pain, migraine headache, ischemic heart disease, intervertebral disk disorders, upper-extremity pain, gout and gouty arthritis, and neuralgia or neuritis. A recent Louis Harris & Associates poll[118] found that pain costs the U.S. economy 50 million lost work days and $3 billion in lost wages per year. The combined expense associated with the treatment of back pain, migraine headaches, and arthritis amounted to an estimated $40 billion annually.[118]

When the reasons persons make visits to physicians' offices were assessed, the data revealed the following painful conditions to be among the top principal reasons: back symptoms, stomach pain, cramps, spasms, headache, chest pain, and knee pain. Depression, which often accompanies pain, was also among the top 20 reasons for office visits.[199,244]

Common Pain Disorders Seen by Primary Care Physicians

Abdominal disorders

Irritable (functional) bowel syndrome

Peptic ulcer disease

Headache disorders

Tension (muscle contraction) headaches

Vascular (migraine or cluster) headaches

Psychogenic conditions

Ischemic disorders

Angina pectoris

Peripheral vascular disease (e.g., claudication)

Musculoskeletal disorders

Low back pain

Rheumatoid or other forms of arthritis

Myofascial pain

Neoplastic disorders

Direct invasion or compression of nerves

Metastases causing invasion or compression of other structures

Neurologic disorders: nerve lesions

Posttraumatic neuritis

Causalgia

Postoperative neurons

Neurologic disorders: nerve lesions—cont'd

Amputation stump (phantom) pain

Coccydynia

Scar pain

Nerve entrapments

Postherpetic neuralgia (shingles)

Trigeminal neuralgia (tic douloureux)

Sympathetic dystrophy (e.g., shoulder-hand syndrome)

Spastic states

Thalamic pain

Psychiatric disorders

Depression, atypical depression

Hypochondriasis

Anxiety, panic disorders

Conversion symptoms

Compensation neurosis

Malingering

Delusions due to psychosis (e.g., dementia, schizophrenia)

Other categories

Temporomandibular joint syndrome (bruxism)

Dental, nasal, sinusoidal, ophthalmologic or otologic pain

Gout

Chronic pancreatitis

Data from Rodgers C, Thompson T. In Tollison CD, Satterwhaite JR, Tollison JW, editors: *Handbook of pain management*, Baltimore, 1994, Williams & Wilkins; Body DB, Merskey H, Nielsen JS. In Smith WL, Merskey H, Gross SC, editors: *Pain: meaning and management*, Jamaica, NY, 1980, SP Medical and Scientific Books; Thompson TL II. In Kaplan HI, Sadock BJ, editors: *Comprehensive textbook of psychiatry*, ed 4, Baltimore, 1985, Williams & Wilkins.

The form of pain associated with cancer is diagnosed in more than one million Americans annually. About eight million U.S. citizens now have cancer or a history of cancer. The incidence of patients with cancer pain depends on the type and stage of disease. Persons with cancer have acute pain associated with diagnostic procedures and therapy, chronic pain associated with disease progression and therapy, pain associated with but not directly caused by the cancer, and pain associated with conditions other than cancer.[74] Estimates of patients with cancer who have moderate to severe pain range from 30% to 45%, and nearly 75% of patients with advanced cancer have pain.[33,141] Breakthrough pain, rated to be severe to excruciating, is estimated to be a problem for 64% of persons with cancer.[180] Cancer patients cared for at home report a higher level of pain than those hospitalized.[72]

Prevalence of moderate to severe pain among hospitalized individuals is also high. Estimates suggest that 58% to 75% of hospitalized adults have excruciating pain.[51,62,145] Among postoperative patients, reports within the 1990s reveal that 74% have moderate to unbearable pain 24 hours after surgery and 65% have moderate to unbearable pain 72 hours after surgery.[4]

Researchers are making progress in learning more about neuroanatomic pathways and the neurophysical and neurochemical mechanisms involved in pain. Yet, the subjective nature of the pain experience in individuals with all types of pain offers specific challenges to those studying pain, as well as to clinicians. Although the basic physiology of pain transmission may be similar, there are individual differences related to genetic makeup, endocrine activity, neural activity, immune system function, stress, psychologic variables, age, gender, environment, and cultural backgrounds.

Despite advances in pharmacology, improvements in modes of delivery of analgesia, development of guidelines for pain management for a number of different populations, and education of physicians and nurses about pain management, the incidence of pain remains stable. Innovative strategies must be tested for effectiveness in reducing the prevalence and incidence of pain among those who have acute and chronic painful conditions and those who have cancer.

Health care involves knowledge of the phenomenon of pain, technical skills to implement pain management guidelines, and an ethical obligation to manage pain. The ethical importance of pain management is enhanced when additional benefits are realized. A review of the literature suggests that CAM therapies which have demonstrated efficacy be considered an integral part of pain management.

CAM THERAPIES FROM THE NURSING PERSPECTIVE

Nursing scholars have a long history of viewing the human being as a whole. Nightingale's work described nursing as a human service mission that focuses on holistic approaches to care. Her nursing care included environmental methods that promoted comfort, pain control, and symptom management. The philosophy of CAM medicine, too, supports a sense of well-being, human integrity, and healing the whole person rather than curing the disease. These concepts are an integral part of science-based nursing practices involving noninvasive, naturalistic care methods and nursing therapeutics that encompass comfort measures, pain reduction, and other symptom management and healing arts to promote well-being and potentiate wholeness and healing.

Specific care methods include guided imagery and other forms of visualization, therapeutic touch, massage, meditation, humor, music, nature, and other aesthetics. These methods overlap therapies currently identified with the field of CAM. [239]

SELECTIVE REVIEW OF ACUTE PAIN OUTCOMES RESEARCH
Acute Postoperative Pain

Approximately 23.3 million operations were performed in the United States in 1989. No matter how skillfully conducted, operations produce tissue damage and pain. Pain is a trigger of the metabolic stress response that increases tissue breakdown, metabolic rate, blood clotting, and water retention. Pain in postoperative patients leads to shallow breathing and cough suppression in an effort to "splint" the traumatized site, causing increased pulmonary secretions and pneumonia. Unrelieved pain also may delay the return of normal gastric and bowel function in the postoperative patient.[4]

The Acute Pain Management Guideline Panel[4] recommended an aggressive and flexible approach to acute pain management incorporating both pharmacologic and nonpharmacologic therapies to control pain and reduce anxiety and stress. Effective pain management not only increases patient comfort and satisfaction, but also may provide additional benefits including earlier mobilization, shortened hospital stays, and reduced costs. Patients differ in their response to postoperative pain and conventional analgesics. Thus it is important to offer CAM therapies as adjuvants to medication to manage discomfort and achieve a balance between analgesia and side effects.[4] The scientific literature provides evidence of the efficacy of relaxation and behavioral therapies, transcutaneous electrical nerve stimulation (TENS), and acupuncture as adjunctive therapies in the treatment of acute postoperative pain.

Relaxation and Behavioral Therapies

Relaxation and behavioral therapies embrace a wide range of therapeutic techniques that are used individually or in combination for pain management. Relaxation, hypnotic, and biofeedback techniques and cognitive-behavioral therapies are among the more common methods in this category of CAM. Relaxation techniques have been categorized as deep methods that include autogenic training, meditation, and progressive muscle relaxation or brief methods that include self-control relaxation, paced respiration, and deep breathing.[164] Hypnotic techniques "induce states of selective attentional focusing or diffusion combined with enhanced imagery" and are often used to induce relaxation.[164] Biofeedback uses monitoring instruments to provide physiologic information that enhances the patient's efforts to influence psychophysiologic responses. Cognitive-behavioral approaches focus on altering negative thoughts and behaviors. When used for pain, the goal of relaxation and behavioral techniques is to assist patients in developing their attentional (cognitive) and physiologic (somatic) self-regulation skills. Presently, relaxation and behavioral therapies may be the least controversial and most widely practiced of all treatments falling under the rubric of CAM therapies. In interdisciplinary pain management programs these strategies are nearly universal and over the past two decades have become one of the few widely practiced alternatives to drugs and surgery. However, these therapies need not be categorized solely as alternatives to medical management of pain, but also may be categorized as strategies for enhancing positive response to other conventional therapies.

Normally such improvements are subjectively experienced as a state of increased general relaxation, which in turn can foster the learning of cognitive (or hypnotic) skills in the suppression of pain. Such states are frequently accompanied by evidence of a reduction in muscle tension and a shift in autonomic activation from sympathetic to parasympathetic dominance. Despite differences in rationale and technique, nearly all self-regulation training begins with instruction in focusing attention and on slow-deep breathing, which may be the key elements in the relaxation response. Self-regulation training does not "cure" pain. However, the successful use of self-regulation of pain may enhance a sense of control and mastery and lead to greater self-efficacy and coping behaviors. Thus the learning of self-regulation skills may lead to positive outcomes in pain management through both direct and indirect routes.

There is strong evidence that such strategies can be useful in pain management.[172] However, while treatment effectiveness, especially in improving mood and behavior of pain patients, is well-established, the mechanism of effect is poorly understood.[203] If—and how—peripheral physiopathology involved in the pain is directly influenced may be unclear. To what degree self-regulation is a centrally acting phenomenon that has much in common with cognitive constructs such as expectancy, self-efficacy, and placebo is also not entirely clear. However, investigations of the neurophysiologic mechanisms of hypnosis show the promise of this approach.[54,118,196]

Relaxation Techniques In the Management of Postoperative Pain. Efficacy of relaxation techniques in the management of postoperative pain has been widely evaluated. Strategies including simple brief relaxation,[99,119,127] imagery,[64,98] and music-assisted relaxation[131,159] have all shown some degree of effectiveness in reducing postoperative pain.[4,80] Table 10-1 lists studies of relaxation techniques and findings.

In a controlled clinical trial Levin et al.[127] investigated the effectiveness of two relaxation techniques in the management of postoperative pain. Forty female patients between the ages of 21 and 65 years who were undergoing elective cholecystectomy were randomly assigned to one of four groups. One treatment group received a taped recording of rhythmic breathing; the second treatment group received a recording of Benson's relaxation technique; an attention-distraction control group received a taped recording of the history of the hospital; the standard care control group received only the perioperative care that was given to all groups. The study controlled statistically for the effects of analgesic medication on pain. Pain sensation and distress were assessed using visual analog scales. Data were collected for the two pain components and for medication usage five times in the first 72 postoperative hours. Only the Benson's relaxation technique group had significantly less pain than the attention-distraction group. No other significant differences were found between groups. The small sample size, which was further reduced by missing data, may have contributed to the lack of additional significant findings.

Mullooly et al.[159] examined the effects of music on postoperative pain and anxiety. Twenty-eight women who underwent elective abdominal hysterectomies were randomly assigned to either an experimental or standard care control group. The experimental group received a 10-minute tape of "easy-listening" music, recorder, and headphones. Pain and anxiety were assessed in all patients on the first and second postoperative day. Patients in the music group reported significantly reduced anxiety on day 1. On day 2, both pain and anxiety were significantly reduced in this group. The findings suggest that easy-listening music may provide a simple therapeutic intervention to reduce postoperative pain and anxiety.

Good[80] systematically reviewed 21 published studies that examined the effects of relaxation and music on postoperative pain. The analysis suggested that relaxation and music were effective in reducing affective pain ratings and observed pain in the majority of the studies, but less effective in reducing pain intensity ratings or opioid intake. The studies were difficult to compare because of differences in study design and methodology, which included differences in surgical procedures, experimental techniques, activities during testing, measurement of pain, and amount of practice using the therapies. There are a number of limitations that could restrict conclusions. Inadequate sample size, lack of random assignment, no assurance of pretest equivalence, delayed posttest administration, and lack of control for opiates at time of testing characterize some of the studies.

Additional studies are needed to compare relaxation techniques to determine the most effective technique for relaxation during postoperative ambulation and rest. The role of individual differences in determining what works for a particular individual requires further investigation. Future research should address design and methodologic shortcomings that characterize some earlier studies.

Although the results of efficacy studies of relaxation techniques and music on postsurgical pain have been mixed, these are low-risk interventions that, when used in conjunction with pharmacologic or other conventional therapies, offer a simple and accessible intervention to reduce anxiety and pain in some postoperative patients.

Hypnosis. Hypnosis is a more complex technique than relaxation therapies that requires specialized training. The scientific literature provides some evidence that suggests hypnosis can be effective for reducing postoperative pain[12,112] (Table 10-1). Additional research is necessary to confirm the findings of these studies and to determine the individual differences that are associated with effectiveness.

Text continued on p. 296

TABLE 10-1   Studies of CAM Therapies in Management of Acute Pain Conditions

Author, Year	Sample Size	Diagnosis	Design	Outcome Variable	Major Findings
Levin et al., 1987	N = 40 women	Elective cholecystectomy	Experimental Random assignment: • Group I: tape recording of rhythmic breathing • Group II: tape of Berson's relaxation technique • Group III: active control (tape of history of hospital to distract attention) • Group IV: standard care control	• Incision pain intensity ratings • Affective pain ratings • Amount of analgesic used during first 72 hours	• Only Benson's relaxation group had significantly less pain than the attention-distraction group • No significant differences in amount of analgesic medication NOTE: Small sample size and missing data may have contributed to lack of additional findings
Mullooly et al., 1988	N = 28 women	Elective abdominal hysterectomy	Experimental Random assignment: • Group I: 10-minute tape, easy-listening music • Group II: control group (standard care)	• Pain intensity ratings × 2 days after surgery • Anxiety ratings × 2 days after surgery	Treatment group reported: • Significant decrease in anxiety, day 1 • Significant decrease in pain and anxiety, day 2

| Good, 1996 | N = 21 studies | Postoperative pain | Systematic literature review of published studies examining effects of relaxation and music | • Self-report of pain intensity
• Self-report of affective pain
• Observed pain
• Amount of opioid analgesia intake | Systematic review revealed
• Relaxation and music effective in reducing affective pain ratings and "observed" pain in majority of studies; less effective in reducing pain intensity ratings or opioid intake
NOTE: Studies difficult to compare because of:
• Differences in design and methodology
• Methodologic limitations |
| Ashton et al., 1997 | N = 32 | Elective coronary artery bypass surgery patients (first-time surgery) | Experimental Stratified randomized assignment, stratified on age < 65 and > 65 years; gender
Hypnotic induction profile (HIP) test:
• Group I: self-hypnosis
• Group II: standard care control | • Intraoperative pharmacologic use
• Amount of analgesic used during 5 postoperative days
• Quality of life assessed using POMS
• Length of intensive care stay
• Length of hospital stay
• Comorbidity
• Extent of patient adherence to self-hypnosis techniques | • Self-hypnosis group showed significant reduction in tension (POMS) following surgery compared to control group
• No significant difference in other POMS categories
• Patients who complied with practice of self-hypnosis technique used significantly less medication than those who did not practice
• No significant difference in medication use between patients practicing self-hypnosis and control group
• No significant difference in intraoperative pharmacologic requirements, length of intensive care and hospital stay, and comorbidity between groups |

Continued

HIP, Hypnotic induction profile test; POMS, profile of mood states; TENS, transcutaneous electrical nerve stimulation.

TABLE 10-1 Studies of CAM Therapies in Management of Acute Pain Conditions—cont'd

Author, Year	Sample Size	Diagnosis	Design	Outcome Variable	Major Findings
					NOTE: Patients in control group practiced a form of relaxation based on the HIP test used for randomization, which could have influenced results
Hargreaves and Lander, 1989	N = 75	Procedure to clean and pack abdominal wounds	Experimental Random assignment: • Group I: active TENS • Group II: placebo TENS • Group III: no treatment	Pain intensity rating on 11-point numeric rating scale	Patients in active TENS group reported significantly lower pain ratings than patients in the other two groups NOTE: No significant difference in narcotic use before procedure that might have influenced results
Warfield et al., 1985	N = 24	Postoperative thoracotomy	Experimental Random assignment: • Group I (N = 12): active TENS • Group II (N = 12): placebo TENS Experimental Random assign-	• Incision pain intensity ratings on 11-point scale at 24 hours and 48 hours after surgery • Tolerance ratings of chest physical therapy • Length of stay in postoperative care unit	• Significantly lower pain intensity ratings in active TENS group during first 24 hours • Significantly shorter stay in postoperative recovery area for active TENS group • Significantly better tolerance of chest physical therapy on postoperative days 1 and 2 for active TENS group • No significant difference in narcotic use or patient report of nausea or vomiting

| Conn et al., 1986 | N = 42 | Postoperative emergency appendectomy | Experimental Stratified random assignment: • Group I: active TENS • Group II: placebo TENS • Group III: control | • Pain intensity ratings at 48 hours after surgery using linear analog scale • Amount of analgesic intake for first and second 24-hour postoperative periods | • Significantly lower pain intensity ratings and analgesic intake in active and placebo TENS groups compared with control group • No significant difference in pain intensity ratings between active and placebo TENS groups • Significant difference in analgesic intake for active TENS group during first 24 hours after surgery
NOTE: Authors concluded placebo effect may have influenced outcomes |
| Benedetti et al., 1997 | N = 324 | Postsurgical patients: • Posterolateral thoracotomy • Muscle-sparing thoracotomy • Costotomy • Sternotomy • Video-assisted thoracoscopy | Experimental Random assignment: • Group I: active TENS • Group II: placebo TENS • Group III: control | • Amount of time from beginning of surgical procedure to time of request for analgesic medication • Amount of analgesic medication intake during first 12 postoperative hours | • TENS not effective in controlling postoperative pain in patients who underwent posterolateral thoracotomy • TENS proved to be useful adjunct to analgesic medication in relieving the moderate pain intensity of muscle-sparing thorocotomy, costotomy, and sternotomy pain • TENS effective in controlling mild pain without any analgesic medication in patients who underwent video-assisted thoracoscopy |

Continued

TABLE 10-1 Studies of CAM Therapies in Management of Acute Pain Conditions—cont'd

Author, Year	Sample Size	Diagnosis	Design	Outcome Variable	Major Findings
Sung YF et al., 1976	N = 40 men	Postoperative dental pain	Experimental Random assignment: • Group I: placebo pill plus placebo acupuncture • Group II: codeine plus placebo acupuncture • Group III: placebo pill plus acupuncture (Ho-Ku point) • Group IV: codeine plus acupuncture (Ho-Ku point)	Pain intensity ratings on 4-point scale every $1/2$ hour $\times$ 3 hours	• Significantly better pain relief from acupuncture at Ho-Ku point than from placebo acupuncture • Quicker relief from acupuncture alone than in combination with codeine • Longer-lasting pain relief with combination acupuncture and codeine
Lee et al., 1992	N = 38 patients seen in emergency department	Acute renal colic	Meta-analysis Assessing effects ment: • Group I: acupuncture • Group II: avafortan (analgesic agent)	Pain intensity ratings on 4-point scale (before treatment and 30 minutes after treatment)	• Significant reduction in pain ratings in both groups; no significant difference between groups • More rapid onset of pain relief with acupuncture • No effect on renal stone passage

Study	N / Design	Condition	Method	Outcome measure	Results
Shekelle et al., 1992	N = 9 randomized, controlled trials	Acute low back pain	of spinal manipulation. Meta-analysis. Assessing effects	Varied; included pain and functional outcomes	Concluded that spinal manipulation hastens recovery from uncomplicated acute low back pain
Anderson et al., 1992	N = 23 randomized, controlled trials	Acute low back pain	of spinal manipulation or mobilization	Varied; included pain and function	Concluded that spinal manipulation reduces pain and has positive short-term effects on daily functioning in patients with acute low back pain without radiculopathy
Hadler et al., 1987	N = 54	Uncomplicated regional lower back pain < 1 month's duration with no prior manipulation	Experimental. Stratified random assignment based on pain duration < 2 weeks or 2 to 4 weeks: • Group I: single long-lever manipulation • Group II: mobilization	Index of disability	• Significant improvement in function for patients having pain for 2 to 4 weeks treated by manipulation (50% reduction in disability within 3 days) • No significant difference in treatment's effect for patient with pain < 2 weeks, but significant improvement with both treatments
MacDonald and Bell, 1990	N = 95	Nonspecific low back pain	Experimental. Random assignment: • Group I: osteopathic manipulation × 5 plus education on posture • Group II: education on posture only	Health status index	• Significant improvement after 1 week of treatment for patients having pain duration of 2 to 4 weeks • No significant treatment effects for patients with pain duration of < 2 weeks or > 4 weeks

Bioelectromagnetic Therapies in Postoperative Pain Management

There is growing interest in the application of electromagnetic and magnetic field therapies for the treatment of pain. Transcutaneous electrical nerve stimulation, which has been in use since the 1970s, is "the technique of applying controlled, low voltage electrical impulses to the nervous system through electrodes attached to the skin."[194] Transcutaneous electrical nerve stimulation is used widely for the control of acute and chronic pain. Two mechanisms of analgesic effect have been proposed. In accordance with the gate control theory,[236] the first mechanism suggests that TENS activates the large myelinated fibers which have a low threshold for electrical stimulation. The increased activity in these fibers blocks the transmission of painful stimuli from the small unmyelinated fibers. The second mechanism suggests that endorphin release is triggered at more intense levels of stimulation activating descending pathways that exert an inhibiting effect on ascending nerve impulses.

Numerous studies have tested the efficacy of TENS therapy in the management of postoperative pain.[4,26,51,86,238] The findings provide evidence that TENS is effective in reducing self-reported mild to moderate pain and analgesic use. For study details see Table 10-1.

A meta-analysis of TENS therapy in postoperative patients conducted by the Agency of Health Care Policy and Research Acute Pain Management Guideline Panel revealed that both TENS and sham TENS significantly reduced pain intensity; no significant differences were reported between the two groups for either analgesic use or pain intensity.[4] Carroll et al.[44] systematically reviewed 36 studies testing the effectiveness of TENS on postoperative pain. In 19 of the studies (1) the trials were not randomized, controlled trials or (2) the reviewers considered the method of randomization inappropriate. Results of 17 of the 19 studies suggested that TENS was effective in controlling postoperative pain. Transcutaneous electrical nerve stimulation therapy was more effective in reducing pain intensity ratings or analgesic use than the control interventions (opioid only and/or sham TENS) in only 2 of the 17 randomized, controlled trials. Carroll et al.[44] concluded that nonrandomized studies overestimated treatment effects.

The findings from the meta-analysis and the systematic review suggest that a placebo effect underlies the reduction of perceived pain, and provide further support for the need to examine individual differences that may account for the nonspecific effects. Further testing of TENS with populations experiencing mild acute pain may be useful.

Transcutaneous electrical nerve stimulation does produce beneficial effects. Thus the clinical guidelines for the management of acute pain[4] recommend the use of TENS as an adjunctive therapy for postoperative pain. The risks are relatively low: TENS may inhibit output of some demand cardiac pacemakers; some patients may have irritation at the electrode site caused by the adhesive or gel. Otherwise, TENS is a safe, noninvasive, inexpensive, and simple method to control mild to moderate pain.

Therapeutic Touch

Nurses and other health care professionals often use therapeutic touch (TT) in hospitals, hospices, community settings, and home settings throughout the United States and the world.[197] Therapeutic touch is endorsed by the National League for Nursing as an appropriate comfort-promoting method.[34] Recent figures suggest that it is taught routinely in more than 80 nursing programs across the country.

Krieger[116] described TT as a natural potential derived from the ancient practice of "laying on of hands." Therapeutic touch differs today in that it is not performed within a religious context, nor does its effectiveness require a professed faith or belief by either the practitioner or the patient.[197] Therapeutic touch does not require direct physical contact between the practitioner and recipient. The intervention begins with the practitioner "centering" (assuming an intentional state of helping the person). Practitioners use the hands as sensors that move 2 to 3 inches above the person's body, assessing energy flow and blockage (deficits). The practitioners' hands redirect areas of accumulated tension and conduct energy to remove excess tension.

Therapeutic touch as an intervention is based on the assumptions that there is a universal energy flow and all living organisms are part of its field. Energy field characteristics of openness, mutual process, dynamic unity, and capacity to establish pattern are fundamental to the understanding of the human-environmental process.[21,139,198]

A growing number of researchers maintain that TT decreases patients' anxiety, promotes relaxation, relieves pain, and decreases depression.*

Quinn[182] replicated the work of Borelli and Heidt,[35] who reported that TT significantly decreased anxiety in hospitalized patients. Quinn and Strelkauskas[182] found that there is a significant increase in positive affect (joy, vigor, contentment, and affection) following TT intervention, and a significant decrease in negative affect (anxiety, guilt, hostility, and depression). Depression is lessened in patients after TT.[197]

Two randomly controlled studies by Meehan[150] and Meehan et al.[151] examined the effects of TT on abdominal and pelvic surgical pain. Although the findings were not statistically significant, the results suggest TT can reduce the need for additional analgesic medication and may have an effect beyond that of a nonspecific placebo effect in the treatment of acute postoperative pain.

Additional study is needed with special emphasis on assessing blockages and changes in body energy following TT. Improved treatment protocols such as lengthening the duration of the intervention should be incorporated.

---

*References 32, 67, 150, 151, 175, 183, 245, 246.

Acupuncture

Acupuncture may be the most well-known traditional medicine therapy, having been in continuous use for more than 23 centuries. Today it is reasonably available as a treatment in the United States.

Acupuncture is based on a philosophy of nature that views the human being as a microcosm or miniature universe. A fundamental assumption of acupuncture is that by observing patterns in the natural world, dynamics of human nature are revealed. Practitioners who use acupuncture view the human body as an ecosystem.

Acupuncture involves stimulating specific anatomic points in the body for therapeutic purposes. These points are most often stimulated using a needle, but practitioners may also use heat, pressure, friction, suction, or impulses of electromagnetic energy to stimulate the points. Basic science research suggests that neurologic pathways are the mechanism by which acupuncture relieves pain.[179]

Acupuncture is among the most researched and documented CAM therapies. An estimated 137 randomized clinical trials on 10 painful conditions have been reported. These studies provide evidence, although not statistically conclusive, of the efficacy of acupuncture in painful conditions such as osteoarthritis,[48,60] fibromyalgia,[57] back pain,[50,83] tennis elbow,[37] painful menstrual cycles,[91] and migraine headaches.[232] The 1997 Consensus Conference on Acupuncture also researched similar conclusions about the efficacy of pain relief with acupuncture on these pain conditions.[166]

There is evidence of efficacy in reducing postoperative dental pain.[166] The authors of two major reviews[187,190] concluded that the study by Sung et al.[220] not only provided considerable support for the short-term efficacy of acupuncture for postoperative pain, but also the significance of point location. Findings from a study of patients with acute renal colic[121] suggest that acupuncture may be an alternative to conventional analgesics in the treatment of renal colic in selected situations, for example, when patients have a history of drug allergy or fail to respond to conventional treatment. See Table 10-1 for study details.

Acute Low Back Pain

On a national scale, back pain is one of the most common, debilitating and expensive pain problems in terms of lost productivity.[95,224] National statistics indicate a general yearly prevalence of low back problems in the U.S. population of 15% to 20%.[8] Low back problems are the most common reason for office visits to primary care physicians and rank third among reasons for surgical procedures.[56] Estimates of total annual societal costs of back pain range from $20 to $50 billion.[161] Therefore, effective treatment for back pain has potential cost-saving implications, not only in terms of reducing time lost from work, but also in avoiding more costly and invasive medical procedures.

Acute low back problems are defined as activity intolerance attributable to back-related symptoms of less than 3 months' duration.[3] Back symptoms include pain in the back as well as back-related leg pain (sciatica).

Spinal Manipulation

Spinal manipulation practiced as a manual healing therapy is based on the understanding that structure and function are interdependent. Dysfunction of any discrete body part can affect the function of other discrete, not necessarily connected, parts of the body.

The clinical guidelines for acute lower back problems in adults[3] recommended that after serious spinal conditions (such as fracture, tumor, infection, or cauda equina) and nonspinal pathologic conditions (vascular, abdominal, urinary, or pelvic disease that can cause referred back pain) are ruled out, spinal manipulation can be used to provide symptomatic relief and improve function. A meta-analysis of the chiropractic literature[117] showed that chiropractic treatment hastened recovery from back strains and sprains.

Evidence of the efficacy of spinal manipulation in uncomplicated acute low back pain is provided by two meta-analyses.[7,201] Shekelle et al.[201] analyzed nine randomized, controlled trials that tested the effects of manipulation against various conservative treatments for patients with acute low back pain. The two studies with the highest-quality scores showed a statistically beneficial effect of manipulation in patients whose pain had been present for 2 to 4 weeks at the time of treatment.[84,138] The meta-analysis of the other seven randomized, controlled trials showed that manipulation significantly increased probability of recovery at 2 or 3 weeks after beginning treatment.[201] Shekelle et al.[201] concluded that spinal manipulation hastens recovery from acute, uncomplicated low back pain.

Twenty-three randomized, controlled trials testing the effectiveness of spinal manipulation or mobilization were meta-analyzed by Anderson et al.[7] The data analysis indicates that manipulation reduces pain and has positive short-term effects on daily functioning for patients with acute low back problems without radiculopathy. See Table 10-1 for spinal manipulation study details. Shekelle et al.[201] also reviewed data to estimate potential risk in lumbar spinal manipulation. Data were limited to case reports, since no systematic report of complications from spinal manipulation has been published. Increasing neurologic deterioration following manipulation has been reported in patients with sciatica. The researchers noted that serious complications from lumbar spinal manipulations, including paraplegia and death, have been reported. However, the authors concluded that the risk of complications is small and may vary by clinical condition.

SELECTIVE REVIEW OF CHRONIC PAIN OUTCOMES RESEARCH
Regional Chronic Pain

Headache. Headache is one of the most common problems among individuals of all ages, and effective treatment remains a great challenge for health care professionals.[169] Among adults, 16% have migraine headaches and 71% have tension-type headaches, the most common form of headache.[168,185] Tension-type headache varies in frequency and severity from rare, brief episodes of discomfort to frequent, long-lasting, or even continuous disabling headaches. Estimates of 1-year prevalence for frequent (more than one a month) tension headache range from 20% to 30%. Migraine is often incapacitating with considerable impact on work and social activities.[130,185] Projections from the American Migraine Study suggest that 8.7 million women and 2.6 million men have migraine headache with moderate to severe disability.[217] Estimates of annual labor costs resulting from lost productivity attributable to migraine disability range from $7 to $15 billion.[215] Effective treatment can reduce the health burden on the individual with headaches by reducing pain and disability and on society by reducing indirect costs.[216]

Relaxation and Behavioral Therapies. There is a large body of research investigating the effectiveness of relaxation and behavioral techniques in the treatment of chronic headaches. A 1995 National Institutes of Health (NIH) technology assessment panel[164] evaluated the scientific evidence and concluded that a number of behavioral and relaxation interventions are useful for the reduction of chronic pain in adults. Based on study designs and consistency of findings, the evidence was rated moderate in support of the conclusion that biofeedback is more effective than relaxation and no treatment in relieving migraine headache. However, the evidence was less clear when biofeedback was compared with psychologic placebo. Both electromyogram (EMG) biofeedback and hypnosis were found to be effective in the treatment of tension headache. In addition, the results from several meta-analyses of clinical trials indicate that multimodal treatments have been effective in the treatment of several categories of regional pain, including chronic headache pain. See Table 10-2 for details of studies.

Holroyd and Penzien[97] compared the efficacy of combined relaxation and thermal feedback training with the most widely used pharmacologic treatment for migraine headache. Results from 25 clinical trials evaluating the effectiveness of propranolol and from 35 clinical trials evaluating the effectiveness of relaxation and thermal feedback training were pooled for analysis. Several relaxation techniques were used in the studies, including progressive muscle relaxation, training in elicitation of the relaxation response, and autogenic training. Relaxation and thermal biofeedback (feedback of skin temperature of the hand) training were administered in combination either concurrently or consecutively in the 35 trials. The meta-analysis findings provide substantial support for the effectiveness of relaxation/biofeedback training and propranolol, but no evidence that the treatments differ in effectiveness.

Hyman et al.[100] examined the effects of relaxation training on a variety of clinical symptoms. The meta-analysis synthesized data from 48 studies, almost half unpublished. Imagery, progressive muscle relaxation, rhythmic breathing, and Benson's relaxation technique were among the therapies studied individually and in combination. The consistently positive effect sizes suggest that relaxation techniques are effective in treating headaches as well as other chronic pain conditions. The findings are only suggestive of efficacy, since the number of studies synthesized for any one clinical condition was relatively small. The results from a meta-analysis of 109 studies that examined nonpharmacologic treatments for chronic pain were also suggestive of the efficacy of relaxation and behavioral techniques for migraine and tension headaches.[140]

Holroyd and Penzien[96] also evaluated the efficacy of relaxation and biofeedback in the treatment of recurrent tension headache. The meta-analysis synthesized 37 studies, all of which reported data from daily patient recordings. Measures of headache activity were similar to those in the previously described study reported by the same authors.

EMG biofeedback, relaxation, and the combination interventions yielded significantly greater improvements in headache activity than either noncontingent biofeedback (false) or headache-monitoring control conditions. No statistically significant differences were found among the treatment groups.

The effect of patient age on treatment outcome was investigated, and a negative relationship was found. Older patients may represent a subgroup of the tension headache population who are less likely to respond to relaxation and behavioral techniques.

Bogaards and ter Kuile[31] examined the effects of relaxation and behavioral interventions on recurrent tension headache and also investigated the relationships between outcome and patient characteristics. Seventy-eight published studies were meta-analyzed. Treatment conditions were classified as one of the following: EMG biofeedback, relaxation, the combination of EMG biofeedback and relaxation, cognitive therapy, pharmacologic therapies, other therapy (e.g., hypnosis), placebo, or control. Treatments were primarily individual and of relatively short duration with a mean of 7 hours in therapist contact, which is comparable to the study of Holroyd and Penzien.[96] Cognitive therapy and EMG biofeedback alone or in combination with relaxation significantly reduced headache activity when compared with placebo and no-treatment conditions. Most cognitive therapies were multimodal and included EMG biofeedback and relaxation. Relaxation therapy and other therapy were more effective than no treatment. The type of outcome measure (daily headache recordings or global ratings) influenced other results. In conditions that used a headache diary, relaxation therapy was also superior to placebo treatment only. Pharmacologic therapy did not differ from placebo or control if data from daily recordings were used, but was more effective than no treatment if both diary and global measures were used in analyses.

The results confirm prior meta-analyses findings[28,96] on the efficacy of EMG biofeedback, relaxation, and a combination in recurrent tension headache. Duration of treatment did not affect treatment outcome, and the data suggest that treatments of short duration are recommended. Duration of headache complaint and age were interrelated and neg-

Text continued on p. 312

TABLE 10-2	Studies of CAM Therapies in Management of Chronic Pain Conditions				
Author, Year	**Sample Size**	**Diagnosis**	**Design**	**Outcome Variable**	**Major Findings**
Holroyd and Penzien, 1990	N = 60 clinical trials	Migraine headaches	Meta-analysis N = 25 trials evaluating propranolol N = 35 trials evaluating: • Relaxation/thermal feedback • Progressive muscle relaxation • Training in elicitation of relaxation response • Autogenic training	Headache activity measured using either Headache Index or composite score formed by averaging headache frequency, duration, intensity	• Significant reduction (43%) in headache from both propranolol and relaxation/biofeedback training; no evidence that the treatments differed in effectiveness • Significant difference in improvements produced by the two treatments from those observed in placebo (14% reduction) and untreated patients (no improvement)
Hyman et al., 1989	N = 48 studies	Headache and variety of clinical symptoms	Meta-analysis Evaluating effects of relaxation therapies used singularly or in combination: • Imagery • Regressive muscle relaxation • Rhythmic breathing • Benson's relaxation technique (almost half of studies unpublished)	Effect sizes for varied outcomes including headache pain	Positive effect sizes suggest effectiveness of relaxation techniques in treating headache and other chronic symptoms NOTE: Number of studies for any one condition was small

Source	N	Condition	Method	Outcome	Results
Malone and Strube, 1988	N = 109 studies	Chronic pain conditions including migraine and tension headaches, chronic back pain	Meta-analysis Examining nonpharmacologic treatment for chronic pain conditions	Effect sizes and proportion of improved patients for a variety of outcomes	Positive effect size suggestive of short-term efficacy of relaxation and behavioral techniques for: • Migraine and tension headaches • Chronic low back pain
Holroyd and Penzien, 1986	N = 37 studies	Recurrent tension headache	Meta-analysis Examining: • EMG biofeedback • Training in progressive muscle relaxation, meditative procedures or autogenic training • Combined EMG biofeedback with relaxation training • Control conditions: noncontingent (false) biofeedback or headache monitoring	Headache activity and proportion of improved patients	• Significantly greater improvements in headache activity with EMG biofeedback, relaxation, and combined interventions than with control • No significant differences were found among the three treatment groups • Negative relationship between age and treatment outcome suggesting older persons with tension headaches less likely to respond to relaxation and behavioral techniques NOTE: Recent studies reported good treatment results with elderly patients
Bogaards and ter Kuile, 1994	N = 78 studies	Recurrent tension headache	Meta-analysis Testing effects of relaxation and behavioral interventions	Headache activity measured by daily headache diary or global ratings	• Significant reduction in headache activity with cognitive therapy and EMG biofeedback alone or in combination compared with placebo and no treatment

Continued

CBT, Cognitive behavioral training; EMG, electromyogram; FIQ, Fibromyalgia Impact Questionnaire; TENS, transcutaneous electrical nerve stimulation; VAS, visual analog scale.

TABLE 10-2	Studies of CAM Therapies in Management of Chronic Pain Conditions—cont'd			
Author, Year	Sample Size	Diagnosis	Design	Outcome Variable	Major Findings
			• EMG biofeedback • Relaxation • Combined EMG biofeedback and relaxation • Cognitive therapy • Pharmacologic therapy • Other therapies Control groups: • Group I: placebo • Group II: no treatment		• Relaxation therapy and other therapy more effective than no treatment • Type outcome measure influenced other results; relaxation therapy superior to placebo treatment only in treatment conditions that used a headache diary • Duration of headache complaint and age were interrelated and negatively related to treatment outcome NOTE: Duration of treatment did not affect treatment outcomes suggesting treatments of short duration may be effective
Keller and Bzdek, 1986	N = 60 (70% college students)	Tension headache	Experimental Random assignment: • Group I: experimental (5 minutes of therapeutic touch) • Group II: control (5 minutes of placebo therapeutic touch)	Pain assessment using McGill-Melzack Pain Questionnaire immediately before treatment, 5 minutes after treatment, 4 hours after treatment	• No significant differences between the two groups in pre-treatment pain scores or patient characteristics • Significant reduction (70%) in pain in experimental group compared with control group (37%) NOTE: The same practitioner administered both interventions, which may have introduced bias

Vincent, 1989	N = 32	Migraine headache	Experimental Random assignment: • Group I: acupuncture • Group II: placebo acupuncture	• Headache activity measured by diary • Amount of medication usage	• True acupuncture significantly more effective in relieving pain than sham acupuncture • 43% reduction in posttreatment pain scores and 38% reduction in medication usage for acupuncture group; maintained at 4-month and 1-year follow-up
Patel et al., 1989	N = 14 clinical trials	Regional pain: • Lower back • Head and neck • Other sites	Meta-analysis Assessing effectiveness of acupuncture compared with placebo or standard care	Number of improved patients	Pooled results suggest effectiveness of acupuncture in low back and chronic headache pain
Coan et al, 1980	N = 50	Low back pain duration of > 24 weeks	Experimental Random assignment: • Group I: immediate treatment • Group II: delayed treatment Acupuncture using nonstandardized needling points	• Pain intensity rating using 10-point scale • Range of motion rated on a 4-point scale	• Significant improvement in 79% of group receiving 10 sessions of traditional acupuncture • Improvements in group receiving traditional acupuncture maintained by 58% of patients at 40-week follow-up • No improvements seen in no-treatment or dropout patients NOTE: While not conclusive, results suggest traditional acupuncture can be beneficial in treatment of low back pain

Continued

CBT, Cognitive behavioral training; EMG, electromyogram; FIQ, Fibromyalgia Impact Questionnaire; TENS, transcutaneous electrical nerve stimulation; VAS, visual analog scale.

TABLE 10-2   Studies of CAM Therapies in Management of Chronic Pain Conditions—cont'd

Author, Year	Sample Size	Diagnosis	Design	Outcome Variable	Major Findings
ter Riet et al., 1990	N = 51 clinical trials	Chronic pain including headache and back pain	Criteria-based meta-analysis Assessing efficacy of acupuncture	Quality measures of studies	Suggests that efficacy of acupuncture for chronic pain remains doubtful based on quality NOTE: Authors deemed many of the studies of poor or mediocre quality
Shekelle et al., 1992	N = 5 controlled studies	Chronic low back pain	Meta-analysis Assessing effects of spinal manipulation	Varied; included pain and functional outcomes	• Insufficient data to support or refute efficacy of spinal manipulation • Study designs varied, and results from studies contradictory
Anderson et al., 1992	N = 23 randomized, controlled clinical trials	Acute and chronic back pain	Meta-analysis Assessing efficacy of spinal manipulation as compared with other forms of treatment	Varied; included pain and functional outcomes	• Consistent trend for spinal manipulation to produce better results than any other form of treatment to which it was compared • Most studies assessed outcomes within first month of treatment, and few assessed outcomes beyond 3 months NOTE: Authors concluded that long-term effects had not been well studied
Abenhaim and Bergeron, 1992	N = 21 randomized clinical trials	Acute and chronic back pain	Review Systematic review assessing efficacy of manipulative therapy	Varied; included pain and functional outcomes	• Some indication of short-term effectiveness in relieving acute and chronic back pain • Long-term effects of treatment had not been adequately evaluated in the trials

Study	N	Condition	Design	Outcome measures	Results
Lehmann et al., 1986	N = 54	Chronic low back pain (work-related disability)	Experimental Random assignment: • Group I: low-intensity TENS (daily × 3 weeks) • Group II: electroacupuncture (twice weekly × 3 weeks) • Group III: placebo TENS (daily × 3 weeks) Each group given multidisciplinary education program and exercise sessions twice daily	• Patient and physician ratings of disability • Pain intensity ratings for peak and average pain • Measures of trunk strength and spine range of motion • Amount of medication use	• No significant difference in groups at entry • Significant improvement in all groups on all outcome measures at 3 weeks • Significant improvement from entry to 6-month follow-up for all groups except average pain intensity ratings and amount of medication used • Significant improvement in average pain intensity ratings for electroacupuncture group at 6-month follow-up NOTE: Results are confounded by dropout rates and failure of large numbers in acupuncture group to return for follow-up
Deyo et al., 1990	N = 149	Chronic low back pain	Experimental Random assignment: • Group I: TENS • Group II: TENS plus exercise program • Group III: placebo TENS plus exercise • Group IV: placebo TENS	• Sickness Impact Profile Score (modified) • Pain intensity ratings • Range of motion	• Significant improvement in all four groups at 2 weeks with progressive improvement to week 4, but not maintained at 8 weeks • No significant treatment effects found in TENS group on any outcome measure • No significant differences between TENS and sham TENS groups

Continued

CBT, Cognitive behavioral training; EMG, electromyogram; FIQ, Fibromyalgia Impact Questionnaire; TENS, transcutaneous electrical nerve stimulation; VAS, visual analog scale.

TABLE 10-2	Studies of CAM Therapies in Management of Chronic Pain Conditions—cont'd				
Author, Year	**Sample Size**	**Diagnosis**	**Design**	**Outcome Variable**	**Major Findings**
					• Significant improvement in groups that included exercise when compared with TENS and sham TENS only NOTE: Authors concluded that TENS adds no benefit to that of exercise alone and was no more effective than placebo in treatment of chronic low back pain
Marchand et al., 1993	N = 42	Chronic back pain (duration > 6 months)	Experimental • Group I: TENS • Group II: placebo TENS • Group III: control; no treatment	• Pain intensity using VAS • Pain unpleasantness using VAS (baseline 3 days before study and before and after treatments at 1 week, 3 and 6 months)	• Pain intensity and unpleasantness reduced in both TENS and sham TENS groups • Significant difference in reduction of pain intensity ratings in TENS group compared with sham TENS, but not pain unpleasantness ratings
Guieu et al., 1991	N = 24	Low back pain (duration > 3 months)	Experimental • Group I: TENS • Group II: vibration stimulation • Group III: TENS plus vibration • Group IV: control	• McGill Pain Questionnaire scores • Numeric pain intensity ratings on 0 to 10 scale	• Significant differences in outcome measures for TENS and combined treatments compared with control group • Combined treatment more effective than vibration stimulation or TENS alone

Burckhardt et al., 1994	N = 99 women	Fibromyalgia	Experimental Random assignment: • Group I: combined education and CBT (6-week self-management course) • Group II: combined education and physical training (6 weeks of self-management training plus 6 hours of exercise training) • Group III: wait-list control	• Self efficacy for function: FIQ • Tender-point pain • Quality of life	Posttreatment: • Significant improvement in both treatment groups in self-efficacy for function (FIQ) and quality of life • Significant reduction in number of tender points in both treatment groups 3-month follow-up: • Combined education and physical training; significantly better outcomes • Significant improvements in one or more outcomes compared with control group after treatment
Buckelew et al., 1992	N = 119	Fibromyalgia	Experimental Random assignment: • Group I: biofeedback • Group II: exercise • Group III: biofeedback and exercise • Group IV: education-attention control	• Self-efficacy for function • Tender-point pain	• Significant improvements in tender points and self-efficacy for function maintained only by biofeedback/exercise group at follow-up

Continued

CBT, Cognitive behavioral training; EMG, electromyogram; FIQ, Fibromyalgia Impact Questionnaire; TENS, transcutaneous electrical nerve stimulation; VAS, visual analog scale.

TABLE 10-2	Studies of CAM Therapies in Management of Chronic Pain Conditions—cont'd			
Author, Year	**Sample Size**	**Diagnosis**	**Design**	**Outcome Variable**	**Major Findings**
Deluze et al., 1992	N = 70 (54 women and 16 men)	Fibromyalgia	Experimental (double-blind) Random assignment: • Group I: electroacupuncture (6 sessions over 2 weeks) • Group II: placebo acupuncture (needling 2 mm from true sites with less current; 6 sessions over 2 weeks)	• Pain threshold • Pain intensity rating • Stiffness • Self-reported analgesic usage • Sleep quality • Perceived general state	• Significant improvement in electroacupuncture group in all but one outcome measure • Significant differences between Group I and Group II in five outcomes including 70% improvement in pain threshold in Group I compared with 4% in Group II
Dworkin et al., 1994	N = 185 (139 completed study)	Temporomandibular disorders	Experimental Random assignment • Group I: CBT • Group II: standard dental care control	• Pain level • Pain interference • Jaw range of motion • Depression • Somatization	• No significant differences in the two groups in improvements in pain level at 3 months; CBT group continued to decrease pain level and pain interference with activity over 3- to 12-month follow-up • Significantly more CBT patients (86.5%) reported improvement in their temporomandibular disorder than patients in standard care group

| Møystad et al., 1990 | N = 19 (Trial I) N = 13 (Trial II) | Temporo-mandibular joint disease | Crossover design (two trials) Trial I:
• Group I: high-frequency TENS
• Group II: placebo TENS (treatments given in random order; two 30-minute treatments with interval of 1 week between treatments Trial II:
• Group I: low-frequency TENS
• Group II: placebo TENS; procedure same as in Trial I | • VAS pain intensity ratings at rest and before and after treatment; every hour on day of treatment and next morning
• Joint tenderness and jaw function | • Significant improvements in pain scores during function and at rest; and in joint tenderness for all treatments
• High-frequency TENS better than placebo in reducing functional pain
• No other significant differences between TENS and placebo |

CBT, Cognitive behavioral training; EMG, electromyogram; FIQ, Fibromyalgia Impact Questionnaire; TENS, transcutaneous electrical nerve stimulation; VAS, visual analog scale.

atively related to treatment outcome. Older subjects and those with headache complaint of longer duration were less responsive to treatment. Although other meta-analyses[96] have reported similar findings, conclusions must be drawn carefully. More recently published studies have reported good treatment results with elderly patients.[9,10,108]

Therapeutic Touch. A number of researchers have reported the effectiveness of TT in relieving anxiety.[77,90,182,205] Anxiety influences pain by increasing muscle tension; hence, therapeutic touch may, by reducing anxiety, facilitate pain relief. There are few controlled studies investigating the efficacy of TT on chronic pain, but there is some support for the hypothesis that TT can be effective in reducing headache pain. Keller and Bzdek[111] compared the effects of TT with a placebo simulation of TT on tension headache pain. Sixty adult volunteers, the majority (70%) college students, were randomly assigned to either an experimental or a control group. No physical contact was involved in the 5-minute TT treatment received by the experimental group or in the 5-minute mimic TT treatment received by the control group. Pain was assessed with the McGill-Melzack Pain Questionnaire immediately before treatment, 5 minutes after the intervention, and 4 hours after treatment. There were no differences between the two groups in pretreatment pain scores or in patient characteristics. The results indicate that subjects who received TT had a significant reduction (70%) in tension headache pain when compared with subjects who received a mimic form of TT (37%). One of the researchers administered the interventions, which may have introduced some bias into the findings. Table 10-2 contains a study summary.

Acupuncture. Evidence on the efficacy of acupuncture in the management of chronic pain is inconclusive, although there is some support for short-term pain relief in several chronic conditions, including headache.[70,166,190] At least one well-controlled study demonstrated long-term effectiveness in the treatment of migraine headache.[232]

Patel et al.[171] examined the effectiveness of acupuncture for chronic pain in a meta-analysis of 14 randomized, controlled trials. For analysis the trials were classified into three subgroups by type of regional pain (lower back, head and neck, and other sites) and into two subgroups by nature of control (placebo or standard care). Two treatment conditions, formula and classic acupuncture, were analyzed. Whereas formula acupuncture uses a set of fixed points repeatedly, the points used in classic acupuncture vary from patient to patient and treatment to treatment. Most trials achieved "Teh Chi" or "needling" (i.e., numbness in the area of the needle, proof that a point had been located correctly). Outcome was measured by the number of improved patients. Although few of the individual trials reported statistically significant results, pooled results suggest that acupuncture was effective in the treatment of chronic low back and head and neck pain. However, potential sources of bias, such as inadequate blinding, preclude definitive conclusions regarding efficacy. A second meta-analysis of 51 trials[225] reported that most of the studies were of mediocre or poor quality with the best studies yielding contradictory results. Thus no definitive conclusions were drawn, and the efficacy of acupuncture on chronic pain, including headache pain, remains doubt-ful based on the 51 trials.

In a systematic review, Richardson and Vincent[190] reported that results from five controlled clinical trials testing the efficacy of acupunture on chronic headache pain were inconclusive. Although findings suggested benefits from acupuncture, method-ologic problems precluded a definitive conclusion. However, in a well-designed, ran-domized clinical trial, which was not included in the review[171,225] or meta-analyses, Vincent[232] compared the effects of acupuncture with sham acupuncture in 32 referred migraine patients. The treatment points included two standard points and two points based on patient headache pattern and palpatory tenderness. The sham treatment con-sisted of surface needling at locations 2 to 3 cm from the identified points. Six treat-ments were administered in a 6-week period. Diary measures of headache and of med-ication intake were recorded throughout the study. Patients were blinded to the treat-ment group, and blinding was confirmed by assessment of credibility of sham and true treatment procedures. Results indicate that the true acupuncture treatment was signif-icantly more effective than the sham procedure in reducing migraine pain. The acupuncture group had a 43% reduction in posttreatment pain scores and a 38% reduc-tion in medication usage. These improvements were maintained at 4-month and 1-year follow-ups.

Using a crossover design and small samples, two studies demonstrated the thera-peutic effects of acupuncture on tension headache.[85,233] In both studies, true acupunc-ture was compared with sham acupuncture. Significant reductions in pain were achieved, and true acupuncture was shown to be superior to sham acupuncture. Results of these studies[85,232,233] suggest the efficacy of acupuncture in the treatment of tension and migraine headache, but additional research is needed to confirm these find-ings. As concluded in the NIH National Technology Assessment Statement on Acupuncture,[166] testing of acupuncture as a therapeutic intervention is complicated by inherent difficulties in the use of appropriate controls, such as placebo and sham acupuncture groups.

Chronic Back Pain. The scientific literature provides some basis for the conclusion that a number of CAM therapies have demonstrated short-term effectiveness in treating chronic back pain. There is less evidence of long-term efficacy.

Relaxation and Behavioral Therapies. A 1995 NIH technology assessment panel[64] recommended the integration of behavioral and relaxation therapies into the treatment of chronic pain and insomnia. The panel reported that a series of well-designed studies demonstrated that cognitive-behavioral therapies were more effective than placebo and routine care for alleviating low back pain. Furthermore, consistently positive results from several meta-analyses indicate that multimodal treatments are also effective in the treatment of chronic back pain.[164] Malone and Strube[140] examined the effects of nonpharmocologic treatments on a variety of chronic conditions in 109 studies. The pattern of positive effects of moderate size suggests the short-term efficacy of behavioral and relaxation therapies for chronic pain, including chronic back pain.

Acupuncture. In a systematic review Richardson and Vincent[190] reported results from controlled trials that suggest the majority of patients derived clinically significant short-term benefits from acupuncture. Evidence of long-term effectiveness was weaker because variable and often nonexistent or inadequate follow-up periods made long-term efficacy difficult to assess. Evidence of the superiority of acupuncture compared with TENS (as a control condition), and of classically determined needling sites compared with theoretically irrelevant sites, was also inconclusive, although the data trends favored classic acupuncture. However, in one unusual study,[50] traditional acupuncturists were given the freedom to assess patients individually and to select needling points rather than follow a standardized intervention, as was done in all of the other studies. Fifty patients with low back pain of at least 24 weeks' duration were randomly assigned to either an immediate-treatment group or a delayed-treatment group. Pain intensity was measured on a 10-point scale, and range of motion was rated on a 4-point scale. Seventy-nine percent of the treated sample had significant improvement after completing a mean of 10 sessions of traditional acupuncture. The improvements were maintained by 58% of the acupuncture patients at the 40-week follow-up. During the same period there was no improvement in the 10 individuals who received no treatment or dropped out before completing treatment. This study is not statistically conclusive, but the results suggest that acupuncture as traditionally practiced can be beneficial in the treatment of chronic back pain.

Findings from the meta-analysis of Patel et al.[171] of 14 randomized, controlled trials suggest the efficacy of acupuncture in the treatment of chronic low back pain. However, Patel et al. cautioned that the conclusions required careful interpretation because of methodologic limitations in the studies. Ter Riet et al.[225] reported that efficacy of acupuncture on chronic pain remains doubtful based on their meta-analysis of 51 trials, many of which were deemed of poor or mediocre quality.

Additional well-designed studies that address patient characteristics, specificity of needling sites, and characteristics of the treatment process are needed before firm conclusions on the efficacy of acupuncture in the treatment of chronic back pain can be drawn. Furthermore, clinicians should be aware that complications of acupuncture, including hematomas, infections (hepatitis B and *Staphylococcus aureus*), pneumothorax, and spinal nerve and spinal cord injuries attributable to buried needles migrating to the spinal cord, have been reported.[3]

Spinal Manipulation. Findings from a meta-analysis and review provide some evidence of short-term effectiveness of spinal manipulation on chronic back pain, although long-term effectiveness has been inadequately investigated[2,7] (see Table 10-2).

Results from two large clinical trials suggest long-term benefits from manipulation for chronic, nonspecific back and neck pain[115] and for low back pain of mechanic origin.[149] However, both studies have been criticized for serious methodologic flaws that make the findings equivocal.[70,208] Further research is still needed to address the question of long-term efficacy of manipulation for chronic low back pain.

Transcutaneous Electrical Nerve Stimulation. Although TENS is widely used in the management of chronic pain,[158] whether TENS offers long-term efficacy greater than placebo remains equivocal.[70] Results from controlled trials suggest clinically beneficial effects for chronic low back pain, but comparisons with other therapies and with placebo TENS have yielded contradictory findings.[59,82,124,142]

Lehmann et al.[124] investigated the efficacy of electroacupuncture and TENS in the rehabilitation of patients with chronic low back pain. Fifty-four patients with work-related disabilities were randomly assigned to one of three groups: low-intensity TENS, electroacupuncture, or sham TENS. After 3 weeks of treatment, all groups showed significant improvement in all outcome measures. Only the acupuncture group showed significant improvement in average pain scores at the 6-month follow-up. However, the results in this study are confounded by high dropout rates during treatment, failure of a large number of patients in the acupuncture group to return for follow-up, and the lack of blinding in the acupuncture group.

In a randomized clinical trial, Deyo et al.[59] compared the effectiveness of TENS, a program of exercises, and a combination of both in the treatment of chronic low back pain in 149 patients. Patients were randomly assigned to one of four groups of equal size: TENS, TENS plus exercises (relaxation, stretching, and flexibility), sham TENS plus exercises, or sham TENS. All four groups showed significant improvement in almost all measures at week 2 with progressive improvement to week 4, but outcomes regressed to baseline at the follow-up. The researchers concluded that TENS adds no benefit to that of exercise alone and was no more effective than placebo in the treatment of chronic back pain.

In a controlled trial, 42 patients with chronic back pain of 6 months' or more duration were assigned to one of three groups: TENS, sham TENS, or no-treatment control.[142] After treatment, pain intensity and unpleasantness were reduced in both the TENS and sham TENS groups, and TENS was significantly better than the placebo in reducing pain intensity, but not unpleasantness of the pain.

Guieu et al.[82] compared the effectiveness of TENS and vibration stimulation for chronic low back pain. Twenty-four patients with low back pain for 3 or more months were assigned to one of four groups: TENS, vibration simulation (VS), TENS and VS, or control. TENS and the combined treatment (TENS and VS) were superior to the control. The combined treatment was more effective than VS or TENS alone. See Table 10-2 for study details.

Disease-Related Chronic Pain

The following section focuses on selected disease-related chronic pain conditions. Specific methods are discussed that have demonstrated some efficacy in treating the pain associated with the particular problem. In the case of arthritis pain, the discussion below is limited to fibromyalgia. Other forms of arthritis are discussed in Chapter 14.

Fibromyalgia

Relaxation and Behavioral Therapies. Fibromyalgia, which affects up to 20% of all patients seen in rheumatology practices, is a syndrome characterized by diffuse musculoskeletal pain, fatigue, stiffness, sleep disturbance, and resistance to treatment.[109,110] Although relatively few controlled trials have been conducted, preliminary results suggest that cognitive-behavioral therapies can be effective in the management of fibromyalgia pain.[110] Findings from a controlled, but not randomized, study suggest that a 10-week stress reduction program incorporating cognitive behavioral techniques was effective in reducing pain and psychologic distress in fibromyalgia patients.[78]

Two randomized clinical trials have tested the combined effects of cognitive behavioral training (CBT) and exercise in the treatment of pain associated with fibromyalgia.[39,41] Burckhardt et al.[41] randomly assigned 99 women with fibromyalgia to one of three groups: combined education and CBT, combined education and physical training; or a waiting list control group. The education/CBT group received a 6-week self-management course. The education/physical training group received the course and 6 hours of training designed to assist the subjects to exercise independently. After treatment the education groups did not differ significantly, and both groups achieved significant improvements in self-efficacy for function and quality of life and significant reductions in tender-point pain. At the 3-month follow-up the combined education/physical training group had significantly better outcomes.

Buckelew et al.[39] compared the effectiveness of biofeedback and exercise. Patients were randomly assigned to one of four groups: biofeedback, exercise, biofeedback and exercise, or an education-attention control group. The three treatment groups had significant improvements in one or more outcomes when compared with the control group. At the follow-up, only the combined biofeedback/exercise group maintained significant improvements in tender-point pain and self-efficacy for function. Although there are limitations in the studies, the results from the randomized, controlled trials suggest that multimodal treatments combining cognitive behavioral therapies with exercise may be effective in the management of fibromyalgia-associated pain. See Table 10-2 for additional study details.

Acupuncture. The effectiveness of acupuncture in the treatment of arthritis pain has also been investigated. Findings from a controlled trial provide some evidence that acupuncture can provide therapeutic benefits for patients with fibromyalgia.

In a randomized clinical trial, Deluze et al.[57] tested the effects of electroacupuncture in the treatment of fibromyalgia. Seventy referred patients (54 women) were randomly assigned to either the electroacupuncture group or a sham acupuncture group. Patients in each group received six sessions of electroacupuncture or sham acupuncture (needling at sites 2 mm from true sites with less current) over a 2-week period. Patients and evaluators were blinded. The eight outcome measures included pain threshold, stiffness, self-reported analgesic usage, pain intensity scores, and sleep quality. The electroacupuncture group showed significant improvements in seven of eight outcome measures with a significant difference between the groups in five outcomes. The results indicate a 70% improvement in pain threshold in the patients receiving treatment with electroacupuncture compared with 4% in the sham group. The study used careful selection criteria and a sample size calculated on the basis of a pilot study to provide sufficient power. However, the findings are limited by the lack of long-term follow-up.

Temporomandibular Disorders

Relaxation and Behavioral Therapies. Temporomandibular disorder (TMD) refers to a collection of medical and dental conditions affecting the temporomandibular joint (TMJ) and/or muscles of mastication, as well as contiguous tissue. Although specific causes such as degenerative arthritis and trauma underlie some cases of TMD, as a group these conditions have no common etiology or biologic explanation and comprise a heterogeneous group of health problems whose signs and symptoms are overlapping, but not identical. The clinical conditions usually classified as TMD include those with pain or dysfunction in the joint or contiguous structures.[165] As with other chronic pain conditions, patients with persistent pain and dysfunction associated with TMD may suffer psychologically and socially. Although the literature base is small, the 1996 NIH consensus panel recommended that relaxation and behavioral therapies be considered in the treatment of TMD.[165]

In a carefully designed, randomized clinical trial, Dworkin et al.[66] compared the effects of a standard dental TMD treatment with the effect of standard dental treatment plus cognitive behavioral therapy. In the study, 185 referred patients were randomly assigned to one of two treatment groups: the CBT or the standard care control group. Analysis of data from 139 patients who completed the study revealed that there were no significant differences in improvement in pain-level at the 3-month follow-up, but only the CBT group continued the decrease in pain level over the 3- to 12-month follow-up. The CBT group also continued a strong decreasing trend in pain interference in daily activity during the follow-up period. Depression, somatization, or clinical measures of jaw range of motion improved, but the differences between groups were not significant. Significantly more patients in the CBT group (86.5%) reported that their TMD condition had improved than patients in the standard care dental treatment group (70.1%).

The data analysis suggests that cognitive behavioral treatment was not effective with dysfunctional patients who were defined as reporting high levels of pain intensity and TMD pain-related interference with daily activities. Results also indicate that somatization tends to correspond with dysfunctional chronic pain status. Additional research is needed to determine whether somatization is a predictor of nonresponsiveness to cognitive behavior therapies.

Transcutaneous Electrical Nerve Stimulation. Using a double-blind crossover design in two trials, Møystad et al.[158] tested the efficacy of TENS in a group of patients with rheumatic disease involving the TMJ. In the first trial, treatments consisted of high-frequency (HF) TENS and placebo TENS given in random order. Nineteen patients received two 30-minute treatments with an interval of 1 week between treatment sessions. In the second trial the same procedures were used with 13 patients who received low-frequency (LF) TENS and placebo TENS. A visual analog scale (VAS) was used to assess pain intensity associated with function and rest pain before and after treatment, every hour throughout the day of treatment and the next morning. The greatest difference between pretreatment and posttreatment pain recordings during the day of treatment was compared for HF TENS and placebo and for LF TENS and placebo. Joint tenderness and jaw function were also assessed. Although no data were shown, Møystad et al.[158] reported that all treatments produced significant improvements in pain scores during function and at rest and in joint tenderness. HF TENS was better than placebo in reducing functional pain of TMJ rheumatic disease. No other significant differences between TENS and placebo were found.

Feine and Lund[70] analyzed review articles and controlled clinical trials for TMD disorders and chronic musculoskeletal pain disorders to evaluate the efficacy of physical therapy and physical methods. Clinical conditions included TMD, low back pain, tension headache, musculoskeletal disorders, osteoarthritis, fibromyalgia, and myofascial pain. The physical methods included the following CAM or alternative therapies: TENS, acupuncture, and spinal manipulation. The authors concluded that the results from the studies provide little evidence of long-term efficacy for any therapy greater than the effect for placebo. However, there was strong evidence that symptoms improved during treatment with most forms of physical treatment, including placebo. Future research is required to investigate the individual differences that influence the efficacy of specific treatment methods.

SELECTIVE REVIEW OF CANCER PAIN OUTCOMES RESEARCH

Persons with cancer can have acute or chronic pain from the disease process, diagnostic procedures, treatment, or preexisting conditions. Cancer pain is dynamic and ever changing and thus requires careful and frequent assessment to establish the etiology and appropriate course of treatment.[49,141] According to Rowlingson and Hamill,[193] "the diagnosis of cancer intensifies the emotional impact of pain, so attention must be given to the psychosocial aspects of the disease." While drug therapies remain the cornerstone of pain management for persons with cancer, nonpharmacologic interventions can be used as adjunctive therapies to provide additional relief of suffering and to enhance the patient's quality of life. Every patient with cancer should have the expectation of pain control as an integral aspect of his or her care throughout the course of the disease.[162] The clinical guidelines for cancer pain control recommended that psychosocial interventions, such as relaxation and behavioral techniques, "be introduced early in the course of illness while patients have sufficient energy and strength to learn and practice these strategies."[141] Physical methods, including TENS and massage, can also provide comfort for patients with cancer pain. A review of scientific literature provides some evidence of the efficacy of these therapies in the management of cancer-related pain. There is also some evidence that traditional Chinese medicine treatment methods may be useful in reducing cancer pain.

Relaxation and Behavioral Therapies

Devine and Westlake[58] meta-analyzed 116 studies to examine the effects of educational and psychosocial interventions, which they referred to as "psychoeducational care," on seven outcomes in adults with cancer. The seven outcomes were pain, nausea, vomiting, anxiety, depression, mood, and patient knowledge of cancer. Relaxation and behavioral therapies constituted the most prevalent interventions and were found effective in reducing pain and relieving other symptoms. See Table 10-3 for study details.

A 1995 NIH technology assessment panel evaluating relaxation and behavioral therapies for chronic pain reduction reported that the "evidence supporting the effects of hypnosis in alleviating chronic pain associated with cancer seems strong."[164] Other data suggest the effectiveness of hypnosis in other chronic painful conditions, including oral mucositis. In a randomized clinical trial Syrjala et al.[221] compared the efficacy of hypnosis and cognitive behavioral training for reducing pain and nausea during cancer treatment. Sixty-seven bone marrow transplantation patients were assigned to the following groups before transplantation conditioning: (1) cognitive behavioral coping skills, (2) hypnosis training, (3) therapist contact control, and (4) standard care control.

Data analysis indicated that only hypnosis was effective in reducing reported oral pain for patients undergoing bone marrow transplantation. Gender differences were consistent across the groups; on average, women reported less pain than men. However, nausea, emesis, and opioid use did not differ significantly between groups. Pre-transplantation risk (low/high based on diagnosis and number of relapses or remissions) and physical dysfunction (measured by Sickness Impact Profile) were significant predictors of oral pain.

Syrjala et al.[221] suggested that the results confirm their clinical experience, which indicates that imagery was the central component in the hypnosis intervention. Lack of

TABLE 10-3	Studies of Complementary Therapies in Management of Cancer-Related Pain				
Author, Year	Sample Size	Diagnosis	Design	Outcome Variable	Major Findings
Devine and Westlake, 1995	N = 116 studies (67% randomly controlled trials)	Cancer	Meta-analysis Assessing effects of educational and psychosocial interventions, primarily relaxation and behavioral therapies	Pain (McGill Pain Questionnaire and VAS) • Nausea • Vomiting • Anxiety • Depression • Mood • Patient knowledge of cancer	• Medium-sized, statistically significant, beneficial effect on cancer-related pain • Significantly larger effect for relaxation-type therapies on pain reduction than for other psychoeducational interventions
Syrjala et al., 1992	N = 67 (45 completed study)	Bone marrow transplantation	Experimental Random assignment: • Group I: cognitive behavioral coping skills • Group II: hypnosis training • Group III: therapist contact control • Group IV: standard care control	SIP score (measure of health status) • Brief Symptom Inventory score (measure of psychologic functioning) • VAS pain ratings for oral mucositis pain and nausea • Presence/absence of emesis • Amount of daily opioid usage	• Only hypnosis effective in reducing oral pain • On average, women reported less pain than men • Significant predictors of oral pain were SIP physical dysfunction score and pretransplant risks—high/low based on diagnosis and number of relapses or remissions

| Li et al., 1994 | N = 16 men | Liver cancer surgery | Experimental
Double-blind, random assignment to various treatments:
• Chinese herbs
• Ear acupuncture
• Epidural morphine
• Placebo herbs
Patients assigned one, two, or all three treatments or placebo | • VAS pain intensity rating (every 2 hours for 24 hours, then every 4 hours for 4 days)
• Amount of narcotic analgesic usage | • Significantly better outcomes in all groups than in placebo group
• Epidural morphine provided better pain relief than other treatments but caused prolonged abdominal distention and urinary retention
• Chinese herbs and ear acupuncture significantly accelerated restoration of bowel peristalsis
NOTE: Authors recommended epidural morphine immediately after surgery and in combination with Chinese herbs or ear acupuncture |

SIP, Sickness Impact Profile; *VAS*, visual analog scale.

significance in the effectiveness of the cognitive behavioral intervention may be attributed to the large number of components and the limited number (two) of training sessions. In addition, the relatively small sample size may lack the power to detect all significant outcomes.

Although not confined to cancer populations, results from several studies provide additional evidence to suggest that relaxation and behavioral therapies can be effective in reducing cancer-related pain. Malone and Strube[140] evaluated the efficacy of nonpharmacologic treatment for chronic pain, including cancer pain, in 109 studies. Forty-eight studies included sufficient information to calculate effect size. Percentage of improvement was used to evaluate effectiveness in the other studies. Treatment interventions included relaxation and behavioral strategies alone or in combination, TENS, and other interventions. The pattern that emerged suggested short-term effectiveness across types of pain, treatment, and outcome measure. The authors concluded that the positive result may be due to improvement in psychologic factors, such as anxiety and mood, that influence pain. Many of the studies were of low quality; thus conclusions should be interpreted cautiously. Fernandez and Turk[71] meta-analyzed 51 studies and demonstrated that cognitive coping strategies significantly reduced the perception of pain. The results largely pertain to acute pain induced in laboratory conditions, but suggest potential efficacy in acute cancer-related pain.

Transcutaneous Electrical Nerve Stimulation

Research on the effectiveness of TENS therapy on cancer-related pain is limited to single-group studies and case reports.[13,24] Cancer pain may be present as either an acute or chronic condition. Thus the research literature on the efficacy of TENS for acute and chronic pain suggests that some cancer patients, particularly those with mild pain, may benefit from this therapy.*

Massage Therapy

References to massage have appeared for centuries, yet it is only in this century that the various styles of massage and standardized techniques have evolved.[228] Massage therapy (including acupressure) has a large body of research documenting its use in pain management, particularly cancer pain.†

The National Cancer Institute and the clinical guidelines for cancer pain control[141] currently recommend massage as a nonpharmacologic method of pain management.

Mechanisms of pain relief using massage include both endorphin release[107] and neural gate control.[61] Other mechanisms are reduction of ischemia via local circulatory stimulation and skeletal muscle relaxation via parasympathetic stimulation.[148] Studies of cerebral blood flow using positron emission tomography provide support for the

---

*References 4, 26, 124, 140, 141, 142.
†References 19, 43, 195, 206, 229, 240, 241.

gate control theory of pain relief using massage.[65] Anticipation of cutaneous stimuli, touching or shocks, decreased blood flow to nonattended areas of the somatosensory cortex surrounding but not including the area at which the stimulus was expected. Thus anticipation of being touched on an area of the skin tends to suppress sensations from other areas, while actual touch increases attention to the area being touched.

Touch plays a crucial role in human health and well-being,[157] and its significance in affective development is supported by primate studies.[87,88] The nursing literature supports a number of beneficial effects of touch in the hospital setting, including communicating a nonverbal message of reassurance, caring, and acceptance for patients who are in pain or isolated; fostering a sense of self-worth and a positive body image for surgical patients whose body image may have been altered; and helping to orient disoriented or confused patients.*

These studies suggest that therapeutic massage, through promoting comfort and relaxation, has physiologic as well as psychologic effects.

An outcome of massage—relaxation—has been found to be an effective adjunct to standard patient care in terms of both surgical preparation and postoperative care.[29,106] Researchers have studied the effects of brief massage compared with a control intervention on cancer pain with some positive outcomes.[207,241] However, these studies have been criticized as methodologically flawed because of small sample sizes, a large number of symptom variables, brief duration of the massage intervention, and nonindividualized massage treatment.[153] Other researchers have found that massages of at least 30 minutes reduced anxiety, as measured by the State-Trait Anxiety Inventory; self-reported pain; and blood pressure, heart and respiratory rates.[19,73] For example, researchers have found that massage decreased self-reported pain by 75%.[19] These cancer outpatients self-selected massage practitioners, and the practitioners used individualized treatments; either variable could have contributed to the relatively high percentage of reported pain relief.

Traditional Chinese Medicine

Traditional Chinese medicine embraces several treatment methods including acupuncture, herbal medicine, moxibustion (heat therapy), Qi Gong (exercises for internal energy), massage, diet therapy, and meditation. Diagnosis focuses on patterns of disease symptoms. Chinese herbs are rarely prescribed individually. Herbal prescriptions are derived from formulas requiring four or more herbs based on symptom patterns. Several studies suggest the therapeutic benefits of Chinese herbal medicine or combined treatments in managing pain associated with advanced stages of cancer.

Yang et al.[247] evaluated the effectiveness of compound analgesic powder for cancer (CAPC) for cancer pain relief in 91 inpatients. CAPC is an analgesic powder consisting of 20 Chinese drugs. The powder is mixed with tea and applied externally to the area

---

*References 17, 20, 36, 42, 81, 125, 229.

of pain or to acupoints around the painful area. Patients were asked to indicate when they felt relief after application. Marked relief, defined as gradual reduction in pain within 20 to 40 minutes after application with sustained relief for 16 to 28 hours, was achieved by 42 patients (46%). For 22 patients (24%) CAPC was fairly effective, gradually reducing pain within 20 to 40 minutes with the analgesic effect sustained for 8 to 15 hours. For 22 other patients pain was gradually reduced within 40 to 60 minutes, and relief was sustained for 4 to 6 hours. CAPC was ineffective for 5 patients (5.5%) who required a Western analgesic within 2 hours. In total, 94.5% of the patients had relief with CAPC, which suggests that the analgesic powder can be useful in relieving pain associated with advanced cancer.

Wang[237] reported that 70 patients with liver carcinoma were treated with Chinese herbs and externally applied Pu Tuo ointment. The treatment provided effective pain relief in 96.7% of the patients, of whom 83.5% reported "remarkable" relief.

In a double-blind, randomized clinical trial, Li et al.[129] investigated the effects of Chinese therapies and a Western analgesic in the relief of postoperative pain and abdominal distention. Three treatment methods were examined individually and in combination: Chinese herbs, ear acupuncture, and epidural morphine. Sixteen male patients who underwent liver cancer surgery were randomly assigned to one, two, or all three treatment conditions or to a placebo that was similar to the Chinese herbs in taste, color, and dosage. All patients receiving treatment fared significantly better than the placebo patients. Epidural morphine prolonged abdominal distention and urinary retention but provided better analgesic effects than Chinese herbs and ear acupuncture. The latter two treatments significantly accelerated restoration of bowel peristalsis. The authors suggested that epidural morphine be given immediately following surgery and in combination with either Chinese herbs or ear acupuncture to enhance the analgesic effect and reduce the side effects of morphine. See Table 10-3 for additional study details.

EMERGING THERAPIES WITHIN PAIN MANAGEMENT
Herbal Therapies

Indigenous cultures around the world have long used herbal therapies for maintaining health and for treating both acute and chronic illnesses. A wealth of folklore and recorded information exists regarding treatment of pain in Ayurvedic medicine, traditional Oriental medicine, Native American medicine, and herbal/natural product therapies from Europe and North America. While some of these herbs have been tested by Western scientists, many plants, especially those from Central and South America, are still unknown and at risk for extinction. Chinese and Indian cultures have a long herbal tradition, and some herbs such as ginseng have established records of benefits in Asian cultures. Recognition and acceptance of such therapies by Western society lags. In Oriental medicine, mixtures of herbs and other remedies make it difficult to determine whether the positive findings are a result of a synergistic effect of the ingredients or a single active ingredient. Some herbs and natural products have been tested using clinical trials and controlled studies for efficacy and safety.[18,156]

In the area of pain management using herbs, both basic research and clinical studies have been conducted. Best known are salicylic acid from the willow family[152] and morphine from opium poppies. When the mechanisms of action of herbs are examined, these often match those described for conventional drugs (e.g., decreased arachidonate metabolism, altered serotonin release). Although the use of marijuana is illegal and pharmaceutic use is controlled, there are anecdotal reports of the use of marijuana for pain management by individuals with chronic painful conditions.[167] A recent editorial in the *British Journal of Anaesthesia* proposed that more clinical trials on cannabinoids be conducted.[63]

Ginger *(Zingiber officinale)* has shown promise in the treatment of arthritis.[212,213] A study of arthritis induced in rats that were then given oral treatment with ginger oil and eugenol (an oil extracted from cloves) found that both have "potent anti-inflammatory and antirheumatic properties."[200] Clove oil has a long folk tradition for topical use in toothache.[185] Willow has been used for rheumatism, gouty arthritis, ankylosing spondylitis, rheumatoid arthritis, and other systemic connective tissue disorders characterized by inflammatory changes.[163] Feverfew *(Tanacetum parthenium)* has shown benefits in the treatment of migraine,[16,160] although no benefits in rheumatoid arthritis.[173] Also, studies have shown that both platelet aggregation and prostaglandin biosynthesis are inhibited by extracts of feverfew.[52,92] Canada's Health Protection Branch has recently granted a Drug Identification Number for British feverfew permitting the distributor to claim that it is effective in the prophylaxis of migraines.[14] Rosemary has traditionally been used for flatulent dyspepsia and headache, and topically for myalgia, sciatica, and intercostal neuralgia.[38] Animal studies have shown that rosemarinic acid suppresses prostaglandin formation and, unlike nonsteroidal antiinflammatory drugs (NSAIDs), does not interfere with cyclooxygenase or prostacyclin synthetase.[40,184]

One plant derivative that has received attention is topically applied capsaicin, an extract of cayenne pepper and other hot peppers.[243] Interest in capsaicin was heightened by the discovery that it depletes local sensory terminals of substance P, which has been implicated in the pathogenesis and modulation of inflammation and pain in arthritis.*

Capsaicin has been shown to be effective in relieving pain in patients with diabetic neuropathy and osteoarthritis in a meta-analysis by Zhang and Po.[248] Basic research on rats has provided valuable details about afferent neuron function. For example, capsaicin has been shown in rats to have an effective desensitization of thin bladder afferents, thus giving further support to its clinical usefulness.[55] Capsaicin has also been shown to reduce C-nociceptor activity, suggesting its usefulness in treating pain triggered by C-fiber input.[137] Other research has elucidated the action of substance P in

---

*References 15, 89, 128, 132, 174, 234.

cluster headache and shown promising results in diminishing the frequency and number of headache attacks.[204]

Three plant oils high in gamma linoleic acid (GLA) are borage seed oil, black currant oil, and evening primrose oil. These have been studied for their antiinflammatory properties in conditions such as rheumatoid arthritis, migraine headache, and mastalgia.*

Kleijnen[114] urged further rigorous clinical trials on GLA and noted that "for some indications it is a promising treatment." In a study of rats where inflammation was induced, a diet enriched with borage seed oil suppressed inflammation markedly compared with a safflower oil–enriched diet.[223] A double-blind, placebo-controlled trial has demonstrated reversal of diabetic neuropathy by GLA.[102] The pineapple plant derived enzyme bromelain was investigated in the 1960s for its use in reducing swelling and inflammation. No recent human studies using bromelain for painful conditions were found, although there are many citations on in vivo animal experiments and in vitro work on this enzyme. In hamsters bromelain "attenuated the development of contraction-induced injury."[235]

Also of note are herbs traditionally used for sedation and relaxation—valerian (*Valeriana edulis* and *V. officinalis*), hops (*Humulus lupulus*), and kava (*Piper methysticum*).[30,163] Hops, in combination with chicory and peppermint, have been shown to relieve pain in patients with cholecystitis.[45] While the potential for benefits in improving comfort is high, these herbs also have the potential for misuse. Valerian can have adverse effects such as hangover, palpitations, central paralysis, and hallucinations.[147] Heavy kava use in Australia was associated with decreased albumin and plasma protein levels, along with changes "suggestive of pulmonary hypertension."[146] Contraindications to kava use are pregnancy, breast-feeding, and endogenous depression.[30] Lobelia (*Lobelia inflata*) extract has also been investigated for its antidepressant properties in mice.[218,219]

Although many herbs are available in health food stores and some have no known adverse effects, patients should be cautioned in using herbs and warned about claims of exaggerated effectiveness to treat chronic conditions (e.g., see Newall et al.[163] for contraindications for herbal medicines).

Therapeutic Magnetic Fields

Electromagnetic field (EMF) therapeutic methods are generally categorized in the following groups: pulsed electromagnetic fields (PEMFs), pulsed radiofrequency (PRF), low-frequency sine waves, and static magnetic fields. Experimental and clinical data suggest that exogenous magnetic fields can profoundly affect a variety of biologic systems[23,143,103,177,178] including analgesic action, vasodilation, antiinflammatory action, antiedema activity, spasmolytic activity, and healing acceleration.

---

*References 25, 104, 114, 126, 181, 209.

Direct and indirect responses to electromagnetic stimulation reveal the basis for the clinical use of static magnetic fields as stimulation therapy. Researchers now accept that EMF can provide a practical, exogenous method for inducing cell and tissue changes that promote healing. That is, magnetic fields (MFs), in principle, can induce selective changes in the microenvironment surrounding cells, as well as within the cell membrane.

The EMF method most often used in the United States for soft tissue applications is short-wave PRF. PRF therapeutic applications have been reported for the reduction of posttraumatic and postoperative pain and edema in soft tissue, wound healing, burn treatment, sprains and strains of the ankle, hand injuries, and nerve regeneration.[144] PEMF therapy was found to be effective in reducing pain and improving function in osteoarthritis patients.[226,227] PEMFs are approved for the management of postoperative dental pain and edema. Evidence of the effectiveness of these devices exists.[11,189] The efficacy of electroacupuncture (electrical stimulation via acupuncture needles) in reducing acute pain associated with renal colic[121] and in reducing chronic pain associated with fibromyalgia[57] has also been demonstrated (see earlier discussions of acute and chronic pain).

There are several possible explanations for MF and EMF not being widely used in the United States. First, there may be a bias against introduction of magnetic therapeutic technologies, stemming, perhaps, from excess of such at the turn of the century. Also, there is little transfer of the latest knowledge about bioelectric aspects of molecular biology to the medical professionals. Consequently, there is no commonly accepted mechanism for EMF bioeffects. Both intrinsic (such as physiologic and psychologic status, gender, and age) and extrinsic factors (such as nutrition and medications) can affect the efficacy of the MF treatment for pain and tissue healing. The cell membrane may be the site of interaction of low-level EMF. Here the rate of binding of calcium ions to enzyme and/or receptor sites is affected. The concept of ions as transducers of information in the regulation of cell structure and function has widespread acceptance. Analgesic action of EMF is explained also through the enhanced endorphin produced, as well as by antiinflammatory and antiedema activity and reduction in spasms.[103]

Little information exists on the effects of static MFs on pain reduction. Most of the available data relate to anecdotal reports and incidental research that has not followed a rigorous scientific approach. However, in a recent double-blind, randomized clinical trial involving 50 patients with polio, static MF therapy produced significant and prompt pain relief.[231] The Center for Study of Complementary and Alternative Therapies at the University of Virginia has implemented a number of studies to evaluate the effects of static MFs in reducing pain. Jerabek and Pawluk's online publication[103] of magnetic therapy research findings from eastern European countries is a valuable contribution to this emerging field.

Music, Music Vibrations, and Sound for Pain Relief

An abundance of research on music and physiologic responses reveals that musical experiences can elicit a variety of physiologic responses, including changes in heart rate, blood pressure, brain waves, and muscle contractions.[93] For nearly 20 years, physicians in Germany have been using anxiolytic music to alleviate pain and anxiety in more than 90,000 patients.[210] They assessed the differences in music and non-music groups in the following areas: cognitive behavioral, physiologic, nonverbal psychomotor behavior, and situational subjective feelings evaluated through patient interviews and questionnaires.[210] In each case, regardless of whether the treatment was a short-term procedure (as in a spinal tap) or pain occurring over a longer period (as in extended 24-hour [or longer] labor), there were significant differences. In addition to reducing stress and anxiety, the music program had the practical effect of reducing drug dosages by as much as 50% and shortening the recovery period significantly.[210]

Music therapy has been used effectively to provide postoperative pain relief.[80,131,159] Clinical studies also provide some evidence of efficacy in the treatment of pain associated with medical and dental procedures,[214] with cancer,[249] and with emergency laceration repair.[154] The mechanism for pain relief is attributed in large part to the distraction/attentional factors of music. Also, release of endorphins can be triggered by a number of experiences, and there is growing evidence that music is one of these. The limbic system contains a large number of opiate receptors that are highly receptive to the presence of endorphins. Because the limbic system is that portion of the brain most closely involved in feeling responses, this may be a partial explanation for why music affects persons so deeply. Music listening may, under some circumstances, stimulate an increase in the release of endorphins that in turn elicit emotional responses in the limbic system. Thus music and other sound therapies are being investigated which suggest that the effects of vibratory responses within the body to music or other sound waves may also provide pain relief.[42,79,123]

The human body responds to vibratory stimuli. Pacinian corpuscles found in the skin, muscle spindles, and tendons are the receptors responsible for vibrotactile sensibility. Stimulation of the skin with mechanical vibration at appropriate frequencies is known to activate large-diameter afferent nerves from these mechanoreceptors.[76,105,155,222] Activation of the nerves appears to inhibit pain transmission from neurons in the dorsal horn[6] and may repress neurotransmitter release of substance P.[94,176] Results from experimental and clinical studies using a single-frequency, single-amplitude mechanical vibration provide some support for this mechanism of pain relief. Experimental pain thresholds have been raised using mechanical vibration.[27,136,202] Descriptive outcomes from large clinical studies suggest the efficacy of vibration in controlling chronic pain.[133-136] In a controlled trial, vibration and TENS were found more effective in combination than individually in the treatment of chronic pain, although individually the therapies were also more effective than placebo[82] (see earlier discussion of chronic pain).

Chesky and Michel[47] developed technology, the Music Vibration Table (MVT), consisting of a vibratory unit and computerized feedback system, designed to transduce musical sound energy into mechanical vibrations that preferentially activate particular mechanoreceptor systems to provide pain relief. The developers reported the effectiveness of controlled music vibration using the MVT with three patients with varied pain conditions. In a controlled trial, Chesky[46] tested the effects of music and music with vibration in rheumatoid arthritis patients. Twenty-seven patients were randomly assigned to one of three groups: music, music with mechanical vibration via the MVT, or a placebo group that heard a 100-Hz sine wave tone with no vibration or music. Sensory, affective, evaluative, and miscellaneous pain dimensions were measured before and after treatment using the McGill Pain Questionnaire. The music-with-vibration group reported a significant improvement in pain relief compared with the music and placebo groups. In addition, data indicated that the music-with-vibration group had relief across all four pain categories with improvement ranging from 55% (evaluative) to 73% (affective). The music group showed substantial improvement only in the affective category (63%). The placebo group showed no improvement. Findings suggest that music with music vibration provides substantial relief from pain associated with rheumatoid arthritis. Research is needed to investigate the duration of treatment effect, efficacy with other pain conditions, and the influence of individual differences.

The physioacoustic method is another application of sound therapy that uses acoustic stimulation to reduce stress, induce relaxation, and provide pain relief.[123] This physioacoustic method uses a computer system to generate low-frequency sinusoidal sound waves that induce sympathetic resonances (i.e., vibrations) in muscles and other body tissues. The amplitudes and frequencies are varied in a controlled time sequence to produce this sympathetic vibration dozens of times during a treatment session. This variation in frequency and amplitude is thought to be more effective in inducing muscle relaxation than continuous stimulation, which has been associated with numbness and fatigue. Although limited in number, results from clinical trials suggest that physioacoustic therapy is effective in reducing anxiety and pain.[122,123]

It is estimated that millions of people are using technology based on binaural beat stimulation for relaxation, pain management, improved sleep quality, and enhanced immune function. These beats are heard when pure tones (sine waves) of two different frequencies are presented, one to each ear, producing the sensation of a third "beat" frequency, perceived as a fluctuating rhythm at the frequency of the difference between the two auditory inputs. There is speculation that binaural beat devices and tapes may serve a function similar to that of the more widely accepted biofeedback training. Binaural beats are thought to exert an effect on brain function through the mechanism of a "frequency-following response." The Center for Study of Complementary and Alternative Therapies at the University of Virginia is conducting studies to assess the efficacy of binaural beats in pain reduction.

SUMMARY

The purpose of this chapter has been to provide clinicians with evidence that supports the efficacy of a number of well-defined CAM therapies used in promoting comfort and reducing pain in persons with acute, chronic, and cancer-related pain. This state-of -the-art review reveals that the most evidence available supports the use of cognitive behavioral approaches, although there is need for replication of many of these studies using rigorous methodology and adequate sample size.

Data are insufficient in some instances to conclude with full confidence that one CAM method is better than another for a given pain condition, although for a given individual, one approach may be more effective than another, emphasizing the importance of considering individual differences in the treatment of individuals with acute, chronic, and cancer-related pain.

Current and future research will reveal additional data to support the appropriateness and adequacy of nonpharmacologic interventions in promoting comfort and reducing pain when used alone or in conjunction with pharmacologic interventions. These investigations should include assessment of physiologic dimensions of pain and the impact of pain and pain reduction on bodily systems. The next decade will bring new discoveries that will enhance our knowledge and skills in promoting comfort and reducing pain in populations across the age span and in all clinical settings.

Challenges to clinicians are to overcome perceived organizational, bureaucratic, financial, and attitudinal barriers to the integration of therapies for which there is demonstrated efficacy and to work with their patients who are eagerly seeking ways to be active and responsible partners in the treatment of their pain.

REFERENCES

1. Abeles RP: Schemas, sense of control, and aging. In Rodin J, Schaie KW, editors: *Self-directedness: causes and effects through the life course*, New Jersey, 1990, Lawrence Erlbaum Associates.
2. Abenhaim L, Bergeron AM: Twenty years of randomized clinical trials of manipulative therapy for back pain: a review, *Clin Invest Med* 15(6):527, 1992.
3. Acute Low Back Problems Guideline Panel: *Acute low back problems in adults. Clinical practice guideline no 14.* AHCPR pub. no. 95-0642, Rockville, Md, December 1994, Agency for Health Care Policy and Research, Public Health Service, U.S. Department of Health and Human Services.
4. Acute Pain Management Guideline Panel: *Acute pain management: operative or medical procedures and trauma. Clinical practice guideline no 1.* AHCPR pub. no. 92-0032, Rockville, Md, February 1992, Agency for Health Care Policy and Research, Public Health Service, U.S. Department of Health and Human Services.
5. Adams PF, Benson V: Current estimates from the National Health Interview Survey, 1991, *Vital Health Stat* 10:184, 1992.
6. Adriasen H et al: Response properties of thin myelinated fibers in human skin nerves, *Vital Health Stat* 49:111, 1983.
7. Anderson R et al: A meta-analysis of clinical trials of spinal manipulation, *J Manipulative Physiol Ther* 15(3):181, 1992.

8. Andersson GBL: The epidemiology of spinal disorders. In Frymoyer W, editor: *The adult spine: principles and practice*, New York, 1991, Raven Press.

9. Arena JG, Hightower NE, Chong GC: Relaxation therapy for tension headache in the elderly: a prospective study, *Psychol Aging* 3:96, 1988.

10. Arena JG et al: Electromyographic biofeedback training for tension headache in the elderly: a prospective study, *Biofeeback Self Regul* 16:370, 1991.

11. Aronofsky DH: Reduction of dental postsurgical symptoms using nonthermal pulsed high-peak-power electromagnetic energy, *Oral Surg, Oral Med, Oral Pathol* 32(5):688, 1971.

12. Ashton C et al: Self-hypnosis reduces anxiety following coronary artery bypass surgery: a prospective, randomized trial, *J Cardiovasc Surg* 38(1):69, 1997.

13. Avellanosa AM, West CR: Experience with transcutaneous electrical nerve stimulation for relief of intractable pain in cancer patients, *J Med* 13(3):203, 1982.

14. Awang DVC: Feverfew fever: a headache for the consumer, *Herbalgram* 29:34, 1993.

15. Badlamente MA, Cherney SA: Periosteal and vascular innervation of the human patella in degenerative joints disease, *Semin Arthritis Rheum* 18:61, 1989.

16. Baldwin CA, Anderson LA, Phillipson JD: What pharmacists should know about feverfew, *Pharm J* 239:237, 1987.

17. Baldwin L: The therapeutic use of touch and the elderly, *Physical and Occupational Therapy in Geriatrics* 4(4):45, 1986.

18. Balick M et al: Herbal medicine. In Berman BM, Larson DB, editors: *Alternative medicine: expanding medical horizons: a report to National Institutes of Health on alternative medical systems and practices in the United States*, Washington, DC, 1995, U.S. Government Printing Office.

19. Barbour L, McGuire DB, Kirchhoff KT: Nonanalgesic methods of pain control used by cancer outpatients, *Oncol Nurs Forum* 13(6):56, 1986.

20. Barnett K: A theoretical construct of the concepts of touch as they relate to nursing. *Nurs Res* 21(2):102, 1972.

21. Barrett E: The continuing revolution of Rogers' science-based nursing education. In Barrett E, editor: *Visions of Rogers' science-based nursing*, New York, 1990, National League for Nursing.

22. Bassett A: Therapeutic uses of electric and magnetic fields in orthopedics. In Karpenter D, Ayrapetyan S, editors: *Biological effects of electric and magnetic fields*, San Diego, 1994, Academic Press.

23. Bassett CAL: Fundamental and practical aspects of therapeutic uses of pulsed electromagnetic fields (PEMFs), *Crit Rev Biomed Eng* 17:451,1989.

24. Bauer W: Electrical treatment of severe head and neck cancer pain, *Arch Otolaryngol* 109(6):382, 1983.

25. BeLieu RM: Mastodynia, *Obstet Gynecol Clin North Am* 21(3):461, 1994.

26. Benedetti F et al: Control of postoperative pain by transcutaneous electrical nerve stimulation after thoracic operations, *Ann Thorac Surg* 63(3):773, 1997.

27. Bini G et al: Analgesic effect of vibration and cooling on pain induced by intraneural electrical stimulation, *Pain* 18:239, 1984.

28. Blanchard EB et al: Migraine and tension headache: a meta-analytic review, *Behav Ther* 11:613, 1980.

29. Blankfield RP: Suggestion, relaxation, and hypnosis as adjuncts in the care of surgery patients: a review of the literature, *Am J Clin Hyp* 33(3):172, 1991.

30. Blumenthal M: *Herbal therapies*. Blumenthal M (conference presentation), Cambridge, Harvard Medical School, 1996.

31. Bogaards MC, ter Kuile MM: Treatment of recurrent tension headache: a meta-analytic review, *Clin J Pain* 10:174, 1994.

32. Bogulawski M: Therapeutic touch: a facilitator of pain relief, *Top Clin Nurs* 2(1):27, 1980.

33. Bonica JJ: Cancer pain. In Bonica JJ, editor: *The management of pain*, Malvern, Penn, 1990, Lea & Febiger.

34. Booth B: Therapeutic touch, *Nurs Times* 89(31):48, 1993.

35. Borelli M, Heidt P: *Therapeutic touch*, New York, 1981, Springer.

36. Brady B, Nesbit S: Using the right touch, *Nursing* 21(5):46, 1996.

37. Brattberg C: Acupuncture therapy for tennis elbow, *Pain* 16:265, 1993.

38. *British Herbal Pharmacopoeia*, Keighley, 1983, British Herbal Medicine Association.

39. Buckelew S et al: The effects of biofeedback and exercise on fibromyalgia: a controlled trial, *Arch Phys Med Rehabil* 73:980, 1992.

40. Bult H et al: Modification of endotoxin-induced haemodynamic and haematological changes in the rabbit by methylprednisolone, F(ab)2 fragments and rosmarinic acid, *Br J Pharmacol* 84:317, 1985.

41. Burckhardt CS, Mannerkorpi K, Hendenber L, Bjelle A: A randomized, controlled clinical trial of education and physical training for women with fibromyalgia, *J Rheumatol* 21:714, 1994.

42. Burnside I: *Nursing and the aged*, St. Louis, 1988, Mosby.

43. Byass, R: Soothing body and soul, *Nurs Times* 84(24):39, 1988.

44. Carroll D et al: Randomization is important in studies with pain outcomes: systematic review of transcutaneous electrical nerve stimulation in acute postoperative pain, *Br J Anaesth* 77:798, 1996.

45. Charkarski I et al: Clinical study of a herb combination consisting of *Humulus lupulus, Chichorium intybus, Mentha piperita* in patients with chronic calculus and non-calculus cholecystitis, *Probl Vatr Med* 10:65, 1982.

46. Chesky KS: *The effects of music vibration using the MVT on the relief of rheumatoid arthritis pain*, PhD dissertation, Denton, 1992, University of North Texas.

47. Chesky KS, Michel DE: The Music Vibration Table (MVT): Developing a technology and conceptual model for pain relief, *Music Therapy Perspectives* 9:32, 1991.

48. Christensen BV et al: Acupuncture treatment of severe knee osteoarthrosis: a long term study, *Acta Anaesthesiol Scand* 36:519, 1992.

49. Cleeland CS, Syrjala KL: How to assess cancer pain. In Turk D, Melzack R, editors: *Pain assessment*, New York, 1992, Guilford Press.

50. Coan RM et al: The acupuncture treatment of low back pain: a randomized controlled study, *Am J Chin Med* 8(2):181, 1980.

51. Cohen FL: Postsurgical pain relief: Patients' status and nurses' medication choices, *Pain* 9(2):265, 1980.

52. Collier HO et al: Extract of feverfew inhibits prostaglandin biosynthesis [Letter], *Lancet* 2(8200):922, 1980.

53. Conn G et al: Transcutaneous electrical nerve stimulation following appendectomy: the placebo effect, *Ann R Coll Surg Engl* 68:191, 1986.

54. Crawford HJ et al: Effects of hypnosis on regional cerebral blood flow during ischemic pain with and without suggested hypnotic analgesia, *Int J Psychophysiol* 15(3):181, 1993.

55. Cruz F, Avelino A, Coimbra A: Desensitization follows excitation of bladder primary afferents by intravesical capsaicin, as shown by c-fos activation in the rat spinal cord, *Pain* 64:553, 1996.

56. Cypress BK: Characteristics of physician visits for back symptoms: a national perspective, *Am J Public Health* 73(4):389, 1983.

57. Deluze C et al: Electroacupuncture in fibromyalgia: Result of a controlled trial, *Br Med J* 305:1249, 1992.

58. Devine EC, Westlake SK: The effects of psychoeducational care provided to adults with cancer: meta-analysis of 116 studies, *Oncol Nurs Forum* 22(9):1369, 1995.

59. Deyo RA et al: A controlled trial of transcutaneous electrical nerve stimulation (TENS) and exercise for chronic low back pain, *N Engl J Med* 322:23, 1990.

60. Dickens E, Lewith G: A single-blind controlled and randomized clinical trial to evaluate the effect of acupuncture in the treatment of trapezio-metarcarpal osteoarthritis, *Complementary Med Res* 3:5, 1989.

61. Doehring KM: Relieving pain through touch, *Advances in Clinical Care* 4(5):32, 1989.

62. Donovan M, Dillon P, McGuire L: Incidence and characteristics of pain in a sample of medical-surgical inpatients, *Pain* 30(1):69, 1987.

63. Doyle E, Spence AA: Cannabis as a medicine? *Br J Anaesth* 74(4):359, 1995.

64. Drake DR, Gueldner SH: Imagery instruction and the control of postsurgical pain, *Appl Nurs Res* 2:114, 1989.

65. Drevets WC et al: Blood flow changes in human somatosensory cortex during anticipated stimulation, *Nature* 373(6511):249, 1995.

66. Dworkin SF et al: Brief group cognitive-behavioral intervention for temporomandibular disorders, *Pain* 59:175, 1994.

67. Egan E: Therapeutic touch. In Snyder M, editor: *Independent nursing interventions*. New York, 1985, Wiley.
68. Eisenberg DM et al: Unconventional medicine in the United States. Prevalence, costs, and patterns of use, *N Engl J Med* 328(4):246, 1993.
69. Erickson P, Wilson R, Shannon I: *Healthy people 2000: statistical notes: years of healthy life*, Washington, DC, 1995, U.S. Department of Health and Human Services, report 7, Centers for Disease Control and Prevention and National Center for Health Statistics.
70. Feine JS, Lund JP: An assessment of the efficacy of physical therapy and physical methods for the control of chronic musculoskeletal pain, *Pain* 71:5, 1997.
71. Fernandez E, Turk DC: The utility of cognitive coping strategies for altering pain perception: a meta-analysis, *Pain* 38:123, 1989.
72. Ferrell BR, Schneider C: Experience and management of cancer pain at home, *Cancer Nurs* 11(2):84, 1988.
73. Ferrell-Torry AT, Glick OJ: The use of therapeutic massage as a nursing intervention to modify anxiety and the perception of cancer pain, *Cancer Nurs* 16(2):93, 1993.
74. Foley, KM: The treatment of cancer pain, *N Engl J Med* 313(2):84, 1985.
75. Fordyce WE: Pain and suffering: A reappraisal, *Am Psychol* 43(4):276, 1988.
76. Freeman AW, Johnson KO: A model accounting for the effects of vibratory amplitude on responses of cutaneous mechanoreceptors in macaque monkey, *J Physiol* 323:43, 1982.
77. Gagne D, Toye RC: The effects of therapeutic touch and relaxation therapy in reducing anxiety, *Arch Psychiatr Nurs* 8(3):184, 1994.
78. Goldenberg DL et al: A controlled study of a stress reduction, cognitive behavioral treatment program in fibromyalgia, *J Musculoskel Pain* 2:53, 1994.
79. Goldstein A: Thrills in response to music and other stimuli, *Physiological Psychology* 8(1):126, 1980.
80. Good M: Effects of relaxation and music on postoperative pain: a review, *J Adv Nurs* 24:905, 1996.
81. Goodykoontz L: Touch: Attitudes and practice, *Nurs Forum* 18(10):4, 1979.
82. Guieu R, Tardy-Gervet, MR, Roll JP: Analgesic effects of vibration and transcutaneous electrical nerve stimulation applied separately and simultaneously to patients with chronic pain, *Can J Neurol Sci* 18(2):113, 1991.
83. Gunn CC et al: Dry needling of muscle motor points for chronic low-back pain: a randomized clinical trial with long-term follow-up, *Spine* 5(3):279, 1980.
84. Hadler NM et al: A benefit of spinal manipulations as adjunctive therapy for acute low-back pain: a stratified controlled trial, *Spine* 12(7):703, 1987.
85. Hansen PE, Hansen JH: Acupuncture therapy for chronic tension headache: a controlled crossover investigation, *Ugeskr Laeger* 146:649, 1984.
86. Hargreaves A, Lander J: Use of Transcutaneous electrical nerve stimulation for postoperative pain, *Nurs Res* 38(3):159, 1989.
87. Harlow H: The nature of love, *Am Psychol* 13:673, 1958.
88. Harlow H, Harlow M, Hansen E: The maternal affectional system of rhesus monkeys. In Rheingold E, editor: *Maternal behavior in mammals*, New York, 1963, Wiley.
89. Harris ED: Rheumatoid arthritis: Pathophysiology and implications for therapy, *N Engl J Med* 322:1277, 1990.
90. Heidt P: Effect of therapeutic touch on anxiety level of hospitalized patients, *Nurs Res* 30:32, 1981.
91. Helms JM: Acupuncture for management of primary dysmenorrhea, *Obstet Gynecol* 69:51, 1987.
92. Heptinstall S et al: Extracts of feverfew inhibit granule secretion in blood platelets and polymorphonuclear leukocytes *Lancet* 1(8437):1071, 1985.
93. Hodges DA: Neuromusical research: a review of the literature. In Hodges DA, editor: *Handbook of music psychology* ed 2, San Antonio, 1996, IMR Press.
94. Hokfelt W et al: Immunohistochemical analysis of peptide pathways possibly related to pain analgesia: enkephalin and substance P. In *Proceedings of the National Academy of Sciences*, New York, 1977, National Academy of Science.
95. Holbrook T: *The frequency of occurrence, impact, and cost of selected musculoskeletal conditions in the United States*, Chicago, 1984, American Academy of Orthopedic Surgeons.

96. Holroyd KA, Penzien DB: Client variables and the behavioral treatment of recurrent tension headache: a meta-analytic review, *J Behav Med* 9(6):515, 1986.

97. Holroyd KA, Penzien DB: Pharmacological versus non-pharmacological prophylaxis of recurrent migrane headache: a meta-analytic review of clinical trials, *Pain* 42:1, 1990.

98. Horan JJ, Laying FC, Pursell, CH: Preliminary study of effects of in vivo emotive imagery on dental discomfort, *Percept Mot Skills* 42:105, 1976.

99. Horowitz BF, Fitzpatrick JJ, Flaherty GG: Relaxation techniques for pain relief after open heart surgery, *Dimens Crit Care Nurs* 3:346, 1984.

100. Hyman RB et al: The effects of relaxation training on clinical symptoms: A meta-analysis, *Nurs Res* 38(4):216, 1989.

101. International Association for the Study of Pain Subcommittee on Taxomy: Pain terms, a list with definitions and notes on usage, *Pain* 8:249, 1979.

102. Jamal GA et al: Gamma-linolenic acid in diabetic neuropathy, *Lancet* 1(8489):1098, 1986.

103. Jerabek J, Pawluk W: *Magnetic therapy: the eastern European research*, 1998, (availability: wpawluk@compuserve.com).

104. Joe LA, Hart LL: Evening primrose oil in rheumatoid arthritis, *Ann Pharmacother* 27(12):1475, 1993.

105. Johansson RS, Landstrom U, Lundstrom R: Responses of mechanoreceptive afferent units in the glabrous skin of the human hand to sinusoidal displacements, *Brain Res* 244:17, 1982.

106. Johnston M, Vogele C: Benefits of psychological preparation for surgery: a meta-analysis, *Annals of Behavioral Medicine* 15(4):245, 1993.

107. Kaada B, Torsteinbo O: Increase of plasma beta-endorphins in connective tissue massage, *General Pharmacol* 20(4):487, 1989.

108. Kabela E et al: Self-regulatory treatment of headache in the elderly, *Biofeedback Self Regul* 14(3):219, 1989.

109. Kaplan KH, Goldenberg DL, Galvin-Nadeau M: The impact of meditation-based stress reduction on fibromyalgia, *Gen Hosp Psychiatry* 15:284, 1993.

110. Keefe FJ, Caldwell DS: Cognitive behavioral control of arthritis pain, *Med Clin North Am* 81(1):277, 1997.

111. Keller E, Bzdek VM: Effects of therapeutic touch on tension headache pain. *Nurs Res* 35(2):101, 1986.

112. Kiefer RC, Hospodarsky J: The use of hypnotic techniques in anesthesia to decrease postoperative meperidine requirements, *J Am Osteopath Assoc* 79:693, 1980.

113. Kiernan BD et al: Hypnotic analgesia reduces r-iii nociceptive reflex: further evidence concerning the multifactorial nature of hypnotic analgesia, *Pain* 60(1):39, 1995.

114. Kleijnen J: Evening primrose oil, *Br Med J* 309(6958):824, 1994.

115. Koes BW et al: Randomized clinical trial of manipulative therapy and physiotherapy for persistent back and neck complaints: results of one year follow-up, *BMJ* 304:601, 1992.

116. Krieger D: *The therapeutic touch*, Englewood Cliffs, NJ, 1979, Prentice Hall, Inc.

117. LaBan MM, Taylor RS: Manipulation: An objective analysis of the literature, *Orthop Clin North Am* 23(3):451, 1992.

118. Langreth R: Science yields powerful new therapies for pain, *The Wall Street Journal*, 1996, b1-b4.

119. Lawlis GF et al: Reduction of postoperative pain parameters by presurgical relaxation instructions for spinal pain patients, *Spine* 10:649, 1985.

120. Lee VC: Office and hospital pain consults. In Tollison CD, Satterthwaite JR, Tollison JW, editors: *Handbook of pain management*, Baltimore, Md, 1994, Williams & Wilkins.

121. Lee YH et al: Acupuncture in the treatment of renal colic, *J Urol* 147:16, 1992.

122. Lehikoinen P: The Physioacoustic method and the management of work related stress, *Helsingin Laararilehti* (Helsinki Physician Magazine), April 1992.

123. Lehikoinen P, Kanstren J: Corporate health care experiment at the Sibelius Academy: a suitability study of the Physioacoustic system as a treatment device in preventive corporate health care, Conference Presentation, Helsinki, 1997.

124. Lehmann TR et al: Efficacy of electroacupuncture and TENS in rehabilitation of chronic low back pain patients, *Pain* 26:277, 1986.

125. LeMay A: The human connection, *Nurs Times* 82(13):28, 1986.

126. Leventhal LJ, Boyce EG, Zurier RB: Treatment of rheumatoid arthritis with gammalinolenic acid, *Ann Intern Med* 119(9):867, 1993.
127. Levin RF, Malloy GB, Hyman RB: Nursing Management of postoperative pain: use of relaxation techniques with female cholecystectomy patients, *J Adv Nurs* 12:463, 1987.
128. Levine JD et al: Intracuronal substance P contributes to the severity of experimental arthritis, *Science* 226:547, 1984.
129. Li QS et al: Combined traditional Chinese medicine and Western medicine: Relieving effects of Chinese herbs, ear acupuncture and epidural morphine on postoperative liver pain, *Chin Med J* (Engl) 107:289, 1994.
130. Lipton RB, Stewart WF, von Korff M: Burden of migraine: societal costs and therapeutic opportunities, *Neurology* 48(suppl 3):S4, 1997.
131. Locin RG: The effect of music on the pain of selected post-operative patients, *J Adv Nurs* 6:19, 1981.
132. Lotz M, Carson DA, Vaughan JH: Substance P activation of rheumatoid synoviocytes: neural pathogenesis of arthritis, *Science* 235:893, 1987.
133. Lundeberg T: Vibratory stimulation for the alleviation of chronic pain, *Acta Physiol Scand* 523(suppl):1, 1983.
134. Lundeberg T: The suppressive effect of vibratory stimulation and transcutaneous electrical nerve stimulation (TENS) as compared to aspirin, *Brain Res* 294:201, 1984b.
135. Lundeberg T: Long-term results of vibratory stimulation as a measure pain, *Pain* 20:13, 1984.
136. Lundeberg T et al: Effect of vibratory stimulation on experimental and clinical pain, *Scand J Rehabil Med* 20:149, 1988.
137. Lynn B: Capsaicin: Actions on nociceptive c-fibres and therapeutic potential, *Pain* 41(1):61, 1990.
138. MacDonald RS, Bell CMJ: An open controlled assessment of osteopathic manipulation in nonspecific low-back pain, *Spine* 15(5):364, 1990.
139. Malinski V, Barrett E: *Martha E. Rogers: Her life and her work*, Philadelphia, PA, 1994, F.A. Davis Co.
140. Malone MD, Strube MJ: Meta-analysis of non-medical treatment for chronic pain, *Pain* 43:231, 1988.
141. Management of Cancer Pain Guideline Panel: *Management of cancer pain. Clinical practice guideline no 9*, AHCPR pub. no. 94-0592, Rockville, Md, March 1994, Agency for Health Care Policy and Research, Public Health Service, U.S. Department of Health and Human Services.
142. Marchand S et al: Is TENS a placebo affect? A controlled study on chronic low back pain, *Pain* 54:99, 1993.
143. Markov M: Biological effects of extremely low frequency magnetic fields. In Ueno S, editor, *Biomagnetic Stimulation*, New York, 1994, Plenum Press.
144. Markov MS, Pilla AA: Electromagnetic field stimulation of soft tissues, *Wounds*, 7:143, 1995.
145. Marks RM, Sachar EJ: Undertreatment of medical inpatients with narcotic analgesics, *Ann Intern Med* 78(2):173, 1973.
146. Mathews JD et al: Effects of the heavy usage of kava on physical health: summary of a pilot survey in an aboriginal community, *Med J Aust* 148(11):548, 1988.
147. McCaleb RS: Herbal therapies. In McCaleb R S: Conference presentation, Cambridge, Harvard Medical School, March 27, 1996.
148. McKechnie et al: Anxiety states: A preliminary report on the value of connective tissue massage, *J Psychosom Res* 27(2):125, 1983.
149. Meade TW et al: Low back pain of mechanical origin: randomized comparison of chiropractic and hospital outpatient treatment, *J Orthop Sports Phys Ther* 13(6):278, 1991.
150. Meehan MTC: Therapeutic touch and post-operative pain: a Rogerian research study, *Nurs Sci Q* 6(2):66, 1993.
151. Meehan MTC et al: Therapeutic touch and surgical patients' stress reactions, abstracted, *J Pain* 5(suppl):149, 1990.
152. Meier B et al: Pharmaceutical aspects of the use of willows in herbal remedies, *Planta Med* 54:559, 1988.
153. Menard M: *Massage therapy for chronic pain: An overview of research and practice* (unpublished manuscript), 1993.

154. Menegazzi et al: A randomized, controlled trial of music during laceration repair, *Ann Emerg Med* 20:348, 1991.

155. Merzenich MM, Harrington T: The sense of flutter-vibration evoked by stimulation of the hairy skin of primates: Comparisons of human sensory capacity with the responses of mechanoreceptive afferents innervating the hairy skin of monkeys, *Exp Brain Res* 9:236, 1969.

156. Meserole L: Western herbalism. In Micozzi MS, editor: *Fundamentals of complementary and alternative medicine*, New York, 1996, Churchill Livingstone.

157. Montague A: *Touching: The human significance of the skin,* ed 2, New York, 1971, Harper & Row.

158. Møystad A, Krogstad BS, Larheim TA: Transcutaneous nerve stimulation in a group of patients with rheumatic disease involving the temporomandibular joint, *J Prosthet Dent* 64:596, 1990.

159. Mullooly VM, Levin RF, Feldman HR: Music for postoperative pain and anxiety, *J NY State Nurses Assoc* 2:267, 1988.

160. Murphy JJ, Heptinstall S, Mitchell JR: Randomised double-blind placebo-controlled trial of feverfew in migraine prevention, *Lancet* 2(8604):189, 1988.

161. Nachemson AL: Newest knowledge of low back pain: a critical look, *Clin Orthop* 279:8,1992.

162. National Cancer Institute: National Cancer Institute Workshop on Cancer Pain, Bethesda, Md, 1990.

163. Newall CA, Anderson LA, Phillipson JD: *Herbal medicines: a guide for health-care professionals*, London, 1996, The Pharmaceutical Press.

164. NIH Technology Assessment Statement: *Integration of Behavioral and Relaxation Approaches into the treatment of chronic pain and insomnia.* NIH Technology Assessment Statement 1995 Oct 16-18; 1-34.

165. NIH Technology Assessment Statement: *Management of temporomandibular disorders.* NIH Technology Assessment Statement 1996 April 29-May 1; [cited 1997 July 19]; 1-22.

166. NIH Technology Assessment Statement: *Acupuncture.* NIH Technology Assessment Statement Nov 3-5, 1997, 1-24 (draft).

167. Notcutt WG: Cannabis as a medicine [Letter], *Br J Anaesth* 75(2):251, 1995.

168. Olesen J, editor: *Headache classification and epidemiology*, New York, 1994, Raven Press.

169. Olesen J, Bonica JJ: Headache. In Bonica JJ: *The management of pain*, Malvern, Penn, 1990, Lea & Febiger.

170. Paramore LC: Uses of alternative therapies: estimates from the 1994 Robert-Wood-Johnson-Foundation National Access to Care Survey, *J Pain Symptom Manage* 13(2):83, 1997.

171. Patel M et al: A meta-analysis of acupuncture for chronic pain, *Int J Epidemiol* 18(4):900, 1989.

172. Patterson DR et al: Hypnosis for treatment of burn pain, *J Clin Consult Psychol* 60(5):713, 1992.

173. Pattrick M, Heptinstall S, Doherty M: Feverfew in rheumatoid arthritis: A double blind, placebo controlled study, *Ann Rheum Dis* 48(7):547, 1989.

174. Payan P: Neuropeptides and inflammation: The role of substance P, *Am Rev Med* 40:341, 1989.

175. Peric-Knowlton W: The understanding and management of acute pain in adults: the nursing contribution, *Int J Nurs Stud* 21(2):131, 1984.

176. Piercey MF, Folders K: Modification of pain threshold by specific tactile receptors, *Acta Physiol Scand* 107:339, 1981.

177. Pilla AA: State of the art in electromagnetic therapeutics. In Blank M, editor: *Electricity and Magnetism in biology and medicine,* San Francisco, 1993, San Francisco Press.

178. Pilla AA, Markov MS: Weak electromagnetic field bioeffects, *Rev Environ Health*, 10:155, 1994.

179. Pomeranz B: Scientific basis of acupuncture. In Stux B, Pomeranz B: editors: *Acupuncture: textbook and atlas*, Berlin, 1986, Springer-Verlag.

180. Portenoy RK, Hagen NA: Breakthrough pain: definition, prevalence and characteristics, *Pain* 41(3):273, 1990.

181. Pye JK et al: Clinical experience of drug treatments for mastalgia, *Lancet* 2(8451):373, 1985.

182. Quinn JF, Strelkauskas AJ: Psychoimmunologic effects of therapeutic touch on practitioners and recently bereaved recipients: a pilot study. *Adv Nurs Sci* 15(4):13, 1993.

183. Quinn JF: Therapeutic touch as energy exchange: testing the theory, *Ann Adv Nurs Sci* 6(2):42, 1984.

184. Rampart M et al: Complement-dependent stimulation of prostacyclin biosynthesis: inhibition by rosmarinic acid, *Biochem Pharmacol* 35:1397, 1986.

185. Rasmussen BK: Epidemiology: tension-type headache, cluster headache, and miscellaneous headaches. In Olesen J, Tfelt-Hansen P, Welch KMA, editors: *The headaches*, New York, 1993, Raven Press.
186. Rasmussen BK, Breslau N: Epidemiology: Migraine. In Olesen J, Tfelt-Hansen P, Welch KMA, editors: *The headaches*, New York, 1993, Raven Press.
187. Reed JC: Review of acute and chronic pain published studies, *J Altern Complement Med* 2(1):129, 1996.
188. Reynolds JEF, editor: *Martindale: the extra pharmacopoeia*, ed 29, London, 1989, Pharmaceutical Press.
189. Rhodes C: The adjunctive utilization of Diapulse (pulsed high peak power electromagnetic energy) in accelerating tissue healing in oral surgery, *Q Nat Dent Assoc* 39:166, 1981.
190. Richardson PH, Vincent CA: Acupuncture for the treatment of pain: a review of evaluative research, *Pain* 24:15, 1986.
191. Rosenburg M: *Conceiving the self*, ed 2, Malabar, Fla, 1986, Krieger.
192. Rowlingson JC et al: Ajunctive therapy for pain. In Hamill RJ, Rowlingson JC, editors: *Handbook of critical care pain management*, New York, 1992, McGraw-Hill.
193. Rowlingson JC, Hamill RJ: Concomitant chronic pain syndromes. In Hamill RJ, Rowlingson JC, editiors: *Handbook of critical care pain management*, New York, 1992, McGraw-Hill.
194. Sabia A: Mainstreaming holism, *Beginnings* 12(2):4, 1992.
195. Sabourin ME et al: EEG correlates of hypnotic susceptibility and hypnotic trance: Spectral analysis and coherence, *Int J Psychophysiol* 10:125,1990.
196. Rowlingson JC: Pain mechanisms and pathways. In Hamill RJ, Rowlingson JC, editors: *Handbook of critical care pain management*, New York, 1992, McGraw-Hill.
197. Samarel N: The experience of receiving therapeutic touch. *J Adv Nurs* 17(6):651, 1992.
198. Sarter B: *The stream of becoming: a study of Martha Rogers' theory*, New York, 1988, National League for Nursing.
199. Schappert SM: National Ambulatory Medical Care Survey: 1992 Summary, *Vital & Health Statistics Advance Data* series 16:26, 1994.
200. Sharma JN, Srivastava KC, Gan EK: Suppressive effects of eugenol and ginger oil on arthritic rats, *Pharmacology* 49(5):314, 1994.
201. Shekelle PG et al: Spinal Manipulation for low-back pain, *Ann Intern Med* 117:590, 1992.
202. Sherer C et al: The effects of two sites of high frequency vibration on cutaneous pain thresholds, *Pain* 25:133, 1986.
203. Shutty MS, DeGood DE: Patient knowledge and beliefs about pain and its treatment. *Rehabilitation Psychology* 35:43, 1990.
204. Sicuteri F et al: Substance P theory: A unique focus on the painful and painless phenomena of cluster headache, *Headache* 30(2):69, 1990.
205. Simmington JA, Laing GP: Effects of therapeutic touch and relaxation therapy on anxiety in the institutionalized elderly, *Clin Nurs Res* 2(4):438, 1993.
206. Simpson J: Massage: Positive strokes in palliative care, *N Z Nurs J* 84(6):15, 1991.
207. Sims S: Slow stroke back massage for cancer patients, *Nurs Times* 82(47):47, 1986.
208. Smidt GL: Research Study Analysis, *J Orthop Sports Phys Ther* 13(6):288, 1991.
209. Smith RS: The cytokine theory of headache, *Med Hypotheses* 39(2):168, 1992.
210. Spingte R: The neurophysiology of emotion and its therapeutic applications in music therapy and music medicine. In Maranto C, editor: *Applications of music in medicine*, Washington, DC, 1992, National Association for Music Therapy.
211. Spingte R, Droh R, editors: *Music medicine*, St Louis, 1992, MMB Music
212. Srivastava KC, Mustafa T: Ginger (*Zingiber officinale*) and rheumatic disorders, *Med Hypotheses* 29(1):25, 1989.
213. Srivastava KC, Mustafa T: Ginger (*Zingiber officinale*) in rheumatism and musculoskeletal disorders, *Med Hypotheses* 39(4):342, 1992.
214. Standley JM: Music research in medical/dental treatment: Meta-analysis and clinical applications, *J Music Ther* 23(2):56, 1986.
215. Stang PE, Osterhaus JT: Impact of migraine in the United States: data from the National Health Interview Survey, *Headache* 33(1):29, 1993.

216. Stewart WF, Lipton RB, Simon D: Work-related disability: results from the American migraine study, *Cephalagia* 16(4):231, 1996.

217. Stewart et al: Prevalence of migraine headache in the United States. Relation to age, income, race, and other sociodemographic factors, *JAMA* 267(1):64, 1992.

218. Subarnas A et al: An antidepressant principle of lobelia inflata l. (*campanulaceae*), *J Pharm Sci* 81(7):620, 1992.

219. Subarnas A et al: Pharmacological properties of beta-amyrin palmitate, a novel centrally acting compound, isolated from lobelia inflata leaves, *J Pharm Pharmacol* 45(6):545, 1993.

220. Sung YF et al: Comparison of effects of acupuncture and codeine on postoperative dental pain, *Anesth Analg* 56:473, 1976.

221. Syrjala KL, Cummings C, Donaldson GW: Hypnosis or cognitive behavioral training for the reduction of pain and nausea during cancer treatment; a controlled clinical trial, *Pain* 48:137, 1992.

222. Talbot WH et al: The sense of flutter-vibration: comparison of the human capacity with response patterns of mechanoreceptive afferents from the monkey hand, *J Neurophysiol* 31:301, 1968.

223. Tate G et al: Suppression of acute and chronic inflammation by dietary gamma linolenic acid, *J Rheumatol* 16(6):729, 1989.

224. Taylor H, editor: *The Nuprin pain report*, New York, 1985, Louis Harris & Associates.

225. ter Riet G, Kleijnen J & Knipschild P: Acupuncture and chronic pain: a criteria-based meta-analysis, *J Clin Epidemiol* 43(11):1191, 1990.

226. Trock DH, Bollet AJ, Markoll R: The effect of pulsed electromagnetic fields in the treatment of osteoarthritis of the knee and cervical spine: report of randomized, double blind, placebo controlled trials, *J Rheumatol* 21(10):1903, 1994.

227. Trock DH et al: A double-blind trial of the clinical effects of pulsed electromagnetic fields in osterarthritis, *J Rheumatol* 20(3):456, 1993.

228. Turk DC, Melzack RD: The measurement of pain and the assessment of people experiencing pain. In Turk DC, Melzack R, editors: *Handbook of pain assessment*, New York, 1992, Guilford Press.

229. Turton P: Touch me, feel me, heal me, *Nurs Times* 85(19):42, 1989.

230. Vasudevan SV: Impairment, disability, and functional capacity assessment. In Turk DC, Melzack R, editors: *Handbook of pain assessment*, New York, 1992, Guilford Press.

231. Vallbona C et al: Response of pain to static magnetic fields in post polio patients: a double-blind pilot study, *Arch Phys Med Rehabil* 78:1200, 1997.

232. Vincent CA: A controlled trial of the treatment of migraine acupuncture, *Clin J Pain* 5:305, 1989.

233. Vincent CA: The treatment of tension headache by acupuncture: a controlled single case design with time series, *J Psychosom Res* 34(5):553, 1990.

234. Virus RM, Gebhart GR: Pharmacologic action of capsaicin: apparent involvement of substance P and serotonin, *Life Sci* 25:1273, 1979.

235. Walker JA et al: Attenuation of contraction-induced skeletal muscle injury by bromelain, *Med Sci Sports Exerc* 24(1):20, 1992.

236. Wall PD, Melzack R, editors: *Textbook of pain,* ed 2, London, 1984, Churchill Livingstone.

237. Wang DL: Analysis of 70 cases of primary liver carcinoma treated by Pu Tuo ointment and herbs, *Chung Hsi i Chieh Ho Tsa Chih* 10:723, 1990.

238. Warfield CA, Stein JM, Frank HA: The effect of Transcutaneous electrical nerve stimulation on pain after thoracotomy, *Ann Thorac Surg* 39(5):562, 1985.

239. Watson J: Nursing's caring-healing paradigm as exemplar for alternative medicine? *Altern Ther Heal Med* 1(3):64, 1995.

240. Wegner DM: Ironic processes of mental control, *Psychol Rev* 101(1):34, 1994.

241. Weinrich SP, Weinrich MC: The effect of massage on pain in cancer patients, *Appl Nurs Res* 3(4):140, 1990.

242. White KP, Nielson WR: Cognitive behavioral treatment of fibromyalgia syndrome: a follow-up assessment, *J Rheumatol* 22:717, 1995.

243. Wood JN, editor: *Capsaicin in the study of pain*, San Diego, 1993, Academic Press.

244. Woodwell DA, Schappert SM: National Ambulatory Medical Care Survey: 1993 Summary, *Vital Health Statistics Advance Data* 16(270), 1995.
245. Wright SM: The use of therapeutic touch in the management of pain, *Nurs Clin North Am* 22(3):705, 1987.
246. Wright SM: Validity of the human energy field assessment form, *West J Nurs Res* 13(5):635, 1991.
247. Yang G et al: Controlling cancerous pain with analgesic powder for cancers, *J Tradit Chin Med* 15:174, 1995.
248. Zhang WY, Po AL: The effectiveness of topically applied capsaicin: a meta-analysis, *Eur J Clin Pharmacol* 46:517, 1994.
249. Zimmerman et al: Effects of music in patients who had chronic cancer pain, *West J Nurs Res* 11:298, 1989.

SUGGESTED READINGS

Bensky D, Barolet R: *Chinese herbal medicine: formulas and strategies*, Seattle, 1990, Eastland Press.

Blumenthal M, Hall T, Rister R, Gruenwald J, Riggins C, editors: *The German Commission E Monographs: Therapeutic monographs on medicinal plants for human use*, Austin, 1996, American Botanical Council.

Boik J: *Cancer and natural medicine: A textbook of basic science and clinical research*, Princeton, Minn, 1995, Oregon Medical Press.

Bonica JJ, editor: *The management of pain*, Malvern, Penn, 1990, Lea & Febiger.

Hammill RJ, Rowlingson JC, editors: *Handbook of critical care pain management*, New York, 1994, McGraw-Hill.

Huang B, Wang Y: *Thousand formulas and thousand herbs of traditional Chinese medicine, vol 2, Formulas*, China, 1993, Heilongjiang Education Press.

Jacobs J: *Encyclopedia of alternative medicine: a complete family guide to complementary therapies*, Boston, 1996, Journey Editions.

McCaffery M, Beebe A: *Pain: Clinical manual for nursing practice*, St Louis, 1989, Mosby.

National Institute of Nursing Research: National Nursing Research Agenda, volume 6, Symptom management: Acute pain, NIH pub. no. 94-2421, Bethesda, Md, June 1994, National Institutes of Health, U.S. Public Health Service, U.S. Department of Health and Human Services.

Newall CA, Anderson LA, Phillipson JD: *Herbal medicines: A guide for health-care professionals*, London, 1996, The Pharmaceutical Press.

Tollison CD, Satterthwaite JR, Tollison JW, editors: *Handbook of pain management*, Baltimore, 1994, Williams & Wilkins.

Turk DC, Melzack R, editors: *Handbook of pain assessment*, New York, 1992, The Guilford Press.

Wood JN, editor: *Capsaicin in the study of pain*, San Diego, 1993, Academic Press.

CHAPTER 11

Complementary/Alternative Therapies in Select Populations: Women

Fredi Kronenberg, Patricia Aikins Murphy, and Christine Wade

Women's health is studied by a broad spectrum of medical and social science disciplines, but as a discrete topic it is difficult to define. A reductive view limits the discussion of women's health to reproductive function, whereas a broader perspective encompasses not only disease states but also normal life events. Women's health is affected by major causes of mortality, morbidity, and disability (e.g., cardiovascular disease or cancer), but women also seek health care in connection with menstruation, pregnancy, childbirth, menopause, and aging.

Medical treatment of women has been characterized by both overintervention and neglect, and research on many topics in women's health is often sparse. In an effort to correct this situation, the National Institutes of Health (NIH) established an Office of Research on Women's Health (ORWH) in 1990 to ensure that appropriate research is conducted to fill gaps in knowledge. Resources are now being brought to bear to establish and implement a research agenda in women's health in order to better understand and promote health, prevent illness, and effectively treat disease.

WOMEN AND CAM

Women are the primary users of conventional medicine. Women are probably also the primary users of complementary and alternative medicine (CAM). As caregivers for their families and, often, for their communities, they have for centuries used "folk medicine" and "home remedies" now being called CAM. Today these remedies are the subject of biomedical research to determine what works, for whom, under what conditions,

The authors thank Judith Jacobson, PhD, for contributions and editorial assistance; Sara Workman, MPH, for contributions; and Carrie Lewis, MPH, for technical assistance. Grant support was received from The National Institutes of Health grant no. U24-HD33199, The Carol Ann Schwartz Cancer Initiative, and the Fetzer Institute.

and at what dose. While women constitute 52% of the U.S. population, they make 57% of visits to doctors, are prescribed 60% of all prescription medication, and undergo 59% of hospital procedures.[10,108,109] The two leading surgeries in the United States are exclusive to women: cesarean section and hysterectomy.[92] Women make 75% of health care decisions and spend two of every three health care dollars.[108,109]

Since women use more conventional medicine services than men do, they may also use CAM more extensively. Although a U.S. national survey did not find that gender predicted CAM use,[37] other studies indicate that women may use CAM more than men. A study of complementary medicine in Germany found that more women than men (44% vs. 32%) were given CAM and that more women than men preferred CAM to mainstream medicine (62% vs. 52%).[57] A study of Chinese medicine practitioners in New York City found more women than men among non-Asian patients (59% vs. 41%).[54] Women are also greater users of homeopathic remedies (66%).[12]

Why do women choose CAM? Despite the achievements of contemporary conventional medicine, reasons are numerous.[37] They include a preference for more "natural" treatment, belief in unconventional medicine, concern about the side effects of conventional treatments, and dissatisfaction with or lack of confidence in conventional medicine.[80] Studies of people who choose alternatives suggest that most are *not* poorly educated or gullible. Indeed, they have been shown to be relatively well educated and middle class.[28,38,80] McGregor and Peay[80] demonstrated that CAM patients have a substantially lower level of confidence in the efficacy of conventional medicine; however, they clearly were not dissatisfied with their medical practitioners. People who choose alternatives speak of conventional medicine's limitations and narrow-mindedness, as well as their desire for control over their health and health care.[38] Patients often use CAM without informing their conventional medical physicians.[38]

In addition to these general reasons, women may turn to CAM when faced with problems for which Western biomedicine offers treatments that may produce undesirable and sometimes unacceptable effects. For example, pregnant women may wish to avoid drugs that could interfere with fetal development. During menopause, although hormone therapy typically provides effective relief of symptoms such as hot flashes, it may be contraindicated for some individuals, and others desire a more natural approach.

Women also seek alternative approaches in an effort to avoid surgery. Hysterectomy is the most common non–pregnancy-related surgical procedure for women in the United States; one third of all women will have had a hysterectomy by 65 years of age.[115] Uterine fibroids are the primary indication in nearly two thirds of black women and in one third of white women who have hysterectomies. In light of the cost and risk associated with surgery, evaluation of the effectiveness of CAM in reducing the need for surgery is an important question in women's health.

A recent survey of three ethnic groups of women in New York City found that 58% used CAM and about 40% have visited at least one CAM practitioner.[42] In addition to seeking the care of CAM practitioners, many women self-medicate in search of suitable remedies. They do so with insufficient information on safety and efficacy to guide them. Not only does this waste time and money, but some types of experimentation may put certain women at risk. For example, herbs are often considered "natural" and assumed to be nontoxic, but they have numerous physiologically active components, some of which may be contraindicated for individuals with particular medical conditions. Remedies taken by pregnant women may have unknown consequences for fetal growth and development.

It is often argued that CAM remedies are natural and therefore safe. Some CAM methods have been used in traditional cultures for centuries without apparent ill effects. Historical use does not necessarily mean safety, however, and these arguments do not eliminate the need for a research agenda on CAM and women's health that includes well-designed studies on safety and efficacy.

Ideally, clinical decisions should be based on systematic and scientific observations drawn from well-designed research studies.[41] In both conventional medicine and CAM there are many areas in which evidence about the risks, benefits, or efficacy of various choices in treatment is lacking.[87] CAM treatments for women's health problems are particularly in need of research.

CAM METHODS FOR WOMEN'S HEALTH

Most CAM methods would find application across the range of women's health concerns, and women are using many of them. However, certain CAM modalities are particularly promising with respect to women's health. The following brief overview of CAM methods covers important indications and applications but is by no means complete. Medical systems from other countries, so-called ethnomedicines or traditional medicines, are particularly promising for treatment of women's gynecologic conditions. Some of these systems, such as Ayurveda, traditional Chinese medicine (TCM), and Tibetan medicine, have complex theoretic structures and empiric, literature-based traditions and have been practiced as medical systems for thousands of years. They have classic gynecologic texts, materia medica with specific herbs for gynecologic conditions, and modern practitioners who claim success in treating women's reproductive and gynecologic problems. Other traditions are primarily oral and are passed along through apprenticeship.

These systems use different diagnostic techniques than does Western medicine. For example, TCM uses pulse and tongue diagnosis, along with other observations to identify patterns in the individual that indicate imbalances. Herbal formulas and/or acupuncture and other techniques are used to restore balance. Treatment of preconditions to disease, as evident in pattern diagnosis, is an important aspect of these systems. For example, careful attention is paid within these medical systems to length, regularity, flow, blood qualities, and other aspects of the menstrual cycle to prevent development of chronic disease. This type of diagnosis is not typical in Western gynecologic practice. Research is needed on its relevance to women's health outcomes.

Folk herbalism has a long history of use for women's health conditions. There are many ethnic expressions of the tradition of folk herbalism, including practices from countries worldwide. The tradition of women folk herbalists is sometimes known as the Wise Woman tradition and has within its practice remedies for women's health conditions that are promising for research. Herbalism, especially as practiced by midwives, is undergoing a revival in the United States. Almost daily, the popular press and other media are deluging women with articles and other reports on herbal medicine. A wealth of new products confront the consumer. For women to be able to make better-informed choices, it is incumbent upon researchers to study the safety and efficacy of these therapies.

Mind-body therapies include a vast array of disciplines ranging from biofeedback and hypnosis to guided imagery. Many women use mind-body therapies primarily as complements to biomedicine and to prevent disease. These therapies are also being explored as treatments for conditions such as hot flashes, immune dysfunction, chronic pain, diabetes, infertility, and complications of pregnancy. These methods usually have minimal side effects, and research has demonstrated the efficacy of these methods for many conditions not specific to women's health.

It is now recognized that nutrition plays a role in maintaining health and, possibly, in the treatment of disease. Although specific details continue to be researched, there are several dietary topics emerging as important to women's health. One such topic is dietary estrogens—plant-based sources of estrogenic substances found in many foods and herbs. The role of these phytoestrogens and their potential role in women's hormone-dependent diseases, such as uterine fibroids and breast cancer, is an area of current interest. Phytoestrogens are found in fruits, vegetables, and legumes such as soy (see later discussions of menopause and breast cancer).

CAM AND WOMEN'S HEALTH CONDITIONS

The following is a summary of CAM research published in the Western scientific literature in three areas of women's health: menopausal hot flashes, nausea and vomiting in pregnancy, and breast cancer. Two of these are self-limiting and, although not life threatening, are common and can cause women appreciable distress. At times, for some women, nausea and vomiting during pregnancy and menopausal hot flashes can be functionally incapacitating. Breast cancer is a serious illness with considerable associated mortality and morbidity. In these three areas there is a research literature of varying quantity and quality. For many women's health problems, such as fibroids and endometriosis, our searches of the English-language literature have yielded results too meager to summarize.

Menopausal Hot Flashes

Women in the perimenopausal and postmenopausal years may have a number of problems that either occur for a limited period of time before resolving or may increase in magnitude with years after menopause. Other problems continue for years at levels ranging from barely perceptible to annoying to intolerable. Of the complaints associated with the menopausal period, there are several for which women have, in increasing numbers, been seeking modes of therapy other than the standard hormone therapy. These include hot flashes, sleep problems, vaginal dryness, joint pain, weight gain, mood swings, and fatigue. Of these, hot flashes, more than any other, cause women to seek treatment. Hormone therapy (estrogen with or without progesterone) is extremely efficacious in the treatment of hot flashes. It significantly ameliorates and in many cases eliminates hot flashes for a large percentage of women. But some women need or desire other options because they have medical conditions or risk factors for which estrogen is contraindicated, have some adverse reaction to hormone therapy, or choose not to take hormones.

There are a number of nonpharmacologic approaches to hot flashes that women have been exploring on their own. These include vitamins (in particular, vitamin E), behavioral therapies (such as yoga, relaxation, and biofeedback), lifestyle changes (exercise, alcohol use, and dietary changes), herbal remedies (black cohosh, ginseng, and dong quai), any of a number of traditional systems of medicine (such as TCM, Ayurveda, and Tibetan medicine), homeopathy, and acupuncture. Although the efficacy of these approaches has not been demonstrated, because of the popularity of CAM since 1994 investigators are now developing studies of CAM therapies for menopausal problems, particularly hot flashes, as described in the following sections.

Medicinal Herbs. Women of many cultures have used herbs to reduce the discomfort of hot flashes. This includes a history of herbal therapy in Western countries. For most herbal remedies there are few clinical studies to draw on for treatment recommendations. We do know that many herbs contain substances that have potent physiologic effects.

Native American women have traditionally used black cohosh (*Cimicifugae racemosa*) to treat amenorrhea, and before, during, and after labor.[43] It has been used in German medicine for about 50 years and is approved by the German Commission E (somewhat comparable to the U.S. Food and Drug Administration [FDA]) for use in premenstrual discomfort, dysmenorrhea, and menopausal symptoms. Studies have found that black cohosh binds to estrogen receptors, and researchers have postulated that the herb has estrogenic effects.[33,67] Recent pharmacologic investigations did not detect estrogenic growth promotion on experimentally induced mammary tumors in ovariectomized rats.[78a]

Dong quai (*Angelica sinensis*) is another herb used by menopausal women, some of whom report that it helps relieve hot flashes.[71] In the first randomized, placebo-controlled clinical trial of dong quai for the treatment of menopausal symptoms (in 71 post-menopausal women) investigators found no statistically significant difference in the number of hot flashes, vaginal maturation index, or Kupperman Index (a combined index of 11 menopausal complaints).[58] The authors concluded that dong quai, when used alone, is not helpful in relieving menopausal symptoms. Dong quai is typically used as one of several components of traditional Chinese herbal formulas; it is not used alone in TCM and would not be prescribed for all women with menopausal symptoms. Dong quai is sold in health food stores in the United States, women buy it for the treatment of menopausal problems, and some find it helpful. Additional studies are needed to clarify the role of dong quai either singly or in herbal mixtures for the treatment of menopausal complaints.

Ginseng has estrogenic actions that have been demonstrated in humans.[60,94] Ginseng is reported by women to be effective in relieving menopausal symptoms. In a recent placebo-controlled trial ginseng (Ginsana G115) provided some symptomatic relief, particularly for depressed mood and improved self-reported general health and well-being. It was less satisfactory for relief of hot flashes.[78]

Dietary Phytoestrogens. Although particular foods (such as coffee and spicy foods) are reported by some women to trigger individual hot flashes, long-term consumption or emphasis on certain foods in the diet may influence hormone levels and thereby affect whether hot flashes occur at all. Many food plants contain physiologically active estrogenic substances (phytoestrogens). The major classes of phytoestrogens are isoflavones, lignins, coumestans, and resorcylic acid lactones. Isoflavones are found in legumes such as soy, clover, and alfalfa. Lignins are found in whole grains, seeds, fruits and vegetables (especially flaxseed [linseed]), and also rye, millet, and legumes.[6]

Grains and soybeans are the most commonly consumed foods with estrogenic activity, but other plants that contain phytoestrogens include chick peas, pinto beans, french beans, pomegranates, lima beans, and clover.[93] Lignin precursors found in the grains, seeds, and the like are broken down by bacteria in the gut to enterolactone and enterodiol (also called mammalian lignins). Bacteria also remove a glycoside from isoflavone precursors to create the active isoflavones genistein, daidzein, and equol. Many whole grains, including wheat, oats, corn, and rye, contain a fungus (*Fusarium* sp.) that produces estrogenic substances called zearalenol and zearalenone[93]; these are much stronger phytoestrogens than those produced by the plants themselves, although they are still quite a bit weaker than endogenous estrogens.

It is now well established that ingestion of plants containing phytoestrogens can cause reproductive disorders in mammals.[100,102] A diet with substantial intake of these foods can produce estrogen-like effects in women as well. For example, ingestion of estrogenic food plants (linseed, clover sprouts) by postmenopausal women produced changes in vaginal maturation values in an Australian study.[114] In a study of a dietary soy intervention in postmenopausal women in the United States there was a slight but not statistically significant estrogenic effect on vaginal epithelium.[16] It is not surprising that results differ among these studies, since the food plants involved contain different classes of estrogenic compounds (lignans in the grasses and oilseeds and isoflavones in soy) with differing degrees of estrogenicity.

Some phytoestrogens are weakly estrogenic, but they are often found in very high levels in the body. In a study comparing American and Finnish women consuming three diets (omnivorous, lactovegetarian, and macrobiotic) excretion of the most abundant phytoestrogen was found to be highest in the macrobiotic group and lowest in the omnivorous group.[4] Postmenopausal women in Japan eating a traditional low-fat diet were found to have 100 to 1000 times higher levels of several urinary phytoestrogens than levels of the endogenous estrogens in the urine of American or Finnish women eating an omnivorous diet.[7] The Asian diets are associated with a high intake of soy products. The high levels of dietary phytoestrogens may offer an explanation for the low level of hot flashes reported by many Japanese women.

In a study designed to examine the effect of soy on hot flashes more directly, Murkies et al.[84] compared the effect of soy flour with wheat flour supplementation in a randomized, double-blind trial. Hot flashes decreased significantly in the soy group by week 6 and in both groups by week 12. There was no change in vaginal maturation index in either group. Excretion of urinary daidzein, an estrogenic isoflavone in soy, had increased significantly at 12 weeks in the soy group, and there was no significant increase in excretion of urinary phytoestrogens in the wheat group. Interpretation of these results is not clear. Wheat flour also contains phytoestrogens, but with less estrogenic potency than soy phytoestrogens. Milling supposedly removes most of the phytoestrogens from wheat (thus the choice for placebo). There is not yet the critical mass of studies on soy phytoestrogens that is required for definitive conclusions.

The studies suggest a role for diet in modulating endocrine actions in the body. As data accumulate to provide evidence that the phytoestrogen content of some foods may affect physiologic function, it is not unreasonable to think that diet would have the potential to influence an individual's hot-flash pattern, or even whether one has hot flashes at all. How big a role diet may play and whether there are biologic (genetic) differences among populations that result in observed differences in hot-flash prevalences remain to be determined.

Vitamin E. There are anecdotal reports of vitamin E's effectiveness for treating hot flashes, but little objective data. A few clinical trials were conducted in the 1940s and 1950s. Some of the studies found vitamin E to be of value in treating hot flashes, but for the most part the studies were not double-blind, placebo-controlled, or of adequate duration, when considering that in most drug studies of hot-flash therapies there is a considerable placebo effect. In a much cited study of Blatt et al.,[23] a double-blind design (no crossover) was used to compare the effect of vitamin E, estrogen, and a placebo on a combined group of 11 symptoms (not on hot flashes specifically). Vitamin E was no more effective than placebo in treating this symptom complex. This study is cited as demonstrating lack of effectiveness of vitamin E for treating hot flashes, a conclusion not justified from these data.

In a postal survey (self-selected subjects) that included 438 women with hot flashes, 57% of these women reported having tried vitamin E specifically for their hot flashes. Of these women, 27% reported that it helped their hot flashes, but dose and duration of treatment are unknown.[72]

Acupuncture. Wyon et al.[116] administered 8 weeks of acupuncture (one to two times per week for 30 minutes) to 24 naturally menopausal women with hot flashes. The authors compared two forms of acupuncture and found that both significantly reduced the daily number of hot flashes. They also found a decrease in urinary calcitonin gene-related peptide (a potent endothelium-dependent vasodilator of systemic blood vessels). Although there is controversy in the acupuncture field about the appropriateness of the controls used, this study is an important first step in the scientific examination of acupuncture for the treatment of menopausal symptoms.

Behavioral Therapies. Behavioral methods for moderating hot flashes have received limited study. Freedman and Woodward[46] compared paced respiration with muscle relaxation and alpha electroencephalogam (EEG) biofeedback and found that paced respiration training reduced the frequency of hot flashes by about 40% as compared with women who received progressive muscle relaxation training or controls (11 women in each group). Freedman et al. [47] obtained similar results in a more recent study with a somewhat larger subject population (N = 24). Elucidation of the relaxation response for 7 weeks in a randomized, controlled study resulted in significant reductions in hot flash intensity but not in hot flash frequency.[65] The results from these studies suggest the need for additional research in this area.

Exercise. Several groups have presented preliminary data suggesting that exercise moderates at least the severity, if not frequency, of hot flashes. Since exercise has demonstrated effects on sex steroids, it is not unreasonable to think that it might influence hot flashes as well. In a study of the relationship between menopausal symptoms and aerobic fitness in healthy volunteers, Wilbur et al.[113] found that of their 375 subjects (mean age, 47 years), 27% reported via a symptom checklist that they were having hot flashes or night sweats. Joint pains and backaches were the most frequently reported symptom. A bicycle ergometric test of aerobic fitness indicated that 54% of the sample had above-average or average, 27% had average, and 19% had low fitness levels. Hot flashes and night sweats were highest in perimenopausal women. Aerobic fitness was negatively related to hot flashes (although the finding was not statistically significant). Hammar et al.[53] reported that women who belonged to a gymnastic club had fewer hot flashes than women who did not belong, but whose physical activity was not reported. Although these data are weak and there is no study demonstrating that physical activity is a substitute for hormone therapy in relieving hot flashes, exercise may help ameliorate hot flashes.

Nausea and Vomiting in Pregnancy

Nausea and vomiting are among the most common complaints during early pregnancy. The symptoms affect more than 50% of women in Western societies. For most women the condition is self-limiting, with symptoms most common and troublesome in early pregnancy and resolving by the beginning of the second trimester. In some women severe symptoms may lead to dehydration, weight loss, and acidosis, requiring hospitalization for fluid replacement. Whether or not the condition becomes this severe, it can cause considerable distress and temporary disability. Nearly half of employed women believe their work efficiency is reduced by this problem, and as many as 25% require time off from work.[111]

There are pharmacologic treatments for this condition, but concerns about the potential teratogenic effects of medication taken during the critical embryogenic stage limit their use. Most available drugs are listed as FDA category C, which means that either there have been adverse effects noted in animal studies and no human studies are available or that there are no studies at all in humans or animals. Other recommendations include dietary advice (e.g., avoidance of fatty or spicy foods) and lifestyle change (such as avoiding cooking), but few women report complete relief with these recommendations.[88] Consequently, many women turn to CAM therapies to treat nausea and vomiting.

A review of both pregnancy self-help books and lay CAM publications suggests that a host of alternatives are used, including vitamins, herbal products, homeopathic agents, acupressure, and acupuncture. There is little Western scientific evidence about the efficacy of these remedies. This review summarizes the available clinical research in this area, which is discussed elsewhere in greater detail.[85]

Acupressure and Related Methods. Acupressure is the best-studied CAM measure for the treatment of nausea and vomiting of pregnancy. The specific intervention involves stimulation of or pressure on an acupuncture point known as P6 or the Nei Guan point, which is on the volar surface of the forearm, two to three finger breadths above the wrist. This point has been shown in other studies of postoperative emesis, chemotherapy-associated emesis, and motion sickness to be important in the relief of nausea and vomiting.[112] In many studies a commercially available wristband designed to prevent motion sickness has been used. These devices (Sea Bands, Sea Band International,

Greensboro, North Carolina), when properly placed, are designed to apply pressure over the Nei Guan point.

Seven clinical trials of acupressure for treating nausea and vomiting of early pregnancy have compared women using acupressure over the Nei Guan point to a variety of comparison groups* (Table 11-1). In five of the seven trials, significant reductions in nausea and vomiting were noted in the women using acupressure. However, it may not be possible to perform a true double-blind, placebo-controlled trial (the gold standard of clinical research) because of the nature of the intervention. In some studies no alternate intervention was used, which raises a concern that any benefit attributable to acupressure could have been the result of the placebo effect. In other studies acupressure was applied to a sham or "dummy" point (one other than the point thought to be important). The correct point, however, can be identified easily in any number of self-help books, so there remains a concern about a placebo effect. In addition, in two studies the group receiving acupressure was further along in pregnancy than the control subjects; because the condition in question resolves spontaneously as pregnancy advances, the observed benefits could have been due to the normal evolution of pregnancy. In two other studies there was a significant loss (30% to 50%) of study subjects, which also compromises findings. The largest clinical trial, which compared acupressure to sham acupressure and to no intervention, found no beneficial effects. Thus the literature is equivocal.

One study[39] evaluated a related method, sensory afferent stimulation, which delivered a continuous electric current to the volar surface of the wrist. The exact location of the stimulation was not described but was verified in another report to have been the P6 point.[112] Such electrical stimulation has been characterized as a form of "electroacupuncture." Those using the device reported significantly more improvement in symptoms of nausea and vomiting than those wearing the placebo unit. However, it was probably possible to determine which was the active unit, since it produced a tingling sensation in the wrist or hand; thus benefits could have been due to a placebo-type effect. Other observational studies have been made but do not meet criteria for randomized, controlled clinical trials, nor has acupuncture been evaluated in controlled trials. Two Chinese case series described such treatment for nausea and vomiting in early pregnancy,[117,118] but there were no control groups, nor was there discussion of outcome measurements.

The clinical trial research on the use of acupressure or related methods has not produced consistent or methodologically sound findings. However, it is clear from these studies that acupressure of the Nei Guan point benefits many women. It could be argued that in studies which did not provide an intervention to the control group or arm of the trial, positive findings might be due only to the "placebo" effect. However,

*References 19, 21, 32, 34, 39, 63, 89.

TABLE 11-1	Randomized Clinical Trials of Acupuncture or Acupressure for Nausea and Vomiting in Pregnancy		
Author, Year	No. in Study	Intervention	Results
Dundee et al., 1988	350	• Manual acupressure over the P6 or a dummy point, compared to control group (no intervention) • Intervention of 4 days' duration	"Severe" or "troublesome" morning sickness noted in 24% using P6 acupressure, 37% using dummy point acupressure, and 56% using no intervention ($p < 0.005$)
Hyde, 1989	16	• Acupressure wristbands vs. no intervention • 5-day intervention, followed by crossover to other group for 5 days	• Relief of morning sickness in 75% using wristbands ($p < l0.025$) • Reduction of anxiety, depression, and behavioral dysfunction as measured by standard psychometric tools ($p < 0.05$)
de Aloysio and Penacchioni, 1992	60	• Unilateral (right or left wrist) or bilateral acupressure wristbands* vs. placebo wristbands (no pressure exerted on P6 point) • Each version of intervention given for 3 days in crossover design	Reduction or elimination of symptoms in 65% to 69% while using acupressure vs. in 29% to 31% while using placebo ($p < 0.05$)
Bayreuther et al., 1994	16	• Acupressure wristbands* vs. placebo wristbands (applied over a dummy point) • 7-day intervention, followed by crossover to the alternate intervention for 7 days	• Nausea score (using a visual acuity scale) was lower in the group using acupressure compared with the placebo ($p = 0.019$) • No effect on vomiting
Belluomini et al., 1994	60	Manual acupressure on the P6 point vs. pressure on a dummy point for 3 days	• Nausea decreased significantly in treatment group ($p = 0.0021$) • No difference in severity or frequency of vomiting
O'Brien et al., 1996	161	• Accupressure wristbands* vs. wristbands over a dummy point vs. a control group with no intervention • 7-day intervention	No differences across groups in nausea or vomiting
Evans et al., 1993	23	• Continuous electric current stimulation at the P6 point vs. no stimulation • 48-hour intervention followed by crossover to alternate intervention	Improvement in symptoms of nausea and vomiting in 87% of experimental group vs. 43% of controls ($p < 0.05$)

Modified from American College of Obstetricians and Gynecologists, *Obstet Gynecol* 91:151, 1998.
*Sea Bands (Sea Band International, Greensboro, North Carolina).

there may be value in mobilizing such a mind-body interaction if the intervention is simple and inexpensive, if it results in reduction of symptoms, and if it is not associated with any risk. The issue of fetal risk has not been addressed in studies. There does not seem to be any theoretic risk of teratogenesis from acupressure or related methods. However, there are acupressure and acupuncture points that are contraindicated in pregnancy because of their potential to produce uterine contractions; these are not near the Nei Guan point.

Ginger. Ginger root is a remedy used in many traditional cultures as a treatment for nausea. It is frequently mentioned in self-help books as a treatment for nausea and vomiting of pregnancy. Its efficacy is thought to be due to its aromatic, carminative, and absorbent properties. Studies of its use with other types of nausea and vomiting (such as motion sickness) confirm its potential as a treatment. Only one trial has examined the efficacy of this intervention in pregnancy.[45] Women who had been admitted to the hospital for treatment of the most severe form of this condition, hyperemesis gravidarum, were randomly assigned to treatment with 250 mg of ginger in a capsule four times a day or with a placebo. There was a significant improvement associated with ginger: it reduced the degree of nausea and the number of attacks of vomiting.

A caution was raised by one scientist, who suggested that since ginger is a thromboxane synthetase inhibitor, it could theoretically affect sex steroid differentiation of the fetal brain.[45] In this study 27 pregnancies were followed: there was one miscarriage and one voluntary termination, and the remaining infants were born in good health and "without evidence of deformities." However, some problems may be too subtle to be detected in a general physical examination. The issue of teratogenesis should be further explored, especially as it relates to dosage of ginger.

In addition, some herbalists describe ginger as a traditional "menstruation promoter"; whether this means it has potential as an abortifacient is unclear. TCM advises caution in the use of dried ginger in pregnancy. However, Bergner[22] pointed out that typical doses in TCM are larger, perhaps 3 g a day or more. The dose used in the study was 1 g, roughly equivalent to an 8-ounce glass of ginger ale or 4 cups of ginger tea.

There has been little research assessment of a remedy that is widely used traditionally and across cultures. Based on work in other areas and the one trial reported here, it is likely that ginger will be of benefit to some women. Concerns have been raised about its teratogenic potential, but directed investigation of this hypothesis has not been performed. Prudence might indicate avoiding intake of ginger in excess of 1 g daily.

Vitamin B₆. Vitamin B_6 (pyridoxine) was included in the original formulation of the drug Bendectin (Merrell Dow Pharmaceuticals, Cincinnati, Ohio), which was the only drug approved by FDA for treatment of nausea and vomiting in pregnancy. The drug (which had 10 mg of doxylamine and 10 mg of pyridoxine) was withdrawn from the market by its manufacturer after several lawsuits alleging birth defects related to its use. Further epidemiologic study has failed to corroborate allegations of teratogenesis from the use of this combination.[90]

Some clinicians questioned whether the benefit seen from Bendectin may have been due to its vitamin content, and two studies have addressed the efficacy of pyridoxine treatment of nausea and vomiting in early pregnancy. Sahakian et al.[97] compared vitamin B_6 to a placebo; the intervention consisted of taking 25 mg of pyridoxine every 8 hours for 3 days. There was little difference in symptoms among patients with mild to moderate nausea; however, there were significant improvements among women with severe nausea and significant overall reduction in vomiting episodes. In another study women took either 30 mg of pyridoxine daily or a placebo in a randomized, double-blind trial.[103] There was a significant decrease in nausea, as well as a nonsignificant trend toward reduction in episodes of vomiting, associated with vitamin use. Of interest is a study that was unable to demonstrate a relationship between serum vitamin B_6 levels and the prevalence or degree of morning sickness.[101] This suggests that if pyridoxine supplementation is efficacious, the mechanism may not be related to levels of pyridoxine in the blood but to some other factor.

Vitamin B_6 is also a common, available, and inexpensive remedy. It apparently benefits some women in doses of 30 to 75 mg per day, which is higher than the Recommended Daily Allowance (RDA) of 2.2 mg per day.[86] There is little evidence to support a teratogenic effect from this supplement in doses up to 40 mg per day. However, issues of appropriate dosage in pregnancy should be addressed, since pyridoxine has been shown to cause neurologic problems in nonpregnant adults when taken in excessive doses.[30,96,99]

Hypnosis, Hypnotherapy, and Behavior Modification. Some authors characterize nausea and vomiting of pregnancy as a psychologic or behavioral disorder; hypnosis is one technique that may be used for treatment of such disorders. Several published reports have addressed the treatment of nausea and vomiting in early pregnancy using hypnotherapy or behavior modification.[48,56,79,103,110] Most are case series dealing with severely ill women (many were hospitalized). Symptoms improved after hypnotherapy, but it is difficult to separate the effects of treatment from longitudinal improvement as pregnancy advances. Thus the benefits of this intervention are unclear.

Overall Considerations

There is a dearth of research literature to support or refute the efficacy of a number of common remedies for a very common problem. The best-studied remedy seems to be acupressure over the Nei Guan point. A systematic review of this literature (that excluded studies of poor methodologic quality and those whose data could not be combined) found the effects of acupressure to be comparable to those of antiemetic medications but cautioned that the evidence is equivocal.[68] Herbal remedies are commonly advised for nausea and vomiting in pregnancy, and the more common ones are readily available over the counter in health food stores and many pharmacies. Many have pharmacologic effects in the body, and a number are contraindicated in pregnancy. Of the many suggestions encountered in various lay publications, only ginger has been studied, and that in only one trial.

Women seeking alternative, nonpharmacologic therapies for nausea and vomiting of early pregnancy may be advised to try acupressure over the Nei Guan point. This can be achieved through the use of commercial wristbands or by applying manual pressure to the appropriate spot on the volar surface of the wrist. Ginger may be recommended as well, in prudent doses. Vitamin B_6 may also be efficacious in doses that do not exceed 75 mg a day. Apart from these few studies, however, there is little evidence to support or refute the benefits or risks of other remedies. Given the prevalence of the problem of nausea and vomiting for pregnant women and the potential for adverse effects from the use of teratogenic or abortifacient remedies, more research in this field is needed.

Breast Cancer

The most common cancers affecting women in the United States are breast cancer, colorectal cancer, cancers of the reproductive organs, and lung cancer.[8] Breast cancer accounts for over 30% of newly diagnosed cancer in women and nearly 20% of cancer deaths.[8] It is the leading cause of cancer death in women aged 40 to 55 years. Recently breast cancer incidence has leveled off at a rate of about 110 new cases per 100,000 women per year.[9] Currently identified risk factors account for only a minority of cases and are generally not modifiable through preventive behavior.[69] Secondary prevention strategies through screening are the current means for improving survival. Breast cancer is a major health issue for women, not only because it is the most common of women's cancers, but also because of its impact on survival, lifestyle, self-image, and quality of life.[61] Research on both prevention and improving survival is a priority of the current health agenda in the United States.

Dietary Estrogens: Estrogens and Antiestrogens for Hormone-Dependent Cancer.
Exposure to estrogens, whether environmental or endogenous, may increase risk for breast cancer, other hormone-dependent cancers, and other hormone-dependent conditions in women, such as uterine fibroids. Eating soybeans and other plants containing estrogenic substances may lower the risk of developing breast and other cancers.[51] Asians who follow traditional diets have lower breast cancer rates than those who adopt a Western diet.[2] Asians eat much less fat and protein, more fiber, and more carbohydrates, and consume high amounts (10 to 30 g) of soy products compared with the American diet.[59] Adlercreutz et al.[5] reported that the mean consumption of soy prod-

ucts in the traditional Japanese diet of men was 39.2 g per day. The increasing popularity of soy and other phytoestrogenic foods in the American diet, especially in certain subgroups such as vegetarians, may soon reach (or may have reached for some women) biologically active levels. The intake of soy products by Americans has increased approximately 40% between 1980 and 1990.[81]

Today women in Western countries are exposed to higher levels of estrogen over their lifetimes than their ancestors. Part of the reason is that they produce more estrogen over their lifetimes: they weigh more (fat increases estrogen levels through peripheral aromatization), begin to menstruate at a younger age, bear fewer children, breastfeed for shorter periods (if at all), and lead relatively sedentary lives. They also eat a lot of animal products; high-fat diets also appear to increase estrogen levels. This higher lifetime exposure to endogenous estrogens has been postulated to be one reason for high breast cancer incidence in these countries.[91]

It is hypothesized that ingestion of plant estrogens may reduce risk because plant estrogens tend to be weak estrogens, the strongest being only 1/200th as strong as human estrogens.[93] These weak estrogens may perform some of the same beneficial functions as endogenous estrogens and may turn down endogenous estrogen production through a negative feedback effect on the production of hypothalamic and pituitary hormones. Thus women who eat plant estrogens every day may have a constantly lower rate of estrogen production, and this may lower their risk of breast cancer. An epidemiologic study of Chinese women in Singapore found that women who ate a diet high in soy had a lower rate of premenopausal (but not postmenopausal) breast cancer. Dietary intake of red meat increased risk, and polyunsaturated fatty acids, beta-carotenes, and soy protein reduced risk.[76]

The best-studied phytoestrogen is genistein, which decreases tyrosine kinase (involved in cell-cycle regulation and control of mitogenesis) and inhibits angiogenesis.[70] One study found that baby rats exposed to a carcinogen had a 40% lower cancer rate if they also received genistein.[74] Genistein may be an active ingredient, but whole soybeans work, too; a previous study showed that rats fed soybean chips had lower rates of mammary tumors.[17]

Several studies have explored possible associations between aspects of the traditional Asian diet and low risk for hormone-based cancers and other hormone-dependent conditions in women.[6,7] In addition to lower fat content, higher fiber-to-protein ratios are also characteristic of traditional Asian diets when compared with typical diets in the West.

Thus dietary factors may influence hormone levels in women and may play a role in the etiology of hormone-dependent disease. Western diets elevate sex hormones and decrease sex hormone binding globulin (SHBG) concentration, thus increasing the availability of the endogenous steroids to peripheral tissues.[6] Increased fat intake decreases fecal excretion of endogenous estrogen, which may contribute to elevated serum levels and increase availability of endogenous estrogen at peripheral sites.[7] Increased fiber intake increases fecal excretion of endogenous estrogen, thus lowering serum levels.[3] High-fiber diets are associated with increased urinary lignans and isoflavones.[5]

Adverse Effects. Phytoestrogens, including those contained in soy, have been associated with infertility in animals. In Australia in the 1940s, infertility that decimated the sheep industry was subsequently linked to clover forage containing phytoestrogens.[100] Captive cheetahs were found to be infertile after being fed a soy-based diet.[102] Whether phytoestrogens could cause infertility, precocious puberty in children, or cancer is an obvious question. To date, the data and observations do not provide an affirmative answer. In Asia, people of all ages consume considerable quantities of soy-based foods. Asians have lower rates of breast and prostate cancers, as well as later onset of puberty and no more infertility than Westerners. Additional research is needed to confirm the long-term safety of dietary phytoestrogens.

Studies on the role of phytoestrogens in the prevention and treatment of hormone-dependent cancers have a clear place in a research agenda on CAM and women's health.

CAM Therapies for Breast Cancer. A search of the Western scientific literature since 1970 found more than 100 studies that examined CAM methods and breast cancer.[66] Sixty-eight of these were studies of treatments in women; the rest were in animals or in vitro. The biomedical literature since 1980 describes mostly favorable results in the in vitro and animal studies of a variety of agents, but it is important to remind patients that these may not result in safe and/or effective treatments in humans.[66] These laboratory studies are not described in this chapter. Many studies in human subjects were case reports or case series, and these also are not described in this chapter. Of the 68 studies in humans, there were only 15 controlled clinical trials that randomly assigned patients to treatment groups.

The outcomes described in this literature include effects on relief of general symptoms, postmastectomy symptoms, side effects of chemotherapy and/or radiation, immune function, and survival. The treatments tested include herbs, nutrition, chemical treatments, acupuncture, mind-body techniques, manual therapies, and psychosocial interventions. By no means do the methods studied represent the range of CAM used by breast cancer patients. Many CAM treatments are used by breast cancer patients even though there are no studies on them in breast cancer populations.

Diet. There is much speculation on the role of diet in prevention and treatment of cancer. There is only one published study of the effect of a dietary program for breast cancer patients. In a study of 795 patients, those enrolled in the Bristol Cancer Help Center diet and counseling program had poorer survival than controls who received only conventional treatment.[14] Differences between the Bristol patients and control subjects at baseline may account for this finding, which remains controversial. A review of 73 studies of dietary fat intake concluded that linoleic acid and its metabolic derivative arachidonic acid enhance metastasis in breast cancer.[95] This finding may have implications for both primary prevention and prevention of disease recurrence.

Another study assessed diet before cancer diagnosis as a predictor of survival and found that beta-carotene and fruit were associated with enhanced survival.[64] Among 100 patients given treatment with ascorbic acid, mean survival time was 300 days longer than among untreated controls.[26] A review of eight studies of ascorbic acid found no clear benefits, although an earlier review of 71 studies suggested substantial benefits.[18,27]

Psychosocial and Mind-Body Therapies. Two retrospective cohort studies found that patients in a support group did not survive longer than controls.[50,83] A 10-year follow-up of a randomized, controlled trial, however, found that self-hypnosis and support group meetings significantly increased the mean survival time by 18 months.[105]

Relaxation techniques, cognitive therapy, biofeedback, music therapy, breathing exercises, hypnosis, and support groups and their effect on pain control, mood control, reduced anxiety, and adaptation have been examined in studies of varied designs.* A randomized clinical trial of biofeedback and cognitive therapy in 12 patients found that cognitive therapy decreased urinary cortisol levels (a biomarker for stress response).[31] Two studies of mind-body interventions reported reduction of cancer-related pain in the treatment groups.[11,104] A nonrandomized crossover study found that relaxation, guided imagery, and biofeedback improved various measures of immune function (natural killer cell activity, mixed lymphocyte responsiveness, and the number of peripheral blood lymphocytes) in 13 patients.[52] These investigations indicate that these types of methods may be very important for the cancer patient, although the results of these studies are not comparable by method or end points, nor is any one study particularly compelling.

Acupuncture. Acupuncture provides some relief from symptoms associated with conventional cancer treatment, in particular, nausea and vomiting associated with chemotherapy.[112] Acupuncture to relieve chemotherapy-induced nausea and vomiting has seldom been studied among breast cancer patients. One nonrandomized, controlled crossover study found that 63% of patients receiving electroacupuncture treatment had reduced vomiting within 8 hours of treatment.[34] Almost half of the subjects in the study were breast cancer patients. A preacupuncture and postacupuncture treatment study found that symptoms were reduced in 52% of breast cancer patients and that 47% had

---

*References 20, 24, 31, 35, 75, 82, 98.

reduced pain.[44] There is considerable literature on the use of acupuncture to control chronic pain, including meta-analyses.[106] Research is needed to determine how well acupuncture can reduce symptoms in breast cancer patients.

In a nonrandomized, controlled study of immune function in 49 patients (of whom 10 had breast cancer) microwave acupuncture raised white blood cell counts slightly.[29]

Herbs. A number of herbal agents used for cancer treatment side effects appear promising enough to warrant further research, although they are not necessarily ready for formal clinical trials.[66]

Mistletoe *(Viscum album)*, also called Iscador, has been found to stimulate immune function. A 1973 review of 11 studies found mistletoe promising for decreasing tumor size and extending survival.[40] A more recent review of three studies found no evidence of mistletoe's effect on immune function.[49] The relationship between immune function and cancer survival in humans is complex. A well-controlled observational study of survival among patients who use mistletoe might begin to address this question.

A randomized, controlled trial found lymphocyte transformation enhanced among patients who received a Chinese herb formula containing gymnostemma, pentphyllum, makino, and radix atragali seu heysari in addition to conventional treatment.[62] However, the number of patients was small, tumor types varied, and conventional treatments were not described. Another Chinese herbal formula, identified as Yi Qi Sheng Xue, was also found to improve white blood cell counts in the morning in a randomized, controlled trial that studied time of day of administration.[77] Again, chemotherapy regimens were not reported.

Whether there are botanic medicine treatments that enhance immune function after chemotherapy is worthy of further study. The effects of these agents on compliance with treatment schedules, other side effects and symptoms of treatment, disease recurrence, and survival are important research questions. Variables in the study of the immune system that have import for breast cancer patients will have to be identified as outcome measures in studies of botanicals in order to develop the science in this area.

SUMMARY

The research to date on CAM and breast cancer, menopausal hot flashes, and nausea and vomiting of pregnancy does not provide sufficient information about safety and efficacy to make clear clinical recommendations to patients. Although cancer survival has improved, cancer patients are increasingly turning to unconventional therapies in addition to conventional treatment or after exhausting conventional treatment.[1,25] Where conventional intervention is limited, as for nausea and vomiting during pregnancy, pregnant women are seeking alternatives that provide relief and are safe for developing fetuses. Where women are dissatisfied with standard treatment or fear ways in which it may put them at risk, as in hormone replacement therapies for menopausal symptoms or hysterectomy for uterine fibroids, women will continue to seek and use CAM. Patients are reading about CAM therapies in the popular press, hearing about them from friends and relatives, learning about them at workshops on women's health, and choosing products at the health food store or even at the local drug store. Many patients are interested in dietary modification, nutritional supplementation, and mind-body approaches such as yoga, meditation, guided imagery, and support groups. Others are using herbs that physicians may never have heard of—agents such as shark cartilage or antineoplastons—and detoxification techniques such as fasts or enemas.

Women are also seeking help from many kinds of CAM practitioners. They pursue treatment from practitioners of herbal medicine such as TCM, Ayurvedic doctors, and Western herbalists, as well as homeopaths and naturopaths. Patients also turn to chiropractors, massage therapists, and other manual therapists.

Because so little scientific information exists on the safety and efficacy of these approaches, advising patients who seek or use CAM presents a professional challenge to conventional medicine providers. A step-by-step approach for proactively discussing the use of these therapies can be employed.[36] Such a strategy involves listening to patients, as well as advising them, and this type of consultation requires time. The responsibility to do so is not different from discussing other issues essential to medical care, such as alcohol or drug use or a patient's preferences for resuscitation.[36] As treatment options broaden, partnership between care providers and patients in making treatment decisions is crucial for optimal health care.

REFERENCES

1. Abu-Realh MH et al: The use of complementary therapies by cancer patients, [review] [30 refs], *Nurs Connections* 9:3, 1996.
2. Adlercreutz H, Honjo H, Higashi A: Urinary excretion of lignans and isoflavonoid phytoestrogens in Japanese men and women consuming a traditional Japanese diet, *Am J Clin Nutr.* 54:1093, 1991.
3. Adlercreutz H et al: Excretion of the lignans enterolactone and enterodiol and of equol in omnivorous and vegetarian postmenopausal women and in women with breast cancer, *Lancet* 2:1295, 1982.
4. Adlercreutz H et al: Urinary estrogen profile determination in young Finnish vegetarian and omnivorous women, *J Steroid Biochem* 24:289, 1986.
5. Adlercreutz H et al: Effect of dietary components, including lignans and phytoestrogens, on enterohepatic circulation and liver metabolism of estrogens and on sex hormone binding globulin (SHBG), *J Steroid Biochem* 27:1135, 1987.
6. Adlercreutz H et al: Dietary phytoestrogens and cancer: in vitro and in vivo studies, *J Steroid Biochem Molec Biol* 41:331, 1992.
7. Adlercreutz H et al: Dietary phytoestrogens and the menopause in Japan, *Lancet* 339:1233, 1992.
8. American Cancer Society: *Cancer Facts and Figures,* Atlanta, 1994, American Cancer Society.
9. American Cancer Society: *Cancer Facts and Figures,* Website, Atlanta, 1997, American Cancer Society.
10. Anonymous: Updates: report on '84 drug sales, *FDA Consumer* 20:2, 1986.

11. Arathuzik D: Effects of cognitive-behavioral strategies on pain in cancer patients, *Cancer Nurs* 17:207, 1994.
12. Avina RL, Schneiderman LJ: Why patients choose homeopathy, *West J Med* 128:366, 1978.
13. Backon J: Ginger in preventing nausea and vomiting of pregnancy; a caveat due to its thromboxane synthetase activity and effect on testosterone binding, *Eur J Obstet Gynecol Reprod Biol* 42:163, 1991.
14. Bagenal FS et al: Survival of patients with breast cancer attending Bristol Cancer Help Centre, *Lancet* 336:606, 1990.
15. Deleted in proofs.
16. Baird D et al: Dietary intervention study to assess estrogenicity of dietary soy among postmenopausal women, *J Clin Endocrinol Metab* 80:1685, 1995.
17. Barnes S et al: Soybeans inhibit mammary tumors in models of breast cancer, *Prog Clin Biol Res* 347:239, 1990.
18. Basu TK: The significance of ascorbic acid, thiamin and retinol in cancer, *Int J Vitam Nutr Res Suppl* 24:105, 1983.
19. Bayreuther J, Lewith GT, Pickering R: A double-blind cross-over study to evaluate the effectiveness of acupressure at pericardium 6 (P6) in the treatment of early morning sickness (EMS), *Compl Therap Med* 2:70, 1994.
20. Beck SL: The therapeutic use of music for cancer-related pain, *Oncol Nurs Forum* 18:1327, 1991.
21. Belluomini J et al: Acupressure for nausea and vomiting of pregnancy: a randomized, blinded study, *Obstet Gynecol* 84:245, 1994.
22. Bergner P: Is ginger safe in pregnancy? *Medical Herbalism* 3:3, 1991.
23. Blatt MHG, Wiesbader H, and Kupperman HS: Vitamin E and climacteric syndrome, *Arch Intern Med* 91:792, 1953.
24. Bridge LR et al: Relaxation and imagery in the treatment of breast cancer, *Br Med J* 297:1169, 1988.
25. Brigden ML: Unproven (questionable) cancer therapies, *West J Med* 163:463, 1995.
26. Cameron E, Pauling L: Supplemental ascorbate in the supportive treatment of cancer: reevaluation of the prolongation of survival times in terminal human cancer, *Proc Natl Acad Sci USA* 75:4538, 1978.
27. Cameron E, Pauling L, Leibovitz B: Ascorbic acid and cancer: a review, *Cancer Res* 39:663, 1979.
28. Cassileth BR et al: Contemporary unorthodox treatments in cancer medicine, *Ann Int Med* 101:105, 1984.
29. Chengjiang H et al: Effects of microwave acupuncture on the immunological function of cancer patients, *J Tradit Chin Med* 7:9, 1987.
30. Cohen M, Bendich A: Safety of pyridoxine: a review of human and animal studies. *Toxicol Lett* 34:129, 1986.
31. Davis H, IV: Effects of biofeedback and cognitive therapy on stress in patients with breast cancer, *Psychol Rep* 59:967, 1986.
32. de Aloysio D, Penacchioni P: Morning sickness control in early pregnancy by Neiguan point acupressure, *Obstet Gynecol* 80:852, 1992.
33. Duker EM et al: Effects of extracts from Cimicifuga racemosa on gonadotropin release in menopausal women and ovariectomized rats, *Planta Med* 57:420, 1991.
34. Dundee JW, Sourial FB, Bell PF: P6 acupressure reduces morning sickness, Acupuncture prophylaxis of cancer chemotherapy-induced sickness, *J R Soc Med* 81:456, 1988.
35. Edgar L, Rosberger Z, Nowlis D: Coping with cancer during the first year after diagnosis: assessment and intervention, *Cancer* 69:817, 1992.
36. Eisenberg DM: Advising patients who seek alternative medical therapies, *Ann Int Med* 127:61, 1997.
37. Eisenberg DM et al: Unconventional medicine in the United States: prevalence, costs, and patterns of use, *N Engl J Med* 328:246, 1993.
38. Elder NC, Gillcrist A, Minz R: Use of alternative health care by family practice patients, *Arch Fam Med* 6:181, 1997.
39. Evans AT et al: Suppression of pregnancy-induced nausea and vomiting with sensory afferent stimulation, *J Reprod Med* 38:603, 1993.
40. Evans MR, Preece AW: Viscum album: a possible treatment for cancer? *Bristol Med Chir J* 88:17, 1973.
41. Evidence-based work group: Evidence-based medicine: a new approach to teaching the practice of medicine, *JAMA* 268:2420, 1997.

42. Factor-Litvak P et al: Complementary and alternative medicine use for women's health conditions: a pilot survey, 1997 (unpublished work).

43. Felter H, Lloyd J: *King's American Dispensatory*, 1898, Sandy, Ore, 1992, Eclectic Medical Publishing.

44. Filshie J, Redman D: Acupuncture and malignant pain problems, *Eur J Surg Oncol* 11:389, 1985.

45. Fischer-Rasmussen W et al: Ginger treatment of hyperemesis gravidarum, *Eur J Obstet Gynecol Reprod Biol* 38:19, 1991.

46. Freedman RR, Woodward S: Behavioral treatment of menopausal hot flushes: evaluation by ambulatory monitoring, *Am J Obstet Gynecol* 167:436, 1992.

47. Freedman RR et al: Biochemical and thermoregulatory effects of behavioral treatment for menopausal hot flashes, *Menopause* 2:211, 1995.

48. Fuchs K et al: Treatment of hyperemesis gravidarum by hypnosis, *Int J Clin Exp Hypn* 28:313, 1980.

49. Gabius HJ et al: From Ill-defined extracts to the immunomodulatory lectin: will there be a reason for oncological application of mistletoe? *Planta Med* 60:2, 1994.

50. Gellert GA, Maxwell RM, Siegel BS: Survival of breast cancer patients receiving adjunctive psychosocial support therapy: a 10-year follow-up study, *J Clin Oncol* 11(1):66, 1993.

51. Goodman MT et al: Association of soy and fiber consumption with the risk of endometrial cancer, *Am J Epidemiol* 146:294, 1997.

52. Gruber BL et al: Immunological responses of breast cancer patients to behavioral interventions, *Biofeedback Self Regul* 18:1, 1993.

53. Hammar M, Berg G, Lindgren R: Does physical exercise influence the frequency of postmenopausal hot flushes? *Acta Obstetrica et Gynecologica Scandinavica* 69:409, 1990.

54. Hare ML: The emergence of an urban U.S. Chinese medicine. *Med Anthropol Q* 7:30, 1993.

55. Deleted in proofs.

56. Henker FO, III: Psychotherapy as adjunct in treatment of vomiting during pregnancy, *South Med J* 69:1585, 1976.

57. Himmel W, Schulte M, Kochen MM: Complementary medicine: are patients' expectations being met by their general practitioners? *Br J Gen Pract* 43:232, 1993.

58. Hirata J et al: Does Dong Quai have estrogenic effects in postmenopausal women? A double-blind, placebo controlled trial, *Menopause* 4:4, 1997.

59. Holt S: *Soya for health: the definitive medical guide*, New York, 1996, Mary Ann Liebert, Inc.

60. Hopkins MP, Androff L, Benninghoff AS: Ginseng face cream and unexplained vaginal bleeding, *Am J Obstet Gynecol* 159:1121, 1988.

61. Horton J, editor: *The women's health data book, a profile of women's health in the United States*, New York, 1992, Elsevier Science.

62. Hou J et al: Effects of *gynostemma pentaphyllum makino* on the immunological function of cancer patients, *J Tradit Chin Med* 11:47, 1991.

63. Hyde E: Acupressure therapy for morning sickness. A controlled clinical trial, *J Nurse Midwifery* 34:171, 1989.

64. Ingram D: Diet and subsequent survival in women with breast cancer, *Br J Cancer* 69:592, 1994.

65. Irvin JH et al: The effects of relaxation response training on menopausal symptoms, *J Psychosom Obstet Gynaecol* 17:202, 1996.

66. Jacobson J, Workman S, Kronenberg F: Complementary and alternative therapies for breast cancer: a review of the biomedical literature, 1997 (unpublished work).

67. Jarry H, Harnischfeger G: Untersuchungen zur endokrinen wirksamkeit von inhaltsstoffen aus cimicifuga racemosa, *Planta Med* 46, 1985.

68. Jewell D et al: *Pregnancy and Childbirth module of the Cochrane Database of Systematic Reviews*, Issue 1, Oxford, 1997, Update Sortware. (CD-ROM)

69. Kelsey J, Bernstein L: Epidemiology and prevention of breast cancer, *Annu Rev Public Health* 17:47, 1996.

70. Knight D, Eden J: Phytoestrogens: a short review, *Maturitas* 22:167, 1995.

71. Kronenberg F, O'Leary Cobb J, McMahon D: Alternative medicine for menopausal problems: results of a survey, *Menopause* 1:171, 1994.

72. Deleted in proofs.

73. Deleted in proofs.

74. Lamartiniere C: Genistein programs against mammary cancer, Presented at conference: Dietary Phyto-estrogens: Cancer Cause or Prevention? Herndon, Va, September 21-23, 1994, National Cancer Institute.

75. Larsson G, Starrin B: Relaxation training as an integral part of caring activities for cancer patients: effects on wellbeing, *Scand J Caring Sci* 6:179, 1992.

76. Lee H et al: Dietary effects on breast-cancer risk in Singapore, *Lancet* 337:1197, 1991.

77. Li Y, Yu G: A comparative clinical study on prevention and treatment with selected chronomedication of leukopenia induced by chemotherapy, *J Tradit Chin Med* 13:257, 1993.

78. Lindgrin R et al: Effects of gingseng on quality of life in postmenopausal women, *Menopause.* 4:4, 1997.

78a. Liske E: personal communication.

79. Long MAD, Simone SS, Tucher JJ: Outpatient treatment of hyperemesis gravidarum with stimulus control and imagery procedures, *J Behav Ther Exp Psychiatry* 17:105, 1986.

80. McGregor KJ, Peay ER: The choice of alternative therapy for health care: testing some propositions, *Soc Sci Med* 43:1317, 1996.

81. Messina M, Barnes S: The role of soy products in reducing risk of cancer, *J Natl Cancer Inst* 83:541, 1991.

82. Mock V et al: A nursing rehabilitation program for women with breast cancer receiving adjuvant chemotherapy, *Oncol Nurs Forum* 21:899, 1994.

83. Morgenstern H et al: The impact of a psychosocial support program on survival with breast cancer: the importance of selection bias in program evaluation, *J Chron Dis* 37:273, 1984.

84. Murkies AL et al: Dietary flour supplementation decreases post-menopausal hot flushes: effect of soy and wheat, *Maturitas* 21:189, 1995.

85. Murphy PA: Alternative therapies for nausea and vomiting of pregnancy, *Obstet Gynecol* 91:149, 1997.

86. National Research Council (NRC): *Recommended daily allowances,* ed 10, Washington, DC, 1989, National Academy Press.

87. Naylor CD: Grey zones of clinical practice: some limits to evidence-based medicine, *Lancet* 345:840, 1995.

88. O'Brien B, Naber S: Nausea and vomiting during pregnancy: effects on the quality of women's lives, *Birth* 19:138, 1992.

89. O'Brien B, Relyea MJ, Taerum T: Efficacy of P6 acupressure in the treatment of nausea and vomiting during pregnancy, *Am J Obstet Gynecol* 174:708-, 1996.

90. Ornstein M, Einarson A, Koren G: Bendectin/Diclectin for morning sickness: a Canadian follow-up of an American tragedy, *Reprod Toxicol* 9:1, 1995.

91. Pike M, Spicer D: The chemoprevention of breast cancer by reducing sex steroid exposure: perspectives from epidemiology, *J Cell Biochem* 17G(suppl):26, 1993.

92. Pinn V: *Unnecessary hysterectomies: the second most common major surgery in the United States,* United States Committee on Labor and Human Resources, 1993, Subcommittee on Aging.

93. Price KR, Fenwick GR: Naturally occurring oestrogens in foods: a review, *Food Addit Contam* 2:73, 1985.

94. Punnonen R, Lukola A: Oestrogen-like effect of ginseng, *Br Med J* 281:1110, 1980.

95. Rose DP, Hatala MA: Dietary fatty acids and breast cancer invasion and metastasis, *Nutr Cancer* 21:103, 1994.

96. Rudman D, Williams PJ: Megadose vitamins: use and misuse, *N Engl J Med* 309:488, 1983.

97. Sahakian V et al: Vitamin B6 is effective therapy for nausea and vomiting of pregnancy: a randomized, double-blind placebo-controlled study, *Obstet Gynecol* 78:33, 1991.

98. Samarel N, Fawcett J, Tulman L: The effects of coaching in breast cancer support groups: a pilot study, *Oncol Nurs Forum* 20:795, 1993.

99. Schaumburg H et al: Sensory neuropathy from pyridoxine abuse: a new megavitamin syndrome, *N Engl J Med* 309:445, 1983.

100. Schinckel P: Infertility in ewes grazing subterranean clover pastures: observations on breeding behavior following transfer to "sound" country, *Austral Vet J* 24:289, 1948.

101. Schuster K et al: Morning sickness and vitamin B6 status of pregnant women, *Hum Nutr Clin Nutr* 39:75, 1985.

102. Setchell K, Gosselin SJ, Welsh MB, et al: Dietary estrogens: a probable cause of infertility and liver disease in captive cheetahs, *Gastroenterol.* 93:225, 1987.

103. Smith BJ: Management of the patient with hyperemesis gravidarum in family therapy with hypnotherapy as an adjunct, *J N Y State Nurses Assoc* 13:17, 1982.

104. Spiegel D, Bloom JR: Group therapy and hypnosis reduce metastatic breast carcinoma pain, *Psychosomat Med* 45:333, 1983.

105. Spiegel D, Bloom JR: Effect of psychosocial treatment on survival of patients with metastatic breast cancer, *Lancet* 888, 1989.

106. ter Riet G, Kleijnen J, Knipschild P: Acupuncture and chronic pain: a criteria-based meta-analysis, *J Clin Epidemiol* 43:1191, 1990.

107. Deleted in proofs.

108. The Commonwealth Fund: Falik M, Collins K, editors: *Women's health: Commonwealth Fund survey,* Baltimore, 1996, Johns Hopkins University Press.

109. The Commonwealth Fund: *Selected facts on US women's health,* New York, 1997, Commonwealth Fund.

110. Torem MS: Hypnotherapeutic techniques in the treatment of hyperemesis gravidarum, *Am J Clin Hypn* 37:1, 1994.

111. Vellacott ID, Cooke EJ, James CE: Nausea and vomiting in early pregnancy, *Int J Gyneacol Obstet* 27:27, 1988.

112. Vickers AJ: Can acupuncture have specific effects on health? A systematic review of acupuncture antiemesis trials, *J R Soc Med* 89:303, 1996.

113. Wilbur J et al: The relationship among menopausal status, menopausal symptoms, and physical activity in midlife women, *Fam Commun Health* 13:67, 1990.

114. Wilcox G et al: Oestrogenic effects of plant foods in postmenopausal women, *BMJ* 301:905, 1990.

115. Wilcox LS, Koonin LM, Pokras R, et al: Hysterectomy in the United States, *Obstet Gynecol.* 83:549, 1994.

116. Wyon Y et al: Effects of acupuncture on climacteric vasomotor symptoms, quality of life, and urinary excretion of neuropeptides among postmenopausal women, *Menopause* 2:3, 1995.

117. Zhao CX: Acupuncture treatment of morning sickness, *J Tradit Chin Med* 8:228, 1988.

118. Zhao RJ: 39 cases of morning sickness treated with acupuncture, *J Tradit Chin Med* 7:25, 1987.

SUGGESTED READING

Tiran D, Mack S: *Complementary therapies for pregnancy and childbirth,* London, 1995, Balliere Tindall.

CHAPTER 12

Complementary/Alternative Therapies in Select Populations: Women With HIV and AIDS

Leanna J. Standish, Roberta C.M. Wines, and Cherie Reeves

EPIDEMIOLOGY OF HUMAN IMMUNODEFICIENCY VIRUS IN WOMEN

In December 1993, the Centers for Disease Control and Prevention (CDC) officially recognized that women manifest symptoms of human immunodeficiency virus (HIV) and acquired immunodeficiency syndrome (AIDS) in ways that differ from men. At that time, invasive cervical cancer, pulmonary tuberculosis, recurring pneumonia, and severe immunosuppression were added to the CDC's list of AIDS-defining illnesses (ADIs).[28] Within 1 year of the expansion of that list there was an increase of 151% in women with a diagnosis of AIDS in the United States; many of these cases were diagnosed retrospectively.[29]

In the United States there were 89,208 women with a diagnosis of AIDS at the end of 1996, representing 15.34% of the total number of AIDS cases.[31] Broken into ethnic categories there were 49,582 (55.58%) blacks, 20,621 (23.11%) whites, 18,187 (20.39%) Hispanics, 456 (< 0.5%) Asians or Pacific Islanders, and 257 (< 0.5%) Native Americans or Alaskan Natives with AIDS.[31] Women, particularly ethnic minorities, are currently the population most at risk for HIV infection.[32]

When the AIDS epidemic began in the United States, HIV was primarily spread through male-to-male sexual contact. In recent years, however, the primary mode of HIV transmission in the United States has begun to shift to heterosexual sex and injection drug use, thus changing the way in which the public, especially women, must think about this epidemic. The risk a woman faces of infection with HIV through sex with an infected partner or sharing needles with an infected person has greatly increased in recent years.

During the 8-year period of 1985 to 1993, the incidence of HIV infection attributable to male-to-male sexual contact decreased by nearly 20%.[31] At the same time, however, there was an increase in infection rates among women and heterosexual men who use injection drugs by roughly 10%. Trends in AIDS-related deaths show that while overall the number of deaths related to AIDS dropped in 1994 and 1995, the number of women who died increased.[31] In recent years HIV has become a leading health issue for women. For example, AIDS is the leading cause of death among black women aged 25 to 44 years and the fifth leading cause of death in white women. Overall, AIDS is the third leading cause of death among all women aged 25 to 44 years in the United States.[12]

Despite these well-known statistics, women are still consistently less likely to be screened for high-risk behaviors or receive a diagnosis of HIV infection when they present symptoms to a health care provider. A study conducted in a Bronx, New York, emergency department showed that women were less likely to be screened for HIV risk factors and that HIV infection was twice as likely to be recognized in men than in women.[21] This evidence begins to shed light on some of the reasons why women receive the diagnosis of HIV infection and/or AIDS at a much later point in the disease process than men. Another reason for later diagnosis is that women tend to delay their own health needs in favor of others for whom they are the primary care givers.

It is widely accepted that an early HIV diagnosis can improve both quality of life and the chance of long-term survival. An early diagnosis can have implications for health status monitoring and treatment decisions. Many people who receive the diagnosis of HIV infection while they are still healthy are able to take steps to maintain their health.

One other obstacle that women must face in the midst of this epidemic is that there are very few opportunities for women to be involved in HIV/AIDS-related research. To date, most treatment and behavioral research studies have focused on men. The rare study that looks at how HIV affects women is usually concerned with the risk of infection to a fetus, not with the effects of the virus in women who are not pregnant.[12] There have, however, been a few studies looking at the relationship between HIV seropositivity and the virulence of pelvic inflammatory disease (PID) and cervical dysplasia.[2,13,18] The primary arena for which research is lacking is in pharmaceutic drug development.[12] Therefore many health care providers are treating HIV in their female patients by trial and error, using guidelines developed from research with men, adjusting dosages of drugs without guidelines to suggest what might be appropriate.

Current State of Research

Although the research picture is limited, there have been a few recent advances in complementary/alternative medicine (CAM) research focused specifically on women. According to published reports, one in three individuals in the United States is currently using some form of CAM.[6] In addition, some reports claim that up to 78% of the HIV-positive population uses some form of CAM.[15]

In light of this evidence, the Bastyr University AIDS Research Center was established in October 1994 through a 3-year cooperative agreement grant with the Office of

Alternative Medicine (OAM) at the National Institutes of Health (NIH) and the National Institute of Allergy and Infectious Disease. The mission of the research center is to describe the patterns of use and to screen CAM practices for effectiveness in HIV disease. The Alternative Medical Care Outcomes in AIDS (AMCOA) study, which began in October 1995, is a longitudinal prospective observational study designed to allow for the comparison of outcomes associated with the use of different CAM treatments in HIV/AIDS. The goal is to develop a clinical database of outcomes associated with the use of various CAM therapies as preliminary evidence to guide future research.

The study is designed to address the following major research questions: (1) Are there particular CAM therapies or combinations of therapies associated with positive or negative outcomes? (2) Do health outcomes differ in subjects using only CAM treatments versus those using a combination of CAM and conventional medicine? The investigators recruited 1675 HIV-positive men and women who use CAM into the study. This cohort is followed for a minimum of 1 year. Data are provided to the center in the form of a 27-page questionnaire completed independently by each subject. In addition, laboratory data are collected from participants' health care providers every 6 months. To recruit a representative sample of women and minorities into the study, additional funding was requested and procured from the Office of Research on Women's Health.

Data analysis will be conducted on outcome variables, which include changes in CD4+ lymphocyte count, disease progression as classified by the CDC, changes in viral load, quality of life, body-mass index, and mortality. Preliminary descriptive analysis of the first 1016 subjects, a sample that includes 19% women, is shown in Table 12-1. Table 12-2 summarizes the variety of CAM therapies used by these women.

Of the first 19% of women enrolled at baseline, 68% indicated that they were using some form of antiretroviral therapy, and 24% stated that they were using protease inhibitors. However, it is important to note that these data were collected before the explosion in the use of protease inhibitors. The investigators intend to further analyze these and additional data to learn more about the role of CAM in women with HIV/AIDS.

A Naturopathic Approach to Treatment

Naturopathic medicine is one treatment option used by women for HIV/AIDS. Although this diagnostic and treatment approach has not been subjected to controlled clinical trial, many of its elements have some scientific evidence that justify their inclusion. Results from the AMCOA study mentioned above will help to evaluate the outcomes of naturopathic care and compare them to outcomes associated with other systems of care, primarily the current standard of multiple antiretroviral therapy (ART) and antibiotic prophylaxis.

TABLE 12-1	Women's Demographics in the Alternative Medical Care Outcomes in AIDS Study	

Demographics	Percentage of women
Ethnicity	
White, non-Hispanic	47%
Black	35%
Hispanic	8%
Asian/Pacific Islander	< 1%
Native American/Alaska Native	< 3%
Mixed/other	7%
Income	
$10,000 or less	49%
$10,000 to $19,999	19%
$20,000 to $29,999	10%
$30,000 to $39,999	6%
$40,000 to $49,000	1%
$50,000 or more	< 1 %
Do not wish to answer	15%

Population size: N = 194
Mean years of education: 13.7
Mean age: 37.6 years

The first step in a naturopathic visit is an intake interview. Necessary intake information consists of elements similar to those of a conventional medical intake. However, some additional questions are asked about health history and behaviors, both physical and emotional. For an HIV-positive woman it is important to obtain information about previous abnormal Pap smear results; occurrence of genital warts (human papillomavirus) or other cofactor viruses such as Epstein-Barr virus (EBV); herpes simplex types 1, 2, 6, and 8; hepatitis A, B, C or E; and a history of sexually transmitted disease (STD) infection and the types of treatments used, including antibiotic use. Patients are also asked about their history of vaginal and gastrointestinal tract infections. A 24-hour diet recall can assist in assessing adequacy of nutritional intake. Exercise patterns are also reviewed, since they, too, are of concern to a naturopathic physician.

Emotional health is an important component in a naturopathic regimen. Therefore a history of psychoemotional trauma and issues such as anxiety and depression are discussed with each patient. Concerns about the woman's spiritual life and her life's ambitions or goals are addressed.

TABLE 12-2	Women's Treatment Selections in the Alternative Medical Care Outcomes in AIDS Study	
Treatment	**Women reporting use at baseline (%)**	
Prayer	66	
Vitamin C	63	
Aerobic exercise	59	
Massage	57	
Garlic	52	
Support groups	52	
Vitamin E	51	
Acupuncture	49	
Multivitamins	45	
Vitamin B_{12}	45	
Meditation	44	

Population size: N = 194
Mean years of education: 13.7
Mean age: 37.6 years

Laboratory work is an important aspect of health care visits for all HIV/AIDS patients. Values of particular interest to a naturopathic clinician are T/B/NK cell immune panel; HIV RNA viral load; complete blood cell count (CBC) with platelet count and erythrocyte sedimentation rate (ESR); full-fasting blood chemistry studies with lipid panel; dehydroepiandrosterone (DHEA) value; *Candida* sp. antibody panel of immunoglobulins A, M, and G (IgA, IgM, and IgG) with titers; *Candida* sp. serum antigen titer; and a recent Pap smear read by a cytopathologist (e.g., the cytopathologist should look for and report koilocytotic changes that indicate human papillomavirus infection and assess bacterial dysbiosis). If indicated by the woman's medical history, additional laboratory tests are ordered. Possible tests include complete digestive stool analysis, serum antigen or antibody titers of cofactor viruses, serum food allergy panels that evaluate presence of immunoglobulin E (IgE) and IgG in serum against panels of common foodstuffs (helpful in evaluating sinusitis), thyroid panel, ferritin value if anemia is indicated, and vitamin B_{12} and folate levels.

Interpretation of the laboratory tests just mentioned helps establish treatment protocols. For example, a high mean corpuscular volume (MCV) may indicate a deficiency in vitamin B_{12} or folate, or both. Cholesterol levels below 140 md/dl may indicate intestinal malabsorption, whereas high cholesterol levels might indicate a hypothyroid condition or response to ART. Blood urea nitrogen (BUN) levels less than 12 mg/100 ml are associated with protein inadequacy. Adrenal "fatigue" and early insufficiency may be indicated by a DHEA value lower than 200 mg/dl. High *Candida* sp. antibody titers or a positive *Candida* sp. antigen test result may indicate candidiasis, even if the patient is asymptomatic.

A naturopathic physician's treatment, although primarily directed by subjective information from the patient and objective assessments of laboratory values, is driven by the following major principles:

1. Reduce oxidative stress.
2. Improve nutritional status (improve gastrointestinal tract absorption, mucosal immunity, and dietary nutrition).
3. Clear cofactor STDs and yeast and viral infections.
4. Provide antiviral botanic and hydrotherapeutic therapy.
5. Support adrenal function.
6. Provide botanic immunomodulation when appropriate.
7. Increase oxidation of tissues.
8. Provide prophylaxis against opportunistic infections.
9. Provide psychoneuroimmunologic support.
10. Provide support for patients receiving pharmaceutic drugs.

Treatment is always individualized, and the values of the laboratory tests mentioned earlier indicate which systems need support and therefore what treatments should be given. The following is a brief outline of a standard naturopathic treatment protocol with references to scientific studies that provide justification for each treatment.

The core protocol given to many female HIV/AIDS patients in a naturopathic physician's care includes beta-carotene (150,000 IU/day),[5,22,23] vitamin C (2000 mg thrice daily), vitamin E (400 IU twice daily), cod liver oil (1 tablespoon daily),[3,4,19] multivitamin supplements (two capsules twice daily with breakfast and lunch),[1,26] aerobic exercise (minimum of 20 minutes, three times a week),[11,24,25] coenzyme Q10 (30 mg thrice daily between meals),[7,27] SPV-30 (one capsule three times a day if HIV viral load is detectable and woman has refused antiretroviral therapy),[9] Maitake mushroom extract (10 drops twice daily),[32] and *Glycyrrhiza glabra* (licorice) solid extract ($1/4$ to $1/2$ teaspoon twice daily [please note that this should not be given to hypertensive women]).[8,14,17] This protocol serves as a foundation for developing a treatment plan for each individual woman.

A naturopathic approach stresses the importance of beta-carotene, vitamin A, and multivitamin supplements for women. Beta-carotene has been associated with significant increases in white blood cell count, percentage of change in CD4 + lymphocyte counts, and percentage of change in CD4 + /CD8 + ratio.[5] Vitamin A deficiency has been associated with increased mortality[21] and an increase in the horizontal transmission of HIV from a mother to her infant.[23] On the other hand, higher doses of vitamin A and zinc have been associated with faster disease progression.[26] Therefore doses should be monitored by a health care provider. Daily multivitamin use has been linked to a reduced risk of AIDS and a reduced baseline risk of a low CD4 cell count.[1]

When warranted, there are several naturopathic techniques for treating many conditions that are specific to and prevalent among HIV-positive women, including vaginal yeast infections, bacterial vaginitis, cervical atypia, cervical dysplasia, cervical cancer in situ, and human papillomavirus infection (evidenced by anogenital warts or koilocytotic changes in a Pap smear). Treatments for these conditions often include the use of both topical and systemic botanic medicines, vitamin therapy, and homeopathy.

SUMMARY

Infection rates and AIDS diagnoses are increasing among women much faster than in any other population. However, there are many promising possibilities for prevention and treatment. Research studies are beginning to recognize the importance of the inclusion of women. Practitioners of conventional medicine and CAM are discovering more effective ways to manage HIV infection and AIDS. For example, the majority of CAM practitioners surveyed by the Bastyr University AIDS Research Center reported that they believe the treatments they use are effective against HIV. Further research into what those treatments are and how and why they are prescribed is needed to understand what interactions may be taking place. In the meantime, women should take steps to protect themselves from infection with HIV, and if infected, they must educate themselves about all possibilities for treatment options. Not every treatment approach, whether it is alternative or conventional, is appropriate for all women. What may be right for an individual woman should be decided by her and her health care providers. All evidence about her current health status should be considered and frequently monitored so that necessary adjustments can be made when appropriate. It is the responsibility of health care workers to be informed and educated about all treatment options and how and when to use them. Until more evidence of the effects of CAM on HIV and AIDS is supplied by carefully conducted research studies, the amount of knowledge available is limited.

REFERENCES

1. Abrams B, Duncan D, Hertz-Picciotto I: A prospective study of dietary intake and AIDS in HIV-seropositive homosexual men, *J AIDS* 6(8):949, 1993.
2. Barbosa C, Macasaet M, Brockman S et al: Pelvic inflammatory disease and human immunodeficiency virus infection, *Obstet Gynecol* 89(1):65, 1997.
3. B'egin M, Das U: A deficiency in dietary gamma-linolenic and/or eicosapentaenoic acids may determine individual susceptibility to AIDS, *Med Hypotheses* 20(1):1, 1986.
4. Constans J et al: Membrane fatty acids and blood antioxidants in 77 patients with HIV infection, *Rev Med Intern* 14(10):1003, 1993.
5. Coodley G et al: β-Carotene in HIV infection, *J AIDS* 6:272, 1991.
6. Eisenberg D et al: Unconventional medicine in the United States: prevalence, costs and patterns of use, *N Engl J Med* 328(4):248, 1993.
7. Folkers K, Morita M, McRee J: The activities of coenzyme Q10 and vitamin B_6 for immune responses, *Biochem Biophys Res Comm* 193(1):88, 1993.

8. Hattori T et al: Preliminary evidence for inhibitory effect of glycyrrhizin on HIV replication in patients with AIDS, *Antiviral Res* 11(5, 6):255, 1989.

9. Impastato D, Jeu G: Boxwood extract shows promise as an HIV antiviral, *Uptown Express* October/November 1995, pp. 36-37.

10. Ito M et al: Inhibitory effect of glycyrrhizin on the in vitro infectivity and cytopathic activity of the human immunodeficiency virus, *Antiviral Res* 7(3):127, 1987.

11. LaPerriere A et al: Exercise intervention attenuates emotional distress and natural killer cell decrements following notification of positive serological status for HIV-1, *Biofeedback Self Regul* 15(3):229, 1990.

12. Legg J, Minkoff H, Wortley P: HIV disease in women: a growing worry, *Patient Care* May, 30(9): 147, 1996.

13. Maiman M et al: Cervical cancer as an AIDS-defining illness, *Obstet Gynecol* 89(1):76, 1997.

14. Masahiko I et al: Mechanism of inhibitory effect of glycyrrhizin on replication of human immunodeficiency virus (HIV), *Antiviral Res* 10:289, 1988.

15. Mason F: The Complementary Treatments Project's treatment survey, Toronto, Ontario, Canada, unpublished manuscript.

16. Nanba H et al: Immunostimulant activity (in vivo) and anti-HIV activity (in vitro) of 3 branched B1.6 glucan extracted from Maitake mushroom *(Grifola frondosa)*, *Int Conf AIDS* 8(3):30, 1992.

17. Numazaki K, Umetsu M, Chiba S: Effect of glycyrrhizin in children with liver dysfunction associated with cytomegalovirus infection, *Tohoku J Exp Med* 172(2):147, 1994.

18. Olaitan A et al: Cervical abnormality and sexually transmitted disease screening in human immunodeficiency virus-positive women, *Obstet Gynecol* 89(1):71, 1997.

19. Passi S et al: Blood deficiency values of polyunsaturated fatty acids of phospholipids, vitamin E and glutathione peroxidase as possible risk factors in the onset of acquired immune deficiency syndrome, *G Ital Dermatol Venereol* 125(4):125, 1990.

20. Passi S et al: Blood levels of vitamin E, polyunsaturated fatty acids of phospholipids, lipoperoxides, glutathione peroxidase activity and serological screen for syphilis and HIV in immigrants from developing countries, *G Ital Dermatol Venereol* 125(11):487, 1990.

21. Schoenbaum E, Webber M: The underrecognition of HIV infection in women in an inner-city emergency room, *Am J Public Health* 83(3):363, 1993.

22. Semba R et al: Increased mortality associated with vitamin A deficiency during human immunodeficiency virus type 1 infection, *Arch Intern Med* 153:2149, 1993.

23. Semba R, Miotti P, Chiphangwi J: Maternal vitamin A deficiency and mother-to-child transmission of HIV-1, *Lancet* 343:1593, 1994.

24. Solomon G: Psychosocial factors, exercise and immunity: athletes, elderly persons and AIDS patients, *Int J Sports Med* 12(suppl 1):S50, 1991.

25. Spence D et al: Progressive resistance exercise: effect on muscle function and anthropometry of select AIDS population, *Arch Phys Med Rehabil* 71(9):644, 1990.

26. Tang A et al: Dietary micronutrient intake and risk of progression to acquired immunodeficiency syndrome (AIDS) in human immunodeficiency virus type I (HIV-1)–infected homosexual men, *Am J Epidemiol* 138(11):937, 1993.

27. Tanner H: Energy transformations in the biosynthesis of the immune system: their relevance to the progression and treatment of AIDS, *Med Hypotheses* 38(4):351, 1992.

28. US Department of Health and Human Services, Centers for Disease Control and Prevention: 1993 Revised classification system for HIV infection and expanded surveillance case definition for AIDS among adolescents and adults, *MMWR* 41(RR17):5, 1992.

29. US Department of Health and Human Services, Centers for Disease Control and Prevention: Heterosexually acquired AIDS—United States, *MMWR* 43(9):155, 1994.

30. US Department of Health and Human Services, Centers for Disease Control and Prevention: Recommendations for human immunodeficiency virus counseling and voluntary testing for pregnant women, *MMWR* 44(RR-7):1, 1995.

31. US Department of Health and Human Services, Public Health Service, *HIV/AIDS surveillance report* 8(2):15, 1996.

32. Yamada Y, Saito H, Oie S et al: Experimental study of the effect of combined treatment of UFT with CDDP on human solid tumor-xenograft in nude mice, *Jap J Cancer Chemother* 17(7):1327, 1990.

CHAPTER 13

Complementary/Alternative Therapies in Select Populations: Children

May Loo

CAM THERAPY USAGE IN CHILDREN

A recent comprehensive survey indicates that there is a rapid rise in the number of children receiving treatment with complementary/alternative medicine (CAM), from approximately 2% in 1992 to 11% in 1994.[159] The increase in the number of CAM practitioners is projected to be 88% between 1994 and 2010, whereas the increase in the number of physicians will be 16%.[32] The major factors that persuaded parents to seek CAM therapies are word-of-mouth recommendations, fear of the side effects of medications, and persistence of chronic conditions not well alleviated with conventional treatment.[159]

Chiropractic is the most common form of CAM treatment used by children. Reports indicate that children made up 1% of chiropractic patients in 1977 and 8% in 1985.[129] Childhood disorders being treated include pain, respiratory tract problems, ear infection, hyperactivity, enuresis, and gastrointestinal tract problems.[129] Homeopathy is the second most popular form of CAM therapy used by children.[159] Homeopathic remedies are readily available from a variety of sources, including some grocery stores. Although homeopathy may be safe and effective in many childhood conditions, many practitioners believe that homeopathic remedies are best used as adjunctive therapy to conventional medicine in chronic conditions and in acute disorders that respond poorly to conventional therapy.[81] Acupuncture is the third most common therapeutic method used in children[159] but has the largest body of scientific data compared with other CAM therapies. Electrical stimulation, laser, heat, magnet methods, and massage are effective alternatives to needles in treatment of children. Acupuncture and traditional Chinese medicine (TCM) have been used in Asia and Europe to treat a wide spectrum of childhood illnesses. Their use in the United States has been recent but is growing rapidly in popularity. Naturopathy ranks with acupuncture as the third most common complementary therapy used by children,[159] although scientific data are sparse.

TABLE 13-1   CAM Therapies for Pediatric Conditions

Condition	Most Common Therapy	Supportive Data	References
Attention deficit hyperactivity disorder	Biofeedback	Improves attention, behavior, cognition Effects last as long as 10 years	19, 108, 113, 170
	Acupuncture	Laser acupuncture (pilot data): improvement in behavior and cognition, but ineffective with severe ADHD	111
	Chinese herbs	Increase urinary neurotransmitter metabolites	168, 190
	Magnesium supplement	200 mg/day decreases hyperactivity	161
Allergies	Nutrition	Breast-feeding decreases atopy	185
	Acupuncture	More effective (greater desensitization) in older teenagers	100
Asthma	Hypnosis	Asthmatic children are more hypnotizable; reduces physician visits	31 95
	Chinese herbs (oral)	Improves symptoms	71
	Chinese herbs (external patch)	Antitussive and antiasthmatic herbal patches (preventative); effective in acute attacks	167
Colic	Chiropractic treatment	Controls colic	92
	Massage therapy (therapeutic touch)	Empirically decreases colic	48
Diarrhea (acute)	Homeopathic remedies	Significant decrease in duration	78
	Shallow acupuncture treatment	Higher therapeutic effect than drugs	107
Diarrhea (chronic)	Chinese herbs (individualized treatment)	Eliminated symptoms, normalized stools	47
Enuresis	Hypnotherapy	High success in uncontrolled studies	9, 30, 34, 130, 131
		Longer dry period than with imipramine	8
	Acupuncture	Effective alone, more effective with DDAVP	20
	Chiropractic treatment	Decreases enuretic symptoms	140
	Oligoantigenic diet	Relapse with reintroduction of foods	120
Immunization	Homeopathic remedies	Parental preference for homeopathic remedies over vaccination	155
Otitis media	Homeopathic remedies	Reduce pain, prevent relapses	55
	Chiropractic treatment	Decreases symptoms (1 chiropractor)	56
Skin rashes	Chinese herbs	Widespread nonexudative eczema	151
	Acupuncture	Effective for acne	188
Upper respiratory tract infection	Nutrition	Breast-feeding is related to less frequent, shorter bouts	112
	Homeopathic remedies	Ineffective in reducing symptoms	102
	Chinese herbs	Effective in infants with upper respiratory tract infection	191

DDAVP, 1-Deamino-8-D-arginine vasopressin.

Other CAM treatments used in children include touch therapy, osteopathy, oligotherapy, and hypnosis. Children have reported the ability to readily feel energy field from touch therapy.[53] The increasing support for this form of therapy has been anecdotal with little scientific data. Approximately 9% of children receiving treatment with CAM therapies seek osteopaths,[159] who claim success in treating many common childhood conditions.[7] Approximately 4% of pediatric CAM visits are to oligotherapists,[159] who administer poorly absorbed trace elements such as copper, manganese, and zinc to improve health. Relaxation training and imagery are forms of hypnosis that have also been effective in children. In fact, children seem to be able to learn relaxation training better and faster than adults.[54]

Table 13-1 summarizes various pediatric conditions and the CAM therapies most commonly used to treat them.

ROLE OF CAM THERAPIES IN COMMON PEDIATRIC CONDITIONS
Immunizations

Vaccination is an essential component of pediatric well-child care and has both public health and educational ramifications, since up-to-date vaccination is required for entering school. However, like all pharmaceutic products, vaccines have risks and can cause rare but serious adverse effects.[42] Controversy is ongoing regarding pediatric immunization schedules[143] and effectiveness of multiple-antigen vaccines.[135]

A British survey conducted between 1987 and 1993 revealed that preference for homeopathic remedies for illnesses and religion were the most common reasons parents refused immunization. Twenty-one percent of parents believed the risk of diseases to be less than the risk of vaccination and would seek homeopathic treatment if any illness develops in their children. Seventeen percent of parents believed that children "are protected by God and not by vaccines."[155] Many homeopaths recommend homeopathic vaccines, which are not yet supported by scientific data.[166] A significant number of chiropractors believe that contracting an infection is safer than immunization[29] and claim that spinal adjustment is a viable alternative. Although data are insufficient on CAM approaches to vaccination today, practitioners should be aware of the slow yet steady trend toward alternatives and properly address parental concerns and questions regarding immunization.[144]

Upper Respiratory Tract Infections

The common cold is the most frequent acute illness in the United States and throughout the industrialized world. A preschool child has an average of 4 to 10 colds per year. Otitis media is the most common complication. Sinusitis complicates 5% to 10% of upper respiratory tract infections (URIs), especially with more recent technologic advances that allow its detection in infancy.[77] Conventional treatment remains controversial and in the majority of instances ineffective. Antihistamine and combinations of antihistamine with decongestants are the ingredients in at least 800 over-the-counter

(OTC) cold remedies. The majority of studies have concluded that antihistamines are of marginal or no benefit in treating cold symptoms.[49,114,157] Medications are often over-prescribed, leading to higher health care costs[44] and dangerous side effects, such as greater antibiotic resistance.[115] More steroids are prescribed, which leads to a myriad of complications.[118] Vaccination is difficult because of the large number of viral serotypes, difficulty in producing durable immunity, and minimal or no secretion of nasal anti-bodies with parenteral immunization. Although Interferon has been shown to produce good protection against infection, the high doses necessary to produce a prophylactic effect were associated with serious undesirable side effects, including nasal stuffiness, bloody mucus, and mucosal erosions.[89]

Scientific data on CAM treatment for the common cold are surprisingly sparse. In 1971 Linus Pauling carried out a meta-analysis of four placebo-controlled trials and con-cluded that vitamin C alleviates cold symptoms, but subsequent reviews indicated that the role of vitamin C in URI is still controversial.[64-66] A nutritional study of 170 healthy newborns followed for 6 months demonstrated that breast-feeding lowers frequency and duration of acute respiratory tract infection compared with formula feeding.[112]

A randomized, double-blind, placebo-controlled study of 170 children with a start-ing median age of 4.2 years in the experimental group and 3.6 years in the placebo group concluded that individually prescribed homeopathic remedies seem to be inef-fective in reducing symptoms or the use of antibiotics in URI.[102] A clinical trial admin-istering a nontoxic Chinese herbal mixture to 305 infants demonstrated more than 95.1% effectiveness in treatment of URI.[191]

Otitis Media

Acute otitis media (AOM) is most prevalent in young children 8 to 24 months of age. Approximately two thirds of all children will have had at least one episode of AOM before age 3 years, and half of them will have recurrences or chronic otitis media with effusion (OME) into early elementary school years.[60] Most common etiologic factors are allergic rhinitis[33,139] and ascending bacterial or viral agents from the nasopharynx attributable to eustachian tube dysfunction. Conventional therapy consists of antipyret-ics and analgesics, oral decongestants, and antibiotics. In a prospective clinical study of children between 1 and 11 years of age, homeopathic treatment of 103 children was compared with conventional treatment of 28 children. Homeopathic remedies were found to be more effective in reducing pain and preventing relapses.[55] A retrospective, nonrandomized study of 46 children under 5 years of age receiving treatment from a single chiropractor reported decrease in otitis symptoms.[56]

Allergies

Allergic rhinitis affects 5% to 9% of children. Perennial rhinitis is related to allergens that children are exposed to continuously, such as animal dander, house dust mite, mold, and feathers. Seasonal rhinitis is related to seasonal pollenosis and rarely affects children under age 4 or 5 years.[43] Allergic diseases are major causes of morbidity in children of all ages,[183] and allergic rhinitis is a significant cause of middle-ear effusion.[33,117,139] Conventional therapy usually consists of avoidance of allergens, use of air-clearing devices, desensitization shots, and medication with antihistamines and, sometimes, steroids, both of which are frequently abused.[76,82] Antihistamines may be beneficial when sneezing and itching are present.[49]

CAM therapy is common among children with allergic diseases in Sweden[69] and is becoming more popular in the United States, although scientific data specifically on children are still lacking. Physicians have become more aware of the importance of nutrition[158,173] and environmental factors in the development of allergic symptomatology in childhood.[124,182] A prospective, longitudinal study of healthy infants followed from birth to 6 years of age concluded that recurrent wheezing is less common in nonatopic children who were breast-fed as infants.[185] Hypnosis has been reported anecdotally to be effective in hayfever.[180]

Homeopathic remedies for children are unsupported by scientific studies at this time. In a randomized study of 143 patients that included older teenagers, desensitization was compared with specific acupuncture treatment for allergic asthma, allergic rhinitis, or chronic urticaria. The study was ridden with multiple, tedious variables. The conclusion that acupuncture was significantly more effective than desensitization in improving symptoms and in reducing recurrence in all three conditions did not give a breakdown in age-groups.[100] In a clinical report of 75 chronic allergic rhinitis cases that included 3 cases in children 6 to 10 years of age and 17 cases in 11- to 20-year-olds, two different acupuncture treatments were administered according to TCM diagnoses. There was a cumulative 40% cure rate without age differentiation.[187]

Asthma

Asthma affects 6.9% of children from 3 to 17 years of age.[131] In the United States 20% to 25% of school absenteeism is due to asthma, and an estimated 12 million days are spent in bed rest and 28 million days in restricted activities.[131] Etiology for this common disorder is still incompletely understood. Causes include atopy, neural reflexes, infection, and emotional sensitivity.[40] The onset of asthma is rare in the first 3 months of life, but 75% of asthmatic children are symptomatic before their third birthday. The mainstay of conventional treatment consists of bronchodilators and steroids. Parents turn to CAM for their asthmatic children because of drug side effects or fear of taking long-term medication, especially steroids.

The relatively abundant studies on CAM therapy in asthma are on adults and have flaws in methodology. Significant improvement[5,130,131] and even complete cure[36] have been demonstrated with hypnosis, although most studies had weak designs. Hypnosis was recommended for children because they were found to be more hypnotizable,[31] but it is unclear whether the efficacy of hypnosis in asthmatic children is a reflection of children's greater suggestibility or a result of a more reversible disease process.[180] In a recent preschool program 25 children ranging in age from 2 to 5 years received treatment with seven hypnotherapy sessions. The number of physician visits were reduced, and parental confidence in self-management skills increased.[95]

TCM has been used to treat bronchial asthma for several centuries. Improvement from acupuncture treatment has been reported,[162,177,189] and in some countries nearly a fourth of general practitioners believe in the efficacy of acupuncture in the treatment of asthma.[94] Its role in the United States is still controversial; some physicians accept its effectiveness,[175] whereas others criticize data based on poorly conducted studies.[3] In a multicenter, double-blind, placebo-controlled study of 303 children classified into three groups according to TCM diagnosis of asthma, three different herbal treatments vs. placebos demonstrated greater improvement in symptomatology and decrease in production of histamine and LTC4 in the herbal treated group.[71] The majority of acupuncture studies were on adult asthmatics. Despite methodologic weaknesses, it still seems that acupuncture may help drug-induced or allergic asthma.[180]

From the pediatric standpoint, it would be worthwhile to follow the development of external TCM approaches and noninvasive acupuncture. A clinical observation of preventive efficacy of external approach to the treatment of asthma in children reported 78% efficacy in 46 cases treated with external application of plasters made of herbal mixtures with antitussive and antiasthmatic properties and 88% efficacy in 17 children given treatment with antiasthmatic herbal patches. Success was also reported with a different herbal patch for acute attacks. The patches were well received by the children.[167] Laser acupuncture also shows promise in pediatrics because it is a safe, painless alternative to needles.[126]

Homeopathic remedies have been reported to be remarkably effective in asthma in adults,[176] and homeopathic doses of allergens have been shown to alleviate allergic symptoms and desensitize patients to allergens.[178] However, there is paucity of scientific data on homeopathy in both children and adults, as well as lack of consensus amongst homeopaths as to the appropriate treatment, administration regimen, or potency for asthma.[180] Two recent, large reviews of the role of homeopathy in clinical medicine concluded that, except for the occasionally demonstrated benefit, there was little scientific evidence to support the use of homeopathy in the majority of clinical settings.[70,180]

In a number of European countries chiropractic is used for treatment of asthma.[79] A Danish survey reported that 92% of parents who sought chiropractic help considered the treatment beneficial for their children.[35] An Australian survey reported that the most common CAM visits are to chiropractors.[38] There is insufficient scientific support for chiropractic treatment in allergic disease.[180] A few studies in adults generated statistically insignificant data.[73,121] One study found subjective but not objective improvements in individuals with asthma who received treatment in a chiropractic clinic.[79]

Diarrhea

Acute diarrhea is a common occurrence in the pediatric population. Each year an estimated 54,000 to 55,000 U.S. children are hospitalized for diarrhea.[62] The most common etiologic agents are viral pathogens such as rotavirus; few cases are due to bacterial or parasitic infections.[60] *Escherichia coli* is increasingly recognized as a cause of severe bacterial diarrhea in the United States.[156]

Replacement of losses and maintenance of fluid and electrolytes remain the most important therapeutic methods in the treatment of diarrhea,[138,147] and nutritional therapy reduces the impact of acute diarrhea.[101] Breast-feeding has been found to lower the frequency and duration of acute diarrhea in infants under 6 months of age.[112] In most cases of childhood diarrhea, treatment with antidiarrheal compounds is not indicated.[137]

A randomized, double-blind clinical trial comparing homeopathic medicine with placebo in the treatment of acute childhood diarrhea was conducted in Nicaragua in 1991. Eighty-one children 6 months to 5 years of age were given treatment with individualized homeopathic medicine. Standard oral rehydration treatment was also given. There was a statistically significant decrease in the duration of diarrhea in the treatment group.[78] Although criticisms of the study include homeopathic theory as being inconsistent with scientific belief[154] and possible toxicity of the dilute homeopathic remedies,[86] it is also praised for being an impressive,[21] well-designed[17] study that paves the way for future research into the efficacy of homeopathy and other CAM therapies.

A randomized study comparing shallow acupuncture treatment (needles inserted superficially and withdrawn swiftly) with drugs in 761 children ranging in age from 1 to 35 months reported significantly higher therapeutic effect in the acupuncture group. The diagnosis and subsequent choice of points were based on TCM principles, not on stool culture results. Unlike the homeopathy study, this investigation grouped together patients with acute and chronic diarrhea.[107] In a clinical trial using one Chinese herbal formula for treatment of acute diarrhea, there was significant reduction of symptoms and duration of diarrhea.[15]

Chronic, nonspecific diarrhea of childhood differs from acute diarrhea in that it is not associated with significant morbidity. Once potentially serious causes are excluded, appropriate diet can be instituted to minimize complications, and reasonable time is then allowed for spontaneous resolution.[171] In a nonrandomized clinical trial involving 30 children ranging in age from 3 months to 8 years with chronic diarrhea of 2 to 4 months duration that has been unresponsive to Western medical treatment and other treatments of Chinese medicine, individualized acupuncture treatment eliminated symptoms and normalized stools.[47]

Colic

Infantile colic is estimated to affect 20% to 30% of all infants under 4 months of age and remains a medical enigma of nature versus nurture. It may represent a heterogeneous expression of developmental variance, unmet biologic needs, psychologic or emotional distress from poor parent-infant interaction, an intrinsic temperamental predisposition, or colonic hypermotility.[119] Although it is self-limiting by 3 to 4 months of age, treatment is mandated because the psychologic consequences may result in disturbed mother-infant relationship.[72,146] Evidence suggests that uncontrollable crying is the precipitating factor in many cases of infant abuse.[75,181]

Treatment is often directed toward behavioral changes in mothers. Antispasmodics are often not efficacious. Herbal teas and acupuncture have not yet been proven to be efficacious.[116] A prospective, uncontrolled study of 316 colicky infants demonstrated efficacy with chiropractic spinal manipulation in controlling colic in 94% of the cases.[92] A retrospective questionnaire study in 1985 revealed satisfactory results of chiropractic treatment in 90% of infants.[128] Massage therapists have found empirically that touch therapy can decrease severity of colic.[48]

Enuresis

Enuresis affects approximately 5 to 7 million children—15% to 30% of school-age children in the United States.[98,120] By age 8 years, 87% to 90% of children should have nighttime dryness.[28] In 85% of primary nocturnal enuresis (PNE) bedwetting is monosymptomatic, with a spontaneous remission rate of 15% per year of age. The pathophysiology is still not well understood. Multiple factors may interplay: genetic and psychologic predispositions, sleep disorder, urinary reservoir abnormalities, and urine production disorders.[18]

Although PNE is benign, treatment is warranted because of adverse personal, family, and psychosocial effects of the disorder.[120,122] Treatment methods are still controversial. Alarms seem to be the treatment of choice,[28,98,122,147] with medication as second-line treatment. Disadvantages to medications include side effects and high regression rate. Imipramine at 25 to 50 mg/day has both an efficacy and a relapse rate of 60% and is highly toxic if taken in an overdose. 1-Deamino-8-D-arginine vasopressin (DDAVP) is an expensive drug with a short-term efficacy also equal to the relapse rate of approximately 60%. Long-term data are sparse. Adjunctive therapy may include bladder-stretching exercises, which have a success rate of 30%, and behavioral conditioning.[147]

Hypnotherapy has been recognized by conventional practitioners as a potentially effective therapy.[122] Uncontrolled studies have reported high rates of success.[9,30,34,130,131] In one controlled trial, both hypnotherapy and imipramine produced 79% dryness. However, 9 months after the initiation of therapy 65% of the children in the hypnotherapy group remained dry, compared with only 24% in the imipramine group.[8] Data on the long-term efficacy of hypnotherapy are lacking. The requirement that the child practice the self-hypnosis technique several times a day limits compliance with the program.[122]

Acupuncture emerged as a possible therapy for enuresis in 1986, and recent studies are supportive of further evaluation of its viability either as primary or an adjunctive therapy.[120] In a clinical report of 54 enuretic children, short-term success in reducing wet nights was 55% with acupuncture compared to 79% with DDAVP, whereas long-term success rates were 40% and 50%, respectively.[18] A self-controlled regulating device operating on the principles of acupuncture was found to be effective in the treatment of nocturnal enuresis attributable to neurogenic bladder dysfunction.[103] A recent placebo-controlled study in Italy demonstrated that acupuncture was effective alone and was more effective when combined with DDAVP.[20]

The efficacy of chiropractic manipulation in enuresis has been inconsistent. One clinical report identified an 8-year-old boy with functional enuresis who had successful treatment with manipulation.[14] In an uncontrolled study, chiropractic manipulation was less than 50% effective,[104] whereas a controlled clinical trial of 57 children without long-term follow-up demonstrated significant decrease in enuretic symptoms.[140] A comprehensive review of the literature revealed that spinal manipulative therapy was no more effective than the natural regression of enuresis with age.[98]

Food allergy as a cause of enuresis has been in the literature for at least three decades.[45] A recent study of children with severe migraine or attention deficit disorder (ADD) included 21 children with enuresis. Oligoantigenic diets were successful in curing 12 children and improving enuresis in 4 others. Relapse of wetting occurred when foods were reintroduced, the most commonly implicated being chocolate, citrus, fruits, and milk from cows.[120] Although there are no studies available on naturopathic approach, which focuses on natural remedies, such as corn silk and tea or tea and honey, physicians should not dismiss parental opinion that these remedies may be safe and effective.[120] The future of treatment for enuresis should combine various methods to increase the probability of treatment success and minimize risk to the child.[120]

Skin Rashes

Atopic dermatitis affects almost 10% of all children[23] and 20% of children aged 3 to 11 years.[84] It accounts for over 30% of outpatient pediatric visits.[40] Most children with atopic dermatitis commonly come to medical attention with cradle cap and facial and extremity rashes by age 2 to 3 months.[40] Despite considerable research, the etiology of allergic disease remains poorly understood.[6] Allergic dermatitis can be thought of as an inherited skin "sensitivity" that reacts to various external allergens and changes in psychologic states.[147] Food causes atopic dermatitis in 50% of infants, 20% to 30% of young children, and 10% to 15% of children after puberty.[164] Topical steroids remain the main therapeutic method. Dermatologists tend to prescribe antibiotics and use potent topical steroids,[142] which are more readily absorbed in children and can result in hypothalamic-pituitary-adrenal axis suppression.[75] New immune modulators have shown promise in severe atopic dermatitis.[23,67,88]

There is growing use of CAM medicine for dermatitis,[57] although most of the information is in clinical reports and research data are limited. Psoriasis was found to worsen with CAM treatments such as herbs, dietary manipulation, and vitamins.[52] Dietary management with evening primrose oil, rich in gamma-linolenic acid, has been found to be inconsistently effective in small studies.[147] Fish oil supplements (enriched in n-3 polyunsaturated fatty acids) have also been used.[147]

Various herbs offer relief for eczema.[57] A placebo-controlled, double-blind trial used a Chinese herbal prescription specifically formulated for widespread nonexudative atopic eczema. Forty-seven children were randomly assigned to 8-week active treatment and placebo, with an intervening 4-week "washout" period. The response to active treatment was significantly superior to placebo without evidence of hematologic, renal, or hepatic toxicity.[151] Acupuncture treatment of acne has been reported to be successful[110] in as many as 91.3% of adolescents given treatment.[188] Other TCM techniques have also been reported to be helpful.[24]

Hypnotherapy has been reported to improve atopic dermatitis in children.[163]

Homeopathy is frequently used to treat dermatitis. In one homeopathic clinic in Israel more than 80% of the patients expressed satisfaction with treatment. However, the authors of the survey believed that homeopathic medicine complements conventional medicine and is not an alternative.[133] Chiropractic treatment has also been sought by children for allergic problems.[129]

Attention Deficit Hyperactivity Disorder

Attention deficit hyperactivity disorder (ADHD) is the most common neurodevelopmental disorder of childhood, with a prevalence rate between 2% and 11%.[149a] It is a chronic, heterogeneous condition with academic, social, and emotional ramifications for the school-age child. The precise etiology is still unknown, and assessment and management remain diverse. Medication continues to be the mainstay of treatment, with Ritalin the treatment of choice.[63] The tricyclic antidepressants were added as an alternative medication in the 1970s,[13] with clonidine, buspirone (Buspar), and other antidepressants and neuroleptics added to the list in the 1980s.[22,25] Although it is generally agreed that drugs are beneficial on a short-term basis, they have not been shown to produce long-term gains academically or socially.[39] Besides pharmacotherapy, a multimodal approach using a combination of drugs and other methods such as cognitive behavioral therapy (CBT), psychotherapy, social skills training, and school interventions is frequently prescribed for ADHD. Cognitive training has been disappointing in its clinical utility.[1] Compelling evidence is still lacking for long-term efficacy of the multimodal approach,[1,2,17,74] which is currently being evaluated by the NIMH in a multisite collaborative study.[70a] Psychotherapy can be an effective adjunct to medication[148,149] but usually requires a long-term commitment to several years of treatment.

Concerns about side effects of medication,[161a,102a] treatment acceptability,[12,138a] and compliance are additional factors that complicate management of the ADHD child. Clearly, there is room to explore safe, acceptable, and relatively easy alternatives.

Studies have demonstrated that there is a significant difference in baseline electroencephalogram (EEG) measurements in children with attention deficit disorder (ADD) as compared with normally achieving preadolescent males. These differences occur mainly in the parietal region for on-task conditions.[80] In 1991 a critical review of 36 studies in which biofeedback was used as a treatment for hyperactivity indicated that biofeedback alone had not been effectively evaluated, and methodologic problems limit generalizations that it may be applicable to the entire hyperactive population.[105] Recent studies using more sophisticated technology have demonstrated that neurofeedback can improve attention, behavior, and intellectual function in the child with ADD.[19,108,113] Its stabilizing effect has also been found to last as long as 10 years after treatment.[170]

Studies using CAM therapy for treating ADHD encompass more than the usual research difficulties because of the subjective evaluation by parents and teachers of a wide range of 18 characteristics that may qualify for several different diagnoses. A clinical trial using Chinese herbs in the treatment of 66 children with a diagnosis of hyperkinesia based on *Diagnostic and Statistical Manual, Third Edition, Revised (DSM-III-R)* criteria demonstrated 84.8% effectiveness in ameliorating hyperactivity and improving attention and school performance. The herbal remedy was prepared according to the TCM diagnosis of common energetic (Qi) imbalance found in these children. Clinical observations were substantiated by laboratory findings of significant increase in urinary content of norepinephrine (NE), dopamine (DA), 3-4 dihydroxyphenylacetic acid (DOPAC), cyclic adenosine monophosphate (cAMP), and creatinine (Cr).[168] In a randomized study, Chinese herbal treatment was found to be comparable to methylphenidate (Ritalin) but had fewer side effects.[190]

In a prospective, randomized, double-blind pilot study funded by the National Institutes of Health that integrated *DSM-IV* diagnostic criteria, conventional theories of frontal lobe dysfunction and neurotransmitter abnormalities with traditional Chinese theories of energetic imbalances, laser acupuncture was used in the treatment of ADHD in 7- to 9-year-old children. Preliminary data on the six children in the treatment group showed promise in reducing signs and symptoms of ADHD. Using the Conners scale as a weekly follow-up measure, improvement in classroom behavior was reflected by substantial drops in the teachers' scores before and after treatment in five of six children. The parents' scores dropped in three children but did not change in the other three children (Figs. 13-1 and 13-2). One child was promoted to the gifted program, and another demonstrated marked improvement in learning disabilities.[111]

Nutritional management of ADD includes elimination diet, megavitamins, and trace element replacement. The well-known Feingold diet eliminates natural salicylates, food colors, and artificial flavors. Studies have demonstrated mixed results.[87] Megavit-

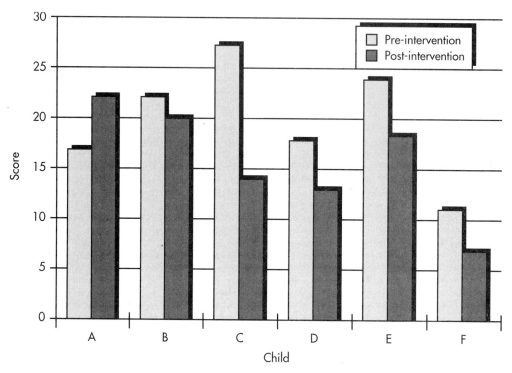

Fig. 13-1 Teachers' scores (Conners scale) for each of six children before and after treatment of attention deficit hyperactivity disorder (ADHD) by laser acupuncture.

amins were demonstrated to be ineffective in the management of ADD in a two-stage study with clinical trial and double-blind crossover. Potential hepatotoxicity is a major concern for use of megavitamins.[68] Oligotherapy focuses on deficiency of trace elements—magnesium, zinc, copper, iron, and calcium—in children with ADD.[96] In a Polish controlled study of 50 7- to 12-year-old hyperactive children with diagnosis based on DSM-IV criteria, magnesium deficiency was found in blood and in hair. Magnesium supplement of 200 mg per day was given for 6 months. Increase in magnesium contents in hair correlated with a significant decrease of hyperactivity in the treatment group.[161] There are no data at this time on homeopathic or chiropractic treatment of ADD, although many practitioners claim anecdotal success with the use of homeopathic nor-pramine and manipulation.

THE FUTURE OF CAM IN CHILDREN

Pediatric usage of CAM therapy is increasing.[160] One major criticism of CAM is the lack of scientific evidence. It is extremely difficult to enforce scientific principles in healing

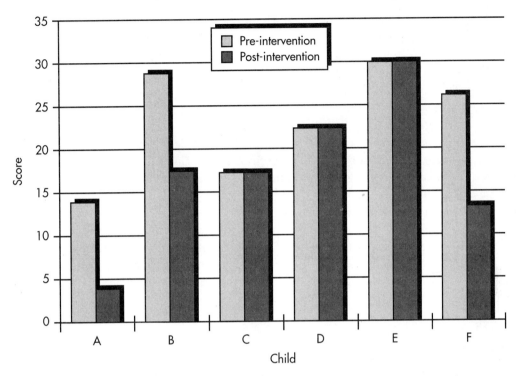

Fig. 13-2 Parents' scores (Conners scale) for each of six children before and after treatment of ADHD by laser acupuncture.

practices that operate within an entirely different paradigm. The scientific method is reductionistic and unifying, whereas CAM therapy is holistic and individualized.[180] Two children with the same diagnosis may be given the same medication but may receive different, more individualized acupuncture treatments or homeopathic remedies. Although the approach to health and disease is different, both conventional medicine and CAM share the common goal of providing safe and effective maintenance of health.

While children are entitled to new therapies,[4] pediatric research in CAM is further complicated by children's vulnerability to violation of their personal rights and to risk exposure.[145] In children of the same age varying cognitive capacity can be required for informed consent.[132,145] Differences in physiologic maturation can change the kinetics, end organ responses, and toxicity of therapy,[4] so data from adult studies cannot be extrapolated for children.[106] Even in conventional medicine, children are often rendered "therapeutic orphans"[153] because of history of abuses in pediatric research, a heightened sensitivity to risks in children—especially since the thalidomide disaster— and a limited market potential.[145] In the United States 80% of drugs have age limits or contain disclaimers for pediatric use.[61] Therefore protecting children by giving them only scientifically proven therapies is counterbalanced by denying them access to possible safe and effective treatment that may not be proven for many years to come.

A second criticism of CAM is that it is unsafe because there are reports of complications. To reject CAM because of these isolated reports is analogous to rejecting all antibiotics because of the gray-baby syndrome associated with chloramphenicol.

A third criticism is that visits to CAM practitioners cause delay in diagnosis.[192] Conventional medicine is endowed with superb technologic support for making physical diagnoses, whereas some CAM practitioners may claim the ability to diagnose a discomfort on an energetic level that is not yet defined biomedically. An integration of these disciplines should provide a better understanding of human health and disease. Patients are often reluctant to inform their physicians of their visits to CAM practitioners.[41] Physicians must be more open-minded and informed and must respect and not denigrate patients' beliefs in healing practices. Currently many medical centers are incorporating courses in CAM. When the gap between conventional medicine and CAM is bridged, delay in diagnosis can be minimized and the common goal of finding safe and effective treatment for children can be achieved.

REFERENCES

1. Abikoff H: Cognitive training in ADHD children: less to it than meets the eye, *J Learning Disabil* 24:205, 1991.
2. Abikoff H, Gittleman R: Hyperactive children treated with stimulants: is cognitive training a useful adjunct? *Arch Gen Psychiatry* 42:953, 1985.
3. Aldrige D, Pietroni PC: Clinical assessment of acupuncture in asthma therapy: discussion paper, *J R Soc Med* 80:222, 1987.
4. American Academy of Pediatrics, Committee on Drugs: Guidelines for the ethical conduct of studies to evaluate drugs in pediatric populations. *Pediatrics* 95:287, 1995.
5. Aronoff GM, Aronoff S, Peck LW: Hypnotherapy in the treatment of bronchial asthma, *Ann Allergy* 34(6):356, 1975.
6. Asher MI et al: International study of asthma and allergies in childhood (ISAAC): rationale and methods, *Eur Respir J* 8(3):483, 1995.
7. Attlee T: Cranio-sacral therapy and the treatment of common childhood conditions, *Health Visitor* 67(7):232, 1994.
8. Banerjee S, Srivastav A, Palan BM: Hypnosis and self-hypnosis in the management of nocturnal enuresis: a comparative study with imipramine therapy, *Am J Clin Hypnosis* 36:113, 1993.
9. Baumann FW, Hinman F: Treatment of incontinent boys with non-obstructive disease, *J Urol* 111:114, 1974.
10. Baumann PH: [Academic medicine and complementary medicine differ from each other in reasoning and evaluation but not in goals], *Schweizerische Rundschau fur Medizin Praxis* 83:1432, 1994.
11. Beasley JW: Chiropractic (letter, comment), *J Fam Pract* 36(4):378, 1993.
12. Bennett DS, Power TJ, Rostain AL, Carr DE: Parent acceptability and feasibility of ADHD interventions: assessment, correlates, and predictive validity, *J Pediatr Psych* 21:643, 1996.
13. Biederman J et al: A double-blind placebo controlled study of desipramine in the treatment of ADD. I. Efficacy. *J Am Acad Child Adolesc Psychiatry* 28:777, 1989.
14. Blomerth PR: Functional nocturnal enuresis, *J Manipulative Physiological Therapeutics* 17(5):335, 1994.
15. Bo MQ, Zhang FR: Xi xie ting in the treatment of infantile diarrhea. *Chung-Kuo Chung Hsi I Chieh Ho Tsa Chih* 13(6):324, 1993.

16. Brown KH: Homeopathy study questions (letter, comment), *Pediatrics* 94(6 Pt 6):964, 1994.
17. Brown RT, Wynne ME, Medenis R: Methylphenidate and cognitive therapy: a comparison of treatment approaches with hyperactive boys, *J Abn Child Psychol* 13:69, 1985.
18. Caione P, Nappo S, Capozza N et al: Primary enuresis in children: which treatment today? *Minerva Pediatrica (Italy)* 46(10):437, 1994.
19. Calhoun G Jr, Fees CK, Bolton JA: Attention-deficit hyperactivity disorder: alternatives for psychotherapy? *Perceptual Motor Skills* 79(1 Pt 2):657, Aug 1994.
20. Capozza N, Greti G, De Gennaro M et al: Trattamento dell'enuresi notturna. Studio comparativo tra desmopressina ed agopunctura, usate singolarmente o in associazione, *Minerva Pediatrica (Italy)* 43:577, 1991.
21. Carlston M: Homeopathic diarrhea trial (letter, comment), *Pediatrics* 1:159, 1995.
22. Casat CD, Pleasants DZ, Schroeder DH, Parler DW: Bupropion in children with attention deficit disorder, *Psychopharmacol Bull* 25(2):198, 1989.
23. Charlesworth EN: Practical approaches to the treatment of atopic dermatitis, *Allergy Proc* 15(6):269, 1994.
24. Chen D, Jiang N, Cong X: Forty-seven cases of acne treated by prick-bloodletting plus cupping, *J Tradit Chin Med* 13(3):185, Sept 1993.
25. Chen SW, Vidt DG: Patient acceptance of transdermal clonidine: a retrospective review of 25 patients, *Cleveland Clin J Med* 56(1):21, 1989.
26. Chen Y, Rennie DC, Dosman JA: Influence of environmental tobacco smoke on asthma in nonallergic and allergic children, *Epidemiology* 7(5):536, 1996.
27. Deleted in proofs.
28. Cochat P, Meunier P, Di Maio M: Enuresis and benign micturition disorders in childhood. I. Diagnosis and management, *Archives de Pediatrie (French)* 2(1):57, 1995.
29. Colley F, Haas M: Attitudes on immunization: a survey of American chiropractors (comments), *J Manipulative Physiological Therapeutics* 17:584, 1994.
30. Collison DR: Hypnotherapy in the management of nocturnal enuresis, *Med J* 1:52, 1970.
31. Collison DR: Which asthmatic patients should be treated by hypnotherapy? *Med J Aust* 1:776, 1975.
32. Cooper RA, Stoflet SJ: Trends in the education and practice of alternative medicine clinicians, *Health Affairs* 15(3):226, 1996.
33. Corey JP, Adham RE, Abbass AH, Seligman I: The role of IgE-mediated hypersensitivity in otitis media with effusion. *Am J Otolaryngol* 15(2):138, Mar-Apr 1994.
34. Crasilneck HB, Hall JA: *Clinical hypnosis: principles and applications,* New York, 1996, Grune & Stratton, pp. 245-246.
35. Danish Public Health Insurance statistics on chiropractic treatment, *Sygesikringens Forhandlingsudvalg, Amstraadsforeningen,* Copenhagen, Denmark, 1980.
36. Diamond HH: Hypnosis in children: complete cure of forty cases of asthma, *Am J Hypnosis* 1:124, 1959.
37. Diamond L et al: A dose-response study of the efficacy and safety of ipratropium bromide nasal spray in the treatment of the common cold, *J Allergy Clin Immunol* 95(5 Pt 2):1139, 1995.
38. Donnelly WJ, Spykerboer JE, Thong YH: Are patients who use alternative medicine dissatisfied with orthodox medicine? *Med J Aust* 142:439, 1985.
39. Dulcan MK: Using psychostimulants to treat behavioral disorders of children and adolescents, *J Child Adolesc Psychopharmacol* 1:7, 1990.
40. Eichinwald H, editor: *Pediatric therapy,* St Louis, 1993, Mosby.
41. Eisenberg DM, Kessler RC, Foster C, et al: Unconventional medicine in the United States: prevalence, costs and patterns of use, *N Engl J Med* 328:246, 1993.
42. Ellenberg SS, Chen RT: The complicated task of monitoring vaccine safety, *Publ Health Rep* 112(1):10, 1997.
43. Elliot FE, Ugazio AG: Allergies. In Eichinwald H, editor: *Pediatric therapy,* St Louis, 1993, Mosby.
44. English JA, Bauman KA: Evidence-based management of upper respiratory infection in a family practice teaching clinic, *Fam Med* 29(1):38, 1997.
45. Esperanca M, Gerrard JW: Nocturnal enuresis: comparison of the effect of imipramine and dietary restriction on bladder capacity, *Can Med Assoc J* 101:721, 1969.
46. Fedoseev GB, Upur KH, et al: The correction of biological defects in bronchial asthma patients by the methods of Chinese medicine, *Terapevticheskii Arkhiv* 68(3):52, 1996.

47. Feng WL: Acupuncture treatment for 30 cases of infantile chronic diarrhea, *J Tradit Chin Med* 9(2):106, June 1989.
48. Field T: Massage therapy for infants and children, *J Develop Behavioral Pediatr* 16(20):105, April 1995.
49. Fireman P: Pathophysiology and pharmacotherapy of common upper respiratory diseases (Review), *Pharmacotherapy* 13(6 Pt 2):101S; 143S, 1993.
50. Fireman P: Diagnosis of allergic disorder (Review), *Pediatr Rev* 16(5):178, 1995.
51. Fisher P et al: Homeopathic treatment of childhood diarrhea (letter, comment), *Pediatrics* 97(5):776, 1996.
52. Fleischer AB Jr, Feldman SR et al: Alternative therapies commonly used within a population of patients with psoriasis, *Cutis* 58(3):216, Sept 1996.
53. France NE: The child's perception of the human energy field using therapeutic touch, *J Holistic Nurs* 11(4):319, Dec 1993.
54. Friebel V: Relaxation training for children—a review of the literature (German), *Praxis der Kinderpsychologie und Kinderpsychiatrie*, 43(1):16, 1994.
55. Friese KH, Kruse S, Moeller H: Acute otitis media in children, comparison between conventional and homeopathic therapy, *HNO* (German) 44(8):462, 1996.
56. Froehle RM: Ear infection: a retrospective study examining improvement from chiropractic care and analyzing for influencing factors, *J Manipulative Physiol Ther* 19(3):169, 1996.
57. Frost J: Complementary treatments for eczema in children, *Professional Nurse* 9(5):330, Feb 1994.
58. Frymann VM, Carney RE, Springall P: Effect of osteopathic medical management on neurologic development in children, *J Am Osteopath Assoc* 92(6):729, 1992.
59. Fung KP, Chow OKW, So SY: Attenuation of exercise-induced asthma by acupuncture, *Lancet* 2:1419, 1986.
60. Gellis & Kagan's *Current pediatric therapy*, Vol. 14, Philadelphia, 1993, W.B. Saunders.
61. Gilman J, Gal P: Pharmacokinetic and pharmacodynamic data collection in children and neonates, *Clin Pharmacokinetics* 23:1, 1992.
62. Glass RC et al: The epidemiology of rotavirus diarrhea in the United States: surveillance and estimates of disease burden, *J Infect Dis* 174(suppl 1):S5, Sept 1996.
63. Greenhill LL: Pharmacologic treatment of attention deficit hyperactivity disorder: pediatric psychopharmacology, *Psychiatr Clin North Am* 15:1, 1992.
64. Hamila H: Vitamin C and common cold incidence: a review of studies with subjects under heavy physical stress, *Int J Sports Med* 17(5):379, July 1996.
65. Hamila H: Vitamin C supplementation and common cold symptoms: problems with inaccurate reviews, *Nutrition* 12(11-12):804, 1996.
66. Hamila H: Vitamin C intake and susceptibility to the common cold, *Br J Nutr* 77(1):59, 1997.
67. Hanifin JM et al: Recombinant interferon gamma therapy for atopic dermatitis, *J Am Acad Dermatol* 28(2 Pt 1):189, 1993.
68. Haslam RA, Dalby JT, Rademaker AW: Megavitamin therapy and attention deficit disorders, *Pediatrics* 74:103, 1984.
69. Hedros CA: Alternative therapy is common among children with allergic diseases (Swedish), *Lakartidningen* 85(43):3580, Oct 26, 1988.
70. Hill C, Doyon F: Review of randomised trials in homeopathy, *Rev Epidemiol Sante Publ* 38:138, 1990.
70a. Hinshaw SP et al: Comprehensive assessment of childhood attention-deficit hyperactivity disorder in the context of a multisite, multimodal clinical trial, *J Atten Deficit* 1:217, 1997.
71. Hsieh KH: Evaluation of efficacy of traditional Chinese medicines in the treatment of childhood bronchial asthma: clinical trial, immunological tests and animal study, Taiwan Asthma Study Group, *Pediatr Allergy Immunol* 7(3):130, August 7, 1996.
72. Hunziker UA, Barr RG: Increased carrying reduces infant crying: a randomized controlled trial, *Pediatrics* 77:641, 1986.
73. Hviid C: A comparison of the effect of chiropractic treatment on respiratory function in patients with respiratory distress symptoms and patients without, *Bull Eur Chiro Union* 26:17, 1978.
74. Ialongo NS et al: The effects of a multimodal intervention with attention deficit hyperactivity disorder children: a 9-month follow-up, *J Am Acad Child Adolesc Psychiatry* 32(1):182, 1993.
75. Illingworth RS: Infantile colic revisited, *Arch Dis Child* 60:981, 1985.

76. Imam AP, Halpern GM: Uses, adverse effects of abuse of corticosteroids, part II, (Review), *Allergologia et Immunopathologia* 23(1):2, 1995.

77. Isaacson G: Sinusitis in childhood, (Review) *Pediatr Clin North Am* 436:1297, Dec 1996.

78. Jacobs J et al: Treatment of acute childhood diarrhea with homeopathic medicine: a randomized clinical trial in Nicaragua, *Pediatrics* 93(5)719, 1994.

79. Jamison JR et al: Asthma in chiropractic clinic: a pilot study, *J Aust Chiro Assoc* 16:137, 1986.

80. Janzen T, Graap K, Stephanson S et al: Differences in baseline EEG measures for ADD and normally achieving preadolescent males, *Biofeedback and Self Regulation* 20(1):65, 1995.

81. Kaplan B: Homeopathy: everyday uses for all the family, *Professional Care of Mother and Child* 4(7):212, Oct 1994.

82. Katcher ML: Cold, cough, and allergy medications: uses and abuses, *Pediatr Rev* 17(1):12, 1996

83. Kay AB: Alternative allergy and the General Medical Council, *Br Med J* 306(6870):122, 1993.

84. Kay J, Gawkrodger DJ, Mortimer MJ, Jaron AG: The prevalence of childhood atopic eczema in a general population, *J Amn Acad Dermatol* 30(1):35, 1994.

85. Keatin JC Jr: Functional nocturnal enuresis (letter; comment), *J Manipulative Physiol Ther* 18(1):44, 1995.

86. Kerr HD: Homeopathy study questions (letter), *Pediatrics* 94(6 Pt 1):964, 1994.

87. Kien CL: Current controversies in nutrition, *Curr Probl Pediatr* 22:351, 1990.

88. Kimata H: High dose gamma-globulin treatment for atopic dermatitis, *Arch Dis Child* 70(4):335, 1994

89. Kirkpatrick G: The common cold: primary care, *Clin Office Pract* 23(4):657, Dec 1996.

90. Kleijnen J: Vitamin E (letter; comment), *Lancet* 345(8951):737, March 18 1995.

91. Kleijnen J, Knipschild P, ter Reit G: Clinical trials of homeopathy, *Br Med J* 302:323, 1991.

92. Klougart N, Nilsson N, Jacobsen J: Infantile colic treated by chiropractors: a prospective study of 316 cases, *J Manipulative Physiol Ther* 12(4):281, Aug 1989.

93. Knipschild P: Searching for alternatives: loser pays, *Lancet* 341:1135, 1993.

94. Knipschild P: Systematic reviews: some examples, *Br Med J* 309(6956):719, 1994.

95. Kohen DP, Wynne E: Applying hypnosis in a preschool family asthma education program: uses of storytelling, imagery, and relaxation, *Am J Clin Hypnosis* 39(3):169, January 1997.

96. Kozielec T, Starobrat-Hermelin B, Kotkoiak L: Deficiency of certain trace elements in children with hyperactivity, *Psychiatria Polska* 28(3):345, May-June 1994.

97. Kramer NA: Comparison of therapeutic touch and casual touch in stress reduction of hospitalized children, *Pediatr Nurs* 16:483, 1990.

98. Kreitz BG, Aker PD: Nocturnal enuresis: treatment implications for the chiropractor, *J Manipulative Physiol Ther* 17(7):465, September 1994.

99. Krieger D: *Therapeutic touch: how to use your hands to help or heal*, Englewood Cliffs, NJ, 1979, Prentice-Hall.

100. Lai X: Observation on the curative effect of acupuncture on type I allergic diseases, *J Tradit Chin Med* 13(4):243, Dec 1993.

101. Laney DW Jr, Cohen MB: Approach to the pediatric patient with diarrhea, *Gastroenterol Clin North Am* 22:499, 1993.

102. Lange de Klerk ES, Blommers J, Kuik DJ, Bezemer PD: Effect of homeopathic medicines on daily burden of symptoms in children with recurrent upper respiratory tract infections, *Br Med J* 309(6965):1329, Nov 19, 1994.

102a. Lawrence JD, Lawrence DB, Carson BS: Optimizing ADHD therapy with sustained release methylphenidate, *Am Fam Physician* 55(5):1705, 1997.

103. Lebedev VA: The treatment of neurogenic bladder dysfunction with enuresis in children using the SKE-NAR apparatus (self-controlled energy-neuroadaptive regulator), *Voprosy Kurortologii, Fizioterapii I Lechebnoi Fizicheskoi Kultury* 4:25-6, Russian July-Aug, 1995.

104. Leboeuf C et al: Chiropractic care of children with nocturnal enuresis: a prospective outcome study, *J Manipulative Physiol Ther* 14(2):110, 1991.

105. Lee SW: Biofeedback as a treatment for childhood hyperactivity: a critical review of the literature, *Psychol Rep* 68(1):163, 1991.

106. Levine R: *Ethics and regulation of clinical research*, ed 2, New Haven, Conn, 1986, Yale University Press.

107. Lin Y et al: Clinical and experimental studies on shallow needling technique for treating childhood diarrhea, *J Tradit Chin Med* 13(2):107, June 1993.

108. Linden M, Habib T, Radojevic V: A controlled study of the effects of EEG biofeedback on cognition and behavior of children with attention deficit disorder and learning disabilities, *Biofeedback and Self Regulation* 21(1):35, 1996.
109. Deleted in proofs.
110. Liu J: Treatment of adolescent acne with acupuncture, *J Tradit Chin Med* 13(3):187, Sept 1993.
111. Loo M, Naeser MA, Hinshaw S, Bay, RB: Laser acupuncture treatment for ADHD. NIH grant #1 RO3 MH56009-01. Presented at 1998 annual American Academy of Medical Acupuncture (AAMA) Symposium, San Diego, Calif, as recipient of Medical Acupuncture Research Foundation (MARF) First Place Research Award.
112. Lopez-Alarcon M, Villalpando S, Fajardo A: Breast-feeding lowers the frequency and duration of acute respiratory infection and diarrhea in infants under six months of age, *J Nutr* 127(3):436, 1997.
113. Lubar JF, Swartwood MO, Swartwood JN, O'Donnell PH: Evaluation of the effectiveness of EEG neurofeedback training for ADHD in a clinical setting as measured by changes in T.O.V.A. scores, behavioral ratings, and WISC-R performance, *Biofeedback Self Regulation* 20(1)83, March 1995.
114. Luks D, Anderson MR: Antihistamines and the common cold: a review and critique of the literature (Review), *J Gen Intern Med* 11(4):240,1996.
115. Mainous AG III, Hueston WJ, Clark JR: Antibiotics and upper respiratory infection: do some folks think there is a cure for the common cold (comments)? *J Fam Pract* 42(4):357, 1996.
116. Matheson I: Infantile colic—what will help? *Tidsskrift for den Norske Laegeforening* (Norwegian) 115(19):2386, August 20, 1995.
117. Mattucci KF, Greenfield BJ: Middle ear effusion—allergy relationships (comments, review), *Ear, Nose, Throat J* 74(11):752, 758, 1995.
118. Meltzer EO, Tyrell RJ, et al: A pharmacologic continuum in the treatment of rhinorrhea: the clinician as economist, *J Allergy Clin Immunol* 95(5):1147, 1995.
119. Miller AR, Barr RG: Infantile colic: is it a gut issue? *Pediatr Clin North Am* 38:1407, 1991.
120. Miller K: Concomitant nonpharmacologic therapy in the treatment of primary nocturnal enuresis, *Clin Pediatr* (spec. ed.):32, July 1993.
121. Miller WD: Treatment of visceral disorders by manipulative therapy. In Goldstein M, editor: The research status of spinal manipulative therapy, *NINCDS Monograph*, Bethesda, Md, 1975, US Department of Health, Education, and Welfare, pp. 295-301.
122. Moffatt ME: Nocturnal enuresis: a review of the efficacy of treatments and practical advice for clinicians, *J Devel Behav Pediatr* 18(1):49, Feb 1997.
123. Morton AR, Fazio SM, Miller D: Efficacy of laser-acupuncture in the prevention of exercise-induced asthma, *Ann Allergy* 70(4):295, 1993.
124. Mudd KE: Indoor environmental allergy: a guide to environmental controls (Review), *Pediatr Nurs* 21(6):534, Nov-Dec 1995.
125. Murray RH, Rubel AJ: Physicians and healers—unwitting partners in health care, *N Engl J Med* 326:61, 1992.
126. Naeser MA, Wei XB: *Laser acupuncture, an introductory textbook*, Boston, 1994, Boston Chinese Medicine.
127. Nagel GA: Naturopathy as metaphor, *Schweizerische Rundschau fur Medizin Praxis* 82(25-26):735, German, June 22, 1993.
128. Nilsson N: Infantile colic and chiropractic, *Eur J Chiro* 33:264, 1985.
129. Nyiendo J, Olsen E: Visi characteristics of 217 children attending a chiropractic college teaching clinic, *J Manipulative Physiol Ther* 11(2):78, April 1988.
130. Olness K: The use of self hypnosis in the treatment of childhood nocturnal enuresis: a report on forty patients, *Clin Pediatrics* 14:273, 1975.
131. Olness K, Kohen DP: *Hypnosis and hypnotherapy with children*, ed 3, New York, 1996, The Guilford Press.
132. Paul M: Informed consent in medical research: children from the age of 5 should be presumed competent (letter), *Br Med J* (clinical research ed.) 314(7092):1480, 1997.
133. Peer O, Bar Dayan Y, Shoenfeld Y: Satisfaction among patients of a homeopathic clinic, *Harefuah* 130(2):86, Jan 15, 1996.
134. Deleted in proofs.
135. Petry LJ: Immunization controversies (editorial, comment), *J Fam Pract* 36(2):141, 1993.
136. Phillips K, Gill L: Acupressure. a point of pressure, *Nurs Times* 89(45):44, 1993.

137. Pickering LK: Therapy for acute infectious diarrhea in children, *J Pediatrics* 118:S118, 1991.
138. Powell DW, Szauter KE: Nonantibiotic therapy and pharmacotherapy of acute infectious diarrhea, *Gastroenterol Clin North Am* 22:683, 1993.
138a. Power TJ, Hess LE, Bennett DS: The acceptability of interventions for attention-deficit hyperactivity disorder among elementary and middle school teachers, *J Dev Behav Pediatr* 16:238, 1995.
139. Pulec JL: Allergy: a commonly neglected etiology of serous otitis media (editorial; comment), *Ear, Nose, Throat J* 74(11):739, 1995.
140. Reed WR, Beavers S, Reddy SK, Kern G: Chiropractic management of primary nocturnal enuresis, *J Manipulative Physiol Ther* 17(9):596, Nov-Dec 1994.
141. Reilly DT, Taylor MA, McSharry C, Atchison T: Is homeopathy a placebo response? Controlled trial of homeopathic potency, with pollen in hayfever as model, *Lancet* 881, Oct 18, 1986.
142. Resnick SD, Hornung R, Konrad TR: A comparison of dermatologists and generalists management of childhood atopic dermatitis, *Arch Dermatol* 132(9):1047, 1996.
143. Robbins AS: Controversies in measles immunization recommendations, *West J Med* 158(1):36, 1993.
144. Roden J: Childhood immunization, homeopathy and community nurses, *Contemp Nurs* 3:34, 1994.
145. Rowell M, Zlotkin S: The ethical boundaries of drug research in pediatrics, *Pediatr Clin North Am* 44(1):27, 1997.
146. Rubin SP, Pendergast M: Infantile colic: incidence and treatment in a Norfolk community, *Child Care Health Dev* 10:219, 1984.
147. Rudoph AM: *Rudoph's pediatrics*, ed 20, Stamford, 1996, Appleton & Lange.
148. Satterfield JH et al: Three year multimodality treatment study of 100 hyperactive boys, *J Pediatrics* 98:650, 1981.
149. Satterfield JH, Cantwell DP, Satterfield BT: Multimodality treatment: a two year evaluation of 61 hyperactive boys, *Arch Gen Psychiatry* 36:965, 1980.
149a. Shaywitz B, Fletcher JM, Shaywitz SE: Attention deficit hyperactivity disorder, *Adv Pediatr* 44:331, 1997.
150. Shaywitz B, Siegel NJ, Pearson HA: Megavitamins for minimal brain dysfunction: a potentially dangerous therapy, *JAMA* 238:1749, 1977.
151. Sheehan MP, Ahterton DJ: A controlled trial of traditional Chinese medicinal plants in widespread nonexudative atopic eczema, *Br J Dermatol* 126:179, 1992.
152. Shields JH: Childhood immunizations: controversy and change, *Pennsylvania Nurse* 48(4):6, 1993.
153. Shirkey H: Therapeutic orphans, *J Pediatr* 72:119, 1968.
154. Shoultz DA: Homeopathic diarrhea trial (letter), *Pediatrics* 95(1):160, 1995.
155. Simpson N, Lenton S, Randall R: Parental refusal to have children immunized: extent and reasons, *Br Med J* (clinical research ed.) 310:227, 1995. (published erratum appears in *Br Med J* 1995 310(6982):777, March 25, 1995 (see comments).
156. Slutsker L et al: *Escherichia coli* 0157:H7 diarrhea in the United States: clinical and epidemiologic features, *Ann Intern Med* 126(7):505, April 1, 1997.
157. Smith MB, Feldman W: Over-the-counter cold medications: a critical review of clinical trials between 1950 and 1991, *JAMA* 269(17):2258, May 5, 1993.
158. Solomon WR: Prevention of allergic disorders, *Ped Rev* 15(8):301, 1994.
159. Spigelblatt LS: The use of alternative medicine by children, *Pediatrics,* 94:811, 1994.
160. Spigelblatt LS: Alternative medicine: should it be used by children? *Curr Probl Pediatr* 25:180, 1995.
161. Starobrat-Hermelin B, Kozielec T: The effects of magnesium physiological supplementation on hyperactivity in children with attention deficit hyperactivity disorder (ADHD): positive response to magnesium oral loading test, *Magnes Res* 10(2):149, 1997.
161a. Stein MA et al: Methylphenidate dosing: twice daily versus three times daily, *Pediatrics* 98(4 pt 1):748, 1996.
162. Sternfield M, Fink A, Bentwich Z, Eliraz A: The role of acupuncture in asthma: changes in airway dynamics and LTC4 induced LAI, *Am J Clin Med* 17:129, 1989.
163. Stewart AC, Thomas SE: Hypnotherapy as a treatment for atopic dermatitis in adults and children, *Br J Dermatol* 132(5):778, 1995.
164. Stogman W, Kurz H: Atopic dermatitis and food allergy in infancy and children, *Wiener Medizinische Wochenschrift* (German) 146(15):411, 1996.

165. Strachan DP, Anderson HR, Johnston ID: Breastfeeding as prophylaxis against atopic disease (letter, comment), *Lancet* 346(8991-8992):1714, Dec 23-30,1995.

166. Sulfaro F, Fasher B, Burgess MA: Homeopathic vaccination: what does it mean? Immunization Interest Group of the Royal Alexandra Hospital for Children, *Med J Austral* 161(5):305, Sept 5, 1994.

167. Sun Y: External approach to the treatment of pediatric asthma, *J Tradit Chin Med* 15(4):290, Dec 1995.

168. Sun Y et al: Clinical observation and treatment of hyperkinesia in children by traditional Chinese medicine, *J Tradit Chin Med* 14(2):105, June 1994.

169. Tandon MK, Soh PF, Wood AT: Acupuncture for bronchial asthma? A double-blind crossover study, *Med J Aust* 154(6)9, 1991.

170. Tansey MA: Ten-year stability of EEG biofeedback results for a hyperactive boy who failed fourth grade perceptually impaired class, *Biofeedback Self Regulation* 18(1):33, Mar 1993.

171. Treem WR: Chronic non-specific diarrhea of childhood, *Clin Pediatrics* 31:413, 1992.

172. United Nations General Assembly: 1960 Declaration of the Rights of the Child: Adopted by the General Assembly of the United Nations, New York, 1959, United Nations.

173. Vidailhet M: Towards preventive dietetics in children (Review), *Revue du Praticien* 43(2):171, Jan 15 1993.

174. Vincent C, Furnham A: Why do patients turn to complementary medicine? An empirical study, *Br J Clin Psychol* 35(pt 1):37, Feb 1996.

175. Vincent CA, Richardson PH: Acupuncture for some common disorders: a review of evaluative research, *J R Coll Gen Pract* 37:77, 1987.

176. Vincenzo F: A clinical case: asthma and Staphysagria and homeo-mesotherapy, *Homeopath Int* 1(2):13, 1987.

177. Virsik K, Kritufek D, Bangha O, Urban S: The effect of acupuncture on bronchial asthma, *Prog Respir Res* 14:271, 1980.

178. Wallace KR: The homeopathic treatment of asthma and allergies, *Br Homeopath J* 75:218, 1986.

179. Walter AA: Megavitamin and megamineral therapy in childhood (letter, comment), *Can Med Assoc J* 146(12):2140, 1992.

180. Watkins AD: The role of alternative therapies in the treatment of allergic diseases, *Clin Exper Allergy* 24(9):813, 1994

181. Weissbluth M, Christoffel KK, Davis AT: Treatment of infantile colic with diclyclomine hydrochloride, *J Pediatr* 104:951, 1984.

182. Wood RA: Environmental control in the prevention and treatment of pediatric allergic diseases, *Curr Opin Pediatr* 5(6):692, Dec 1993.

183. Wood RA: Prospects for the prevention of allergy in children, *Curr Opin Pediatr* 8(6):601, Dec 1996.

184. Wood RA, Doran TF: Atopic disease, rhinitis and conjunctivitis, and upper respiratory infections, *Currt Opin Pediatr* 7(5):615, Oct 1995.

185. Wright AL, Holberg CJ, Taussig LM, Martinez FD: Relationship of infant feeding to recurrent wheezing at age 6 years, *Arch Pediatr Adolesct Med* 149(7):758, 1995.

186. Wright DN, Huang SW: Current treatment of allergic rhinitis and sinusitis, *J Florida Med Assoc* 83(6):389, Jun-Jul 1996.

187. Xu Y: Treatment of acne with ear acupuncture—a clinical observation of 80 cases, *J Tradit Chin Med* 9(4):238, 1989.

188. Yu S, Cao J, Yu Z: Acupuncture treatment of chronic rhinitis in 75 cases: *J Tradit Chin Med* 13(2):103, June 1993.

189. Zang J: Immediate antiasthmatic effect of acupuncture in 192 cases of bronchial asthma, *J Tradit Chin Med* 10:89, 1990.

190. Zhang H, Huang J: Preliminary study of traditional Chinese medicine treatment of minimal brain dysfunction: analysis of 100 cases, *Chung Hsi I Chieh Ho Tsa Chih* (Chinese) 10(5):278, 1990.

191. Zhang XP: Clinical and experimental study on yifei jianshen mixture in preventing and treating infantile repetitive respiratory infection, *Chung-kuo Chung Hsi I Chieh Ho Tsa Chih* (Chinese) 13(1):23, 1993.

192. Zimmer G, Miltner E, Mattern R: Life threatening complications in alternative medicine—problems in patient education, *Versicherungsmedizin* (German) 46(5):171, 1994.

CHAPTER 14

Complementary/Alternative Therapies in Select Populations: Elderly Persons

Frederic M. Luskin, Ellen M. DiNucci, Kathryn A. Newell, and William L. Haskell

In this chapter we evaluate the use of complementary/alternative medicine (CAM) approaches to the treatment of Alzheimer's disease and osteoarthritis. We have chosen these two chronic conditions because they are responsible for disability in a great number of people over the age of 65 years and because current medical management is often inadequate. In neither case is there a cure or even a clearly proven treatment. Therefore these conditions can lead to costly medical care that is often palliative at best, and each deserves a careful exploration of the efficacy of alternative treatment methods.

ALZHEIMER'S DISEASE

Alzheimer's disease is a degenerative disorder that alters memory, cognition, and behavior. Ten percent of individuals in the United States who are 65 years of age and older have Alzheimer's disease, and up to 50% of those 85 and older have the disease in some form.[4] In 1995, approximately four million individuals in the United States had Alzheimer's disease, with the number estimated to triple by the year 2050. Current U.S. costs for the care of patients with Alzheimer's disease is calculated to be between $90 and $100 billion per year.[78]

Diagnosis

The only definitive method for diagnosing Alzheimer's disease is through patient autopsy. During autopsy, brain tissue is examined for the presence of neurofibrillary tangles and neuritic plaques. What makes diagnosis difficult is that such plaques and tangles also exist in smaller numbers in elderly persons with normal health. In patients with Alzheimer's disease, brain tissue plaque may be composed of unusual formations or may contain an overabundance of proteins such as microtubule-associated protein (MAP), tau protein, and amyloid protein. In addition to brain tissue abnormalities, lower quantities of neurotransmitters such as serotonin, acetylcholine, norepinephrine, somatostatin, and corticotrophin-releasing factor are often found. In some individuals with Alzheimer's disease, larger than normal quantities of aluminum have been discovered in the brain. It has not been proved, however, that prolonged exposure to aluminum is the cause of Alzheimer's disease.[71]

According to the *Diagnostic and Statistical Manual of Mental Disorders, Fourth Edition (DSM-IV)* of the American Psychiatric Association,[10] the criteria for determining whether one has Alzheimer's disease include the following:

1. Cognitive impairment indicted by inadequate memory.
2. One or more of the following conditions: aphasia, apraxia, agnosia, and/or an inability to plan and organize one's life.
3. Inability to function in social or occupational settings.
4. Slow onset of and steady decrease in cognitive abilities.
5. Other conditions, such as Parkinson's disease, brain tumor, nutritional deficiencies, hypothyroidism, and substance abuse, must be ruled out.

Normally there are three stages in the progression of Alzheimer's disease. As with most diseases that occur in stages, progress from one stage to another is often uneven and is not inevitable. The first stage includes such symptoms as recent memory impairment affecting work-related duties, confusion about directions to commonly traveled locations, and changes in behavior and mood. During the second stage, patients with Alzheimer's disease may have auditory or visual hallucinations, difficulty in reading and writing, and behaviors that require that they be monitored constantly. In the third stage the patient may become mute, lose control of the excretory processes, and have limited capabilities for self-care.[52]

One's genes have been linked to the development of Alzheimer's disease. People whose parents have the disease are at higher risk for developing it.[9] However, even if a person has one or more family members who have the disease, this does not necessarily mean that the individual will develop it.[71] In addition to genetic predisposition, other risk factors include aging, past serious head trauma that produced an unconscious state,[78] Down syndrome, and little or no formal education.[17]

In a study using Catholic nuns as subjects, the importance of lifestyle factors on the prevention and manifestation of Alzheimer's disease is suggested.[89] In this study some of those who on autopsy exhibited the tangles and plaques associated with Alzheimer's disease never developed the disease while alive. The critical finding was that nuns who had had a stroke were more likely to show symptoms of the disease. There is also some corollary evidence linking atherosclerosis with the development of Alzheimer's disease.[8]

The rate of Alzheimer's disease development tends to be higher in those who are less educated, suggesting that cognitive abilities developed earlier in life may protect older individuals from the ravages of the disease. In the study using Catholic nuns, researchers examined their early adult diaries. Nuns who used less complex sentences and less descriptive prose showed a decline in cognitive abilities and a concomitant tendency to develop Alzheimer's disease later in life.[89]

Conventional Medical Management

Although there is no cure for the disease, there are conventional treatments that alleviate some memory difficulties as well as other symptoms in those with mild to moderate forms of Alzheimer's disease. As of December 1996, there were two U.S. Food and Drug Administration (FDA)–approved drugs specifically for treating the disease, both of which include significant risk for side effects.[5,6]

Other conventional treatments include hormone replacement therapy in women and the use of antiinflammatory drugs such as ibuprofen. To treat behavioral disturbance and psychotic symptoms, neuroleptic drugs are typically used.[33] However, a 2-year, prospective, longitudinal study reported that the use of neuroleptic substances may hasten cognitive deterioration in those with dementia.[75]

Nonpharmacologic treatment of Alzheimer's disease includes behavioral therapies, physical and mental stimulation, reality orientation therapy, memory training programs, psychotherapy, and physical stimulation through physical exercise, occupational therapy, and positive interactions therapy.[19]

CAM Therapies for Alzheimer's Disease

In a survey, 101 primary caregivers for people with Alzheimer's disease and those who attended support groups were questioned about their use of CAM therapies. Fifty-five percent administered at least one CAM therapy to enhance memory of the patient; 20% gave three or more treatments, including vitamins (84%), health foods (27%), herbal medicines (11%), "smart" pills (9%), and home remedies (7%).[28] This survey corroborates the one by Eisenberg that documented that CAM therapies are widely used.[35]

In this chapter we review the CAM therapies that have solid research to substantiate their continued use. For Alzheimer's disease the three with the greatest scientific efficacy are *Ginkgo biloba*, vitamin E, and music therapy. At present all three treatments appear to be useful for different aspects of the disease, and each has minimal side effects when compared with conventional drug treatments.

Ginkgo biloba. *Ginkgo biloba* extract (GBE) is a prevalent, legal, over-the-counter medicine in Europe. In 1994 the German government approved *G. biloba* for use with dementia patients. In the United States the extract has not yet been approved by FDA. However, it can be bought in the United States as an over-the-counter nutritional supplement at health food and grocery stores.

GBE was tested in a randomized, placebo-controlled study on 40 patients with medium-severity Alzheimer's disease. After 1 month, attention, memory, psychopathologic symptoms, functional performance, and psychomotor ability improved in the treatment group. During the study no adverse reactions to the extract were observed. Members of the placebo group showed either no change or some deterioration.[56]

In a 24-week, prospective, randomized, double-blind study, Alzheimer's dementia and multiinfarct dementia outpatients received either GBE or placebo. The GBE was found to be highly effective with few side effects. The adverse effects, which were reported by a small percentage of subjects, included headache, allergic skin reactions, and gastrointestinal tract complaints.[59]

In a review of 44 randomized, placebo-controlled, double-blind studies, *Ginkgo biloba* special extract (GBSE) was examined along with the drugs nimodipine and tacrine for treatment of the following conditions: Alzheimer-type dementia, vascular dementia, and a combination of the two dementias and cerebral function impairment not diagnosed as dementia. *G. biloba* was included in 25 of the 44 studies. The review confirmed the clinical efficacy of all three substances as valuable for improving behavior, psychometrics, and psychopathologic symptoms. A significantly higher percentage of patients receiving the drugs nimodipine and tacrine had adverse side effects.[66]

In a pilot study in the United States researchers compared three different GBEs commonly distributed in the United States (Ginkgo Power, Ginkgold, and Super Ginkgo). They found that Ginkgold increased alpha waves related to enhanced cognition in the greatest number of subjects. Ginkgold was suggested as a potential candidate for classification as a cognitive activator, although more studies of this compound are still needed.[57]

In another study it was found that the administration of a 120-mg daily dosage of *G. biloba* (EGb 761) did not lead to significant results when subjects' Global Deterioration Scale score was greater than 4 points and their Mini Mental State Examination score was less than 15. The authors of the study noted a German study in which patients with degenerative dementia were treated with 240 mg of EGb 761 and showed notable improvement compared with those receiving placebo. The authors contended that EGb 761 may be useful in ridding the body of free radicals, which harm cell membranes, and in augmenting the replacement rate of acetylcholine, one of the neurotransmitters that is found to be diminished in patients with Alzheimer's disease.[57]

In one review article, the authors stated that proclaiming *G. biloba* a cognitive enhancer may be premature, since too few controlled studies have been conducted. However, they believe the current findings support continuing research to determine the efficacy of treating dementia with GBE.[87]

At present, most of the studies on GBE have been conducted in Germany. There is at least suggestive evidence that for patients with mild to moderate Alzheimer's disease the product has utility. GBE has been shown to have effects similar to those achieved with conventional medical pharmacology but with fewer side effects.

Vitamin E. Vitamin E has been studied as a treatment designed to inhibit the progression of Alzheimer's disease because of its utility as a free-radical scavenger.[14] Some researchers have theorized that free radicals play a role in the damaging effects of Alzheimer's disease.[34,58] It is unclear whether this is because of the body's inability to repair free-radical damage or because of the excessive production of free radicals.[38] Free radicals do not pose a threat to health until they are out of balance with antioxidants.[100] Vitamin E, as an antioxidant, may protect the body from free-radical injury.

A laboratory study of animal cortical nerve cell cultures examined the effects of vitamin E on the amyloid beta protein (AβP), an amino acid found in Alzheimer's disease plaques. This investigation reported that vitamin E was influential in deterring cell destruction caused by AβP. Researchers believed that cellular death may be due to oxidative processes and free-radical proliferation and that usage of vitamin E and other antioxidants may reduce damage and inhibit the course of Alzheimer's disease.[14]

A 2-year, randomized, controlled study examined the effects of vitamin E and several other treatments of 341 moderate cases of Alzheimer's disease. The subjects received either 2000 IU of vitamin E, 10 mg of selegiline (a drug treatment for Parkinson's disease), vitamin E and selegiline, or placebo. The results of the study showed that the vitamin E treatment group had a 670-day median delay of disease progression; the selegiline group had a 655-day delay; the group receiving both selegiline and vitamin E had a 585-day delay; and the placebo group had a 440-day delay[84] (Fig. 14-1).

Researchers in a case-control study determined that both Alzheimer's disease and multiinfarct dementia subjects had notably lower plasma concentrations of vitamin E and beta-carotene than the control subjects. The researchers concluded that lower levels of these antioxidants may hasten progression of Alzheimer's disease and that further study of these substances may be beneficial in discovering their possible disease-inhibiting effects.[106]

In a study that compared plasma vitamin E levels of community-dwelling early Alzheimer's disease subjects to those of normal spouses and age-matched control subjects, Alzheimer's disease patients were reported to have lower levels of vitamin E.[80] Lower blood levels of vitamin E suggest a potential for higher levels of free-radical damage. Although little has been mentioned about the possible side effects of vitamin E, Alzheimer's researchers noted that a 1994 study cited a higher risk for hemorrhagic stroke for those ingesting vitamin E; however, the authors mentioned that not enough data exist to uphold this finding.[38] Vitamin E and other antioxidants in general may be beneficial in slowing the progression of Alzheimer's disease and are clearly worthy of further studies to determine efficacy and optimal dosage.

Music Therapy. Music therapy is a noninvasive method for treating various psychologic symptoms of Alzheimer's disease, including depression, feelings of isolation, agitation, wandering behaviors, and loss of sense of self.[1] It also has potential for use as a substi-

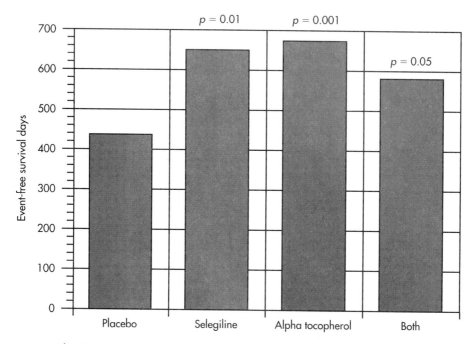

Fig. 14-1 Median number of days of event-free survival in patients with Alzheimer's disease treated with selegiline, alpha tocopherol (vitamin E), or both. Event-free survival is defined as survival until the occurence of death, institutionalization, inability to perform activities of daily living, or severe dementia. *P* values are for the differences in event-free survival between the placebo group and each of the treatment groups.

tute for restraints for those whose disease causes them to wander away from where they are safe.[40]

A case study of five Alzheimer's disease patients at the University of Oklahoma Health Sciences Center noted that a number of cognitive skills remain intact in Alzheimer's patients, despite the typical decline in ability. Among the retained skills was the ability to play a musical instrument.[13]

Music therapy interventions were used in a case study of three subjects with Alzheimer's disease who exhibited repetitive disruptive vocalization behavior. The study reported that this behavior improved in two of the three subjects.[25] In another case study using music therapy it was observed that use of individually selected music was helpful in controlling agitation behaviors in confused patients.[44]

A 6-month, randomized, controlled study of 60 Alzheimer's disease patients used three groups, one of which listened to Big Band music. The mood and ability to recall past events improved more in the music activity group than in the other two groups.[67]

A study of 20 long-term care center residents with Alzheimer's disease found that music therapy reduced the patients' level of agitation.[23]

In a small study researchers evaluated the effect of the use of participatory music on the sociability and reality orientation of Alzheimer's disease patients. According to the study, the music created a positive outcome.[88] In a study of 30 patients with Alzheimer's disease who wandered, the subjects were randomly placed in either a music group or a reading group. Those who received the music therapy sat in or remained near the sessions for longer periods than did those in the reading sessions.[51]

Researchers have noted that, since many patients with Alzheimer's disease have prolonged bouts of depression and other negative emotions, psychosocial interventions such as music therapy would be beneficial. The researchers also state, however, that most of these conclusions come from case studies[20] and that further work is needed to definitively establish the way in which music can benefit persons with Alzheimer's disease.

Other CAM Therapies

As suggested by the research, many factors such as strokes, atherosclerosis, limited education, isolation, and oxidative damage are linked to Alzheimer's disease. Because of the broad spectrum of links to the disease, there are a wide variety of treatments that have suggestive evidence of efficacy. A few of these areas are briefly reviewed. In each of these domains, although the evidence is suggestive, it is not yet established that the treatment is effective for Alzheimer's disease patients.

Phytoestrogens. Recent studies have indicated that hormone replacement therapy improves cognitive ability and mood in women with Alzheimer's disease.[7] It is suggested that lower levels of estrogen in postmenopausal women may be associated with the incidence of dementia[15] and that estrogen replacement therapy in postmenopausal women may lower the risk of Alzheimer's disease.[55] Some studies have indicated that estrogen may guard against beta amyloid toxicity. Thus estrogen may be useful in inhibiting or preventing Alzheimer's disease[50] and enhancing the memory of women who already have the disease.[11] There is reason to suggest that phytoestrogens, or plant-derived estrogens, which are found predominantly in soy products, may produce similarly favorable outcomes through similar mechanisms as hormone replacement therapy, with lower risk.

Bioelectromagnetics. Bioelectromagnetics is the science of how electrical systems within the body are influenced by external electromagnetic fields (EMFs) and how alterations in the body's EMFs may modify physiologic, cognitive, and psychologic states.[92] It is hypothesized that taking precautions in the usage of and exposure to electrical equipment (e.g., power lines and other machinery) may be helpful in preventing cellular disturbances in the brain. However, findings are preliminary and more research is needed.

The Reagan Research Institute has reported that specific EMFs may disturb calcium ions within the brain cells.[8] In another study researchers noted that those exposed to frequent and concentrated amounts of EMFs in the workplace were three times more prone to dementia than those who were exposed to smaller amounts.[92] Even more provocative are studies that examine how EMFs can be used for healing. Placebo-controlled clinical trials point to the possibility that EMFs may be influential in healing wounds and specific bone fractures.[12]

Essential Fatty Acids. Essential fatty acids (EFAs), both alone and in combination with antioxidants, are hypothesized as possible treatments for Alzheimer's disease. In a double-blind, placebo-controlled trial that treated Alzheimer's disease patients with EFAs and antioxidants, the EFA and placebo groups both showed improvement in mood and cognitive ability, with greater levels of improvement in the EFA group.[30]

Dehydroepiandrosterone. There is some evidence to suggest that diminishing reserves of dehydroepiandrosterone (DHEA) may be linked to Alzheimer's disease, particularly with regard to the amyloid precursor protein (APP),[31] and could also be related to other forms of dementia.[105] Researchers also reported that DHEA deficiencies are found not only in those with Alzheimer's disease but also in those with atherosclerosis and cancer.[86]

Massage. Massage has been used as a form of relaxation for dementia patients. In one study of patients in an Alzheimer's disease unit, patients were assigned to one of three groups: those who received hand massage, those who received therapeutic touch, and those in the control group, who were simply watched by another person. Although hand massage was more relaxing than therapeutic touch, both had greater efficacy than simple presence.[90] In another study by the same researchers, it was found that hand massage was beneficial in reducing agitation. However, study results were not always consistent.[91]

Social Support. Social support for patients with early-stage Alzheimer's disease can provide emotional support, offer modeling, and enhance coping ability.[32] The effect of social support increases a sense of belonging, allows for information interchanges, and provides an outlet for the expression of grief.[104] Social support has been shown to be beneficial for cancer patients[93] and for patients with heart disease[2]; therefore it is reasonable to suggest that it may be a useful adjunctive treatment for both patients with Alzheimer's disease and their caregivers.

OSTEOARTHRITIS

Osteoarthritis (OA), the most common form of arthritis, is a degenerative joint disease characterized by the inflammation, breakdown, and eventual loss of the cartilage in weight-bearing joints. Cartilage is the protein substance that serves as a "cushion" between the bones of the joints; when damaged, it can cause severe joint pain, stiffness, and physical disability. The hips, knees, ankles, neck, lower back, and hands are the joints most commonly affected. Hip pain can be especially severe, making walking difficult; however, OA of the knee results in the greatest number of elderly individuals with disability.[22]

Osteoarthritis affects an estimated 16 million persons in the United States, mostly elderly women, and is the second leading cause of disability in adults over 65 years of age.[72] About 5% of the U.S. population has hip or knee OA. With age, that percentage increases until almost 10% of all adults over age 62 years have OA of the knee.[39] Because of its frequency, OA accounts for much of the disability caused by affliction to the lower extremities in elderly individuals. Hip and knee OA accounts for at least 70% of the more than 200,000 total hip and knee replacement surgeries performed each year in the United States.[39]

Diagnosis

Osteoarthritis is difficult to diagnose definitively for two significant reasons: (1) no laboratory tests are specifically designed for the diagnosis of OA and (2) radiographic findings often do not match patient reports of pain (e.g., when joint destruction is demonstrated, it does not necessarily follow that a patient will have severe pain; conversely, a patient may have severe pain with only minor radiographic findings).

Symptoms of OA vary greatly from patient to patient. Some patients can be debilitated by their symptoms (e.g., pain, disfigurement), whereas others may be completely unaware of the disease. With normal aging, cartilage degenerates, making the incidence of OA partly a function of age. Other precursors to the development of OA include infections; past fractures; history of other types of arthritis (e.g., rheumatoid arthritis); stress on joints caused by obesity, poor posture and occupational abuse; metabolic disorders affecting the joints; the influence of heredity; and hormonal disturbances.[72]

In advanced cases of OA the cartilage cushion between the bones of the joints can be completely lost. Often, this leads to pain and the limitation of joint mobility. Inflammation of the cartilage can also stimulate new bone outgrowths (e.g., spurs, bunions) to form around the joints, further limiting mobility.

Conventional Medical Management

Currently there is no known cure for OA. Treatment is aimed primarily at pain relief and the reduction of disability caused by loss of joint mobility.[103] Common treatments include the following:

- Weight loss
- Rest
- Exercise (e.g., swimming, walking)

- Physical and occupational therapy
- Use of mechanical support devices (e.g., splints, canes, walkers)
- Pain relievers such as aspirin and acetaminophen
- Medications injected into the joints (e.g., cortisone)
- Topical creams (e.g., capsaicin)
- Nonsteroidal antiinflammatory drugs (NSAIDs)
- Surgery (e.g., arthrocentesis, arthroscopy, osteotomy, total knee or hip replacement)

In elderly individuals the use of NSAIDs poses a significant risk for gastrointestinal tract distress, as well as liver and kidney problems, which can cause discomfort equal to that of the OA symptoms themselves.[22] NSAIDs are also expensive, and their efficacy is unproved.[103] The use of medication injected into the joints can diminish pain for periods of time, but long-term use of medications such as cortisone can be damaging to tissues and bones, and, as with the use of NSAIDs, the efficacy is unproved. Topical creams like capsaicin can provide temporary relief from joint pain, but the need for constant use (recommended use is four times daily) can be difficult for patients to manage. In addition, side effects such as burning and stinging are common.[72] The use of surgery has the potential to dramatically reduce pain and restore joint mobility, but the risks are the high cost and the complications inherent in any surgery.

Exercise for OA patients, when performed at moderate levels, is beneficial in two ways. First, it can promote the mobility of joints simply by use, and, second, it aids in weight loss that minimizes strain on the joints. There are few exercise programs that have been proven to be appropriate for this population. However, strength training, resistance training, and aerobic activity have been shown to benefit patients with OA.[26,37,76,77,85]

CAM Therapies for Osteoarthritis

Studies suggest that CAM therapies are widely used by OA patients. The Arthritis Foundation estimated in 1982 that $1.8 billion had been spent on "unproven remedies."[54] One study in Austria surveyed more than 100 arthritis sufferers, the majority with OA, and found that 64% had used some form of "self-therapy" (including heat treatments and folk remedies) and that one fourth of respondents had employed the services of CAM providers, mostly chiropractors and acupuncturists.[49] Respondents reported chiropractors to be the most helpful of all practitioners consulted, including general practitioners. Two other studies are cited in a report on nontraditional treatments of arthritis.[54] One found that of 384 arthritis patients surveyed, one third used nontraditional treatments; the other found through interviews that CAM use was as high as 94%. These data are in line with information collected in the U.S. survey on CAM therapy use conducted by Eisenberg et al.[35] in the early 1990s.

To determine the efficacy of CAM therapies for OA, which are summarized in Table 14-1, a thorough search was conducted. This included books,[29,41,47,73] the Internet, literature reviews,[70] and peer-reviewed scientific journals. Clearly, the use of rigorous standards to evaluate alternative approaches to OA is in its infancy. While there are many anecdotal reports of effectiveness, only the CAM therapies found efficacious in the scientific literature are discussed in detail in this chapter.

Diet. There is little argument that making sensible dietary changes can be beneficial to a person's overall health. The use of general practices of good nutrition, such as eating a diet low in fat and high in complex carbohydrates and avoiding specific foods such as coffee, red meat, vinegar, vegetables that contain high levels of plant acids (e.g., toma-

TABLE 14-1 Efficacy of CAM Therapies for Osteoarthritis			
Therapy	Level of Supporting Evidence		
	Significant	Moderate	Anecdotal Only
Diet and alternative pharmacologic therapies	Nutritional • Supplements[24] • Glucosamine[74,83]	• Reconstructive therapy[47] • Hormone replacement therapy[79] • Diet • Herbals[65]	• Chelation therapy • Cell therapy • Enzyme therapy
Alternative systems and methods	Traditional Chinese medicine[101] • Herbs • Acupuncture[37,43,96,108] • Acupressure	• Pulsed electromagnetic fields[98,107] • Transcutaneous electrical stimulation[94]	Osteopathy[47]
Mind-body control	• Self-management and education[68,69] • Cognitive behavioral therapy[60,64]	• Social support[45,46,99,102] • Yoga • Relaxation	• T'ai chi • Qi Gong • Guided imagery • Meditation • Aromatherapy • Music therapy • Shiatsu • Reflexology • Massage • Rolfing • Craniosacral • Applied kinesiology
Manual healing	N/A	Chiropractic[48]	

toes, rhubarb), berries rich in fruit acids, white sugar, white flour, and artificial additives and flavorings, have all been suggested to help with OA. However, there is little scientific literature substantiating the claims that these special diets, including the restriction of certain foods, is beneficial to individuals with OA.

Nutritional Supplements. Some nutritional supplements have been studied with positive outcomes in the treatment of OA; a few of these have been adopted as part of standard treatment in countries outside the United States. Glucosamine is a naturally occurring chemical in the body that helps stimulate the production of collagen, one of the main components of cartilage. Proponents of oral glucosamine suggest that it not only reduces pain but can reverse degenerative joint disorders.[95] Compared with a placebo and ibuprofen in a double-blind, randomized trial, glucosamine was found to be as effective as ibuprofen, with fewer adverse reactions, and more effective than placebo,[83] whereas a multicenter, randomized, double-blind study with 155 patients with knee OA found glucosamine sulfate to be as effective as NSAIDs without the risks. Other researchers who have found similar results suggest that glucosamine has been neglected in the United States as a front-line therapy for OA.[74] An Italian study published in the *American Journal of Medicine* compared S-adenosylmethionine, another nutritional measure supporting proteoglycan synthesis, with naproxen and a placebo in 734 patients with degenerative joint disease. The S-adenosylmethionine provided the same analgesic effect as naproxen but was better tolerated.[24] Both glucosamine and S-adenosylmethionine have been suggested for use in treatment as well as in the prevention of OA.[74,83]

Hormone Replacement Therapy. There is some evidence that women may be at lower risk for OA when receiving hormone replacement therapy (HRT). Researchers at the University of California, San Francisco, found that the women who were currently receiving estrogen therapy had nearly a 40% lower risk of having hip OA compared with women who had never used estrogen.[79] The risk of developing moderate to severe OA was even lower in the former group. Although HRT is currently used as standard treatment for the prevention of heart disease, osteoporosis, and various symptoms of menopause in a vast number of postmenopausal women in the United States, it has not been considered a stand-alone treatment for OA and comes with the increased risk of breast and reproductive cancers.

Reconstructive Therapy. Reconstructive therapy has been used for large numbers of pain sufferers in countries other than the United States. Two studies, one completed in the early 1950s with 1600 patients and one completed in 1987 with 88 patients, found reconstructive injections to be helpful in cases of sacroiliac sprain and low back pain.[47] Although no studies were found that examined OA specifically, it appears that reconstructive treatments are commonly used in other countries and warrant investigation in the United States.

Herbals. The treatment of OA with a combination of herbal formulas was examined in a double-blind, placebo-controlled, crossover study. A combination of *Boswellian serrata, Curcuma longa, Withania somnifera,* and zinc was shown to significantly reduce pain severity and disability in 42 OA patients.[65] These, along with many other herbal products used for a multitude of disease conditions, pose a particularly difficult challenge for investigators. Most are unregulated and thus vary in potency, purity, and dose. There is also an inherent risk of unknown drug interactions.

Other alternative pharmacologic approaches such as chelation therapy, cell therapy, and enzyme therapy are suggested by guidebooks to CAM but were not evaluated in peer-reviewed medical journals.

Traditional Chinese Medicine. Traditional Chinese medicine (TCM), including the use of Chinese herbs, acupuncture, and acupressure, has been explored for use with OA patients, perhaps more than any other CAM therapy. One study of TCM for OA of the knee joint used oral administration of herbal remedies in conjunction with steaming, washing, and gentle joint manipulation and obtained significant results with patients 42 to 86 years of age.[101] Of the 28 patients, 7 were cured (had no remaining symptoms), 13 showed marked effect (symptoms were gone and reappeared only occasionally, when the patient was tired or cold), and 6 were improved (symptoms were markedly improved but not gone altogether); only 2 patients had no effect.

Acupuncture alone has been tested in multiple studies of pain and OA with mixed results. In one retrospective study of acupuncture for knee joint pain on specific acupuncture points called Bachmann points, 71% of patients were helped.[108] A randomized, wait-list–controlled trial with 29 patients with OA of the knee reported significant reduction in pain and joint mobility with the treatment of acupuncture, as well as a $63,000 cost savings attributable to these patients' no longer requiring surgery.[27] These positive results are consistent with a recent pilot study of 12 patients with OA of the knee.[18] Two separate controlled trials examined the effects of acupuncture and diazepam, which is believed to inhibit the effects of acupuncture. The results suggested acupuncture to be effective in pain relief even with the antagonistic effect of the diazepam.[36,96] However, in both studies sham acupuncture was used as a control and was also found to be effective for pain relief. Similar results were found in another randomized, controlled trial of 40 patients with OA pain.[43] In studies using placebo (in this case, sham acupuncture), follow-up after treatment becomes an important research issue. Other investigators have found a placebo to be equally effective during treatment and yet not have lasting effects comparable to the "active" therapy months after treatment has ended. In these cases, the placebo effect is hypothesized to explain the value of sham acupuncture during and on completion of treatment. Clearly, physician and patient beliefs are important factors in explaining the ways in which healing can occur without a clear understanding of the mechanisms involved.

Osteopathy. Osteopathy, a unique system of medicine, integrates many of the manipulative CAM therapies noted in Table 14-1 (e.g., physical manipulation, craniosacral work, relaxation, and nutritional guidance) and claims to have therapeutic benefit to arthritis sufferers.[47] However, no studies of its efficacy specifically for OA were found.

Pulsed Electromagnetic Fields. Pulsed electromagnetic fields (PEMFs) in the treatment of OA of the knee (N = 86) and cervical spine (N = 81) were explored in a randomized, double-blind, controlled trial with positive results for OA patients.[98] Statistical significance was found in both PEMF groups as compared with placebo groups on measures of pain, pain during motion, patient overall assessment, and physician global assessment. The placebo groups showed significance at the posttest, but results dropped off after 1-month follow-up, whereas significance remained in the PEMF groups for patients with knee OA and cervical spine OA. These results replicate an earlier pilot study by the same investigators in 27 patients with OA of the knee[97] and indicate PEMF to have therapeutic benefit to patients with OA of the knee and cervical spine. Another randomized, double-blind, placebo-controlled trial attained similar results with 78 patients with OA of the knee, resulting in significant improvement in a number of clinical measures.[107] Researchers suggest that more trials are needed to assess long-term effects, as well as use in other areas of OA.

Transcutaneous Electrical Stimulation. Transcutaneous electrical stimulation (TENS), which has been shown to minimize postoperative pain in several controlled studies, was used in 10 patients with OA of the knee in a pilot study.[94] Results indicated the TENS device to be effective in short-term pain relief; however, results were also significant using a placebo device. A more recent controlled study of 36 patients with OA of the knee corroborates the results of this earlier pilot study and, again, raises the confounding issue of how important the placebo is in the treatment of pain.

Other CAM Therapies

CAM therapies that are grouped under the umbrella of mind-body treatments usually contain one or both of the following core components: patient education and training in relaxation skills. The mind-body therapies suggested for use with OA patients include, but are not limited to, cognitive behavioral therapy, social support, Eastern forms of exercise, meditation, guided imagery, aromatherapy, and music therapy. Some of these therapies reduce suffering, in part because they induce the relaxation response.[16] However, only very few of these therapies have been studied directly with OA sufferers.

Cognitive Behavioral Therapy. A number of studies conducted by Keefe et al.[60-64] have used cognitive behavioral therapy (CBT) to treat OA sufferers. Results from these randomized, controlled trials suggest that CBT is effective in the reduction of pain, psychologic disability, and pain-related behaviors. Results have demonstrated CBT to be effective in diminishing physical disability. Other studies using CBT and other self-management techniques have had similar results, although it must be noted that many of these studies have used small samples.[21]

Self-Management. Kate Lorig created the Arthritis Self-Management Program (ASP) at Stanford University. This program, supported by the National Arthritis Foundation, is a widely used program of education, exercise, and relaxation. Interestingly, evaluations of this program from 1981 through 1984 found patients reporting only minimal pain reduction.[68] However, in a recent report, significant pain reduction, a decline in number of visits to the physician, and a $189 per-patient cost benefit for OA patients were found.[69] Other studies find self-management programs to be helpful but more difficult to manage for older individuals.[53]

Social Support. Social support has been shown to be especially helpful for elderly individuals with health problems.[45,46,99] One study, which used biweekly telephone calls for 6 months to 193 OA sufferers, reported significant improvement in physical disability, psychologic disability, and pain.[102] Although few studies of social support have been directed specifically at OA, social support has been shown to improve the quality of life in older individuals faced with other debilitating disease conditions.[2,70] It can be a low-cost adjunct to treatment with great potential for benefit and no risk.

Eastern Forms of Exercise. Yoga is the only form of Eastern exercise that has been systematically studied with patients with OA in a randomized, controlled trial.[42] After 8 weeks of yoga practice, 17 subjects with OA of the hands improved significantly in measures of pain during activity, tenderness, and finger range of motion. T'ai chi and Qi Gong, both gentle exercises of Chinese origin and similar to yoga in terms of safety and relaxation, have been practiced by older people outside the United States for hundreds of years. To date there are no studies that attest to their effectiveness for OA patients.

Chiropractic. Chiropractic is one of the more popular CAM therapies used by patients with arthritis.[49] Surprisingly, there have been few controlled trials conducted on its efficacy for OA patients. However, one recent review of the literature in this area has suggested its use, in conjunction with nutritional supplementation and exercise rehabilitation, as a first line of therapy, over the use of NSAIDs, for OA of the spine.[48]

Unlike chiropractic, other areas of manual healing, such as shiatsu massage, reflexology, Swedish massage, rolfing, craniosacral manipulation, and applied kinesiology, are not yet being used widely and, again, have no randomized controlled trials to attest to their efficacy.

Research indicates that some CAM treatments have clear indications of efficacy for use with OA patients, such as the use of nutritional supplements, acupuncture, CBT, self-management programs, and social support. Where there is the suggestion of efficacy, as with yoga, TENS, and PEMFs, further work must investigate treatment efficacy and help determine whether there are contraindications. Where there is minimal or no controlled research, but case study and anecdotal reports indicate that a therapy may be appropriate for OA, as with reconstructive therapy, osteopathy, and Eastern forms of exercises like T'ai chi and Qi Gong, CAM providers may be well situated to serve as both critical investigator and care provider.

Recently interest has emerged for the use of self-report measures of patient satisfaction and symptom evaluation as a way to track the effectiveness of treatment. By this process the care provider can involve the patient in ongoing evaluation of his or her personal care, as well as investigate the general efficacy of the treatments provided.[82]

SUMMARY

There are many CAM treatments for arthritis and Alzheimer's disease. With the dramatic rise in the number of elderly people, in particular those living past the age of 85, the incidence of these diseases will increase. Current medical treatment for either condition is not adequate to control the human suffering and, often, is not cost effective. Although there is some excellent research into the effectiveness of CAM treatments for these conditions, it is insufficient and rarely definitive. Since surveys reliably show that people use CAM methods to manage their health, it seems only responsible to systematically evaluate the care that people are already receiving.

REFERENCES

1. Aldridge D: Alzheimer's disease: rhythm, timing and music as therapy, *Biomed Pharmacother* 48:275, 1994.
2. Anderson D, Deshaies G, Jobin J: Social support: social networks and coronary artery disease rehabilitation: a review, *Can J Cardiol* 12(8):739, 1996.
3. Alzheimer's Association: Alzheimer's conference success, Greater San Francisco Bay Area Chapter Newsletter, 6, Winter 1997.
4. Alzheimer's Association: Alzheimer's disease and related disorders fact sheet: an overview of the dementias, *Fact Sheet*, 1990.
5. Alzheimer's Association: Facts about Cognex and Alzheimer's disease, *Fact Sheet*, June 1993.
6. Alzheimer's Association: Facts about donepezil hydrochloride and Alzheimer's disease, *Fact Sheet*, December 1996.
7. Alzheimer's Association: Facts about a study of estrogen and Alzheimer's disease, *Fact Sheet*, January 1997.

8. Alzheimer's Association and Ronald and Nancy Reagan Research Institute: Research roundup: advances in Alzheimer's research, 7(1):4, Spring 1997.

9. Alzheimer's Disease Education and Referral Center: Genes and APO E, *Connections* 5(1):3, 1996.

10. American Psychiatric Association: *Diagnostic and statistical manual of mental disorders,* ed 4, Washington, DC, 1994, The Association.

11. Asthana S, Craft S, Baker LD, et al: Transdermal estrogen improves memory in women with Alzheimer's disease, *Soc Neurosci Abstr* 22(1):200, 1996,

12. Baker M: The force may be with you, *Stanford Med* 13(4):18, 1996.

13. Beatty WW, Winn P, Adams RL, et al: Preserved cognitive skills in dementia of the Alzheimer's type, *Arch Neurol* 51:1040, 1994.

14. Behl C, Davis J, Cole GM, Schubert D: Vitamin E protects nerve cells from amyloid B protein toxicity, *Biochem Biophys Res Comm* 186(2):944, 1992.

15. Behl C, Widmann M, Trapp T, Holsboer F: 17-B Estradiol protects neurons from oxidative stress-induced cell death in vitro, *Biochem Biophys Res Comm* 216(2):473, 1995.

16. Benson H: *The relaxation response,* New York, 1975, Morrow.

17. Berg L: *Advances in biomedical research, MD Minute,* St Louis, 1996, Washington University Alzheimer's Disease Research Center.

18. Berman BM, Lao L, Greene M, et al: Efficacy of traditional Chinese acupuncture in the treatment of symptomatic knee osteoarthritis: a pilot study, *Osteoarthritis Cartilage* 3(1):1, 1994.

19. Bohorquez A, Liano E, Fernandez de Araoz G, Guillen F: Non-pharmacological treatments for Alzheimer's disease, *Mood Cognitive Dis* Facts and Research in Gerontology supplement, 109, 1995.

20. Bonder BR: Psychotherapy for individuals with Alzheimer's disease, *Alz Dis Assoc Dis* 8(suppl 3):75, 1994.

21. Bradley LA, Young LD, Anderson KO, et al: Psychological approaches to the management of arthritis pain, *Soc Sci Med* 19(12):1353, 1984.

22. Brandt KD: Nonsurgical management of osteoarthritis, with an emphasis on nonpharmacologic measures, *Arch Fam Med* 4(Dec):1057, 1095.

23. Brotons M, Pickett-Cooper PK: The effects of music therapy intervention on agitation behaviors of Alzheimer's disease patients, *J Music Ther* 33(1):2, 1996.

24. Caruso I, Pietrogrande V: Italian double-blind multicenter study comparing S-adrenosylmethionine, naproxen, and placebo in the treatment of degenerative joint disease, *Am J Med* 83(5A)66, 1987.

25. Casby JA, Holm MB: The effect of music on repetitive disruptive vocalizations of persons with dementia, *Am J Occup Ther* 48(10):883, 1994.

26. Chamberlain M, Care G, Harfield B: Physiotherapy in osteoarthritis of the knees, *Int Rehab Med* 4:101, 1982.

27. Christensen B, Iuhl I, Vilbeck H, et al: Acupuncture treatment of severe knee osteoarthritis: a long-term study, *Acta Anaesthesiol Scand* 36:519, 1992.

28. Coleman LM, Fowler LI, Williams ME: The use of unproven therapies by people with Alzheimer's disease, *J Am Geriatr Assoc* 43(7):747, 1995.

29. Collinge W: *The American Holistic Health Association complete guide to alternative medicine,* New York, 1996, Warner Books.

30. Corrigan FM, Van Rijn AV, Horrobin DF: Essential fatty acids in Alzheimer's disease, *Ann NY Acad Sci* 640:250, 1991.

31. Danenberg HD, Haring R, Fisher A, et al: DHEA increases production and release of Alzheimer's amyloid precursor protein, *Life Sci* 59(19):1651, 1996.

32. Davies H, Robinson D: Supportive group experiences for patients with early-stage Alzheimer's disease, *J Am Geriatr Soc* 43(9):1068, 1995.

33. Devanand DP, Levy SR: Neuroleptic treatment of agitation and psychosis in dementia, *J Geriatr Psych Neurol* 8(suppl 1):18, 1995.

34. Edelberg HK, Wei JY: The biology of Alzheimer's disease, *Mechanisms Aging Dev* 91:95, 1996.

35. Eisenberg D, Kessler R, Foster C, et al: Unconventional medicine in the United States: prevalence, costs, and patterns of use, *N Engl J Med* 328:246, 1993.

36. Eriksson S, Lundeberg T, Lundeberg S: Interaction of diazepam and naloxone on acupuncture induced pain relief, *Am J Chin Med* 19(1):1, 1991.
37. Ettinger WH, Burns R, Messier SP: A randomized trial comparing aerobic exercise and resistance exercise with a health education program in older adults with knee osteoarthritis, *JAMA* 277(1):25, 1997.
38. Evans DA, Morris MC: Is a randomized trial of antioxidants in the primary prevention of Alzheimer's disease warranted? *Alz Dis Assoc Dis* 10(suppl 1):45, 1996.
39. Felson DT: Weight and osteoarthritis, *Am J Clin Nutr* 63(3):430S, 1996.
40. Fitzgerald-Clouthier ML: The use of music therapy to decrease wandering: an alternative to restraints, *Music Ther Persp* 11(1):32, 1993.
41. Fugh-Berman A: *Alternative medicine: what works: a comprehensive easy-to-read review of the scientific evidence, pro and con*, Tucson, 1996, Odonian Press.
42. Garfinkel M, Schumacher RH, Husain A, et al: Evaluation of a yoga based regimen for treatment of osteoarthritis of the hands, *J Rheumatol* 21:2341, 1994.
43. Gaw AC, Chang LW, Shaw L-C: Efficacy of acupuncture on osteoarthritic pain: a controlled double-blind study, *N Engl J Med* 293(8):275, 1975.
44. Gerdner LA: Effects of individualized music on confused and agitated elderly patients, *Arch Psychiatr Nurs* 7(5):284, 1993.
45. Gerin W, Pieper C, Levy R, Pickering T: Social support and social interaction: a moderator of cardiovascular reactivity, *Psychosomat Med* 54(3):324, 1992.
46. Gliksman M, Lazarus R, Wilson A, Leeder S: Social support, marital status, and living arrangement correlates of cardiovascular disease risk factors in the elderly, *Soc Sci Med* 40:811, 1995.
47. Goldberg B: *Alternative medicine: the definitive guide*, Fife, Wa, 1993, Future Medicine Publishing.
48. Gotlieb M: Conservative management of spinal osteoarthritis with glucosamine sulfate and chiropractic treatment, *J Manipulative Physiol Ther* 20(6):400, 1997.
49. Gray D: The treatment strategies of arthritis sufferers, *Soc Sci Med* 21(5):507, 1985.
50. Green PS, Gridley KE, Simpkins JW: Estradiol protects against beta-amyloid induced toxicity in SK-N-SH human neuroblastoma cells, *Neurosci Lett* 218(3):165, 1996.
51. Groene RW: Effectiveness of music therapy in 1-1 intervention with individuals having senile dementia of the Alzheimer's type, *J Music Ther* 30(3):138, 1993.
52. Gwyther LP: *Stages of progression in Alzheimer's disease: care of Alzheimer's patients: a manual for nursing home staff*, Washington, DC, 1985, American Health Care Association.
53. Hampson SE, Glasgow RE, Zeiss AM, et al: Self-management of osteoarthritis, *Arth Care Res* 6(1):17, 1993.
54. Hawley DJ: Nontraditional treatment of arthritis, *Nurs Clin North Am* 19(4):663, 1984.
55. Henderson VW, Paganini-Hill A, Emanuel CK, et al: Estrogen replacement therapy in older women: comparisons between Alzheimer's disease cases and nondemented control subjects, *Arch Neurol* 51:896, 1994.
56. Hofferberth B: The effect of EGb 761 in patients with senile dementia of the Alzheimer's type: a double-blind placebo-controlled study on different levels of investigation, *Hum Psychopharmacol* 9:215, 1994.
57. Itil T, Martorano D: Natural substances in psychiatry (*Ginkgo biloba* in dementia), *Psychopharmacol Bull* 31(1):147, 1995.
58. Jeandel C, Nicholas MB, Dubois F, et al: Lipid peroxidation and free radical scavengers in Alzheimer's disease, *Gerontology* 35:275, 1989.
59. Kanowski S, Hermann WM, Stephan K, et al: Proof of efficacy of the *Ginkgo biloba* special extract EGb 761 in outpatients suffering from mild to moderate primary degenerative dementia of the Alzheimer's type or multi-infarct dementia, *Pharmacopsychiatry* 29(2):47, 1996.
60. Keefe F, Caldwell D: Cognitive behavioral control of arthritis, *Adv Rheumatol* 81(1):277, 1997.
61. Keefe F, Caldwell D, Queen K: Osteoarthritic knee pain: a behavioral analysis, *Pain* 28:309, 1987.
62. Keefe F, Caldwell D, Queen K: Pain coping strategies in osteoarthritis patients, *J Consult Clin Psychol* 55:208, 1987.
63. Keefe F, Caldwell D, Williams D: Pain coping skills training in the management of osteoarthritic knee pain. II. Follow-up results, *Behav Ther* 1:435, 1990.

64. Keefe F, Dunsmore J, Burnett R: Behavioral and cognitive-behavioral approaches to chronic pain: recent advances and future directions, *J Consult Clin Psychol* 60:528, 1992.
65. Kulkarni R: Treatment of osteoarthritis with a combination herbomineral formulation: a double-blind, placebo-controlled, cross-over study, *J Ethnopharmacol* 33(1-2):91, 1991.
66. Letzel H, Haan J, Feil WB: Nootropics: efficacy and tolerability of products from three active substance classes, *J Drug Devel Clin Pract* 8(2):77, 1996.
67. Lord TR, Garner JE: Effects of music on Alzheimer's patients, *Percept Motor Skills,* 76(2):451, 1993.
68. Lorig K, Laurin J, Gines G: Arthritis self-management, *Nurs Clin North Am* 19(4):637, 1984.
69. Lorig K, Mazonson PD, Holman HR: Evidence suggesting that health education for self-management in patients with chronic arthritis has sustained health benefits while reducing health care costs, *Arth Rheumatism* 35(4):439, 1993.
70. Luskin FM, Newell KA, Griffith M, et al: A review of mind/body therapies in the treatment of cardio-vascular disease. Part I: implications for the elderly, *Alt Ther* 4(3):46, 1998.
71. Mace NL, Rabins PV: *The 36-hour day,* Baltimore, 1991, Johns Hopkins University Press.
72. March LM: Osteoarthritis, *Rheumatology* 166(1):98, 1997.
73. Marti JE: *The alternative health and medicine encyclopedia,* Detroit, 1995, Visible Ink Press.
74. McCarty M: The neglect of glucosamine as a treatment for osteoarthritis: a personal perspective, *Med Hypotheses* 42(5):323, 1994.
75. McShane R, Keene J, Gedling K, et al: Do neuroleptic drugs hasten cognitive decline in dementia? prospective study with necropsy follow up, *Br Med J* 314(706):266, 1997.
76. Minor M: Exercise in the management of osteoarthritis of the knee and hip, *Arthritis Care Res* 7(4):198, 1994.
77. Minor M, Sanford M: Physical interventions in the management of pain and arthritis, *Arthritis Care Res* 6(4):197, 1993.
78. National Advisory Council on Aging: Report to Congress on the scientific opportunities for developing treatments for Alzheimer's disease, Bethesda, Md, 1995, National Institue of Health/National Institute on Aging.
79. Nevitt MC, Cummings SR, Lane NE, et al: Association of estrogen replacement therapy with the risk of osteoarthritis of the hip in elderly white women: study of Osteoporotic Fractures Research Group, *Arch Intern Med* 156(18):2073, 1996.
80. Osmand AP: Plasma levels of antioxidant vitamins in patients with Alzheimer's disease, *Neurobiol Aging* 11(Abstract 270):318, 1990.
81. Paganini-Hill A: Estrogen replacement therapy and risk of Alzheimer's disease, *Arch Intern Med* 156(19):2213, 1996.
82. Pincus T: Analyzing long term outcomes of clinical care without randomized controlled clinical trials: the consecutive patient questionnaire database, *Advances: J Mind Body Health* 13(2):3, 1997.
83. Rovat L: Clinical research in osteoarthritis design and results of short-term and long-term trials with dis-ease modifying drugs, *Int J Tissue React* 14(5):243, 1992.
84. Sano M, Ernesto C, Thomas RG, Klauber MR: A controlled trial of selegiline, alpha tocopherol or both as treatment for Alzheimer's disease, *N Engl J Med* 336(17):1216, 1997.
85. Schilke JM, Johnson GO, Housh TJ, O'Dell JR: Effects of muscle-strength training on the functional sta-tus of patients with osteoarthritis of the knee joint, *Nurs Res* 45(2):68, 1996.
86. Shealy CN: A review of DHEA, *Integrative Physiol Behavioral Sci* 30(4):318, 1995.
87. Smith PF, Maclenennan K, Darlington C: The neuroprotective properties of the *Ginkgo biloba* leaf: a review of the possible relationship to platelet-activating factor (PAF), *J Ethnopharmacol* 50:131, 1996.
88. Smith-Marchese K: The effects of participatory music on the reality orientation and social ability of Alzheimer's residents in a long term care setting, *Activities, Adaptation, Aging* 18(2):41, 1994.
89. Snowdon DA, Kemper SJ, Mortimer JA, et al: Linguistic ability in early life and cognitive function and Alzheimer's disease in late life: findings from the nun study, *JAMA* 275(7):528, 1996.
90. Snyder M, Egan EC, Burns KR: Efficacy of hand massage in decreasing agitation behaviors associated with care activities in persons with dementia, *Geriatr Nurs* March/April, 60, 1995.
91. Snyder M, Egan EC, Burns KR: Interventions for decreasing agitation behaviors in persons with demen-tia, *J Gerontol Nurs* 34, July 1995.

92. Sobel E, Dunn M, Davanipour Z, et al: Elevated risk of Alzheimer's disease among workers with likely electromagnetic field exposure, *Neurology* 47(6):1477, 1996.

93. Spiegel D: Health caring: psychosocial support for patients with cancer, *Cancer* 74(4 suppl):1453, 1994.

94. Taylor P, Jallett M, Flaherty L: Treatment of osteoarthritis of the knee with transcutaneous electrical nerve stimulation, *Pain* 11:233, 1981.

95. Theodosakis J: *The arthritis cure,* New York, 1997, St. Martin's Press.

96. Thomas M, Eriksson S, Lundeberg T: A comparative study of diazepam and acupuncture in patients with osteoarthritis pain: a placebo controlled trial, *Am J Chin Med* 19(2):95, 1991.

97. Trock DH, Bollet AJ, Dyer RH, et al: A double-blind trial of the clinical effects of pulsed electromagnetic fields in osteoarthritis, *J Rheumatol* 20:456, 1993

98. Trock DH, Bollet AJ, Markoll R: The effect of pulsed electromagnetic fields in the treatment of osteoarthritis of the knee and cervical spine: report of randomized double blind placebo controlled trials, *J Rheumatol* 21:1903, 1994.

99. Uchino N, Cacioppo J, Keicolt-Glaser J: The relationship between social support and physiological processes: a review with an emphasis on underlying mechanisms and implications for health, *Psychosocial Bull* 119(3):488, 1996.

100. Veris Research Information Service: *Carotenoids fact book,* La Grange, Ill, 1997, The Service.

101. Weiheng C, Zuoxu L, Jin Z: Treating osteoarthritis of the knee joint by traditional Chinese medicine, *Am J Tradit Chin Med* 14(4)279, 1994.

102. Weinberger M, Hiner SL, Tierney WM: Improving functional status in arthritis: the effect of social support, *Soc Sci Med* 23(9):899, 1986.

103. What can be done about osteoarthritis? *Drug Ther Bull* 34(5):33, 1996.

104. Yale R: Support groups for newly diagnosed Alzheimer's clients, *Clin Gerontol* 8(3):86, 1989.

105. Yanase T, Fukahori M, Taniguchi S, et al: Serum DHEA and DHEA sulfate in Alzheimer's disease and in cerebrovascular dementia, *Endocrine J* 43(1):119, 1996.

106. Zaman Z, Roche S, Fielden P, et al: Plasma concentrations of vitamins A and E and carotenoids in Alzheimer's disease, *Age Aging* 21:91, 1992.

107. Zizic T, Hoffman K, Holt P, et al: The treatment of osteoarthritis of the knee with pulsed electrical stimulation, *J Rheumatol* 22(9):1757, 1995.

108. Zwolfer W, Grubhofer G, Cartellieri M, Sapcek A: Acupuncture in gonarthrotic pain "Bachmann's knee program," *Am J Chin Med* 20(3-4):325, 1992.

SUGGESTED READINGS

Goldberg B: *Alternative medicine: the definitive guide,* Puyallup, Wash, 1993, Future Medicine Publishers.

Kahn RL, Rowe JW: *Successful aging,* New York, 1998, Pantheon Books.

Klein WC, Bloom M: *Successful aging: strategies for healthy living,* New York, 1997, Plenum Press.

Lorrig K, Fries J: *The arthritis helpbook,* Reading, Mass, 1990, Addison-Wesley.

Luskin FM, Newell KA: Mind body approaches to successful aging. In Watkins A, editor: *Mind body medicine: a clinician's guide to psychoneuroimmunology,* New York, 1997, Churchill Livingstone.

Mace NL, Rabins PV: *The 36-hour day: a family guide to caring for persons with Alzheimer's disease, related dementing illnesses, and memory loss in later life,* Baltimore, 1991, Johns Hopkins University Press.

Murray MT, Pizzorno JE: *Encyclopedia of natural medicine,* ed 2, Rocklin, Calif, 1998, Prima Publications.

Tappen RM: *Interventions for Alzheimer's disease: a caregiver's complete reference,* Baltimore, 1997, Health Professions Press.

Complementary/Alternative Medicine in the Twenty-First Century

Joseph J. Jacobs

This book began with a discussion of the major issues, along with the role of preclinical studies, which define the field of complementary/alternative medicine (CAM), followed by separate chapters on clinical research on CAM therapies in the treatment of specific medical conditions. To complete our scientific assessment of CAM, a brief discussion of the *consumer* and the *marketplace* is warranted, as these variables will ultimately shape health care policy as much as, if not more than, clinical research in the twenty-first century. Each of these variables—*consumer, marketplace,* and *clinical research*—will develop its own relevant focus, but they will also work together to shape CAM research and practices and their potential integration with conventional medicine in the next century.

The Consumer and CAM

The emergence of CAM as a social phenomenon has been viewed as a paradigm shift in medicine in the United States. It is one of several indicators of a changing health care market. One of the changes is occurring in the patient-doctor relationship. The traditionally held views of provider-patient relationships are evolving from a willing, passive, dependent patient to an activist health consumer who demands and seeks out timely and accurate health information. The new patient, who is also a health care consumer, is prepared to seek, lobby for, and be critical of health information and medical care practice in general. These patients no longer accept with blind faith their doctors' pronouncements or recommendations.

Health consumers, armed with unprecedented access to information from numerous venues—self-help books, the Internet, seminars, and word of mouth—are becoming more "empowered" to take control of their health care destinies. The lack of information and attempts by their physicians to explain CAM as placebo response or that it is without much scientific merit become a barrier. From the consumer's perspective,

CAM is plausible, especially since it is derived from seemingly age-old principles. The patient comes out of the transactional relationship feeling relatively powerless to have any control over his or her own delivery of care. Turning to a CAM practitioner is a predictable and overt expression of empowerment—the ability to choose one's own healing paradigm despite what the physician might suggest. One good example of this empowerment can be found in a survey on the use of CAM that was published in 1998 in the *Journal of the American Medical Association.*[1] It was reported that most individuals who use CAM do so because of a "congruence with their own values, beliefs and philosophical orientations toward health and life." Variables relevant to predicting CAM usage in a sample of 1035 patients using a mail survey with a 69% return rate were more education, poorer health status, a more holistic orientation toward health, and a "transformational" change in health that influenced their own personal view. Approximately 40% said they had used some form of CAM during the past year for health conditions including chronic pain (37%), anxiety and "other health problems" (31%), sprains/muscle strains (26%), addictive problems (25%), and arthritis (25%). The most common therapies included chiropractic, life-style, diet, exercise and movement, and relaxation. Noteworthy was the finding that most of these individuals used CAM not because they felt dissatisfied with conventional medicine but rather because CAM was closer to their own beliefs about health. Only a small percentage (4.4%) relied solely on CAM for treatment.

Empowerment shifts the burden of health care decision making to the patient. The patient becomes responsible for gaining access to and participating in a health care system, which includes diagnosis and treatment planning. The Dietary Supplement Health and Education Act of 1994 states that "consumers should be empowered to make informed choices about preventative health care programs based on scientific studies relating to dietary supplements."

Access is one component of empowerment. An underlying principle of the free-market system is that all of its participants have equal access to all information. The health care marketplace must meet the imperative to supply information that helps health consumers make informed, rational choices about their health care.

Another option suggests developing a strategy that offers an opportunity for sharing information between health care provider/physician and patient. Eisenberg[2] has suggested a step-by-step approach to shared decision making between provider and patient. Following a conventional medical evaluation and discussion of conventional therapeutic options with or without consultation (depending on the patient's choice), address the following points—before a CAM consultation:

- Ensure that the patient recognizes and understands his or her symptoms.
- Maintain a record of all symptoms including the patient's own opinions and assumptions.

- Review any potential for harmful interactions, which include risks and benefits that might occur.
- Plan for follow-up to review CAM effectiveness of treatment.

This approach helps to keep communication channels open between patient and practitioner so that the patient receives the most effective and safest treatment for his or her condition(s).

From the conventional physician's perspective, it is important to be knowledgeable about the various types of CAM therapies to ensure a level of trust with the patient. Patients have a stronger sense of confidence when their providers give advice from a position of knowledge. Part of the information-gathering process for the clinician is to periodically survey patient attitudes and preferences for CAM therapies. The choices made by the patients may lead to the healing of their condition(s) as they focus more on improving their quality of life and less on a cure.

A second component of empowerment is the formation of self-help groups—a consumer-driven operation. Self-help groups assist patients who want to work in a socially supportive environment. Patients need to talk about their fears and anxieties associated with their condition(s) and their treatment options, including CAM, in a nonhostile, open, and accepting group setting. One such group, SHARE, offers support groups in English and Spanish, a hotline in several languages, and a broad spectrum of educational programs dealing with conventional and CAM treatments. SHARE's overall goals are to enlighten, empower, educate, be an advocate for, and support patients who have breast or ovarian cancer. It does not offer medical advice, but only attempts to promote harmonious relationships between medical caregivers and patients. More self-help groups that promote discussions, at least, about CAM are expected to grow and continue to be advocates for patients.

The Market and CAM

Retail Products. The use of CAM by both providers and consumers has been directed at acute and chronic diseases, health promotion, and disease prevention. Two classes of retail products that have figured most prominently are nutritional supplements and herbal therapies. The nutraceutic industry promotes vitamins and herbs to enhance feelings of well-being and provide therapeutic benefit. In addition, there are many products that enhance or facilitate ambulation or performance of tasks that enable a more normal daily life. For example, "hardware" products that are not nutritional may be purchased in health food stores or pharmacies. A new chain of stores called ALIVE offers products that go beyond nutritional supplements; these include tapes for relaxation, devices for personal massage, various "natural" skin and beauty products, and services that assess posture and provide chiropractic-designed devices to enhance posture (i.e., devices that electronically scan the foot soles to provide customized shoe insoles).

New Paradigm Venture, a market research company, conducted a survey of consumer spending on health-related retail products and found that in 1994, consumers in the United States spent more than $100 billion on various products not ordinarily considered to be part of the medical mainstream.[3] Tables 1 through 3 display consumer spending on products ranging from CAM pills to wellness products. Table 4 shows the number of products that were marketed in 1994 to address specific medical conditions. Consumer spending and usage of these products clearly reflect a strong belief in health care products outside of the conventional medical mainstream.

The health consumer is caught in the natural tension between the market that is promoting CAM and the medical directors who monitor the attitudes of the conventional medical community. More integrated networks between alternative and conventional markets are expected to occur with or without clear research findings. It is likely that as the market-driven health care economy evolves, a $100 billion complementary care expenditure could be predicted by the year 2000 or early next century.

An entirely different "product"—a data bibliographic and archive system (see Chapter 1)—once completely developed, will have ramifications across the field of CAM. This system includes data sets from research studies, questionnaires, and protocols used in the data sets and software programed to answer specific questions about

TABLE 1   **1994 Expenditures on CAM Pills in the United States**

Alternative Pills	Amount Spent (in Billions of Dollars)
Vitamins	$3.745
Herbal remedies	$0.874
Homeopathy	$0.15
TOTAL	$4.8

From New Paradigm Ventures, Inc: *Complementary medicine research project,* South Norwalk, Conn, 1996, internal publication.

TABLE 2   **1994 Expenditures on Nutraceutic Products in the United States**

Nutraceutic Products	Amount spent (in Billions of Dollars)
Diet, lactose, fiber aids	$0.510
Vitamins, minerals, herbal products	$5.7
Sports, herbal, and fortified beverages	$20.9
Meals, snacks, meal replacements	$37.3
TOTAL	$64.4

From New Paradigm Ventures, Inc: *Complementary medicine research project,* South Norwalk, Conn, 1996, internal publication.

CAM. Potential customers include health researchers, social scientists, educators, students, and policymakers. Perhaps the greatest number of potential customers will be the direct-response buyers who will use CAM information products to explore and answer questions on specific CAM treatments and their potential efficacy. This type of either primary or secondary analysis extends and defines the original work. If offered on the Internet, which can then be downloaded in multimedia formats such as CD-ROMs, its availability can be maximized.

Integration With Managed Care. The increase in consumer usage of CAM has led both medical insurers and hospitals to reexamine their own practices and policies. Recently

TABLE 3	1994 Expenditures on Wellness Products in the United States
Wellness Products	**Amount spent (in Billions of Dollars)**
Miscellaneous home products	$2.5
Supplements	$3.5
Health and beauty aids	$14.0
Specialty foods and diets	$22.0
Fitness products	$24.5
Smoking cessation products, water and air filtration systems	$0.5
TOTAL	$67.0

From New Paradigm Ventures, Inc: *Complementary medicine research project,* South Norwalk, Conn, 1996, internal publication.

TABLE 4	Number of Products Available in the United States (by Medical Category)
Category	**Number of Products**
Arthritis	82
Asthma and allergies	16
Backache and headache	60
Cancer survivors	11
Diabetes	42
Diet and exercise	18
Eye care	30
New mothers	31
Osteoporosis	31
Sports medicine	38
TOTAL	359

From New Paradigm Ventures, Inc: *Complementary medicine research project,* South Norwalk, Conn, 1996, internal publication.

Pelletier et al.[4] surveyed 18 insurers and 7 hospitals regarding which of 34 different CAM therapies were most often covered or used. It was reported that the insurance companies in this study mainly selected CAM therapies such as acupuncture, biofeedback, chiropractic, and nutrition and not so much others, such as herbal medicine, Ayurveda, and craniosacral therapy. Hospitals have started to integrate CAM therapies such as acupuncture, massage, and meditation. The biggest reported obstacle for insurance companies and hospitals to include CAM was the lack of information concerning its usefulness. The evaluation for cost-effectiveness and longer-term benefits of CAM are important variables for further study.

As research continues to reveal the prevalence of CAM, health care providers are repositioning themselves to succeed in this health-driven economy. They are actively learning more about the managed-care industry and how to participate in it. Research shows that many people still rely on indigenous healing systems for spiritual, emotional, and physical health needs. Thus many managed-care organizations are grappling with how to financially integrate indigenous care as part of their benefits package because they want to retain this unique marketing opportunity to increase their market share. Before any strategy of integration occurs, there will need to be changes in the perception of CAM by conventional health care providers and vice versa.

Changes can be seen in hospitals that have begun to apply conventional technologies in a "holistic" manner. For example, the Griffin Hospital in Derby, Connecticut, a 160-bed, Yale-affiliated hospital, has instituted a patient-oriented approach to the delivery of hospital care based on the Plane Tree philosophy. It has implemented community-oriented programs to address health care issues and concerns, including the use of CAM therapies. As Griffin Health Services Corporation, which includes a health-maintenance organization (HMO), and other managed-care organizations reposition themselves in this new health care environment, how might CAM fit into their strategic plans? A unique opportunity exists for the development of a system of care, rather than CAM and conventional medicine merely being competing providers in a crowded market. A vertically integrated provider/payer system may easily integrate CAM practitioners into a complementary system of care.

To be competitive in a market-driven health care economy, managed-care providers are focusing on the following objectives: (1) to increase market share, (2) to decrease costs, and (3) to maintain quality.

Increase Market Share. To increase market share, managed-care organizations must offer a broad range of health care products and services that add clinical value to attract potential subscribers. Therapies like acupuncture, massage therapy, and chiropractic manipulation may be considered to have "clinical value adaptivity" to conventional care. Clinical value may be seen in a situation where acupuncture is an integral part of a low back pain management program and provides a cheaper, more cost-effective treatment for pain management in some patients. Clinical value may also been seen in the development of wellness centers to meet the needs of clients wanting to use different strategies to prevent the onset of diabetes, heart disease, or cancer. This strategy helps to develop a chain of wellness centers that would feature a major role for CAM. This may result in enhanced patient referrals and, at the same time, provide a source of revenue for managed-care organizations.

Interest from health insurance providers such as American Western Life Insurance Company, Oxford Health Plans, Pacific Health & Life, and, to some extent, Mutual of Omaha has focused primarily on financial reimbursement through the development of policy riders to cover usage of CAM. A significant gap remains in determining how CAM clinical practices may be included under an umbrella of a more comprehensive, integrated health care system. Managed-care organizations should play a major role in providing information on safe and effective medications and treatments. The large number of original prescription drugs now sold over the counter, not to mention the increase in usage of CAM, has shifted the burden of health care decision making to the consumers of these products. Managed-care organizations must declare themselves to be patient advocates to attract potential clients to their programs.

Decrease Costs. Managed-care organizations must provide a comparative analysis of different treatment approaches to specific conditions. Cost-effective treatment options will result in attracting new clients. How, then, is cost reduction achieved? Part of the answer lies in offering affordable products that are attractive to potential policyholders. Cost-benefit programs must compare CAM with conventional medical interventions (i.e., surgery), not only to provide patients with an overview of treatments options, along with cost, but also to identify the most cost-effective treatment option.

For example, for several years a program developed by Dr. Dean Ornish to reverse the progression of cardiac disease was evaluated by the Mutual of Omaha insurance company. The evaluation was relatively risk free because physicians have been trying to get their cardiac patients to decrease their fat intake, exercise more, decrease stress in their lives, and obtain mutual support to get them through the process. The clinical methodology used was not outside medical mainstream opinion. Mutual of Omaha was able to accomplish its rather straightforward objectives with minimal controversy. The evaluation of other CAM therapies such as determining the benefits of prayer or magnetic therapy presents more challenging obstacles.

Although 34% of the patients in Eisenberg's survey (see Chapter 1) were using some form of CAM, 66% were not. People who pay premiums for health care want assurance that their premium dollars are being expended in a cost-effective way. Most people do not want to abandon conventional care; that is why a team approach is important. Collaboration between conventional medicine and CAM must occur in a clinical setting and through the process of clinical evaluation for efficacy.

Maintain Quality. Consumers want a managed-care organization to maintain quality, especially if CAM medical practices are offered. It is necessary for managed-care organizations to provide a high-quality network of CAM providers. Conventional practitioners must have confidence in the CAM providers for referral purposes. It has been suggested[2] that when patients visit a CAM provider, they should attempt to elicit answers to questions such as the following:

- The provider's belief in his or her therapy's effectiveness based on other patients' experiences with the same treatment: Are these patients available to speak with?
- What does the therapy(s) consist of?
- How frequently is it given?
- How are decisions reached (and by whom) regarding whether the treatment is beneficial?
- Are there side effects to the therapy? If so, what are those side effects?
- How much time will the therapy take?
- Is insurance reimbursement available?
- Will the CAM provider give findings, plans, and follow-up information back to the patient?

With quality control in place, managed-care organizations can shift their energy to the development of compensated services provided by CAM providers. Much of this development is rooted in basic business decisions in the marketplace. It represents changes in attitudes not only by conventional providers but also by employers and worker groups. States now provide mandates for change within individual markets. This has led to the state of Washington's recent mandate for CAM reimbursement. Managed-care organizations must "catch up" on their knowledge of CAM. To what extent this may hasten CAM integration with conventional medicine more universally can only be conjecture at present. It is likely that CAM will not disappear from the health care scene and that integration with conventional medicine will need to be more completely addressed in the twenty-first century.

Clinical Research and CAM

Chapter 1 framed the debate regarding usage of CAM within the United States. The evidence presented throughout this book shows that proof of both safety and treatment efficacy of CAM is still needed for all medical conditions. Treatment approaches that cannot demonstrate their effectiveness would not be expected to be in demand by the public. However, consumers use and promote CAM therapies not by what clinical research demonstrates, but more by personal experiences. The physician in many cases may know very little about these therapies and may never be informed by the patient of their usage, which could cause multiple unclear and potentially dangerous treatment outcomes.

Patient usage of CAM will continue to increase for various reasons. For some patients prevention will be the major focus; for others, control of pain. Current studies in both areas are promising. It is proposed that scientific research and the clinician work together for the integration of CAM within the U.S. health care system. Many CAM therapies will not be evaluated, in part because of (1) the huge cost associated with clinical trials, (2) unclear and questionable scientific assumptions, and (3) personal or scientific bias against CAM.

The U.S. Food and Drug Administration (FDA) has been instrumental in furthering CAM research in the right direction. It encouraged the focus to be on issues of safety, and it sponsored and facilitated scientific workshops devoted to exploring necessary steps and processes for regulation in a more timely fashion. Current legislation is promising (see Chapter 1). Still more linkages and communication between the FDA and other health care agencies, including the National Institutes of Health (NIH), the Health Care Financing Administration (HCF), the Health Resource Service Administration (HRS), and the Department of Veterans Affairs (VA), would help coordinate and implement various program needs.

Conventional medicine will accept the integration of certain CAM therapies based in part on research findings and in part on marketplace demand through continued consumer pressure. To hasten the process, it is proposed that partnerships be introduced between industry, third-party payers, private foundations, and the federal government directed at funding treatment outcome studies, innovative diagnostic procedures, and novel treatment interventions. Clinical practice audits with certain limitations would also be a possible mechanism for the evaluation of CAM. When a spirit of cooperation and trust develops between conventional medicine and CAM, the health care consumer will ultimately benefit from a much-improved health care system in the twenty-first century.

REFERENCES

1. Astin JA: Why patients use alternative medicine: results of a national study, *JAMA* 279(19):1548, 1998.
2. Eisenberg DM: Advising patients who seek alternative medical therapies, *Ann Intern Med* 127:61, 1997.
3. New Paradigm Ventures, Inc: *Complementary medicine research project,* South Norwalk, Conn, 1996, internal publication.
4. Pelletier KR et al: Current trends in the integration and reimbursement of complementary and alternative medicine by managed care, insurance carriers and hospital providers, *Am J Health Promotion* 12(2):112, 1997.

Definitions of Complementary/Alternative Therapies Described in the Text

Acupuncture

Thin needles are inserted superficially on the skin at locations throughout the body. These points are located along "channels" of energy. Heat can be applied by burning (moxibustion), electric current (electroacupuncture), or pressure (acupressure). Healing is proposed by the restoration of a balance of energy flow called "Qi." Another explanation suggests that, possibly, the stimulation activates endorphin receptors.

Alexander technique

A bodywork technique in which rebalancing of "postural sets" (i.e., physical alignment) is taught by mentally focusing on the way correct alignments should look and feel and through verbal and tactile guidance by the practitioner.

Antineoplastons

Naturally occurring peptides, amino acid derivatives, and carboxylic acids are proposed to control neoplastic cell growth using the patient's own "biochemical defense system," which works jointly with the immune system (see Chapter 6).

Applied kinesiology

A form of treatment that uses nutrition, physical manipulation, vitamins, diets, and exercise for the purpose of restoring and energizing the body. Weak muscles are proposed to be a source of dysfunctional health.

Aromatherapy

A form of herbal medicine that uses various oils from plants. Route of administration can be through absorption in the skin or inhalation. The action of antiviral and antibacterial agents is proposed to aid in healing. The aromatic biochemical structures of certain herbs are thought to act in areas of the brain related to past experiences and emotions (e.g., limbic system).

Ayurveda

A major health system that emphasizes a preventive approach to health by focusing on an inner state of harmony and spiritual realization for self-healing. Includes special types of diets, herbs, and mineral parts and changes based on a system of constitutional categories in lifestyle. The use of enemas and purgation is for the purpose of cleansing the body of excess toxins.

Biofeedback

A mind-body therapy procedure in which sensors are placed on the body for the purpose of measuring muscle, heart rate, and sweat responses or neural activity. Information is provided by visual, auditory, or body-muscle cell activation for the purpose of teaching to either increase or decrease physiologic activity which, when reconstituted, is proposed to improve health problems (i.e., pain, anxiety, or high blood pressure). In some cases relaxation exercises complement this procedure.

Brachytherapy

Ionizing radiation therapy with the source applied to the surface of the body or located a short distance from the treated area.

Bristol Cancer Help Center (BCHC) diet

A stringent diet of raw and partly cooked vegetables with proteins from soy; claimed to enhance the quality of life and attitude toward illness in cancer patients.

Cell therapy

Healthy cellular material from fetuses, embryos, or organs of animals is directly injected into human patients for the purpose of stimulating healing in dysfunctional organs. May also include blood transfusions or bone marrow transplantations.

Chelation therapy

Involves the removal—through intravenous

infusion of a chelating agent (synthetic amino acid ethylenediamine tetraacetic acid [EDTA])—of metal, toxins, lead, mercury, nickel, copper, cadmium, and plaque for the purpose of treating certain diseases (e.g., cardiovascular). Ancillary treatments include the use of vitamins, changes in diet, and exercise.

Cognitive therapy

Psychologic therapy in which the major focus is on altering and changing irrational beliefs through a type of "socratic" dialogue and self-evaluation of certain illogical thoughts. Conditioning and learning are important components of this therapy.

Craniosacral therapy

A form of gentle manual manipulation used for diagnosis and for making corrections in a system made up of cerebrospinal fluid, cranial and dural membranes, cranial bones, and sacrum. This system is proposed to be dynamic with its own physiologic frequency. Through touch and pressure, tension is proposed to be reduced and cranial rhythms normalized, leading to improvement in health and disease.

Dance therapy

A movement-based therapy that aids in promoting feeling and awareness. The goal is to integrate body, mind, and self-esteem. It uses different parts of the body such as fingers, wrists, and arms to respond to music.

Diathermy

The use of high-frequency electrical currents as a form of physical therapy and in surgical procedures. The term "diathermy," derived from the Greek words *dia* and *therma*, literally means "heating through." The three forms of diathermy employed by physical therapists are short-wave, ultrasound, and microwave.

Dimethylaminoethanol (DMAE)

Pharmacologic therapy that uses a natural substance found in certain foods and the human brain. Is a precursor to the transmitter acetylcholine. It is proposed to have a stimulant effect on the central nervous system if used as a supplement.

Electrochemical treatment (ECT)

A method using direct current to treat cancer. It involves inserting platinum electrodes into tumors and applying a constant voltage of less than 10 V to produce a 40- to 80-mA current between the anodes and cathodes for 30 minutes to several hours.

Electroencephalographic normalization

Gross neural activity is recorded from the scalp as an electroencephalogram (EEG) to assist in "restoring a balance in health" by training patients to produce more uniform and consistent EEG frequencies throughout certain or all areas of the brain (occipital, frontal, temporal, and parietal).

Environmental medicine

A practice of medicine in which the major focus in on cause-and-effect relationships in health. Evaluations are made of such factors as eating and living habits and types of air breathed. Testing in the patient's own environment is performed to determine what precipitators are present that may be related to disease or other health problems. A treatment protocol is developed from this information.

Eye movement desensitization and reprocessing (EMDR)

A technique that proposes to remove painful memories by behavioral techniques. Rhythmic, multisaccadic eye movements are produced by allowing the patient to track and follow a moving object while imaging a stressful memory or event. By using deconditioning, including verbal interaction with the therapist, the painful memory is extinguished and health improved.

Feldenkrais method

A bodywork technique in which its founder used the integration of physics, judo, and yoga. The practitioner directs sequences of movement using verbal or hands-on techniques or teaches a system of self-directed exercise to treat physical impairments through the learning of new movement patterns.

Hallucinogens

The use of lysergic acid diethylamide (LSD) to produce at certain doses anticraving for certain illicit drugs such as cocaine, or ibogaine, a stimulant, to assist in developing tolerance and decreasing symptoms of dependence.

Hatha yoga

The branch of yoga practice that involves physical exercise, breathing practices, and movement. These exercises are designed to have a salutary effect on posture, flexibility, and strength for the ultimate purpose of preparing the body to remain still for long periods of meditation.

Hellerwork

A bodywork technique that treats and improves proper body alignment through the development of a more complete awareness of the physical body. The goal is to realign fascia for improvement in standing, sitting, and breathing using " body energy," verbal feedback, and changing emotions and attitudes.

Herbal medicine

Herbs are used to treat various health conditions. Herbal medicine is a major form of treatment for more than 70% of the world's population.

Homeopathy

A form of treatment in which substances (minerals, plant extracts, chemicals, or disease-producing germs), which in sufficient doses would produce a set of illness symptoms in healthy individuals, are given in microdoses to produce a "cure" of those same symptoms. The *symptom* is not thought to be part of the illness but part of a curative process.

Hydergine

A phytotherapeutic method that combines extracts from the ergot fungus. Originally proposed to be used as an antihypertensive agent.

Hydrazine sulfate

A pharmacologic treatment proposed to treat certain cancers (see Chapter 6).

Hyperbaric oxygen

A therapy in which 100% oxygen is given at or above atmospheric pressure. An increase in oxygen in the tissue is proposed to increase blood circulation and improve healing and health and influence the course of disease.

Hyperthermia

The use of various heating methods (such as electromagnetic therapy) to produce temperature elevations of a few degrees in cells and tissues, leading to a proposed antitumor effect This is often used in conjunction with radiotherapy or chemotherapy for cancer treatment.

Immunoaugmentative therapy

A cancer treatment which proposes that cancer cells can be arrested by the use of four different blood proteins; this approach is also proposed to restore the immune system. Can be used as an adjunctive therapy.

Jin Shin Jyutsu

A bodywork technique that uses specific "healing points" at the body surface, which are proposed to overlie energy flowing (Qi). The therapist's fingers are used to "redirect, balance, and provide a more efficient energy flow" to and throughout the body.

Laetrile

A pharmacologic treatment using apricot pits that has been proposed to treat certain cancers (see Chapter 6).

Light therapy

Natural light or light of specified wavelengths is used to treat disease. This may include ultraviolet light, colored light, or low-intensity laser light. The eye generally is the initial entry point for the light because of its direct connection to the brain.

Magnetic therapy

Magnets are directly placed on the skin, stimulating living cells and increasing blood flow by ionic currents that are created from polarities on the magnets. Both acute and chronic health conditions are suggested to be treatable by this procedure.

Manual manipulation

A group of therapies with different assumptions and, in part, different areas of treatment. The major focus includes both stimulation and body manipulation, which are proposed to improve health or arrest disease, or both. Includes soft tissue manipulation through stroking, kneading, friction, and vibration. Types include *massage,* adjustment of the spinal column *(chiropractic),* and tissue and musculoskeletal *(osteopathic)* manipulation.

Mediterranean diet

A diet that is thought to provide optimal distribution of daily caloric intake of different nutrients and includes 50% to 60% carbohydrates, 30% fats, and 10% proteins. The diet is derived from the eating habits of people in the Mediterranean area, who were shown to have reduced rates of cardiovascular disease.

Mind-body therapies

A group of therapies that emphasize using the mind or brain in conjunction with the body to assist the healing process. Mind-body therapies can involve varying degrees of levels of consciousness, including *hypnosis,* in which selective attention is used to induce a specific altered state (trance) for memory retrieval, relaxation, or suggestion; *visual imagery,* in which the focus is on a target visual stimulus; *yoga,* which involves integration of posture and controlled breathing, relaxation, and or meditation; *relaxation,* which includes lighter levels of altered states of consciousness through indirect or direct focus; and *medita-*

tion, in which there is an intentional use of posture, concentration, contemplation, and visualization.

Muscle energy technique

A manual therapy with components of both passive mobilization and muscle reeducation. Diagnosis of somatic dysfunction is performed by the practitioner after which the patient is guided to provide corrective muscle contraction. This is followed by further testing and correction.

Music therapy

The use of music either in an active or passive mode. Proposed to help allow for the expression of feelings, which helps to reduce stress. Other types of "vibratory" sounds can be used mainly to reduce stress, anxiety, and pain.

Native American therapies

Therapies used by many Native American Indian tribes, including their own healing herbs and ceremonies that use components with a spiritual emphasis.

Naturopathy

A major health system that includes practices which emphasize diet, nutrition, homeopathy, acupuncture, herbal medicine, manipulation, and various mind-body therapies. Focal points include self-healing and treatment through changes in lifestyle and emphasis on health prevention (see Chapter 12).

Neuroelectric Therapy

Transcranial or cranial neuroelectric stimulation (TENS), once called "electrosleep"; originally used in the 1950s for the treatment of insomnia. In a typical TENS session, surface electrodes are placed in the mastoid region (behind the ear) and, similar to electroacupuncture, stimulated using a low-amperage, low-frequency alternating current. It has been suggested that TENS stimulates endogenous neurotransmitters such as endorphins that produce symptomatic relief.

Ornish diet

A life-choice program based on eating a vegetarian diet containing less that 10% fat. The diet is high in complex carbohydrates and fiber. Animal products and oils are avoided.

Orthomolecular therapy

A therapeutic approach that uses naturally occurring substances within the body such as proteins, fat, and water which promote restoration or balance (or both) by using vitamins, minerals, or other forms of nutrition to subsequently treat disease or promote healing, or both.

Oslo diet

An eating plan that emphasizes increased intake of fish and reduced total fat intake. Diet is combined with regular endurance exercise.

Pilates

An educational and excerise approach using the proper body mechanics, movements, truncal and pelvic stabilization, coordinated breathing, and muscle contractions to promote strengthening. Attention is paid to the entire musculoskeletal system.

Piracetam

A pharmacologic treatment proposed to be useful in the treatment of dementia. Uses a cyclic relative of the transmitter gamma-aminobutyric acid (GABA).

Prayer

The use of prayer(s) that are offered to "some higher being" or authority for the purpose of healing and/or arresting disease. May be practiced by the individual patient, by groups, or by other(s) with or without the patient's knowledge (e.g., intercessory).

Pritikin diet

A weight management plan that is based on a vegetarian framework. Meals are low in fat, high in fiber, and high in complex carbohydrates.

Qi Gong

A form of Chinese exercise-stimulation therapy that proposes to improve health by redirecting mental focus, breathing, coordination, and relaxation. The goal is to "rebalance" the body's own healing capacities by activating proposed electrical or energetic currents that flow along meridians located throughout the body. These meridians, however, do not follow conventional nerve or muscle pathways. In Chinese medical training and practice this therapy includes "external Qi," which is energy transmitted from one person to another for the purpose of healing.

Raja yoga

Yoga practice that includes all of the other forms of yoga practice. The practitioner is instructed to follow moral directives, physical exercises, breathing exercises, meditation, devotion, and service to others to facilitate religious awakening.

Reconstructive therapy

A nonsurgical therapy for arthritis that involves the injection of nutritional substances into the supporting tissues around an injured joint. The intent is to cause the dilation of blood vessels, which will allow fibroblasts to form around the injury and begin the healing process.

Reflexology

A bodywork technique that uses reflex points on the hands and feet. Pressure is applied at points that correspond to various body parts with the intention of eliminating blockages thought to produce pain or disease. The goal is to bring the body into balance.

Reiki

Comes from the Japanese word meaning "universal life force energy." The practitioner serves as a conduit for healing energy directed into the body or energy field of the recipient without physical contact with the body.

Restricted environmental stimulation therapy (REST)

A procedure which uses a completely sensory-deprived environment for the purpose of increasing physical or mental healing through a nonreactive state.

Rolfing

A bodywork technique that involves the myofascia. The body is realigned by using the hands to apply a deep pressure and friction that allows more sufficient posture, movement, and the "release" of emotions from the body.

Shark cartilage

A cancer therapy which proposes that shark cartilage can interrupt blood supply to a tumor(s) and subsequently "starves" it of any nutrients by using the antiangiogenic properties and other substances contained in the cartilage (see Chapter 6).

Shiatsu

A bodywork technique involving finger pressure at specific points on the body mainly for the purpose of balancing "energy" in the body. The major focus is on prevention by keeping the body healthy. The therapy uses more than 600 points on the skin which are proposed to be connected to pathways through which energy flows. A Japanese form of acupressure.

T'ai chi

A technique that uses slow, purposeful motor-physical movements of the body for the purpose of control and achieving a more balanced physiologic and psychologic state.

Therapeutic riding

A form of animal-assisted therapy in which either passive or active movements are produced to aid in approximating the human gait. In certain cases physiotherapeutic exercises are performed.

Therapeutic touch

A body energy field technique in which hands are passed over the body without actually touching to recreate and change proposed "energy imbalances" for restoring innate healing forces. Verbal interaction between patient and therapist helps to maximize effects.

Traditional Chinese medicine

An ancient form of medicine that focuses on prevention and secondarily treats disease with an emphasis on maintaining balance through the body by stimulating a constant, smooth-flowing Qi energy. Herbs, acupuncture, massage, diet, and exercise are also used.

Trager psychophysical integration

A bodywork technique in which the practitioner enters a meditative state and guides the client through gentle, light, rhythmic nonintrusive movements. "Mentastics" exercises using self-healing movements are taught to the clients.

Transcranial electrostimulation

Pulsed electrical stimulation of 50 microamperes or less is applied between two electrodes attached to the ear. The stimulation is proposed to activate endogenous opioid activity, which may assist in the treatment of certain health problems such as substance abuse and physical pain.

Twelve-Step Program

A program such as Alcoholics Anonymous that is based on a series of 12 steps, or tasks, which participants are asked to complete. As members progress through the 12 steps, they are expected to gain courage to attempt personal change and develop a greater acceptance of themselves. Programs emphasize the group process through the sharing of stories and experiences and through social interactions with other group members. Most 12-step programs incorporate a spiritual component and ask members to turn their lives over to a higher power.

The definitions listed above are not complete; for additional information, the interested reader should consult books such as Micozzi's *Fundamentals of Complementary and Alternative Medicine* (see other Suggested Readings in Chapter 1).

APPENDIX B

Selected Resources for Complementary/ Alternative Medicine

ORGANIZATIONS

American Academy of Medical Acupuncturists
5820 Wilshire Blvd., Suite 500
Los Angeles, CA 90032
Phone: (213) 937-5514

American Association of Naturopathic Physicians
601 Valley St., Suite 105
Seattle, WA 98109
Phone: (206) 328-8510

American Chiropractic Association
1701 Clarendon Blvd.
Arlington, VA 22209
Phone: (703) 276-8800

American Massage Therapy Association
820 Davis St., Suite 100
Evanston, IL 60201
Phone: (847) 864-0123

PUBLICATIONS

Advances: The Journal of Mind-Body Health
John E. Fetzer Institute
9292 West KL Avenue
Kalamazoo, MI 49009
Phone: (616) 375-2000

Alternative Therapies in Health and Medicine
InnoVision Communications
101 Columbia Street
Aliso Viejo, CA 92656
Phone: (800) 899-1712

HerbalGram
American Botanical Council
P.O. Box 2016600
Austin, TX 78720

Journal of Alternative and Complementary Medicine: Research on Paradigm, Practice and Policy
Mary Ann Liebert, Inc.
2 Madison Ave.

Larchmont, NY 10538
Phone: (914) 834-3100; (800) MLIEBERT

OTHER RESOURCES

American Botanical Council
P.O. Box 201660
Austin, TX 78720-1660
(512) 331-8861; (800) 373-7105
Commission E monographs (monographs published by the German government's Commission E, an expert committee of physicians, pharmacologists, toxicologists and other authorities, charged with writing monographs on a number of commonly used herbal medicines) have been translated by and are available from the Council.
Web site: **http://www.herbalgram.org/ commission_e/index.html**

Centers for the Study of Complementary and Alternative Medicine
Addictions
Center for Addiction and Alternative Medicine Research (CAMMR)
University of Minnesota Medical School
914 S 8th St., Suite D917
Minneapolis, MN 55404
Thomas J. Kiresuk, PhD, Principal Investigator
Web site: **http://www.winternet.com/~caamr/**

Aging
Complementary and Alternative Medicine Program at Stanford University (CAMPS)
730 Welch Road, Suite B
Palo Alto, CA 94304-1583
William L. Haskell, PhD, Principal Investigator
Web site: **http://scrdp.stanford.edu/camps.html**

Asthma, Allergy, and Immunology
Center for Alternative Medicine Research in Asthma and Immunology
University of California at Davis

425

TB 192, Division of Rheumatology-Clinical
Immunology
Davis, CA 95616
Merrill Gershwin, MD, Principal Investigator
Web site: **http://www-camra.ucdavis.edu**

Cancer
University of Texas Center for Alternative and
Complementary Medicine Research in Cancer
P.O. Box 20186, No. W430
Houston, TX 77225
Guy Parcel, PhD, Principal Investigator
Web site: **http://www.sph.uth.tmc.edu/utcam**

Chiropractic
Consortorial Center for Chiropractic Research
741 Brady St.
Davenport, IA 52803-5260
William Meeker, DC, MPH, Principal Investigator
Web site: **http://www.c3r.org**

General Medical Conditions
Center for Alternative Medicine Research at Beth
Israel Hospital/Deaconess Medical Center
330 Brookline Ave.
Boston, MA 02215
David Eisenberg, MD, Principal Investigator
Web site:
http://www.bidmc.harvard.edu/medicine/camr

Human Immunodeficiency Virus/Acquired Immunodeficiency Syndrome
Bastyr University AIDS Research Center
14500 Juanita Dr., NE
Bothell, WA 98011
Leanna Standish, ND, PhD, Principal Investigator
Web site:
http://www.bastyr.edu/research/research.html

Pain
Center for Alternative Medicine Pain Research
and Evaluation
Kernan Hospital Mansion
2200 Kernan Dr.
Baltimore, MD 21207
Brian Berman, MD, Principal Investigator
Web site: **www.compmed.ummc.ab.umd.edu**

University of Virginia Center for the Study of
Complementary and Alternative Therapies
University of Virginia School of Nursing
McLeod Hall
15th and Lane St.
Charlottesville, VA 22903-3395
Ann Gill Taylor, EdD, Principal Investigator
Web site:
http://www.med.virginia.edu/nursing/centers/alt-ther.html

Stroke and Neurologic Conditions
Center for Research in Complementary and Alternative Medicine for Stroke and Neurological Disorders
Kessler Medical Rehabilitation Research and Education Corporation (KMRREC)
1199 Pleasant Valley Way
West Orange, NJ 07052
Samual Schiflett, PhD, Principal Investigator
Web site: **http://www.umdnj.edu/altmdweb**

Women's Health
Center for Complementary/Alternative Medicine
Research in Women's Health
Columbia University College of Physicians and
Surgeons
630 West 168th St., Box 75
New York, NY 10032
Fredi Kronenberg, PhD, Principal Investigator
Web site:
http://cpmcnet.columbia.edu/dept/rosenthal/

APPENDIX C

Research Databases

Databases from the Richard and Hinda Rosenthal Center for Complementary and Alternative Medicine
College of Physicians and Surgeons
630 West 168 St.
New York, NY 10032
Web site:
http://cpmcnet.columbia.edu/dept/rosenthal/
Contains 56 databases; 36 of these are available through the Internet and 17 are available to the public. Many areas of complementary/alternative medicine are represented.

Herb Research Foundation
1007 Pearl St., Suite 200
Boulder, CO 80302
Web site: **http://www.herbs.org**
Private library of papers covering botanic issues. Fee for searching plus a per-page charge.

NAPRALERT
College of Pharmacy
The University of Illinois at Chicago
Phone: (312) 996-2246
Web site:
http://pcog8.pmmp.uic.edu/mcp/MCP.html

Contains information from more than 120,000 articles on ethnomedical data of plants.

Office of Alternative Medicine
(National Institute of Health)
P.O. Box 8218
Silver Spring, MD 20907-8218
Web site: **http://altmed.od.nih.gov**
Describes, among other things, scientific program areas, information resources, and a CAM citation index.

University of Texas Center for CAM Research in Cancer
Web site: **http://www.sph.uth.tmc.edu/utcm/**
A listing of the latest research findings regarding herbal, biologic, and chemical agents used in the treatment of cancer can be accessed by clicking on "reviews of agents."

U.S. Department of Agriculture
Web site: **http://probe.nalusda.gov**
Contains a database of 80,000 items on herbs used throughout the world. For access to records on taxonomy and use of herbs.

For a more complete listing of other databases see Wooton JC: Directory of databases for research into alternative and complementary medicine, *J Alternat Complement Med* 3:179, 1997.

Glossary

American Diabetes Association guidelines

Clinical practice recommendations dealing with prevention, screening, and diagnosis of diabetes. In addition, standards of medical care for patients with diabetes mellitus are established and published.

Acquired immunodeficiency syndrome (AIDS)

A condition associated with the infection of the human immunodeficiency virus (HIV).

Anecdotal health reports

Impressionistic information that may or may not be collaborated by other sources regarding whether a health intervention was useful.

Angiogenesis

Formation of new blood vessels.

Antioxidant

A chemical that inhibits oxidation, a process that causes deterioration of DNA in cells. Oxidation of low-density cholesterol particles in the artery wall appears to be a key process in the development of atherosclerosis, and there is some evidence that selected antioxidants reduce the rate of initiation or progression of atherosclerosis.

Autoimmune process

Antibodies are produced within a person's body that attack specific cells and cell functions. In the case of diabetes, the beta cells of the pancreas are attacked by antibodies and are eventually destroyed.

Bacille Calmette-Guérin (BCG)

A product of the treatment of tuberculosis organisms that is used as a vaccine against this disease, causing an increase in immune reactivity.

Barthel index

A standardized instrument for the assessment of functional outcomes such as independence in self-care and mobility. This reliable, well-validated index is widely used in U.S. medical rehabilitation settings.

Beck Anxiety and Depression Scales

The Beck Anxiety Inventory (BAI) has 21 items, each representing an anxiety symptom rated on a four-point scale (0-3) ranging from "Not at all" to "Severely, I could barely stand it." The Beck Depression Inventory (BDI) is designed to assess the severity of depression in adolescents and adults and also uses a 21-item inventory assessing an individual's complaints, symptoms, and concerns related to his or her current level of depression.

Boston Motor Inventory

Developed for use in studies of patients with hemiplegia or paralysis; measures isolated, active range of motion for four leg movements and three arm movements.

Brief Psychiatric Rating Scale

A multisymptom category rating tool originally designed for use by clinical observers of inpatient psychiatric populations in pharmacologic outcome studies The items are rated on a one- to seven-point severity scale and assess psychotic symptoms such as hallucinations, unusual thought content, conceptual disorganization, bizarre behavior, self-neglect, and suicidality. Administration is by a trained interviewer. Symptoms can be readily graphed over time, so baseline changes can be detected and interventions mounted.

Brief Social Phobia Scale

An observer-rated scale designed to assess the characteristic symptoms of social phobia using three subscales: fear, avoidance, and physiologic arousal. Results are then combined for a total score.

CAM

Complementary/alternative medicine.

Carcinogenesis
Formation of cancer.

Cervical dysplasia
The appearance of abnormal cells on the cervix, possibly a precursor to cervical cancer, usually associated with the human papillomavirus (HPV), which causes genital warts.

Clinical practice guidelines
Statements and official guidelines for patient health care and treatment.

Clusters
In epidemiologic research, groupings of people or tendencies within a population.

Coenzyme Q10
A naturally occurring, fat-soluble antioxidant that is used for energy production in body cells. Coenzyme Q10 occurs in the lipid core of inner mitochondrial membranes. It functions in the electron transport chain that produces adenosine triphosphate (ATP), the basic cellular energy-producing molecule. It is also known as ubiquinone. It has been promoted for a variety of cardiovascular disorders.

Conductivity
Refers to electrical conductivity; in the body, the higher the water content the higher the conductivity.

Contract-relax-antagonist-contract technique
A proprioceptive neural facilitation (PNF) technique used to facilitate muscle relaxation and lengthening in the agonist muscle (see Proprioceptive Neural Facilitation in Chapter 7).

Cytochrome P-450 enzymes
Oxygenating catalysts for a wide variety of reactions responsible for detoxification of many drugs.

Derailment
The moving in random fashion from one topic, thought, or behavior to another. A psychotic state descriptive term used in a mental status examination.

Dong quai *(Angelica senensis)* (also spelled dang gui, tang kuei)
A root used in traditional Chinese medicine (TCM) formulas for menopausal symptoms and other conditions in patients who meet specific criteria in TCM diagnosis. Currently it is being sold as a single-ingredient product in U.S. health food stores and used by women for menopausal symptoms.

Double-blind study
An experimental clinical research technique in which neither the patient nor the researcher is aware of whether treatment given is active (medicinal) or inactive (nonmedicinal).

Drug courts
A special court given the responsibility to handle cases involving less serious drug-related offenses. Offenders are given the opportunity to complete a treatment program under intensive supervision in lieu of harsher penalties such as incarceration. The judge wipes clean all record of arrest if the offender graduates from the program; otherwise, the client may have to serve his or her sentence in full. The design and structure of drug court programs are developed at the local level, to reflect the unique strengths and needs of each community.

DSM IV
The DSM IV (*Diagnostic and Statistical Manual of Mental Disorders, Fourth Edition*) (American Psychological Association Press, 1994) is a standardized classification and diagnostic manual of mental disorders.

Dysplasia
Abnormal size, shape, and organization of adult cells.

Echinacea
A narrow-leafed perennial member of the daisy family native to the central U.S. Originally used by Native Americans, its rhizome and roots seem to exert an immune-stimulant effect.

Eicosanoid
Biologically active substances derived from arachidonic acid.

Electrolysis
A process in which electrical energy causes a chemical change in a conducting medium, usually a solution or a molten substance. Electrodes, usually pieces of metal, induce the flow of electric energy through the medium. Electrons enter the solution through the cathode and leave the solution through the anode. Negatively charged ions, or anions, are attracted to the anode; positively charged ions, or cations, are attracted to the cathode.

Electroosmosis
The movement of fluids through diaphragms as a result of the application of an electric current.

Electrophoresis
The migration of the electrically charged solute particles present in a colloidal solution toward the electrode with an opposite charge when two electrodes are placed. This technique is widely

employed in biochemical analysis, for example, in the separation and study of plasma protein.

Endorphins

Any of a group of proteins with potent analgesic (pain killing) properties that occur naturally in the brain.

Enkephalins

Pentapeptides are molecular chains of amino acids containing five amino acid residues; the enkephalins have a marked affinity for opioid receptors and thus have opiate and analgesic activity. They occur naturally in the brain and spinal cord.

Epidemiology

The study and reporting of the presence, spread, and cause of disease within a population.

Epstein-Barr virus (EBV)

Member of the herpes family of viruses. Causes mononucleosis and may be involved in some forms of chronic fatigue syndrome.

Eysenck Personality Inventory (EPI)

A self-report questionnaire used to measure the personality dimension of neuroticism-stability (N) and extraversion-introversion (E), including a lie scale (L). The EPI consists of two parallel forms, thus making possible retesting after experimental treatment without interference from memory factors.

Flexner Report

A report written in the early twentieth century concerning strengths and weaknesses of medical education in the United States.

Fluoxetine, sertraline, and ritanserin

Fluoxetine (Prozac) and sertraline (Zoloft) are orally administered antidepressants. The drugs are presumed to inhibit the central nervous system (CNS) neuronal uptake of serotonin. Ritanserin (Ondansetron) is a 5HT-3 antagonist. It is used clinically as an antiemetic (to treat nausea and vomiting).

Genotype

The genetic constituents of the organism.

Hamilton Anxiety and Depression Scale

Rating scales that have been used for decades in the assessment of anxiety and depression. They are completed by clinician interviewers and use a semistructured interview format with the patient. Hamilton scales are thought to be more systematic in evaluating neurovegetative symptoms than cognitive symptoms, a strength of Beck rating scales.

Heating pattern

The distribution of rate of temperature rise in a human body or model. The unit of measure is degrees Celsius per minute per watt.

Human immunodeficiency virus (HIV)

A retrovirus believed to be a contributing cause of acquired immunodeficiency syndrome (AIDS).

hypnotic induction profile test

Evaluates hypnotic capacity—the degree to which an individual can control dissociation, become absorbed, and accept suggestion.

Immunoglobulin A (IgA)

An immunoglobulin found in body fluids. IgA protects the body's mucosal surfaces from infection.

Immunoglobulin G (IgG)

A prominent type of immunoglobulin existing in the blood. Also called gamma globulin.

Intermittent claudication

A complex of symptoms characterized by an absence of pain or discomfort in a limb when at rest and the commencement of pain, tension, or weakness after the limb is put to use, attributable to reduced blood flow through narrowed arteries. The symptoms can intensify to become disabling but subside again after a period of rest.

In vitro

In an artificial environment outside of the organism.

In vivo

In the organism itself.

Iridology

The study of the iris of the eye to define the disease entity in the body.

Isocyanates

Compounds with a functionality group (N = C = O). Such compounds have been found to elicit an asthmatic response in some individuals and to help reduce the asthmatic response in others.

Isoflavones, lignans, and coumestans

Three main classes of phytoestrogens, which are plant compounds with estrogen-like biologic activity.

Jenkins Activity Survey

A self-report, multiple-choice inventory designed to assess the coronary-prone behavior pattern known as type A behavior. Type A behavior has been implicated as an independent risk factor in the etiology of coronary heart disease, including both myocardial infarction and coronary atherosclerosis.

Kampo formulations

Combinations of herbal components used in Japan, which have free-radical scavenging activity with efficacy that shows concentration-dependent properties. Kampo has been evaluated with regard to cerebral ischemia and brain damage.

Leukotrienes

Biologically active compounds consisting of 20-carbon carboxylic acids formed from arachidonic acid, which function as regulators of allergic and inflammatory reactions.

Likert Self-Report

A self-report method for measuring attitudes, the scale provides options on a continuum of various numbers (e.g., strongly disagree, 1, to strongly agree, 7). It is suitable for measuring the strength and dimensionality of attitudes.

Locus of control

A concept that describes how patients attribute responsibility for disease management. Patients with diabetes may believe that control of their illness depends on themselves (internal) or powerful others (external) or is governed by chance.

Low-density lipoprotein cholesterol

Cholesterol is produced in the liver and is needed to form cell membranes, nerve coating, and certain hormones. When a lipoprotein contains more fat than protein, it is called a low-density lipoprotein (LDL) and increases the risk of atherosclerosis because it contributes to a fatty buildup in the arteries.

Mesh terms

Individual words or terms used to access, through database and computer searches, research information related to particular health issues. For example, in CAM such terms might include "acupuncture," "homeopathy," or "alternative medicine."

Meta-analysis

A technique in which scientific data from several unrelated clinical trials are reviewed by interpreting treatment effects as to consistency and magnitude of effect.

Metaplasia

Change in type of adult cells.

National Acupuncture Detoxification Association

Formed in 1985 as a membership and training organization. At present, NADA trainers have taught more than 4000 acupuncturists, counselors, nurses, and physicians how to perform acupuncture for substance abuse in the United States and almost that many in Europe.

National Health and Nutrition Examination Survey (NHANES)

An ongoing survey conducted by the National Center for Health Statistics. NHANES III was conducted from 1988 to 1994 and contains data on 33,994 persons 2 months of age and older. Five domains of data are monitored: household adult, household youth, medical examination, laboratory, and dietary recall data.

Nei Guan point

An acupuncture point (also called point P6 or Inner Gate) above the inner wrist, which is used in treating nausea and vomiting. In traditional Chinese medicine practice it is used in conjunction with other points.

N-1 design

A type of an evaluation in which goals, diagnosis, treatment, and outcomes are directed and assessed for one specific patient under study.

Nottingham Health Profile

A brief self-assessment of physical, emotional, and social health, with emphasis on evaluating patients' subjective perception of their health status.

Nurses Observation Scale for Inpatient Evaluation

Psychometric tool that assesses the ward behavior of psychiatric inpatients. Nursing personnel use a 30-item paper-and-pencil observational inventory to evaluate patient status and change. The six factors measured are social competence, social interest, personal neatness, irritability, manifest psychosis, and psychomotor retardation.

Pelvic inflammatory disease

A condition usually brought on by untreated gonorrhea and chlamydial infection. Symptoms include severe pelvic pain and high fever.

Perceived Guilt Index (PGI)

A self-report measure of guilt experienced by an individual based in part on his or her own interpretation of emotions such as anxiety, guilt, or obsessions and their intensity in everyday life.

Persimmon tannin

A condensed derivative isolated from persimmon. These condensed tannins exhibit concentration-dependent free-radical scavenging activity.

Placebo

A substance or intervention that contains no active medicinal ingredient.

Poultice

A soft, moist mass, about the consistency of cooked cereal, spread between layers of muslin, linen, gauze, or towels and applied hot to a given area to create moist local heat and/or to cause absorption of bioactive compounds from the mass into the skin and surrounding areas.

Power analysis

A statistical technique used to determine the number of patients required to accurately reject the hypothesis that no differences exist between experimental or control groups.

Preclinical studies

Experiments to determine the value of treatments. They include basic studies, which study the effects and mechanisms, and clinical trials, which consist of Phases I to III trials.

Pritikin Longevity Center

Teaches the principles of the Pritikin diet, as well as exercise and stress management, in 1- to 4-week residential programs.

Profile of mood state

A tool that assesses dimensions of affect or mood in individuals 18 years of age and older. It is used to measure outpatients' response to various therapeutic approaches, including drug evaluation studies. The 65-item paper-and-pencil test measures the following dimensions of mood: tension-anxiety, depression-dejection, anger-hostility, vigor-activity, fatigue-inertia, and confusion-bewilderment.

Prooxidant

An agent that causes oxidation in the cell, a process often harmful to DNA.

Proprioceptive neural facilitation

A system of evaluation and treatment of neuro-musculoskeletal dysfunction based on neurophysiologic principles. The practitioner uses sensory stimulation from manual contacts and verbal and visual cues to elicit efficient and functional movement.

Prostaglandins

Compounds derived from arachidonic acid via the cyclooxygenase pathway that regulate a diverse group of physiologic processes.

Provider practice acts

Descriptions of scope of practice and licensing/certification requirements for health providers generally enacted through individual state legislatures.

Psychoneuroimmunology

Field of medical research that explores linkages between behavior, the nervous system, and the immune system.

Purpose in Life

A test that measures the degree to which an individual has found meaning in life. It is useful with addicted, retired, handicapped, and philosophically confused individuals for purposes of clinical assessment, student counseling, vocational guidance, and rehabilitation. Subjects rate 20 statements, complete 13 sentence stems, and write an original paragraph describing their ambitions in life. The test is based on Victor Frankl's *Will to Meaning* and embraces his logotherapeutic orientation.

Randomization

An experimental procedure in which subjects are assigned to either a treatment or nontreatment group purely on chance.

Resorcylic acid lactones

Phytoestrogens produced by molds that commonly contaminate cereal crops.

Retinoids

Compounds similar to vitamin A.

Scarification

Production in the skin of many small, superficial scratches or punctures, as for introduction of a vaccine.

Sishencong points

A group of four acupuncture points located on the highest point of the head. According to ancient Chinese belief these points function to "tranquilize" the mind and regulate the CNS to promote sleep.

State-Trait Anxiety Inventory

A commonly used, short (40-item) measurement tool that provides information about a person's level of both state and trait anxiety. Anxiety has been viewed as having two distinct forms. The *state* form of anxiety is the transitory feeling of fear or worry that most of us experience from time to time. The *trait* form of anxiety is the relatively stable tendency of an individual to respond anxiously to a stressful situation. Thus the level of trait anxiety reflects the proneness to exhibit state anxiety.

State-Trait Anxiety Inventory for Children

A short, 40-item self-report measurement tool that provides information about a child's level of both state and trait anxiety.

Structural equations

A comprehensive statistical approach that deals with complex, multidimensional relationships between research variables.

Succussion

A procedure in which shaking of a dilute solution reduces its medicinal and biochemical concentration. Used quite often in the practice of homeopathy.

Sulfonylurea drugs

A type of medicine, taken orally, that stimulates the pancreas to produce and secrete more insulin. These drugs are used to lower blood glucose in type 2 diabetes mellitus. The first- and second-generation sulfonylureas are similar in lowering blood glucose by decreasing insulin resistance and increasing insulin secretion. The second-generation drugs are more potent and more effective but have an increased risk of hypoglycemia.

Symptom checklist 90R

A 90-item self-report inventory designed to assess the psychologic symptoms of psychiatric and medical patients. The inventory measures somatization, obsessive-compulsive symptoms, interpersonal sensitivity, depression, anxiety, phobic anxiety, psychoticism, paranoid ideation, hostility, and global indices of psychopathologic conditions.

Syncytial virus

A virus in the multinucleated mass of protoplasm produced by the merging of cells.

Thermogram

A photographic record of the amount of heat radiated from the surface of the body, obtained by an infrared sensing device, revealing a "hot spot" of potential tumors or other disorders. This technique has been used in conjunction with phantoms to study heating patterns inside the human body.

Thromboxane

One of two compounds that are potent inducers of platelet aggregation.

Type 1 (insulin-dependent) diabetes mellitus

An autoimmune disorder of metabolism. Antibodies are produced that damage the insulin-producing beta cells of the pancreas. Insulin becomes deficient, and the cells cannot use glucose efficiently. Blood glucose levels are elevated, and injected insulin is necessary to control blood glucose.

Type 2 (non–insulin-dependent) diabetes mellitus

A disorder of metabolism that is characterized by tissue resistance to insulin and hyperglycemia. The beta cells of the pancreas become unable to secrete enough insulin to counteract decreased sensitivity (resistance) of the tissues to insulin. Oral medications and diet may be sufficient to normalize blood glucose, but a significant percentage of patients eventually need insulin for adequate control.

U.S. National Health Interview Survey (NHIS)

A 1991 survey conducted by the National Center for Health Statistics containing more than 900,000 records including five core areas (condition, doctor visit, hospital, household, and person) and six supplemental areas (AIDS knowledge and attitudes, cancer control, cancer epidemiology, health insurance, immunization, and youth risk behavior).

Venesection

Phlebotomy; incision of a vein.

Word salad

A symptom of a psychotic state exemplified by complete incoherence of speech, with a mixture of words lacking meaning and logical coherence.

Yale Brown Obsessive-Compulsive scale

A 10-question scale with severity options ranging from 0 to 4; useful for quantifying the level of obsessive-compulsive disorder symptoms.

Index

A

Acamprosate for alcohol addiction, 251

N-Acetylcysteine in cancer prevention, 136

Acquired immunodeficiency syndrome; *see* HIV/AIDS

Acupressure
for nausea and vomiting in pregnancy, 348-349, 350*t*, 351
for neurologic disorders, research overview, 172*t*

Acupuncture
for acute pain
research, 294*t*, 298
for addiction, 253, 254*t*-257*t*, 257-260
for alcohol addiction, 261-262
for allergic rhinitis, 82-83
for allergies, 84*t*, 372*t*, 375
for anxiety, 237
for ADHD, 372*t*, 381, *383*
for benzodiazepine abuse, 271
for breast cancer, 356-357
for breathlessness in cancer patients, 155-156
for cancer, 138
for cancer-related pain, 323-324
CAM therapy outcomes research findings, 321*t*
for children, 371, 373
for chronic pain, 312-317
for cocaine addiction, 265
complications of, 314
database citations for, 210
for depression, 220
for diabetic neuropathy, 110
for diarrhea in children, 372*t*, 377
for enuresis, 372*t*, 379
FDA regulations for, 29
for headache, 312-313
research findings, 305*t*-307*t*, 310*t*
for heroin addiction, 260
for hot flashes, 344, 347
for insomnia, 223-224
for lowering blood glucose, 112
for methamphetamine abuse, 271
for multiple sclerosis, 195
for nausea and vomiting in cancer patients, 156
for neurologic disorders, 177-178

research overview, 172*t*
for nicotine abuse, 270*t*
for opiate addiction, 260
for osteoarthritis, 403-404
for Parkinson's disease, 197
provider practice acts for, 17
for radiation-induced xerostomia, 157
for rashes in children, 372*t*
research on, 19
safety issues, 15
for schizophrenia, 229
for side effects of chemotherapy, 138
for spinal cord injury, 192
for stroke, 180, 183-186
WHO safety guidelines for, 16

Addiction, 248-281; *see also* specific addictions
CAM therapies for, 252-260
acupuncture, 253, 254*t*-257*t*, 257-260
future of, 271
hypnosis, 268-269
nutrition, 262-264
economic impacts of, 249
epidemiology of, 249
standard treatments, 251-252
theories of, 250-251
treatment efficacy, 249-250

s-Adenosyl-L-methionine for depression, 214-215

Adhatoda vasica for asthma, 75

Adolescents with diabetes mellitus, 108

Adrenocorticotropic hormone, levels before and after Qi Gong, 233

African herbs for asthma, 75-76

AIDS; *see* HIV/AIDS in women

AIDS-defining illnesses, 363

Alcohol addiction
CAM therapies for, 254*t*-256*t*, 260-265, 261*t*, 266*t*-267*t*
pharmacologic treatments of, 251
research conclusions, 266*t*-267*t*

Alexander technique for neurologic disorders, research overview, 172*t*

Alfalfa, potential toxicity, 129*t*

Algae; *see Chlorella pyrenoidosa*

Alisma orientale for for allergies, 81

Allergic rhinitis, acupuncture for, 82-83

Allergy(ies)

CAM treatments for, 79-84
in children, 372*t*, 374-375
enuresis due to, 379

Allopathic medicine; *see* Conventional medicine

Aloe vera, potential toxicity, 129*t*

L-Alpha-acetyl-methadol for opiate addiction, 251

Alpha-methyltryptophan for depression, 215

Alpha-tocopherol in cancer treatment, 135

Alternative Medical Care Outcomes in AIDS, 365

Alzheimer's disease, 391-398
CAM therapies for, 393-398
conventional management, 393
diagnosis, 391-393

Ambroxol for asthma, 75

Amenorrhea, black cohosh for, 344

Amino acids, supplementary, for addiction, 264

Amphetamine abuse, 252, 271

AMPT for depression, 215

Amygdalin (laetrile) in cancer treatment, 152

Angina pectoris
plant-based diets and, 100
precipitating events, 91

Anthrosophic diet in cancer therapy, 141

Antibiotics, development of, 8

Anticonvulsant drugs, nonconventional use of, 181

Antidepressant medications for depressive disorders, 213

Antihistamines for upper respiratory tract infections, 373

Antiinflammatory drugs for Alzheimer's disease, 393

Antineoplastons in cancer therapy, 138-140

Antioxidants
for asthma, 71
in lung cancer treatment, 135
for preventing AVD, 101
for preventing cancer, 135
for stroke prevention, 188-189
types of, 101

Anxiety, 209, 234-240
acupuncture for, 237
CAM therapies for, 234-240, 240*t*, 312

Page numbers in italics indicate illustrations; *t* following a page number indicates a table.

Dermatitis, atopic, CAM therapies for, 379-380

Desmodium adscendens for asthma, 75-76

D'hatura for asthma, 75

DHEA; *see* Dehydroepiandrosterone

Diabetes mellitus, 107-122; *see also* Blood glucose
  acupuncture for, 112
  in adolescents, 108
  biofeedback for, 114-118
  emotional and spiritual factors in, 114
  herbal medicine for, 112-113, 113*t*
  incidence of, 107
  insulin-dependent, 107-109
  non-insulin-dependent, 107-115, 119
  self-care in, 108-109
  types of, 107
  yoga for, 114

Diabetic neuropathy, acupuncture for, 110

Diabetic retinopathy, magnesium deficit and, 111

Diagnostic and Statistical Manual of Mental Disorders, major depressive order defined by, 211

Diarrhea in children, CAM therapies for, 377
  research findings, 372*t*

Diet(s); *see also* Nutrition therapy
  for cancer prevention, 131-133
  for diabetes mellitus, 110-111
  diabetic, 107-108
  elimination, for asthma, 71
  estrogen levels and, 345-346
  for multiple sclerosis, 196
  plant-based, 99-100
  for stroke prevention, 188-189
  Western, hormone levels and, 354-355

Diet therapy; *see* Nutrition therapy; specific therapies

Dietary fiber for preventing AVD, 100-101

Dietary supplements; *see* Nutritional supplements; specific supplements

Dietary Supplements Health and Education Act, 28

Dimethyl amino ethanol for neurologic disorders, research, 175*t*

Dimethyl sulfoxide for neurologic disorders, research overview, 175*t*

Ding Jing Hong Pill for schizophrenia, 230

Disease
  culture and, 9, 109
  recovery from, explanations, 21-22

Distraction therapies
  in cancer treatment, 149
  for nausea and vomiting in cancer patients, 156

Disulfiram for alcohol addiction, 251

DMAE for neurologic disorders, research overview, 175*t*

DMSO for neurologic disorders, research overview, 175*t*

Docosahexaenoic acid for asthma, 72-73

Dong quai for hot flashes, 344-345

Dopamine supplements for schizophrenia, 230

Drug(s); *see* Medications

Dysthymic disorder
  defined, 211
  treatment of, 212-213

E

Eastern exercise; *see also* Qi Gong; T'ai chi; Yoga
  for AVD, 96

Echinacea, contraindications to, 196

ECT; *see* Electrochemical treatment

Eczema, 79-81, 380

EDTA chelation for neurologic disorders, research overview, 175*t*

Education, CAM, 29, 30*t*, 31

Eicosanoids, 132-133
  prostate cancer and, 132-133

Eicosapentaenoic acid
  asthma and, 72
  for preventing recurrence of colon cancer, 133

Elderly persons, CAM therapies for, 391-410; *see also* Alzheimer's disease; Osteoarthritis

Electrochemical treatment
  for breast cancer, 49
  for cancer, 37
  in China, 40
  clinical trials, 48-49
  dosage of, 43-45
  for laryngeal carcinoma, 48-49
  for lung cancer, 49
  mechanism studies, 46-47
  methodology studies, 41-45
  for osteosarcoma, 49
  preclinical issues, 40-41
  preclinical safety and toxicity test, 43-46
  preclinical studies of, 40-49
  procedure for, 40

Electroconvulsive therapy for depression, 212

Electrolysis, antitumor effects of, 46

Electromagnetic field methods for pain, 326-327

Electromagnetic therapies, 182; *see also* Transcutaneous electrical nerve stimulation

Electromyography for diabetic patients, 114-115

Electroosmosis, antitumor effects, 46

Electrosleep for anxiety, 239

Electrostimulation, cranial, for insomnia, 224-225

Elimination diets for asthma, 71

EMDR for alcohol abuse, research conclusions, 267*t*

Emotional factors in diabetes mellitus, 114

Empowerment, consumer, through CAM, 411-413

Endorphins, 22, 328

Enemas, coffee, potential toxicity, 129*t*

Energy healing, 188, 194

Enuresis
  CAM therapies for, 378-379
  research findings for CAM therapies in children, 372*t*

Enzyme therapy for osteoarthritis, 403

EPA; *see* Eicosapentaenoic acid

Epilepsy, 178, 198-199

Epipodophyllotoxins in cancer therapy, 143

Epithalamin in cancer therapy, 152

Escherichia coli, diarrhea due to, 377

Esophageal cancer, CAM therapy for, 139*t*, 144

Essential fatty acids for Alzheimer's disease, 398

Essiac in cancer therapy, 142

Estradiol, fat intake and, 132

Estrogen(s); *see also* Phytoestrogens
  breast cancer and, 132
  dietary, breast cancer and, 353-355
  food sources for, 345-346
  from plant sources, 102, 354
  for preventing AVD, 102

Estrogen therapy for hot flashes, 344

Estrone, fat intake and, 132

Ethylenediaminetetraacetic acid in chelation therapy, 92-93

Evening primrose oil
  in cancer therapy, 146
  for multiple sclerosis, 195-196
  for pain, 326
  for psoriasis in children, 380

Evidence-based analysis, assumptions of, 3-4

Exercise; *see* Qi Gong; T'ai chi; Yoga
  for Alzheimer's disease, 393
  asthma linked with, 67, 72
  for chronic pain in fibromyalgia, 316
  eastern, for AVD, 96
  for headache, research findings, 309*t*
  for hot flashes, 347-348
  for women with HIV/AIDS, 368

External electromagnetic fields for Alzheimer's disease, 397-398

F

Fat(s), dietary
  breast cancer and, 132
  colon cancer and, 131-132
  controversy over, 132
  prostate cancer and, 133

Fatty acids, 72, 132, 398

Feingold diet for ADHD, 381-382

Feldenkrais method for neurologic disorders, research overview, 173*t*

Fenugreek seed powder for diabetic patients, 113

Ferromagnetic seed implants for hyperthermia, 53

Feverfew for migraine, 325

Fiber, dietary, 100-101, 137

Fibromyalgia
  CAM therapies for, research findings, 309*t*-310*t*
  chronic pain in, 316-317